ACP | MKSAP® 17

Medical Knowledge Self Assessment Program®

General Internal Medicine

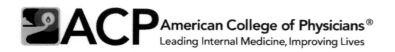

American College of Physicians®
Leading Internal Medicine, Improving Lives

Welcome to the General Internal Medicine Section of MKSAP 17!

In these pages, you will find updated information on routine care of the healthy patient; patient safety and quality improvement; professionalism and ethics; palliative care; common symptoms, including chronic pain, cough, dizziness, and insomnia; musculoskeletal pain; dyslipidemia; obesity; men's and women's health; eye, ear, nose, mouth, and throat disorders; mental and behavioral health; geriatric medicine; perioperative medicine; and many other clinical challenges. All of these topics are uniquely focused on the needs of both generalists and those who practice subspecialty internal medicine.

The publication of the 17th edition of Medical Knowledge Self-Assessment Program (MKSAP) represents nearly a half-century of serving as the gold-standard resource for internal medicine education. It also marks its evolution into an innovative learning system to better meet the changing educational needs and learning styles of all internists.

The core content of MKSAP has been developed as in previous editions—newly generated, essential information in 11 topic areas of internal medicine created by dozens of leading generalists and subspecialists and guided by certification and recertification requirements, emerging knowledge in the field, and user feedback. MKSAP 17 also contains 1200 all-new, psychometrically validated, and peer-reviewed multiple-choice questions (MCQs) for self-assessment and study, including 168 in General Internal Medicine. MKSAP 17 continues to include *High Value Care* (HVC) recommendations, based on the concept of balancing clinical benefit with costs and harms, with links to MCQs that illustrate these principles. In addition, HVC Key Points are highlighted in the text. Also highlighted, with blue text, are *Hospitalist*-focused content and MCQs that directly address the learning needs of internists who work in the hospital setting.

MKSAP 17 Digital provides access to additional tools allowing you to customize your learning experience, including regular text updates with practice-changing, new information and 200 new self-assessment questions; a board-style pretest to help direct your learning; and enhanced custom-quiz options. And, with MKSAP Complete, learners can access 1200 electronic flashcards for quick review of important concepts or review the updated and enhanced version of Virtual Dx, an image-based self-assessment tool.

As before, MKSAP 17 is optimized for use on your mobile devices, with iOS- and Android-based apps allowing you to sync your work between your apps and online account and submit for CME credits and MOC points online.

Please visit us at the MKSAP Resource Site (mksap.acponline.org) to find out how we can help you study, earn CME credit and MOC points, and stay up to date.

Whether you prefer to use the traditional print version or take advantage of the features available through the digital version, we hope you enjoy MKSAP 17 and that it meets and exceeds your personal learning needs.

On behalf of the many internists who have offered their time and expertise to create the content for MKSAP 17 and the editorial staff who work to bring this material to you in the best possible way, we are honored that you have chosen to use MKSAP 17 and appreciate any feedback about the program you may have. Please feel free to send us any comments to mksap_editors@acponline.org.

Sincerely,

Philip A. Masters, MD, FACP
Editor-in-Chief
Senior Physician Educator
Director, Clinical Content Development
Medical Education Division
American College of Physicians

General Internal Medicine

Committee

Karen F. Mauck, MD, MSc, FACP, Section Editor[2]
Associate Professor of Medicine
Firm Chief, Internal Medicine Residency Program
Consultant and Chair of Faculty Development
Division of General Internal Medicine
Mayo Clinic
Rochester, Minnesota

Jack Ende, MD, MACP, Associate Editor[1]
The Schaeffer Professor of Medicine
Perelman School of Medicine at the University of
    Pennsylvania
Philadelphia, Pennsylvania

Thomas J. Beckman, MD, FACP[2]
Professor of Medicine and Medical Education
Associate Director, Internal Medicine Residency Program
Consultant and Chair for Education
Division of General Internal Medicine
Mayo Clinic
Rochester, Minnesota

Molly A. Feely, MD, FACP[1]
Assistant Professor of Medicine
Consultant, Division of General Internal Medicine, Section
    of Palliative Medicine
Program Director, Hospice Palliative Medicine
    Fellowship
Mayo Clinic
Rochester, Minnesota

Rosanne Granieri, MD, FACP[1]
Professor of Medicine
Division of General Internal Medicine
Department of Medicine
University of Pittsburgh School of Medicine
Pittsburgh, Pennsylvania

Scott Herrle, MD, MS, FACP[1]
Assistant Professor of Medicine
Division of General Internal Medicine
Department of Medicine
University of Pittsburgh School of Medicine
Veterans Affairs Pittsburgh Healthcare System
Pittsburgh, Pennsylvania

Wendy S. Klein, MD, MACP[2]
Associate Professor Emeritus of Medicine, Obstetrics
    and Gynecology
Department of Internal Medicine
Virginia Commonwealth University School of Medicine
Richmond, Virginia

Paul S. Mueller, MD, MPH, FACP[2]
Professor of Medicine and Professor of Biomedical Ethics
Consultant and Chair
Division of General Internal Medicine
Mayo Clinic
Rochester, Minnesota

Kurt J. Pfeifer, MD, FACP[1]
Professor of Medicine
Division of General Internal Medicine
Department of Medicine
Medical College of Wisconsin
Milwaukee, Wisconsin

Amy Tu Wang, MD, FACP[2]
Assistant Professor of Medicine
Division of General Internal Medicine
Harbor-UCLA Medical Center
Torrance, California

Christopher M. Wittich, MD, PharmD, FACP[1]
Associate Professor of Medicine
Associate Director, Internal Medicine Residency Program
Consultant and Practice Chair
Division of General Internal Medicine
Mayo Clinic
Rochester, Minnesota

Editor-in-Chief

Philip A. Masters, MD, FACP[1]
Senior Physician Educator
Director, Clinical Content Development
American College of Physicians
Philadelphia, Pennsylvania

Director, Clinical Program Development

Cynthia D. Smith, MD, FACP[2]
American College of Physicians
Philadelphia, Pennsylvania

General Internal Medicine Reviewers

Leslie F. Blum, MD, FACP[1]
Ravi Gupta, MD, FACP[1]
Kouta Ito, MD, MS, FACP[1]
Richard J. Lin, MD, PhD, FACP[1]
Lia Logio, MD, FACP[1]
George Moxley, MD[2]
Steven Ricanati, MD, FACP[1]
Adrian Sequeira, MD, FACP[2]
Susan Wolver, MD, FACP[1]

General Internal Medicine ACP Editorial Staff

Jackie Twomey[1], Staff Editor
Megan Zborowski[1], Senior Staff Editor
Margaret Wells[1], Director, Self-Assessment and Educational Programs
Becky Krumm[1], Managing Editor

ACP Principal Staff

Patrick C. Alguire, MD, FACP[2]
Senior Vice President, Medical Education

Sean McKinney[1]
Vice President, Medical Education

Margaret Wells[1]
Director, Self-Assessment and Educational Programs

Becky Krumm[1]
Managing Editor

Katie Idell[1]
Manager, Clinical Skills Program and Digital Products

Valerie A. Dangovetsky[1]
Administrator

Ellen McDonald, PhD[1]
Senior Staff Editor

Megan Zborowski[1]
Senior Staff Editor

Randy Hendrickson[1]
Production Administrator/Editor

Linnea Donnarumma[1]
Staff Editor

Susan Galeone[1]
Staff Editor

Jackie Twomey[1]
Staff Editor

Julia Nawrocki[1]
Staff Editor

Kimberly Kerns[1]
Administrative Coordinator

Rosemarie Houton[1]
Administrative Representative

---

1. Has no relationships with any entity producing, marketing, reselling, or distributing health care goods or services consumed by, or used on, patients.

2. Has disclosed relationship(s) with any entity producing, marketing, reselling, or distributing health care goods or services consumed by, or used on, patients.

Disclosure of Relationships with any entity producing, marketing, reselling, or distributing health care goods or services consumed by, or used on, patients.

Patrick C. Alguire, MD, FACP
Consultantship
National Board of Medical Examiners
Royalties
UpToDate
Stock Options/Holdings
Amgen Inc., Bristol-Myers Squibb, GlaxoSmithKline, Stryker Corporation, Zimmer Orthopedics, Teva Pharmaceuticals, Medtronic, Covidien Inc., Express Scripts

Thomas J. Beckman, MD, FACP
Research/Grants/Contracts
Pfizer Medical Education Group
Other (Associate Editor)
Mayo Clinic Proceedings

Wendy S. Klein, MD, MACP
Consultantship
Pfizer

Karen F. Mauck, MD, MSc, FACP
Research/Grants/Contracts
Pfizer
Stock Options/Holdings
Exact Sciences

George Moxley, MD
Employment
Virginia Commonwealth University

Paul S. Mueller, MD, MPH, FACP
Board Member
Boston Scientific Patient Safety Advisory Board
Other (Associate Editor)
NEJM Journal Watch General Medicine, Massachusetts Medical Society

Adrian Sequeira, MD, FACP
Employment
Louisiana State University Health Shreveport School of Medicine

Cynthia D. Smith, MD, FACP
Stock Options/Holdings
Merck and Co.; spousal employment at Merck

Amy Tu Wang, MD, FACP

Consultantship

Agency for Healthcare Research and Quality–funded
  Evidence-based Practice Center – The Technology
  Evaluation Center of Blue Cross Blue Shield of America

Acknowledgments

The American College of Physicians (ACP) gratefully acknowledges the special contributions to the development and production of the 17th edition of the Medical Knowledge Self-Assessment Program® (MKSAP® 17) made by the following people:

Graphic Design: Michael Ripca (Graphics Technical Administrator) and WFGD Studio (Graphic Designers).

Production/Systems: Dan Hoffmann (Director, Web Services & Systems Development), Neil Kohl (Senior Architect), Chris Patterson (Senior Architect), and Scott Hurd (Manager, Web Projects & CMS Services).

MKSAP 17 Digital: Under the direction of Steven Spadt, Vice President, Digital Products & Services, the digital version of MKSAP 17 was developed within the ACP's Digital Product Development Department, led by Brian Sweigard (Director). Other members of the team included Dan Barron (Senior Web Application Developer/Architect), Chris Forrest (Senior Software Developer/Design Lead), Kara Kronenwetter (Senior Web Developer), Brad Lord (Senior Web Application Developer), John McKnight (Senior Web Developer), and Nate Pershall (Senior Web Developer).

The College also wishes to acknowledge that many other persons, too numerous to mention, have contributed to the production of this program. Without their dedicated efforts, this program would not have been possible.

MKSAP Resource Site (mksap.acponline.org)

The MKSAP Resource Site (mksap.acponline.org) is a continually updated site that provides links to MKSAP 17 online answer sheets for print subscribers; the latest details on Continuing Medical Education (CME) and Maintenance of Certification (MOC) in the United States, Canada, and Australia; errata; and other new information.

ABIM Maintenance of Certification

Check the MKSAP Resource Site (mksap.acponline.org) for the latest information on how MKSAP tests can be used to apply to the American Board of Internal Medicine for Maintenance of Certification (MOC) points.

Royal College Maintenance of Certification

In Canada, MKSAP 17 is an Accredited Self-Assessment Program (Section 3) as defined by the Maintenance of Certification (MOC) Program of The Royal College of Physicians and Surgeons of Canada and approved by the Canadian Society of Internal Medicine on December 9, 2014. Approval extends from July 31, 2015 until July 31, 2018 for the Part A sections. Approval extends from December 31, 2015 to December 31, 2018 for the Part B sections.

Fellows of the Royal College may earn three credits per hour for participating in MKSAP 17 under Section 3. MKSAP 17 also meets multiple CanMEDS Roles, including that of Medical Expert, Communicator, Collaborator, Manager, Health Advocate, Scholar, and Professional. For information on how to apply MKSAP 17 Continuing Medical Education (CME) credits to the Royal College MOC Program, visit the MKSAP Resource Site at mksap.acponline.org.

The Royal Australasian College of Physicians CPD Program

In Australia, MKSAP 17 is a Category 3 program that may be used by Fellows of The Royal Australasian College of Physicians (RACP) to meet mandatory Continuing Professional Development (CPD) points. Two CPD credits are awarded for each of the 200 *AMA PRA Category 1 Credits*™ available in MKSAP 17. More information about using MKSAP 17 for this purpose is available at the MKSAP Resource Site at mksap.acponline.org and at www.racp.edu.au. CPD credits earned through MKSAP 17 should be reported at the MyCPD site at www.racp.edu.au/mycpd.

Continuing Medical Education

The American College of Physicians (ACP) is accredited by the Accreditation Council for Continuing Medical Education (ACCME) to provide continuing medical education for physicians.

The ACP designates this enduring material, MKSAP 17, for a maximum of 200 *AMA PRA Category 1 Credits*™. Physicians should claim only the credit commensurate with the extent of their participation in the activity.

Up to 26 *AMA PRA Category 1 Credits*™ are available from December 31, 2015, to December 31, 2018, for the MKSAP 17 General Internal Medicine section.

Learning Objectives

The learning objectives of MKSAP 17 are to:
- Close gaps between actual care in your practice and preferred standards of care, based on best evidence

- Diagnose disease states that are less common and sometimes overlooked or confusing
- Improve management of comorbid conditions that can complicate patient care
- Determine when to refer patients for surgery or care by subspecialists
- Pass the ABIM Certification Examination
- Pass the ABIM Maintenance of Certification Examination

Target Audience

- General internists and primary care physicians
- Subspecialists who need to remain up-to-date in internal medicine and in areas outside of their own subspecialty area
- Residents preparing for the certification examination in internal medicine
- Physicians preparing for maintenance of certification in internal medicine (recertification)

Earn "Instantaneous" CME Credits Online

Print subscribers can enter their answers online to earn instantaneous Continuing Medical Education (CME) credits. You can submit your answers using online answer sheets that are provided at mksap.acponline.org, where a record of your MKSAP 17 credits will be available. To earn CME credits, you need to answer all of the questions in a test and earn a score of at least 50% correct (number of correct answers divided by the total number of questions). Take any of the following approaches:

1. Use the printed answer sheet at the back of this book to record your answers. Go to mksap.acponline.org, access the appropriate online answer sheet, transcribe your answers, and submit your test for instantaneous CME credits. There is no additional fee for this service.

2. Go to mksap.acponline.org, access the appropriate online answer sheet, directly enter your answers, and submit your test for instantaneous CME credits. There is no additional fee for this service.

3. Pay a $15 processing fee per answer sheet and submit the printed answer sheet at the back of this book by mail or fax, as instructed on the answer sheet. Make sure you calculate your score and fax the answer sheet to 215-351-2799 or mail the answer sheet to Member and Customer Service, American College of Physicians, 190 N. Independence Mall West, Philadelphia, PA 19106-1572, using the courtesy envelope provided in your MKSAP 17 slipcase. You will need your 10-digit order number and 8-digit ACP ID number, which are printed on your packing slip. Please allow 4 to 6 weeks for your score report to be

emailed back to you. Be sure to include your email address for a response.

If you do not have a 10-digit order number and 8-digit ACP ID number or if you need help creating a user name and password to access the MKSAP 17 online answer sheets, go to mksap.acponline.org or email custserv@acponline.org.

Disclosure Policy

It is the policy of the American College of Physicians (ACP) to ensure balance, independence, objectivity, and scientific rigor in all of its educational activities. To this end, and consistent with the policies of the ACP and the Accreditation Council for Continuing Medical Education (ACCME), contributors to all ACP continuing medical education activities are required to disclose all relevant financial relationships with any entity producing, marketing, re-selling, or distributing health care goods or services consumed by, or used on, patients. Contributors are required to use generic names in the discussion of therapeutic options and are required to identify any unapproved, off-label, or investigative use of commercial products or devices. Where a trade name is used, all available trade names for the same product type are also included. If trade-name products manufactured by companies with whom contributors have relationships are discussed, contributors are asked to provide evidence-based citations in support of the discussion. The information is reviewed by the committee responsible for producing this text. If necessary, adjustments to topics or contributors' roles in content development are made to balance the discussion. Further, all readers of this text are asked to evaluate the content for evidence of commercial bias and send any relevant comments to mksap_editors@acponline.org so that future decisions about content and contributors can be made in light of this information.

Resolution of Conflicts

To resolve all conflicts of interest and influences of vested interests, the American College of Physicians (ACP) precluded members of the content-creation committee from deciding on any content issues that involved generic or trade-name products associated with proprietary entities with which these committee members had relationships. In addition, content was based on best evidence and updated clinical care guidelines, when such evidence and guidelines were available. Contributors' disclosure information can be found with the list of contributors' names and those of ACP principal staff listed in the beginning of this book.

Hospital-Based Medicine

For the convenience of subscribers who provide care in hospital settings, content that is specific to the hospital setting has been highlighted in blue. Hospital icons (H) highlight where the hospital-based content begins, continues over more than one page, and ends.

High Value Care Key Points

Key Points in the text that relate to High Value Care concepts (that is, concepts that discuss balancing clinical benefit with costs and harms) are designated by the HVC icon (HVC).

Educational Disclaimer

The editors and publisher of MKSAP 17 recognize that the development of new material offers many opportunities for error. Despite our best efforts, some errors may persist in print. Drug dosage schedules are, we believe, accurate and in accordance with current standards. Readers are advised, however, to ensure that the recommended dosages in MKSAP 17 concur with the information provided in the product information material. This is especially important in cases of new, infrequently used, or highly toxic drugs. Application of the information in MKSAP 17 remains the professional responsibility of the practitioner.

The primary purpose of MKSAP 17 is educational. Information presented, as well as publications, technologies, products, and/or services discussed, is intended to inform subscribers about the knowledge, techniques, and experiences of the contributors. A diversity of professional opinion exists, and the views of the contributors are their own and not those of the American College of Physicians (ACP). Inclusion of any material in the program does not constitute endorsement or recommendation by the ACP. The ACP does not warrant the safety, reliability, accuracy, completeness, or usefulness of and disclaims any and all liability for damages and claims that may result from the use of information, publications, technologies, products, and/or services discussed in this program.

Errata

Errata for MKSAP 17 will be available through the MKSAP Resource Site at mksap.acponline.org as new information becomes known to the editors.

Table of Contents

Perioperative Medicine

General Internal Medicine High Value Care Recommendations

The American College of Physicians, in collaboration with multiple other organizations, is engaged in a worldwide initiative to promote the practice of High Value Care (HVC). The goals of the HVC initiative are to improve health care outcomes by providing care of proven benefit and reducing costs by avoiding unnecessary and even harmful interventions. The initiative comprises several programs that integrate the important concept of health care value (balancing clinical benefit with costs and harms) for a given intervention into a broad range of educational materials to address the needs of trainees, practicing physicians, and patients.

HVC content has been integrated into MKSAP 17 in several important ways. MKSAP 17 now includes HVC-identified key points in the text, HVC-focused multiple choice questions, and, for subscribers to MKSAP Digital, an HVC custom quiz. From the text and questions, we have generated the following list of HVC recommendations that meet the definition below of high value care and bring us closer to our goal of improving patient outcomes while conserving finite resources.

High Value Care Recommendation: A recommendation to choose diagnostic and management strategies for patients in specific clinical situations that balance clinical benefit with cost and harms with the goal of improving patient outcomes.

Below are the High Value Care Recommendations for the General Internal Medicine section of MKSAP 17.

- Statistical significance does not equal clinical importance, especially for large studies with uncommon outcomes.
- Relative risk comparisons tend to exaggerate outcomes relative to absolute risk measures; whenever possible, absolute risk should be used when explaining risk to patients (see Item 129).
- Numbers needed are estimates of the number of patients who must receive an intervention to cause one patient to experience the outcome being studied; numbers needed are useful indicators of the clinical impact of an intervention because they provide a sense of magnitude of benefit/harm expected from the intervention (see Item 162).
- Although the periodic health examination has been associated with increased delivery of preventive services, multiple studies have failed to show a beneficial effect of the periodic health examination on morbidity or mortality.

- A condition is amenable to screening if it is sufficiently common, will cause significant morbidity and mortality if left untreated, has a preclinical stage to allow for detection, and has an effective, available treatment that can improve prognosis if given early.
- Screening based on clinical guidelines needs to be individualized to account for patient circumstances; shared decision-making discussions should be documented and include the rationale for not providing screening that might otherwise be recommended.
- Although providing the appropriate preventive services is vital for optimal medical care, it is equally important to recognize what screening tests should not be performed and when screening should be discontinued.
- Women should have a life expectancy of at least 10 years to benefit from screening mammography (see Item 9).
- The U.S. Preventive Services Task Force recommends that all adults be screened for obesity, hypertension, tobacco use, alcohol misuse, and depression (if adequate resources are available to provide support and treatment for depression).
- The U.S. Preventive Services Task Force recommends against using prostate-specific antigen level to screen average-risk men for prostate cancer.
- Patients who have no genetic family history available (for example, due to adoption) should not undergo genetic testing without other reason.
- Although pharmacogenetic testing is available for many drug-metabolizing enzymes, its use has been clinically limited and is not routinely recommended.
- Providing age- and risk-appropriate vaccination is one of the most cost-effective preventive health measures available and is essential to the practice of high value care.
- Influenza vaccination is recommended for all persons aged 6 months and older unless specifically contraindicated.
- Pneumococcal vaccination with the 23-valent pneumococcal polysaccharide vaccine (PPSV23) and 13-valent pneumococcal conjugate vaccine (PCV13) is indicated for all adults aged 65 years and older and for certain high-risk persons younger than 65 years.
- Bivalent, quadrivalent, and nine-valent vaccines for human papillomavirus are approved for use in females and quadrivalent and nine-valent vaccines for males between the ages of 11 and 26 years to prevent cancer.
- Vaccination with herpes zoster vaccine is recommended for individuals aged 60 years and older, including patients with a previous episode of zoster.

- Annual vaccination against influenza and one-time vaccination against pertussis with the tetanus toxoid, reduced diphtheria toxoid, and acellular pertussis (Tdap) vaccine is recommended for all health care workers.
- Smokers should receive pneumococcal vaccination and annual influenza vaccination.
- Given small potential effect, time limitations, and opportunity costs, the U.S. Preventive Services Task Force recommends offering dietary and exercise behavioral counseling based only on individual patient circumstances (grade C).
- Hospital-to-primary provider communication at discharge, predischarge patient education, medication reconciliation, and timely post-hospitalization follow-up are all necessary to improve patient safety during transitions of care.
- The Model for Improvement involves defining the goal of the project (aim), measuring the baseline to see if interventions lead to improvement (measures), determining what changes can be made to improve quality (ideas), and implementing and testing the change in a process called a Plan-Do-Study-Act cycle.
- The Lean model focuses on closely examining a system's processes and eliminating non-value-added activities, or waste, within that system (see Item 6).
- The Six Sigma model has an emphasis on reducing cost, variation, or defects within a process to make the process more effective.
- A cause-and-effect diagram, also known as a fishbone or Ishikawa diagram, is a quality improvement tool that is used to list and organize root causes of a problem (see Item 57).
- Physicians are not ethically obliged to grant patient requests for ineffective tests and treatments; they should advise patients that using an ineffective intervention does not promote patient well-being, may cause harm, and violates the profession's commitment to stewardship of health care resources.
- Palliative medicine maximizes quality of life for patients with serious illness through meticulous symptom management and by aligning comprehensive care to meet the patients' goals as much as possible.
- Palliative care may be provided concurrently with life-prolonging therapies or with therapies with curative intent; hospice is palliative care that is reserved for patients in the terminal phase of their disease.
- When bad news is communicated in a skillful and empathic manner using the SPIKES (Setting, Perception, Invitation, Knowledge, Empathy, Strategize) protocol, patient satisfaction is increased, and depression and anxiety are decreased (see Item 21).
- Studies indicate that approximately 85% of diagnoses are correctly made simply by performing a detailed history and physical examination.
- Diagnostic testing beyond the history and physical examination should be used in an intentional, logical, and stepwise fashion; nearly 30% of all health care costs are spent on unnecessary tests and treatments.
- Reasonable quality evidence refutes the commonly held belief that ordering additional, unnecessary diagnostic testing alleviates patient fears and concerns.
- Nonpharmacologic modalities that can be effective when part of a multimodal approach to pain management include exercise, ice and heat therapy, transcutaneous electric nerve stimulation, massage, acupuncture, and chiropractic manipulation.
- There is no evidence to support the efficacy of long-term opioids in managing chronic pain, and there are significant harms associated with their use.
- Evidence that further diagnostic testing helps reassure patients with medically unexplained symptoms or improves outcomes is limited; negative test results may, in fact, increase patient anxiety over a potentially missed diagnosis (see Item 95).
- In patients with medically unexplained symptoms, the point of aborting diagnostic testing and unsuccessful therapy and shifting primary attention toward symptom management (and if indicated, mental health care) requires clinical judgment on an individualized basis and patient engagement in the conversation.
- Consistent follow-up visits with brief focused history and physical examination are the cornerstone of management of patients with medically unexplained symptoms (see Item 122).
- Cognitive-behavioral therapy may be beneficial in the management of medically unexplained symptoms and should be considered in place of additional testing (see Item 16).
- Routine antibiotic treatment of uncomplicated upper respiratory tract infections and acute bronchitis in the nonelderly immunocompetent patient is not indicated because of lack of efficacy and associated harms and costs (see Item 63).
- Most cases of otitis media with effusion resolve spontaneously; observation and symptomatic treatment of conditions contributing to eustachian tube dysfunction are appropriate (see Item 11).
- The Dix-Hallpike maneuver can be used to distinguish central from peripheral causes of vertigo; for peripheral causes, the Epley maneuver is an effective and safe treatment; neuroimaging is not necessary in patients with peripheral vertigo (see Item 3).
- Management of patients with disequilibrium involves physical therapy, visual and auditory screening followed by correction of impairment, and mobility aids that stabilize ambulation; extensive imaging and testing is unnecessary (see Item 18).
- The initial treatment of insomnia is nonpharmacologic and focuses on implementing good sleep hygiene via

- patient education or brief cognitive-behavioral therapy (see Item 139).
- Although effective for short-term treatment of insomnia, the use of benzodiazepines is limited by dependence, tolerance, and the side effects of daytime somnolence, falls, cognitive impairment, and anterograde amnesia.
- The most valuable diagnostic and management test in patients with syncope is postural blood pressure measurement; extensive additional testing, including telemetry, cardiac enzyme testing, CT of the head, echocardiography, carotid ultrasonography, and electroencephalography, aided diagnosis in less than 2% of patients and altered management decisions in less than 5% of patients.
- The American College of Physicians does not recommend brain imaging, either with CT or MRI, in the evaluation of a patient with simple syncope and a normal neurologic examination.
- Most patients with syncope can be safely managed as outpatients; indications for hospital admission for patients with syncope include presence of severe traumatic injuries or a high short-term risk for adverse cardiovascular outcomes.
- Diagnostic testing for low back pain should be reserved for patients with severe or progressive neurologic deficits, patients for whom a serious underlying condition is suspected, or patients who do not have symptom improvement after 4 to 6 weeks of conservative management (see Item 109).
- Most patients with acute musculoskeletal low back pain have an excellent prognosis no matter what therapeutic intervention is used; therapeutic interventions should focus on symptom management and maintaining function.
- Massage therapy for low back pain is likely to be helpful in patients with subacute or chronic symptoms and no abnormal neurologic findings (see Item 51).
- Surgery has been shown to have definite benefits only for patients with low back pain due to disk herniation causing persistent radiculopathy, patients with painful spinal stenosis, and those with cauda equina syndrome.
- Imaging studies and laboratory testing are not needed for most patients with neck pain; patients with a history of trauma, presence of neurologic signs or symptoms, fever, weight loss, or immunosuppression may require additional testing (see Item 167).
- Most patients with neck pain recover with conservative therapy, including mobilization, exercise, analgesic agents, and physical therapy.
- Although most rotator cuff tears can be managed conservatively, immediate surgery is indicated for younger patients with an acute full-thickness tear, and surgery may be indicated for patients with partial tears who do not respond to conservative therapy.

- Imaging studies are not indicated for patients with clinical findings consistent with epicondylosis; treatment of epicondylosis should focus on avoidance of activities that cause pain (see Item 5).
- Surgery in carpal tunnel syndrome is reserved for patients who do not respond to conservative measures, have intolerable pain, have severe disease on nerve conduction testing, or have evidence of muscle wasting on examination.
- In patients with acute knee pain, plain radiographs are generally needed only if a traumatic fracture is suspected.
- Patellofemoral pain syndrome is characterized by anterior knee pain that is usually gradual in onset and worsens with running, prolonged sitting, and climbing stairs; this is a clinical diagnosis and imaging studies are not usually needed.
- The Ottawa ankle and foot rules are useful in excluding ankle fractures, with an extremely high sensitivity (>95%); if these rules are not met, obtaining radiographs is not necessary, as the probability of an ankle fracture is exceedingly low.
- Initial treatment of plantar faciitis is multimodal and consists of patient education, activity modification, application of ice, correcting improper mechanics, and heel stretches.
- There is insufficient evidence to support the routine measurement of lipoprotein(a), apolipoprotein B, and LDL particles in the evaluation or management of dyslipidemia.
- Baseline creatine kinase measurement is not routinely indicated before starting statin therapy or for monitoring therapy in the absence of symptoms of muscle disease.
- Current guidelines recommend against screening for androgen deficiency in asymptomatic men, regardless of age.
- Because pregnancy commonly causes changes in the normal bleeding pattern, pregnancy testing must be performed in all women with abnormal uterine bleeding before more extensive testing is ordered.
- Because most symptoms of cyclic mastalgia are self-limited, management usually requires only education, reassurance, and appropriate breast support (see Item 106).
- Healthy women of reproductive age generally do not require a pelvic examination or other studies before beginning hormonal contraception.
- In a patient with dysmenorrhea, if pelvic pathology is not suspected and a diagnosis of primary dysmenorrhea is made, symptomatic treatment may begin without additional evaluation.
- Hormone measurements during perimenopause are imprecise, cannot predict onset of menopause, and are therefore not recommended.
- Viral conjunctivitis is often acute, unilateral, and associated with antecedent upper respiratory tract infection

- and exposure to infected persons; treatment is supportive and should not include topical antibiotics.
- Intranasal glucocorticoids, antihistamines, and topical decongestants are all appropriate for initial treatment of acute sinusitis; antibiotics should not be used initially (see Item 55).
- In patients with symptoms of acute sinusitis, antibiotics are recommended only for those with severe symptoms (fever, purulent drainage, and facial pain) of 3 to 4 days' duration, worsening of symptoms that were initially improving, or failure to improve after 10 days of supportive therapy.
- Whispered voice test, finger rub test, hearing loss questionnaire, and hand-held audiometry are all reasonable screening tests for hearing loss.
- Interventions that decrease fall risk in community-dwelling older adults include implementing individualized exercise programs (physical therapy, tai chi), limiting polypharmacy, addressing orthostasis, assessing footwear, and adding vitamin D supplementation.
- Pelvic floor muscle training is recommended as first-line therapy for stress urinary incontinence (see Item 43).
- Behavioral therapy utilizing prompted voiding has been shown to reduce urinary incontinence in older patients with dementia (see Item 85).
- Bladder training is recommended as first-line therapy for urge urinary incontinence.
- Weight loss and exercise are recommended for obese women with urinary incontinence.
- Advanced static mattresses or overlays reduce the risk of pressure ulcers in at-risk patients (see Item 8).
- Several organizations recommend against obtaining routine preoperative laboratory studies or chest radiography in healthy, asymptomatic patients undergoing elective or low-risk surgery (see Item 34).
- Patients without coronary artery disease (CAD) or CAD risk factors with an estimated major adverse cardiac event risk of less than 1% or with a functional capacity of 4 or more metabolic equivalents do not require preoperative coronary evaluation (see Item 58).
- In asymptomatic patients at low risk for cardiovascular disease, cardiac testing is unnecessary (see Item 46).
- Preoperative coronary revascularization in asymptomatic patients has not been shown to reduce postoperative cardiac complications and should be reserved for the same indications as in the general setting.
- Preoperative spirometry should be performed only for dyspnea or hypoxia of uncertain cause (see Item 4).
- The mainstay of perioperative pulmonary risk management is lung expansion maneuvers, including deep breathing exercises and incentive spirometry.
- Conservative postoperative measures that may reduce the risk of pulmonary complications from suspected obstructive sleep apnea include nonsupine positioning, careful use of sedatives and opioids, and continuous pulse oximetry (see Item 33).
- Preoperatively, for patients with low thromboembolic risk, warfarin therapy is stopped with no bridging anticoagulation, whereas high-risk patients should receive bridging anticoagulation.
- For patients with cardiovascular disease and postoperative anemia, transfusion of red blood cells is recommended if the patient has symptoms attributable to anemia or a hemoglobin level less than 7 to 8 g/dL (70-80 g/L) (see Item 19).
- First-line therapy for erectile dysfunction includes lifestyle modification (weight loss, exercise, smoking cessation), psychotherapy as needed, and phosphodiesterase type 5 inhibitors, provided the patient has no contraindications (see Item 24).
- Older patients who present with symptoms of a mood disorder or cognitive dysfunction should be screened for hearing loss (see Item 27).
- Direct-to-consumer genetic tests have questionable clinical validity and may lead to patient misinterpretation of test results and unnecessary anxiety (see Item 29).
- Decision-making capacity exists when a patient demonstrates an ability to understand relevant information, appreciate the situation and its possible consequences, manipulate information rationally, and make a reasoned choice (see Item 41).
- When a patient lacks decision-making capacity, a surrogate who best knows the patient's health care values, goals, and preferences must make decisions (see Item 82 and Item 128).
- Men with low or low-normal testosterone levels should have confirmatory morning serum total testosterone testing before initiating testosterone therapy, and further evaluation of the cause of hypogonadism should be pursued before treatment is started (see Item 49).
- The diagnostic cognitive error of anchoring can be avoided by being willing to reconsider the initial diagnosis and act on the appearance of new clinical information; close clinical observation is often an important high value intervention (see Item 54).
- Proton pump inhibitor therapy can be initiated without 24-hour esophageal pH monitoring in patients with chronic cough who have a normal chest radiograph and symptoms suggestive of gastroesophageal reflux disease (see Item 67).
- Palpating the pulse is an effective, low-risk, and inexpensive way to screen adults aged 65 years and older for atrial fibrillation (see Item 68).
- All overweight and obese patients should be offered a comprehensive lifestyle intervention for weight loss including diet, physical activity, and behavioral therapy (see Item 73).
- Genetic testing for BRCA gene mutations should only be performed in patients with a family history that is suggestive of an increased genetic risk (see Item 76).
- Antipsychotic medications, individualized exercise programs, and skilled nursing facility placement have not been shown to be beneficial in reducing fall risk in cognitively impaired patients (see Item 77).

- Inactivated influenza vaccine can be safely administered to patients with an egg allergy who have only experienced hives upon exposure to eggs (see Item 78).
- Patients with a family history suggestive of an inherited disorder should receive genetic counseling before undergoing genetic testing so that they understand the ramifications of testing; genetic testing is expensive and may impact a patient's ability to obtain health and life insurance (see Item 81).
- The diagnosis of lower extremity edema due to chronic venous insufficiency usually may be made based on a consistent clinical presentation and minimal laboratory testing (see Item 84).
- Artificial nutrition and pharmacologic agents do not improve morbidity and mortality or quality of life in cancer patients with cachexia (see Item 100).
- It is reasonable to proceed with elective noncardiac surgery without extensive additional testing in patients with asymptomatic severe aortic stenosis; these patients should undergo appropriate intraoperative and postoperative hemodynamic monitoring (see Item 104).
- Treatment of drug-induced lower extremity edema is discontinuation of the offending agent (see Item 105).
- Imaging of the shoulder is typically not needed to diagnose rotator cuff tendinitis but should be considered if a full-thickness rotator cuff tear is suspected or if there is diagnostic uncertainty (see Item 108).
- In patients with mild lower urinary tract symptoms caused by benign prostatic hyperplasia, observation with conservative therapy measures is appropriate (see Item 110).
- Vitamin supplementation, either with a multivitamin or with a single- or paired-vitamin preparation, has not been shown to reduce the risk for cardiovascular disease or cancer (see Item 114).
- Central adiposity increases risk for hypertension, type 2 diabetes mellitus, and coronary heart disease; in obese and overweight patients, measuring waist circumference is a cost-effective way to risk stratify patients (see Item 124).
- Screening for cervical cancer can be stopped in women age 65 years and older who have had three consecutive negative Pap smears or two consecutive negative Pap smears plus human papillomavirus test results within the last 10 years, with the most recent test performed within 5 years (see Item 126).
- In the absence of suspicious symptoms, physical examination findings, or family history in a patient undergoing a preparticipation sports evaluation, additional testing with either cardiovascular imaging or electrocardiography to exclude hypertrophic cardiomyopathy is not indicated (see Item 131).
- In patients with hyperlipidemia but without clinical atherosclerotic cardiovascular disease (ASCVD), diabetes mellitus, an LDL cholesterol level of 190 mg/dL (4.92 mmol/L) or higher, or elevated 10-year risk for developing ASCVD,

- therapeutic lifestyle modification is the primary intervention for prevention of ASCVD (see Item 133).
- Intranasal glucocorticoids are first-line therapy for patients with upper airway cough syndrome due to allergic rhinitis; antibiotics should not be used without clear evidence of bacterial infection (see Item 136).
- The mainstay of obesity treatment is lifestyle modification that includes diet for weight loss, increased physical activity, and behavioral therapy (see Item 137).
- In patients with usual symptoms of benign prostatic hyperplasia (BPH), a careful history and physical examination can usually render the diagnosis; a urinalysis is also indicated in evaluating BPH to exclude infection, malignancy, or postobstructive nephropathy (see Item 138).
- Treatment of cerumen impaction is indicated only in symptomatic patients or if the tympanic membrane needs to be visualized (see Item 140).
- Palliative care that is initiated early and integrated throughout the disease trajectory results in prolonged life of higher quality in patients with serious illness when compared with patients who do not receive palliative care (see Item 143).
- In older patients who require posthospital rehabilitation but cannot tolerate active, intensive therapy (3 hours per day, 5 days per week), rehabilitation services may be performed in a skilled nursing facility (see Item 144).
- In the case of a patient who refuses life-prolonging treatment, the physician's duty is to understand the rationale for the decision and ensure that it is informed; provided that the decision meets these criteria, the physician must honor it (see Item 146).
- In patients with insomnia in whom sleep hygiene techniques are ineffective, sleep restriction may be beneficial; sleep restriction limits and then gradually increases the time in bed for sleep (see Item 151).
- Patients with intact decision-making capacity have the right to request the withdrawal of any treatment, even those that are life prolonging (see Item 155).
- There is no specific objective laboratory test to diagnose systemic exertion intolerance disease (formerly known as chronic fatigue syndrome); recommended value-based tests to rule out this disease include complete blood count, glucose level, and thyroid function tests (see Item 157).
- In patients with cardiac risk factors undergoing elevated-risk procedures, preoperative coronary evaluation is not required if the patient has a good functional capacity (≥4 metabolic equivalents) (see Item 163).
- All adults aged 50 to 75 years should be screened for colorectal cancer using high-sensitivity fecal occult blood testing every year, flexible sigmoidoscopy every 5 years, combined flexible sigmoidoscopy every 5 years with high-sensitivity fecal occult blood testing every 3 years, or colonoscopy every 10 years; discontinuation of screening should be considered in patients with life expectancy of less than 10 years (see Item 168).

General Internal Medicine

High Value Care in Internal Medicine

An economically unsustainable amount of money is spent on health care in the United States–18% of the U.S. gross domestic product–leaving less money to pay for other essential services such as public health and safety, infrastructure, and education. Despite spending more on health care than any other country, the United States has health outcomes, including mortality, survival, and life expectancy, that rank at or near the bottom when compared with other high-income countries.

Misuse and overuse of medical interventions contribute significantly to this untenable health care spending. Physicians are uniquely positioned to take the lead in addressing these problems by partnering with patients and other health care providers to reduce the use of medical interventions (tests and treatments) that offer minimal or no benefit and may lead to unintended harm.

High value care is care that balances the clinical benefit of a given medical intervention with its harms and costs, with the goal of improving patient outcomes. High value care represents a paradigm shift away from the belief that more care is better care toward the idea that evidence-based, individualized care is better care. High value care places patients and their outcomes, values, and concerns at the center of every major clinical decision, using cost-effective and low-risk tools (for example, history and physical examination) and patient-centered communication to improve patient outcomes. This approach helps lay a foundation for dealing with the psychological burden that accompanies diagnostic uncertainty and allows both patients and physicians to be more comfortable with a conservative course of care. New drugs, devices, procedures, and tests are the primary drivers of increased health care spending; however, it is critical that physicians use testing and medical technology judiciously and selectively assess whether potential benefits justify the costs.

The Alliance for Academic Internal Medicine and the American College of Physicians (ACP) have developed a simple stepwise framework to help providers incorporate high value care into daily practice (**Table 1**). The ACP has also developed clinical recommendations and physician resources to help physicians practice high value care (available at http://hvc. acponline.org/index.html). Additionally, over 72 medical specialty societies and Consumer Reports (an independent product testing organization) have participated in the American Board of Internal Medicine Foundation's Choosing Wisely campaign, which promotes stewardship of medical resources

TABLE 1. High Value Care Framework: Steps Toward High Value Care

Step 1: Understand the benefits, harms, and relative costs of the interventions that you are considering.

Step 2: Decrease or eliminate the use of interventions that provide no benefits and/or may be harmful.

Step 3: Choose interventions and care settings that maximize benefits, minimize harms, and reduce costs (using comparative effectiveness and cost-effectiveness data).

Step 4: Customize a care plan with patients that incorporates their values and addresses their concerns.

Step 5: Identify system-level opportunities to improve outcomes, minimize harms, and reduce health care waste.

Reprinted with permission from Smith CD; Alliance for Academic Internal Medicine-American College of Physicians High Value, Cost-Conscious Care Curriculum Development Committee. Teaching high-value, cost-conscious care to residents: the Alliance for Academic Internal Medicine-American College of Physicians Curriculum. Ann Intern Med. 2012 Aug 21;157(4):284-6. [PMID: 22777503]

by asking societies to create evidence-based lists of tests and procedures whose necessity should be questioned. The Choosing Wisely lists and accompanying patient educational information are available at www.choosingwisely.org.

KEY POINT

- High value care is care that balances the clinical benefit of a given medical intervention with its harms and costs, with the goal of improving patient outcomes.

Interpretation of the Medical Literature

Introduction

Physicians must be familiar with an ever-expanding knowledge base that is founded on published research. Consequently, physicians must understand the basic principles of research to be able to independently interpret the literature, remain current in their medical knowledge, and apply the results of studies to provide high value care for their patients.

Study Designs

Many research study designs exist, and it is important to recognize the strengths and weaknesses of each and the appropriate application of information derived from these studies to clinical situations.

Experimental Studies

In an experimental study, subjects and interventions are determined at the study outset, and investigators and subjects are often blinded to the intervention to minimize biased outcomes. In the most common type of experimental study, a randomized controlled trial (RCT), subjects are randomly assigned to either an intervention or control group to equally distribute predictive factors and minimize confounding among the groups. Although RCTs are considered the most rigorous study design and have the greatest ability to draw causal inferences, these studies usually involve detailed protocols and patients with a narrow disease spectrum–conditions that are challenging to replicate in ordinary practice settings. Consequently, RCTs often have limited generalizability. A variation of an RCT is a cluster-randomized trial, in which groups (or clusters) of study subjects are randomized to a treatment or control group; this design is helpful in evaluating interventions directed toward specific groups of people instead of individual patients. A less rigorous experimental design is the quasi-experimental study, in which investigators assign patients to intervention and control groups in a nonrandom manner. This type of design is typically used when randomization would be impractical or unethical. The different types of experimental studies and observational studies are compared in **Table 2**.

Observational Studies

An observational study does not employ interventions or patient assignment to groups; alternatively, researchers compare two or more naturally existing groups. Observational studies are often less rigorous than experimental studies, thus reducing the ability to draw causal inferences. Advantages of observational studies include the capacity to utilize natural practice settings and to involve patients with wider ranges of illnesses and exposures. A disadvantage of observational studies is that they are more subject to confounding and bias than experimental studies.

Observational designs include cohort studies, case-control studies, cross-sectional studies, and case series. A cohort study investigates the outcomes of groups (cohorts) with or without certain exposures or treatments. An example is a study that examines the rates of type 2 diabetes mellitus among patients with high socioeconomic status versus patients with low socioeconomic status. In prospective cohort studies, patients are observed for outcomes going forward in time, whereas retrospective cohort studies look at patients' histories, often after an outcome has occurred. Prospective cohort studies are more rigorous than retrospective cohort studies because they reduce bias by selecting patients and statistical methods a priori. The standard outcome measure for a cohort study is relative risk.

A case-control study, which is usually retrospective, compares the outcomes of patients with a disease (cases) to those without a disease (controls). For instance, patients with and without type 2 diabetes could be compared with respect to exposure to high-calorie, fast-food diets. Case-control studies can be particularly valuable in the study of rare diseases. To reduce bias in case-control studies, investigators carefully match selected cases to controls in terms of demographic and prognostic factors. Additionally, investigators often increase statistical power by recruiting more controls than cases. For case-control studies, the standard estimate of risk is the odds ratio.

Cross-sectional studies examine associations between diseases and exposures within a group of patients at one point in time. This study design is most commonly used to determine disease prevalence and infer causation. Survey studies are generally cross-sectional studies. Case series include only patients with the condition of interest. These patients are evaluated, either prospectively or retrospectively, to identify exposures or outcomes. Cross-sectional and case series designs are limited, based on the absence of control groups.

Systematic Reviews

Systematic reviews provide a comprehensive summary, synthesis, and analysis of the literature that pertains to a focused research question. Systematic reviews involve exhaustive literature searches, systematic data abstraction, multiple reviewers, and a narrative summary regarding the strengths and limitations of the analysis. Systematic reviews minimize error by combining results from many studies. They may also include meta-analysis, which involves the statistical analysis of pooled data from the studies identified in a systematic review meeting certain predefined criteria for adequacy. The purpose of meta-analysis is to draw conclusions using a greater amount of data than is available in each of the individual studies. The limitations of systematic reviews and meta-analysis result from variability in the identification and selection of studies and from the inclusion of weak studies. However, a systematic review with meta-analysis that is based on the rigorous selection of numerous, high-quality RCTs could be considered the highest level of evidence.

KEY POINTS

- In a randomized controlled trial, subjects are randomly allocated to an intervention or control group, and investigators and subjects are often blinded to the intervention to minimize biased outcomes.

- Observational designs include cohort studies, case-control studies, cross-sectional studies, and case series; patients are not randomly allocated to an intervention or control group, thus reducing the ability to draw causal inferences.

- A systematic review provides a comprehensive summary, synthesis, and analysis of the literature that pertains to a focused research question and may or may not include meta-analysis; systematic reviews minimize errors by combining results from many studies but may be limited by variability in the identification and selection of studies and from the inclusion of weak studies.

TABLE 2. Types of Study Designs

Study Design	Description	Strengths	Weaknesses	Key Threats to Validity
Experimental Studies				
Randomized controlled trial (RCT)	Subjects are randomly allocated to a treatment group or a control group	Strongest design for determining causation	Expensive, time consuming, not practical for many clinical situations Limited follow-up duration Limited number of outcomes that can be assessed Limited generalizability	If randomization is ineffective If data are not analyzed according to initially assigned group If key individuals are aware of group assignment (not blinded) If follow-up is incomplete
Cluster-randomized trial	Subjects are randomized by clusters (e.g., nursing unit) rather than as individuals	Same as for RCTs Can be used if randomization of patients is not ethical or feasible	Same as for RCTs Challenging to analyze	Same as for RCTs If analysis does not account for clustering
Quasi-experimental design	Review of data collected before and after an intervention	Can be used if randomization of patients is not ethical or feasible	Patients not randomized	If no adjustment for possible confounding
Observational Studies				
Cohort study	Studies outcomes of groups using observed assignment	Able to detect associations, but these are not always cause-effect relationships Able to study multiple outcomes over a long period of time Large sample size	Requires complicated statistical techniques to minimize confounding Prospective designs can be expensive and take many years before results are available	Selection bias in cohort Bias in measurement of exposures and outcomes If important confounders not accounted for
Case-control study	Compares past exposures in patients with and without disease	Useful for rare diseases or exposures Inexpensive	High risk for bias High risk for confounding Cannot assess incidence/prevalence	Selection bias, especially in controls Measurement bias, especially recall bias
Cross-sectional study	Determines prevalence of disease (e.g., survey studies)	Can be completed quickly Inexpensive	May result in misleading information Provides information on only one point in time High risk for bias	Selection bias, response bias If sample is not representative
Case series	Describes the characteristics of a group (or series) of patients (or cases)	Hypothesis generating Observations may be useful in designing a study to evaluate possible explanations or causes for the observed findings	High risk for bias Cannot infer causation	Multiple biases related to subject selection and the characteristics observed

Validity of a Study

Validity, or the trustworthiness of a study's results, can be threatened by many factors, including errors in sampling, measurement, and data analysis. Internal validity is the extent to which a study's results are true and supported by the study. External validity is the degree to which a study's findings are generalizable to other settings.

Study errors can be random or systematic. Random error, which is due to chance, can be reduced by increasing the sample size and measurement precision. Systematic error results from bias and influences the study findings in a certain direction. Systematic error cannot be improved by increasing the sample size; it must be addressed by eliminating bias. For example, a study randomizes two groups of patients with

H
CONT.

diabetes to receive a new medication that lowers blood glucose levels (intervention group) or a placebo (control group), with the study outcome being self-monitored blood glucose (SMBG) measurements. If it were found that most of the intervention group patients recorded fasting morning SMBG levels and most of the control group recorded SMBG levels following the evening meal, any overall differences in glycemic control between the two study groups would be biased by the systematic, between-group differences in SMBG monitoring. When designing studies, systematic error is minimized by ensuring that the comparison groups are sampled, measured, and analyzed in the same way.

Confounding occurs when the hidden effect of an extraneous variable (the confounding variable) influences the outcome of a study. For example, early research indicated that coffee drinkers were more likely to develop pancreatic cancer. However, coffee drinkers are also more likely to be smokers. It was later demonstrated that the outcome of pancreatic cancer in these studies was attributable to smoking (confounding variable), not coffee consumption. Confounding can be decreased through the use of matching, randomization, and statistical methods such as multivariate analysis.

Statistical Analysis

Confidence Intervals and *P* Values

Every research finding reflects some amount of error, which is often expressed as a 95% confidence interval (CI). The 95% CI indicates that the researcher can be 95% certain that the value expressed in a study truly lies within that interval. The sample size of a study can influence the CI; larger samples will tend to allow more precise estimates and a narrower CI, whereas smaller sample sizes tend to yield wider CIs. Sample size is also directly proportional to a study's power, which is the probability of detecting an association between variables or a difference between groups when the association or difference truly exists. Statistical power can be used to determine the minimum sample size required for a study to demonstrate a specified effect.

The *P* value is another statistical indicator that indicates the likelihood of the study result being caused by chance alone. A *P* value of less than 0.05, which is a commonly used cut-off for statistical significance, represents a 1 in 20 chance of obtaining the observed results by chance, assuming that there is no difference between the study groups. Similarly to CIs, the *P* value is also related to the degree of difference between groups and the study's sample size; studies with large samples are more likely to produce statistically significant results. It is important not to confuse statistical significance with clinical importance, because a study that reports statistically significant *P* values may not be clinically relevant. This is particularly true for studies with large sample sizes or uncommon events of interest.

P values offer less information than CIs, because CIs can demonstrate the plausible range of an event or outcome, whereas *P* values indicate only statistical significance. Specifically, the lower and upper limits of a CI reveal, in discrete terms, the range of values around a given point, which allows readers to determine a plausible range of clinical significance and to apply study results to patients in clinical settings. For example, a study showed an association between influenza vaccination and development of Guillain-Barré syndrome (GBS), with a *P* value of 0.02 and a relative incidence of 1.45 (CI, 1.05 to 1.99). Considering the baseline GBS risk of 10 cases per million, influenza vaccination might result in 14.5 cases per million persons. However, the CI indicates that the risk of GBS from influenza vaccination ranges from only 5% increased risk to doubling of the risk. Accordingly, the worst-case risk would yield an absolute risk increase of 10 cases per million and a number needed to harm of 100,000. More strikingly, the best-case risk would yield an absolute increase of 0.5 cases per million and a number needed to harm of 2 million.

Calculations for Diagnostic Tests and Medical Therapeutics

Sensitivity, Specificity, and Predictive Values

Sensitivity is the ability of a test to detect patients with a disease when it is truly present. Specificity is the ability of a test to exclude disease in patients truly without the disease. The sensitivity and specificity are characteristics of a specific diagnostic test and do not change with the prevalence of disease in the population of patients to which they are applied (**Table 3**).

Compared with sensitivity and specificity, predictive values indicate the likelihood that a positive test result (positive predictive value [PPV]) or negative test result (negative predictive value [NPV]) truly reflects the presence or absence of disease in a specific patient population to which the test is applied. They are generated when applying tests of known sensitivity and specificity to a particular group of patients and are therefore dependent on the prevalence of the disease in that population. Because a positive test is more likely to be truly positive in a patient population with a high prevalence of disease, the PPV is directly related to prevalence. Conversely, a negative test is more likely to be truly negative when the prevalence of disease in the tested population is low; therefore, the NPV is inversely related to prevalence.

Likelihood Ratios

Likelihood ratios are a newer statistical tool that greatly simplifies applying diagnostic test results to patient care. The likelihood ratio (LR) is the ratio of the probability of a given test result (positive or negative) among patients with a disease to the probability of the same test result among patients without the disease. The posttest odds of a disease are equal to the pretest odds of the disease multiplied by the LR; the posttest odds can then be converted to a percentage to yield the more commonly recognized posttest probability. A major benefit of LRs is that they can be determined for any test for which the sensitivity and specificity are known, allowing clinicians to apply them to patients based on the clinically assessed pretest

TABLE 3. Common Terms Used in the Interpretation of the Medical Literature for Diagnostic Tests

Term	Definition	Calculation	Notes
Prevalence (Prev)	Proportion of patients with the disease in the population	Prev = (TP + FN) / (TP + FP + FN + TN)	
Sensitivity (Sn)	Proportion of patients with the disease who have a positive test	Sn = TP / (TP + FN)	
Specificity (Sp)	Proportion of patients without the disease who have a negative test	Sp = TN / (FP + TN)	
Positive predictive value (PPV)	Proportion of patients with a positive test who have the disease	PPV = TP / (TP + FP)	Increases with *increasing* prevalence
Negative predictive value (NPV)	Proportion of patients with a negative test who do not have the disease	NPV = TN / (TN + FN)	Increases with *decreasing* prevalence
Positive likelihood ratio (LR+)	The ratio of the probability of a positive test result among patients with the disease to the probability of a positive result among patients without the disease	LR+ = Sn / (1 − Sp)	
Negative likelihood ratio (LR−)	The ratio of the probability of a negative test result among patients with the disease to the probability of a negative result in patients without the disease	LR− = (1 − Sn) / Sp	
Pretest odds	The odds that a patient has the disease before the test is performed	Pretest odds = pretest probability / (1 − pretest probability)	
Posttest odds	The odds that a patient has the disease after a test is performed	Posttest odds = pretest odds × LR	LR+ is used if result of test is positive; LR− is used if result of test is negative. A nomogram is available to calculate posttest probability using pretest probability and LR without having to convert pretest probability to odds (see Figure 1)
Pretest probability	Proportion of patients with the disease before a test is performed	Pretest probability can be estimated from population prevalence, clinical risk calculators, or clinical experience if no evidence-based tools exist	
Posttest probability	Proportion of patients with the disease after a test is performed	Posttest probability = posttest odds / (1 + posttest odds)	

FN = false negative; FP = false positive; TN = true negative; TP = true positive.

probability of disease to generate a posttest likelihood of the presence or absence of the condition being tested. **Figure 1** shows a nomogram that may be used to estimate the posttest probability when the pretest probability and likelihood ratio are known.

Separate LRs are calculated for use when a test result is positive (LR+) or when a test result is negative (LR−). Larger positive LRs and smaller negative LRs are more apt to affect clinical decisions. For ease of clinical use, several general LR rules apply. LR+ values of 2, 5, and 10 correspond to an increase in disease probability of 15%, 30%, and 45%, respectively; LR− values of 0.5, 0.2, and 0.1 correspond to a decrease in disease probability of 15%, 30%, and 45%, respectively.

Relative and Absolute Risk

The effectiveness of different therapeutic interventions is frequently reported as relative or absolute risk differences between study groups. Relative comparisons compare the

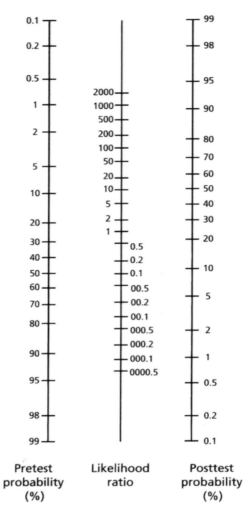

FIGURE 1. Nomogram for interpreting diagnostic test results. In this nomogram, a straight line drawn from a patient's pretest probability of disease (which is estimated from experience, local data, or published literature) through the likelihood ratio for the test result will point to the posttest probability of disease.

Reprinted with permission from Fagan TJ. Letter: Nomogram for Bayes theorem. N Engl J Med. 1975 Jul 31;293(5):257. [PMID: 1143310] Copyright 1975, Massachusetts Medical Society.

CONT. rates of events, such as death or complications, in two study groups using measures that include relative risk, odds ratios, and hazard ratios (**Table 4**). Absolute comparisons, on the other hand, represent absolute (that is, total) differences in outcomes between two groups.

A disadvantage of relative comparisons is the potential for exaggerated outcomes, especially if the outcomes are uncommon. For instance, interventions that reduce the rate of a disease from 40% to 20% and 4% to 2% each have a relative risk reduction of 50%. However, the absolute risk reduction (ARR) for the first case is 20%, whereas the ARR for the second case is 2%.

Numbers Needed

Numbers needed are estimates of the number of patients who must receive an intervention to cause one patient to experience the outcome being studied; if beneficial, it is termed the number needed to treat (NNT), and if detrimental, the number needed to harm (NNH). Numbers needed are useful indicators of the clinical impact of an intervention because they provide a sense of magnitude expected from the intervention. Numbers needed are calculated by taking the reciprocal of the change in absolute risk. For example, for the two interventions previously discussed, the NNT in the first case is 5 (1/0.2) and in the second case 50 (1/0.02) (see Table 4). **H**

KEY POINTS

- Confidence intervals provide more information than P values because they reveal the plausible range of an event, allowing clinical significance to be estimated.

- Statistical significance does not equal clinical importance, especially for large studies with uncommon outcomes.

- Relative risk comparisons tend to exaggerate outcomes relative to absolute risk measures; whenever possible, absolute risk should be used when explaining risk to patients.

- Numbers needed are estimates of the number of patients who must receive an intervention to cause one patient to experience the outcome being studied; numbers needed are useful indicators of the clinical impact of an intervention by providing a sense of magnitude of benefit/harm expected from the intervention.

Levels of Evidence and Recommendations

Physicians make clinical decisions about patients by interpreting evidence from the published literature; however, not all evidence is developed with the same rigor. Therefore, the U.S. Preventive Services Task Force has identified levels of evidence that reflect the rigor of methods used in a study (**Table 5**). Additionally, grades of recommendations for providing a clinical service were created by balancing the level of evidence with the risk versus benefit of the service (**Table 6**).

Routine Care of the Healthy Patient

History and Physical Examination
Periodic Health Examination

Although the periodic health examination has been associated with increased delivery of preventive services, multiple studies have failed to show a beneficial effect of the periodic health examination on morbidity or mortality; however, many of these trials were older, limited in scope, and assessed out-of-date interventions. Many physicians argue that the periodic health examination builds physician-patient relationships, which may promote improved adherence to physician recommendations.

TABLE 4. Common Terms Used in the Interpretation of the Medical Literature for Therapeutics

Term	Definition	Calculation	Notes
Absolute risk (AR)	The probability of an event occurring in a group during a specified time period	AR = patients with event in group / total patients in group	Also known as event rate; can be for benefits or harms. Often, an experimental event rate (EER) is compared with a control event rate (CER)
Relative risk (RR)	The ratio of the probability of developing a disease with a risk factor present to the probability of developing the disease without the risk factor present	RR = EER / CER	Used in cohort studies and randomized controlled trials
Absolute risk reduction (ARR)	The difference in rates of events between experimental group (EER) and control group (CER)	ARR = | EER − CER |	
Relative risk reduction (RRR)	The ratio of absolute risk reduction to the event rate among controls	RRR = | EER − CER | / CER	
Number needed to treat (NNT)	Number of patients needed to receive a treatment for one additional patient to benefit	NNT = 1 / ARR	A good estimate of the effect size
Number needed to harm (NNH)	Number of patients needed to receive a treatment for one additional patient to be harmed	NNH = 1 / ARI	ARI = absolute risk increase and equals | EER − CER | when the event is an unfavorable outcome (e.g., drug side effect)

TABLE 5. U.S. Preventive Services Task Force Hierarchy of Research Design

Level	Description
I	Properly powered and conducted RCT; well-conducted systematic review or meta-analysis of homogeneous RCTs
II-1	Well-designed controlled trial without randomization
II-2	Well-designed cohort or case-control analytic study
II-3	Multiple time series with or without the intervention; dramatic results from uncontrolled experiments
III	Opinions of respected authorities, based on clinical experience; descriptive studies or case reports; reports of expert committees

RCT = randomized controlled trial.

Reprinted from U.S. Preventive Services Task Force. U.S. Preventive Services Task Force Procedure Manual. Agency for Healthcare Research and Quality Publication No. 08-05118-EF. www.uspreventiveservicestaskforce.org/Page/Name/procedure-manual. Published July 2008. Accessed June 24, 2015.

TABLE 6. U.S. Preventive Services Task Force Grade Definitions

Grade	Definition and Suggestion for Practice
A	There is high certainty that the net benefit is substantial. Offer or provide this service.
B	There is high certainty that the net benefit is moderate. Offer or provide this service.
C	There is at least moderate certainty that the net benefit is small. Offer or provide this service for selected patients depending on the individual circumstances.
D	There is moderate or high certainty that the service has no net benefit or that the harms outweigh the benefits. Discourage use of this service.
I (Insufficient)	Evidence is lacking, of poor quality, or conflicting, and the balance of benefits and harms cannot be determined. If the service is offered, patients should understand the uncertainty about the balance of benefits and harms.

Adapted from U.S. Preventive Services Task Force. Grade definitions. www.uspreventiveservicestaskforce.org/uspstf/grades.htm. Updated February 2013. Accessed June 24, 2015.

In patients who do have regularly scheduled examinations, some aspects of preventive care are optimally addressed over several visits; thus, preventive care should be considered at every visit when feasible and an effort made to prioritize recommendations based on the patient's needs.

Routine History and Physical Examination

The history and physical examination can help identify those who are at risk for disease and who may benefit from additional screening tests or counseling. In patients who have positive findings on a detailed history, including a review of systems, a relevant physical examination pertinent to those concerns should be performed. The physical examination should include measurement of height and weight (to calculate BMI) and assessment of blood pressure. In persons with a BMI of 30 or more, the physician should assess for signs and symptoms of obstructive sleep apnea, as this condition is known to be underrecognized in primary care practices and has a high prevalence among obese persons. Heart rate should also be evaluated, as checking the pulse has been shown to increase detection of atrial fibrillation. The U.S. Preventive Services Task Force (USPSTF) recommends against routine abdominal and testicular examination for the purposes of cancer screening, and both the USPSTF and the American College of Physicians (ACP) recommend against screening pelvic examinations. Abdominal palpation for detection of abdominal aortic aneurysm and carotid auscultation for detection of carotid stenosis have both been shown to have poor reliability. Although all of the benefits of a comprehensive physical examination may not be clearly defined in regards to patient outcomes, the comprehensive physical examination is not directly associated with increased harm, may have less tangible benefits related to the physician-patient relationship, and is generally accepted as a standard of care. There is no evidence to support a routine panel of laboratory tests in all adult patients.

Internists are commonly asked to perform preparticipation sports examinations. The American Academy of Family Physicians (AAFP) and American Academy of Pediatrics, with several national sports medicine organizations, created a monograph on the approach to preparticipation physical evaluations, including free history and physical examination forms (available at www.aap.org/en-us/about-the-aap/Committees-Councils-Sections/Council-on-sports-medicine-and-fitness/Pages/PPE.aspx). Current American Heart Association (AHA) guidelines on preparticipation screening consist of a 12-step clinical history and physical examination focused on cardiovascular screening. The elements of this examination include evaluating the family history for evidence of heart disease or premature death, cardiac-related symptoms (such as unexplained near-syncope/syncope or exertional dyspnea or fatigue), and physical examination findings (including hypertension and murmurs). Additional testing, with either cardiovascular imaging or electrocardiography, is not indicated in the absence of suspicious symptoms, physical findings, or family history.

KEY POINT

HVC
- Although the periodic health examination has been associated with increased delivery of preventive services, multiple studies have failed to show a beneficial effect of the periodic health examination on morbidity or mortality.

Screening

Principles of Screening

Primary prevention is preventing disease or injury before it occurs, with the goal of decreasing the incidence of disease.

Secondary prevention is early detection of disease in asymptomatic patients to promote early intervention and reduce complications of disease. Most screening tests fall into the category of secondary prevention. Tertiary prevention is optimizing care of patients with established disease to improve function and reduce complications.

A condition is amenable to screening if it is sufficiently common, will cause significant morbidity and mortality if left untreated, has a preclinical stage to allow for detection, and has an effective, available treatment that can improve prognosis if given early. An ideal screening test must be widely available, safe, acceptable to the patient, of reasonable cost, and highly sensitive and specific for the disease of interest or have a complementary confirmatory test that has high specificity. The screened patient should be at risk for the condition and have adequate quality of life and life expectancy to benefit from screening.

Individuals who are likely to benefit from screening are often determined by the results of randomized controlled trials, but the results of these studies can be affected by commonly encountered biases. Selection (volunteer) bias occurs when patients who volunteer or comply with screening are healthier than those who do not undergo screening. The possibility of selection bias highlights the need for screening trials to use intention-to-treat analysis, which evaluates patient outcomes based on their initial group assignment in a randomized controlled trial instead of by the intervention they ultimately received; this minimizes selection bias. Lead-time bias occurs when survival time (time from diagnosis to death) appears to be lengthened because the screened patient is diagnosed earlier during the preclinical phase but does not live longer in actuality. As a result, disease-specific mortality rates rather than survival time should be used as an outcome. Screening is also more likely to detect indolent disease, which has a long latent period, than aggressive disease, which has a short latent period and is most often detected with onset of symptoms. This causes length-time bias, in which a screen-detected cohort will have overrepresentation of indolent disease, whereas a symptom-detected cohort will have overrepresentation of aggressive disease. Consequently, the screen-detected cohort falsely appears to have a better prognosis. A drastic type of length-time bias that has been increasingly recognized, especially in prostate, breast, and thyroid cancers, is overdiagnosis. Overdiagnosis occurs when disease that would not otherwise have been clinically significant during a patient's lifespan is detected.

KEY POINT

- A condition is amenable to screening if it is sufficiently common, will cause significant morbidity and mortality if left untreated, has a preclinical stage to allow for detection, and has an effective, available treatment that can improve prognosis if given early.

Screening Recommendations for Adults

Recommendations on which screening tests to use are frequently based on clinical practice guidelines. The USPSTF systematically reviews the available evidence and issues recommendations for clinicians and health care systems on screening, counseling, and preventive medicine based on the strength of evidence of benefit or harm of these interventions. **Table 7** provides a summary of the USPSTF screening recommendations. The ACP also publishes evidence-based clinical practice guidelines, guidance statements, and best practice advice (which recommend a clinical approach in areas where there may be insufficient or conflicting evidence). The National Guideline Clearinghouse provides a convenient online resource (www.guideline.gov) to compare clinical practice guidelines. Recommendations also change periodically as evidence emerges from large population-based trials. Therefore, clinicians should maintain awareness of these changes as they emerge, reflect upon the rationale and literature supporting the changes, and consider how to best incorporate new screening recommendations into practice.

Clinical guidelines are also sometimes used to develop quality performance measures, although this is an imperfect process given the need to individualize the appropriateness of screening in individual patient circumstances. Consequently, the medical record should reflect a shared decision-making discussion with the patient and the rationale for not providing screening that might normally be recommended.

To ensure that patients are receiving appropriate screening, many electronic health record (EHR) systems include features such as tracking and reminder systems for both providers and patients. This has been shown to improve adherence to evidence-based screening guidelines. Providing patients with electronic access to their health records may also help engaged patients facilitate appropriate screening. An additional resource for screening recommendations is the Electronic Preventive Services Selector (ePSS) developed by the Agency for Healthcare Research and Quality (AHRQ), available at http://epss.ahrq.gov/PDA/index.jsp. It is a point-of-care web- and mobile-based application that provides patient-specific clinical preventive services recommendations based on USPSTF guidelines.

Although providing the appropriate preventive services is vital for optimal medical care, it is equally important to recognize which screening tests should not be performed. **Table 8** provides a summary of screening interventions not routinely recommended by the USPSTF, many of which the USPSTF recommends against.

Specific Screening Tests
Screening for Chronic Diseases
The USPSTF strongly recommends screening all men 35 years of age and older for lipid disorders. Screening is also recommended in men 20 to 34 years of age and older if risk factors for atherosclerotic cardiovascular disease (ASCVD) are present (diabetes mellitus, personal history of coronary heart disease

or noncoronary atherosclerosis, family history of cardiovascular disease before age 50 years in male relatives or age 60 years in female relatives, tobacco use, hypertension, obesity [BMI ≥30]). The USPSTF makes no recommendation for or against routine screening for lipid disorders in men aged 20 to 34 years or in women aged 20 years and older who do not have risk factors for ASCVD. However, lipid screening is recommended in women aged 20 years and older if any of the aforementioned risk factors are present. Although the optimal screening interval is undetermined, the USPSTF states that it is reasonable to rescreen every 5 years, or at a shorter interval if the patient's lipid levels are approaching those that would indicate therapy. The 2013 American College of Cardiology/American Heart Association (ACC/AHA) cardiovascular risk guideline recommends assessment of cardiovascular risk in all adults 20 to 79 years of age every 4 to 6 years, evaluating for the ASCVD risk factors noted previously, with measurement of total cholesterol and HDL cholesterol levels. As part of this assessment in patients aged 40 to 79 years, calculation of the 10-year risk for ASCVD using the Pooled Cohort Equations is also recommended. (An online ASCVD risk calculator is available at http://tools.cardiosource.org/ASCVD-Risk-Estimator).

All adults should be screened for hypertension. The USPSTF cites the recommendation of the Seventh Report of the Joint National Committee on Prevention, Detection, Evaluation, and Treatment of High Blood Pressure to screen every 2 years for those with blood pressure below 120/80 mm Hg and yearly for those with systolic blood pressure of 120 to 139 mm Hg or diastolic blood pressure of 80 to 89 mm Hg. The report of the committee members of the Eighth Joint National Committee addressed management but not detection of hypertension.

In 2008, the USPSTF recommended screening for type 2 diabetes only in asymptomatic adults with sustained blood pressure higher than 135/80 mm Hg. An updated draft guideline, issued in October 2014, recommends screening for abnormal blood glucose and type 2 diabetes in adults with risk factors, including age 45 years or older, obesity or overweight, first-degree relative with diabetes, history of gestational diabetes or polycystic ovary syndrome, and certain high-risk ethnic backgrounds (African Americans, American Indians/Alaska Natives, Asian Americans, Hispanics/Latinos, and Native Hawaiians/Pacific Islanders). Recommended screening tests include fasting plasma glucose level, hemoglobin A_{1c}, or 2-hour oral glucose tolerance test. The American Diabetes Association recommends screening every 3 years if test results are normal.

According to the USPSTF, all adults should be screened for obesity using BMI. A 2013 joint guideline from the AHA, ACC, and The Obesity Society recommends screening for obesity at least annually. Adults with BMI of 30 or higher should be referred for intensive behavioral interventions.

The USPSTF recommends one-time screening for abdominal aortic aneurysm (AAA) with abdominal ultrasonography in all men aged 65 to 75 years who have smoked

TABLE 7. Summary of USPSTF Screening Recommendations[a]

Condition	Screening Recommendation
Chronic Diseases	
Abdominal aortic aneurysm	One-time abdominal ultrasonography in all men ages 65-75 y who have ever smoked[b]; selective screening in all men ages 65-75 y who have never smoked
Depression	All adults, when staff-assisted depression care support is available
Diabetes mellitus	All adults with sustained blood pressure >135/80 mm Hg according to 2008 recommendation; all adults at increased risk according to 2014 draft recommendation
Hypertension	All adults
Lipid disorders	All men age ≥35 y; all women age ≥45 y at increased risk; start at age 20 y for adults at increased cardiovascular risk
Obesity	All adults
Osteoporosis	Women age ≥65 y; women <65 y of age when 10-year fracture risk is ≥9.3%
Thyroid disease	Insufficient evidence to recommend for or against screening for thyroid disease (grade I)
Infectious Diseases	
Chlamydia	All sexually active women age ≤24 y; all sexually active women at increased risk of infection[c]
Gonorrhea	All sexually active women at increased risk of infection[c]
Hepatitis B virus	All adults at high risk[d]
Hepatitis C virus	One-time screening for adults born between 1945 and 1965; all adults at high risk[e]
HIV infection	One-time screening for all adults ages 15-65 y; repeated screening for adults at high risk[f]
Syphilis	All adults at increased risk of infection[g]
Tuberculosis	USPSTF defers to CDC guidelines, which recommend screening for high-risk individuals[h]
Substance Abuse	
Alcohol misuse	All adults
Tobacco use	All adults
Cancer	
Breast cancer	Biennial screening mammography for women ages 50-74 y; initiation of screening before age 50 y should be individualized (grade C).
Cervical cancer	Women ages 21-65 y with cytology (Pap smear) every 3 y; in women ages 30-65 y who want to lengthen screening, screen with cytology and HPV testing every 5 y.
Colorectal cancer	All adults ages 50-75 y using annual high-sensitivity FOBT, flexible sigmoidoscopy every 5 y, combined high-sensitivity FOBT (every 3 y) plus flexible sigmoidoscopy (every 5 y), or colonoscopy every 10 y
Lung cancer	Not recommended for the average-risk patient; annual low-dose CT in high-risk patients (adults ages 55-80 y with a 30-pack-year smoking history, including former smokers who have quit in the last 15 years) (see MKSAP 17 Pulmonary and Critical Care Medicine)
Skin cancer	Insufficient evidence for skin cancer screening examinations (grade I)

CDC = Centers for Disease Control and Prevention; FOBT = fecal occult blood testing; HPV = human papillomavirus; USPSTF = U.S. Preventive Services Task Force.

[a]Unless otherwise specified, all recommendations listed are grade A or B, for which the USPSTF suggests providing this service in practice. Grade C recommendations are offered for selected patients depending on individual circumstances. Grade D services should be discouraged. Grade I indicates that there is insufficient evidence to assess the balance of benefits and harms for a service.

[b]In the USPSTF recommendation, an "ever-smoker" is a person who has smoked at least 100 cigarettes in his or her lifetime.

[c]Women who are at increased risk of infection include those with a history of sexually transmitted infection (STI), those with new or multiple sexual partners, those who use condoms inconsistently, and commercial sex workers.

[d]Persons at high risk of hepatitis B virus (HBV) infection include those born in countries with at least a 2% prevalence of HBV infection, persons receiving dialysis or cytotoxic or immunosuppressive treatments, HIV-positive persons, injection drug users, men who have sex with men (MSM), and household contacts or sexual partners of persons with HBV infection.

[e]Persons at high risk of hepatitis C virus infection include injection and intranasal drug users, persons who received a blood transfusion before 1992, persons on long-term hemodialysis, prisoners, and persons who received unregulated tattoos.

[f]Persons at high risk of HIV infection include MSM, active injection drug users, persons with behavioral risk factors (those who have unprotected vaginal or anal intercourse; have sexual partners who are HIV-infected, bisexual, or injection drug users; or exchange sex for drugs or money), persons who have acquired other STIs, and persons who live and receive care in a high-prevalence setting (HIV seroprevalence of ≥1%).

[g]Persons at increased risk for syphilis infection include prisoners, MSM, and persons who exchange sex for money or drugs.

[h]Persons at high risk for tuberculosis infection include injection drug users, HIV-positive persons, those who have close contact with persons with known or suspected tuberculosis, those who live or work in high-risk settings, and recent immigrants from countries with a high prevalence of tuberculosis.

TABLE 8. Screening Interventions Not Routinely Recommended by the USPSTF for Asymptomatic, Average-Risk Adults[a]

Routine urine tests (grade D)[b]

Resting or exercise electrocardiography for CHD screening in asymptomatic adults at low risk for CHD events (grade D)[b,c]

Nontraditional risk factors (including CT coronary artery calcium score[b], high-sensitivity C-reactive protein, ankle-brachial index, carotid intima-media thickness, lipoprotein(a), and homocysteine) in screening asymptomatic adults with no history of CHD to prevent CHD events (grade I)

Screening for asymptomatic carotid stenosis (grade D)[b]

Screening for AAA in women who have never smoked (grade D)

PSA screening for prostate cancer (grade D)[b]

CA-125 measurement or pelvic ultrasonography for ovarian cancer screening (grade D)[b]

Abdominal palpation, serologic markers, or ultrasonography for pancreatic cancer screening (grade D)

Screening for testicular cancer (grade D)

Spirometry in asymptomatic individuals (including asymptomatic smokers) for COPD screening (grade D)[c]

Genetic screening tests for hereditary hemochromatosis (grade D)

Screening for chronic hepatitis B virus infection (grade D)[c]

AAA = abdominal aortic aneurysm; CHD = coronary heart disease; PSA = prostate-specific antigen; USPSTF = U.S. Preventive Services Task Force.

[a]Grade D services should be discouraged. Grade I indicates that there is insufficient evidence to assess the balance of benefits and harms for a service.

[b]Also recommended against in the American Board of Internal Medicine Foundation's Choosing Wisely initiative.

[c]Also recommended against in the American College of Physicians' High Value Care initiative.

at least 100 cigarettes in their lifetime and selective screening in men in this age group who have never smoked. There is insufficient evidence to recommend for or against screening for AAA in women aged 65 to 75 years who have ever smoked. Women who have never smoked should not be screened for AAA.

The USPSTF recommends screening for osteoporosis by measurement of bone mineral density in women aged 65 years and older and in younger women who have a fracture risk equal to or higher than a 65-year-old white woman (9.3%). The physician can use the Fracture Risk Assessment Tool (FRAX) (www.shef.ac.uk/FRAX/) to determine if the 10-year fracture risk for younger women is greater than or equal to 9.3%. The USPSTF concludes that the current evidence is insufficient to recommend routine screening for osteoporosis in men. The ACP recommends periodic individualized assessment of risk factors for osteoporosis in older men. By age 65 years, at least 6% of men have dual-energy x-ray absorptiometry (DEXA)–determined osteoporosis, so risk factor assessment before this age is reasonable. Risk assessment and screening guidelines are further discussed in MKSAP 17 Endocrinology and Metabolism.

The USPSTF concludes that there is insufficient evidence to recommend for or against screening for thyroid disease. The ACP recommends screening women over age 50 years who have at least one symptom that can be attributed to thyroid disease. The American Thyroid Association and the American Association of Clinical Endocrinologists recommend measuring thyroid-stimulating hormone (TSH) in individuals with risk factors for hypothyroidism (for example, personal history of autoimmune disease, neck radiation, or thyroid surgery) and consideration of TSH testing in adults age 60 years and older.

According to the USPSTF, all adults should be screened for depression if adequate resources are available to provide support and treatment. A useful clinical tool for screening is the two-item Patient Health Questionnaire (PHQ-2), which has an 83% sensitivity and 90% specificity for depression, which is comparable to longer, more complex screening instruments. Using this tool, the clinician asks, "During the past 2 weeks, how often have you been bothered by any of the following problems: (1) little interest or pleasure in doing things, or (2) feeling down, depressed, or hopeless?" If the patient responds positively to either question, further evaluation is indicated.

Screening for Infectious Diseases

The USPSTF recommends screening for chlamydia in all sexually active women age 24 years and younger and in women older than 24 years who are at increased risk of infection. Women who are at increased risk include those with a history of sexually transmitted infection (STI), those with new or multiple sexual partners, those who use condoms inconsistently, and commercial sex workers. The USPSTF concludes that there is insufficient evidence to recommend for or against chlamydia screening in men. Nucleic acid amplification tests can be performed on first-voided urine or vaginal or endocervical swabs. The Centers for Disease Control and Prevention (CDC) recommends that any patient who has a positive test result be retested 3 months after treatment.

Screening for gonorrhea is recommended by the USPSTF for all pregnant and nonpregnant sexually active women who are at increased risk of infection (same risk factors as with chlamydia). The USPSTF has not determined that there is sufficient evidence to recommend for or against screening for gonorrhea in men at high risk, and the task force recommends against screening for men and women who are at low risk. Nucleic acid amplification tests can be performed on first-voided urine or urethral swabs from men and vaginal or endocervical swabs from women. The CDC recommends that any patient who has a positive test result be retested 3 months after treatment.

The USPSTF recommends one-time HIV screening for all adults aged 15 to 65 years. Individuals with risk factors for HIV should be screened regardless of age, and repeated screening is recommended in this population. Based on prevalence data, men who have sex with men (MSM) and active injection drug users have a very high risk for HIV infection. Other individuals at risk for HIV include those with behavioral risk factors (those who have unprotected vaginal or anal intercourse; have sexual partners who are HIV-infected, bisexual, or injection drug users; or exchange sex for drugs or money), those who have acquired other STIs, and those who live and receive care in a high-prevalence setting (HIV seroprevalence of ≥1%). The USPSTF also recommends screening all pregnant women for HIV. Combined HIV antibody immunoassay/p24 antigen testing is the preferred screening test for HIV infection. Diagnosis of HIV is discussed in MKSAP 17 Infectious Disease.

The USPSTF also recommends screening for hepatitis B virus (HBV) in all adults at high risk, which includes persons born in countries with at least a 2% prevalence of HBV infection, persons receiving dialysis or cytotoxic or immunosuppressive treatments, HIV-positive persons, injection drug users, MSM, and household contacts or sexual partners of persons with HBV infection. Screening is performed with hepatitis B surface antigen (HBsAg) serologic studies; antibodies to hepatitis B antigens (anti-HBs and anti-HBc) are also obtained to differentiate between immunity and infection. All pregnant women should also be screened for HBV.

According to the USPSTF, all adults born between 1945 and 1965 should receive one-time screening for hepatitis C virus (HCV) with anti-HCV antibody testing. Additionally, all adults at high risk (injection and intranasal drug users, persons who received a blood transfusion before 1992, persons on long-term hemodialysis, prisoners, and persons who received unregulated tattoos) should receive HCV screening. The CDC recommends that HIV-positive patients undergo annual HCV screening. Screening is performed with anti-HCV antibody followed by polymerase chain reaction (PCR) viral load testing if positive (see MKSAP 17 Gastroenterology and Hepatology).

The USPSTF recommends syphilis screening for all pregnant women and all adults at increased risk for infection. Populations at risk are prisoners, MSM, and persons who exchange sex for money or drugs. Initial screening tests include the VDRL test and rapid plasma reagin (RPR) test.

The CDC has issued guidelines for tuberculosis (TB) screening that recommend screening in high-risk individuals, including injection drug users, persons who are positive for HIV, those who have close contact with persons with known or suspected TB, those who live or work in high-risk settings, and recent immigrants from countries with a high prevalence of TB. Appropriate screening tests include tuberculin skin testing or the interferon-γ release assay.

Screening for Substance Use Disorders

According to the USPSTF, all adults should be screened for alcohol misuse. The Alcohol Use Disorders Identification Test (AUDIT) is the most validated screening test for identifying hazardous and harmful drinking in primary care patients (available at http://pubs.niaaa.nih.gov/publications/Audit. pdf). Shorter tests that are comparable to AUDIT include the AUDIT-C test (three items from AUDIT) and single-item screening ("How many times in the past year have you had five [four for women] or more drinks in one day?"). The physician also should provide persons engaged in risky or hazardous drinking with brief behavioral counseling.

The USPSTF recommends that all adults be screened for tobacco use. To engage patients, physicians should consider using the 5 A's (Ask, Advise, Assess, Assist, and Arrange) (see Behavioral Counseling).

Although the USPSTF has concluded that there is not enough evidence to recommend for or against illicit drug screening, there are several questionnaires that are valid and reliable in screening for drug use. The Drug Abuse Screening Test (DAST-10) (available at https://www.drugabuse.gov/sites/ default/files/files/DAST-10.pdf) is a 10-item survey similar to the AUDIT tool used for alcohol screening. A single-item screening question ("How many times in the past year have you used an illegal drug or used prescription medications for nonmedical reasons?") has been shown to be highly sensitive and may be used for screening.

Screening for Cancer

Cancer screening guidelines have evolved significantly in recent years based on accumulating evidence of the potential benefits and harms associated with screening, diagnosis, and treatment. As a result, guidelines issued by organizations may differ significantly, and some recommendations may be controversial. This highlights the need to understand the evidence underlying the different guidelines and to engage in shared decision-making when deciding on an appropriate cancer screening strategy for an individual patient.

There is also sparse evidence on when to stop screening for cancer. In general, it is recommended that individuals with fewer than 10 years of quality life expectancy not receive most cancer screening.

Breast Cancer

Breast cancer screening discussed in this section applies to asymptomatic average-risk women. Women with significant risk factors for breast cancer, including family history of breast or ovarian cancer or personal history of atypia or lobular carcinoma in situ, should undergo a formal breast cancer risk assessment. Screening for breast cancer in women with increased risk is discussed in MKSAP 17 Hematology and Oncology.

In 2009, the USPSTF updated its recommendations for breast cancer screening to endorse biennial screening mammography for all women aged 50 to 74 years. Additionally, routine mammographic screening for women younger than 50 years is no longer recommended; rather, the USPSTF recommends individualized screening decisions for women younger than 50 years based on patient context and values regarding specific benefits and harms. The USPSTF reasons that while the benefit of screening may be similar in women ages 40 to 49 years (1 breast cancer death avoided per 1900 invited to screen, 15% relative risk reduction) compared with women ages 50 to 59 years (1 breast cancer death avoided per

1300 invited to screen, 14% relative risk reduction), there is a lower incidence of breast cancer and higher risk of harms in the younger age group. Harms can include false-positive screening results, which may lead to unnecessary emotional stress, biopsies, and unnecessary treatment. The ACP, AAFP, and Kaiser Permanente Care Management Institute concur with these guidelines; however, specialty organizations including the American Cancer Society (ACS), National Comprehensive Cancer Network, American Congress of Obstetricians and Gynecologists (ACOG), American College of Surgeons, American College of Radiology, and Society of Breast Imaging continue to recommend annual screening mammography starting at age 40 years. The ACP advises against screening average-risk women younger than 40 years for breast cancer.

For women age 75 years and older, the USPSTF found insufficient evidence to recommend for or against screening mammography, and other organizations recommend shared decision-making for this age group to develop an individualized approach. The ACP advises against screening for breast cancer in average-risk women age 75 years and older. As with other cancer screening tests, studies have suggested that women should have a life expectancy of at least 10 years to benefit from screening mammography.

The USPSTF does not recommend for or against clinical breast examination (CBE) and cites potential harms of CBE, including false-positive test results that lead to anxiety and additional imaging and biopsies. The ACS and ACOG recommend CBE every 3 years for women ages 20 to 39 years and yearly for women older than 40 years. The USPSTF recommends against breast self-examination (BSE), citing two trials showing increased imaging and biopsies for women who performed BSE. The ACS and ACOG have shifted towards recommending breast self-awareness, encouraging women to know how their breasts normally look and feel, with BSE as an option.

Breast density is an increasingly recognized risk factor for breast cancer. In addition to increasing breast cancer risk, high breast density is common (present in up to 50% of women) and also decreases the sensitivity of mammography. Evidence has shown that digital mammography may be better than film mammography in women with high breast density; however, currently, high breast density alone does not necessitate additional breast imaging other than routine screening mammography.

Prostate Cancer
In 2012, the USPSTF issued updated guidelines recommending against prostate-specific antigen (PSA) screening for prostate cancer. The USPSTF outlined harms associated with PSA screening, including those resulting directly from screening and diagnostic procedures (anxiety, additional testing including biopsies, overdiagnosis), and harms related to treatment of screen-detected cancer (surgical complications, urinary incontinence, erectile dysfunction, radiotherapy-induced bowel dysfunction). The benefit of PSA screening and associated

early treatment is prevention of between 0 and 1 prostate cancer deaths per 1000 men screened. Therefore, the USPSTF concluded that the benefits of PSA screening do not outweigh the harms. Most other organizations recommend a shared decision-making approach for men in the age group most likely to benefit (50-69 years of age according to the ACP, 50 years of age to 10 years of life expectancy according to the ACS, and 55-69 years of age according to the American Urological Association [AUA]). As a high value care intervention, the ACP recommends that clinicians have a one-time discussion (more if the patient requests) with average-risk men aged 50 to 69 years who inquire about PSA-based prostate cancer screening to inform them about the limited potential benefits and substantial harms of screening for prostate cancer using the PSA test. The ACP and AUA do not recommend PSA screening for men older than 69 years or those with less than a 10- to 15-year life expectancy.

Many organizations, including the ACP, ACS, and the American College of Preventive Medicine, recommend earlier thresholds for discussing prostate cancer screening in men at increased risk. In general, PSA discussions are recommended to start at age 45 years for black men or men who have a first-degree relative younger than 65 years with prostate cancer, and at age 40 years for men with several family members younger than 65 years with prostate cancer or men who have known or suspected *BRCA1* or *BRCA2* mutations. Although the USPSTF acknowledges that certain groups are at increased risk for prostate cancer, the task force concluded that there was not enough evidence to make separate recommendations. The current USPSTF recommendations do not apply to men with known *BRCA1* or *BRCA2* mutations.

The digital rectal examination (DRE) in combination with PSA screening has been shown to increase prostate cancer detection; however, no studies have suggested benefit of DRE for patient-important outcomes. Therefore, both the USPSTF and AUA do not make a recommendation for or against the use of DRE for screening purposes.

Additional Cancer Screening Tests
According to the USPSTF, women ages 21 to 65 years should be screened for cervical cancer every 3 years with cytology (Pap smear). In women ages 30 to 65 years who want to lengthen the screening interval, a combination of cytology and human papillomavirus (HPV) testing can be performed every 5 years. Screening for cervical cancer is not recommended in women younger than 21 years, women age 65 years and older who are not at high risk and have had adequate prior Pap smears (three consecutive negative cytology results or two consecutive negative cytology results and HPV testing within the past 10 years, with the most recent test performed within 5 years), and women who have had a hysterectomy with removal of the cervix with no history of a precancerous lesion.

The USPSTF recommends screening all adults ages 50 to 75 years for colorectal cancer using high-sensitivity fecal occult blood testing (FOBT) every year, flexible sigmoidoscopy every 5 years, combined high-sensitivity FOBT (every 3 years) plus flexible sigmoidoscopy (every 5 years), or colonoscopy every 10 years. According to a guidance statement issued by the ACP in 2012, patient preference, availability, and benefit and harms should guide the choice of test. The ACS, U.S. Multi-Society Task Force on Colorectal Cancer, and the American College of Gastroenterology (ACG) prefer the use of cancer prevention tests (colonoscopy, flexible sigmoidoscopy, double contrast barium enema, or CT colonography) to cancer detection tests (guaiac FOBT or fecal immunochemical testing). Given higher mortality rates, the ACP recommends that screening start at age 40 years for black persons, whereas the ACG recommends that screening begin at age 45 years in this population. Most guidelines recommend stopping screening if life expectancy is less than 10 years, and the USPSTF recommends against screening after age 85 years. For a discussion on screening recommendations for patients at high risk, see MKSAP 17 Gastroenterology and Hepatology.

The USPSTF concludes that there is insufficient evidence to recommend for or against whole-body skin examinations for the early detection of skin cancer; however, the USPSTF did not examine outcomes in patients at high risk for skin cancer. The ACS recommends monthly skin self-examinations as well as skin examination as part of a periodic health examination for adults age 20 years and older. Behavioral counseling on minimizing exposure to ultraviolet radiation is recommended by the USPSTF for persons younger than 24 years who have fair skin.

Lung cancer screening is not recommended for the average-risk patient. Annual low-dose CT is recommended for high-risk patients, defined as adults ages 55 to 80 years with a 30-pack-year smoking history, including former smokers who have quit in the last 15 years. Refer to MKSAP 17 Pulmonary and Critical Care Medicine for a more detailed discussion on screening in high-risk patients.

KEY POINTS

HVC • Screening based on clinical guidelines needs to be individualized to account for patient circumstances; shared decision-making discussions should be documented and include the rationale for not providing screening that might otherwise be recommended.

HVC • Although providing the appropriate preventive services is vital for optimal medical care, it is equally important to recognize what screening tests should not be performed.

HVC • The U.S. Preventive Services Task Force recommends that all adults be screened for obesity, hypertension, tobacco use, alcohol misuse, and depression (if adequate resources are available to provide support and treatment for depression).

• The U.S. Preventive Services Task Force and the American College of Physicians recommend biennial screening mammography for all women aged 50 to 74 years to screen for breast cancer.

(Continued)

KEY POINTS *(continued)*

• The U.S. Preventive Services Task Force recommends against using prostate-specific antigen level to screen for prostate cancer.

• According to the U.S. Preventive Services Task Force, women ages 21 to 65 years should be screened for cervical cancer every 3 years with a Pap smear.

• The U.S. Preventive Services Task Force recommends screening all adults ages 50 to 75 years for colorectal cancer using high-sensitivity fecal occult blood testing (FOBT) every year, flexible sigmoidoscopy every 5 years, combined high-sensitivity FOBT (every 3 years) plus flexible sigmoidoscopy (every 5 years), or colonoscopy every 10 years.

Genetics and Genetic Testing

Clinical genetics has traditionally focused on identification of specific disease-causing mutations that follow a mendelian pattern of inheritance; however, an increasing number of identifiable genetic variants or groups of specific genetic polymorphisms that do not follow a mendelian pattern of inheritance have been associated with the development of complex diseases. The understanding of the role of these genetic factors in predisposing an individual to certain diseases is rapidly evolving, although the predictive accuracy and appropriate use of this form of genetic testing remain to be established. Additionally, genetic information is increasingly used to individualize treatment for specific patients, such as those with blood disorders and tumors, and to predict individual response to specific medications. The increasing availability and lowering cost of direct-to-consumer genetic testing require clinicians to understand the basics of detecting, diagnosing, and managing genetic diseases.

Taking a Family History

Historical clues, including characteristics of the family history, can suggest the presence of an inherited condition and can be used by clinicians to help guide the appropriateness of obtaining genetic testing (**Table 9**). Despite this recognition, there is no standardized definition as to what constitutes an appropriate family history, and there is also no consensus on how to properly obtain and collect family history information for use in assessing risk for genetic diseases.

A reasonable approach is to obtain a three-generation family history, including information on grandparents, parents, aunts, uncles, siblings, cousins, children, nieces, and nephews. The sex, age, relationship to patient, and presence of any birth defects or medical conditions, including age of onset, should be elicited for each family member. Evidence suggests that persons are better at reporting absence rather than presence of disease in relatives, and accuracy may be increased by asking the patient to confer with other family members. Drawing a pedigree or family tree is often helpful in recognizing patterns of inheritance.

TABLE 9. "Red Flags" Suggesting an Increased Genetic Risk in an Individual or Family

"Red Flag"	Description	Example
Family history of multiple affected family members with the same or related disorders	Such a pattern indicates increased risk, whether through genetic or environmental risk factors or a combination of genes and environment.	Three family members in two generations with cardiovascular disease
Earlier age at onset of disease than expected	Disorders that arise at a younger age than expected may occur because of a genetic predisposition that makes an individual more susceptible to environmental exposures.	Cardiovascular disease occurring in the fourth decade of life
Condition in the less-often-affected sex	A disorder that occurs in the less common sex may occur because of a genetic predisposition that overrides other hormonal, developmental, and environmental factors that contribute to its occurrence.	Breast cancer in a male
Disease in the absence of known risk factors	Genetic predisposition may lead to the occurrence of a disorder in the absence of obvious environmental factors.	Hyperlipidemia in an individual with an ideal diet and exercise regimen
Ethnic predisposition to certain genetic disorders	Some genetic disorders are more common in certain ethnic groups. Awareness of a patient's ethnicity or ancestral background can aid in recommending genetic testing and evaluation of genetic conditions.	Lactose intolerance in an individual of African ancestry
Close biologic relationship between parents	Consanguinity is a relationship by blood or a common ancestor. Because relatives are more likely to share the same genes, children from a consanguineous couple related as first cousins or closer have an increased risk of having an autosomal recessive condition.	Cystic fibrosis

Based on National Coalition for Health Professional Education in Genetics. Core principles in family history: Interpretation. www.nchpeg.org/index.php?option=com_content&view=article&id=199:principles-for-interpretation&catid=64:core-principles-in-family-history&Itemid=126. Accessed May 29, 2015.

Patients who have no genetic family history available (for example, due to adoption) should not undergo genetic testing without other reason.

Genetic Tests and Testing Strategies

Cytogenetic tests are used to detect structural chromosomal abnormalities. Giemsa staining of chromosomes produces a banding pattern that allows karyotyping and aids in detecting structural abnormalities, and fluorescence in situ hybridization and microarray analysis can both be used to detect more subtle chromosomal abnormalities. Direct DNA tests are designed to detect specific genetic mutations. Examples of direct DNA tests include enzyme-linked immunosorbent assay, polymerase chain reaction, and Southern blot analysis. Linkage analysis is an indirect DNA test used when the responsible gene location is known but the precise gene or genetic mutation is not. Biochemical testing relies on measuring the levels of metabolites involved in biochemical pathways to assess enzymatic activity. When an enzymatic defect is present, metabolite levels may be either increased or decreased.

There are several strategies that clinicians may use in genetic testing. Predictive genetic testing uses a genetic test to determine whether or not an individual will develop a condition at some point in his or her lifetime. Diagnostic genetic testing is the use of a genetic test to diagnose or to rule out a condition that is suspected based on results of clinical findings. Pharmacogenetic testing is used to predict a patient's response to a medication. Although pharmacogenetic testing is available for many drug-metabolizing enzymes, its use has been clinically limited and is not routinely recommended. **Table 10** compares the different genetic testing strategies.

Direct-to-consumer genetic testing allows patients to obtain testing without the assistance of a health care provider. Direct-to-consumer testing is based on identifying genetic differences between individuals with a condition and those without the condition. In a case-control–based approach, single-nucleotide polymorphisms (SNPs) that are disproportionately found in affected individuals are identified, and odds ratios are determined for each SNP. Unfortunately, most SNPs have very low odds ratios and contribute only a small proportion to total disease burden. Direct-to-consumer testing has many potential drawbacks, including the validity of the tests themselves. Because of a lack of pretest counseling, patients often misinterpret test results, leading to unnecessary angst. Patients also frequently bring the test results to their physicians, many of whom are not properly prepared to interpret the results. Results can also lead to additional testing, which may be unnecessary.

Genetic testing raises many ethical questions, as the results affect not only the patient but also other members of the family. Testing can also lead to possible discrimination. The Genetic Information Nondiscrimination Act of 2008 protects against genetic discrimination in regard to both health insurance and employment but does not provide any protection against discrimination involving disability, life, or long-term care insurance.

Referral for Genetic Counseling

Genetic counseling should always occur before any genetic test is performed. The essential components of counseling include informing the patient of the test purpose, implications of diagnosis, alternative testing options (including foregoing testing), and

TABLE 10. Types of Genetic Testing and Indications

Genetic Testing Type	Indication
Diagnostic testing	Used to confirm or support a diagnosis in a patient with clinical disease (for example, cystic fibrosis, sickle cell disease)
Predictive testing	Used to identify individuals at risk for heritable disease: *Presymptomatic tests* evaluate for conditions caused by single genes with a high degree of penetrance that will likely eventually cause disease (for example, Huntington disease). *Predisposition tests* evaluate for genetic alterations known to significantly increase the risk of disease (for example, *BRCA* mutation). *Susceptibility tests* evaluate for different genetic markers associated with complex diseases (for example, coronary artery disease).
Pharmacogenetic testing	Tests for genetic factors influencing drug metabolism (for example, TPMT assay for azathioprine)
Tumor (somatic cell) testing	Involves testing tissue (usually cancer) for nonheritable mutations (for example, *HER2*, *KRAS*) for diagnostic purposes or to assist in selecting a specific treatment
Carrier testing	Used to identify a specific genetic mutation in an asymptomatic family member, frequently for reproductive decision making; typically for the heterozygous state of a disease that presents with disease when homozygous (for example, cystic fibrosis, sickle cell disease)
Prenatal (antenatal) testing	Testing during pregnancy (by amniocentesis or chorionic villus sampling) to identify congenital conditions (for example, Down syndrome, Turner syndrome)
Newborn (neonatal) screening	Testing after birth for presence of disease for which preventive measures or treatment exist (for example, phenylketonuria); often legally mandated and varies by state

BRCA = breast cancer susceptibility genes 1 and 2; HER2 = human epidermal growth factor receptor 2; KRAS = Kirsten rat sarcoma viral oncogene; TPMT = thiopurine methyltransferase.

any possible risks and benefits. Approximately 1 hour of counseling is considered standard for each genetic test performed. Ultimately, the decision of whether or not to be tested rests with the patient. Although genetic counseling can be provided by internists, most do not feel adequately equipped or trained to do so; therefore, referral to a genetic counselor in most situations in which genetic testing is being considered is appropriate. The National Society of Genetic Counselors website (http://nsgc.org) can be used by providers to locate a genetic counselor in their area.

KEY POINTS

HVC
- Patients who have no genetic family history available (for example, due to adoption) should not undergo genetic testing without other reason.
- Predictive genetic testing is used to determine whether a person has genetic mutations that are associated with higher risk of certain disorders.
- Diagnostic genetic testing is used to diagnose or to rule out a condition that is suspected based on results of clinical findings.

HVC
- Although pharmacogenetic testing is available for many drug-metabolizing enzymes, its use has been clinically limited and is not routinely recommended.

Immunization

Even though vaccines are one of the most cost-effective preventive health measures available, immunization rates remain unacceptably low. Vaccination recommendations for adults are published on a yearly basis by the Centers for Disease Control and Prevention's Advisory Committee on Immunization Practices (ACIP) at www.cdc.gov/vaccines/acip/index.html (**Table 11**). The American College of Physicians offers a free downloadable Immunization Advisor mobile application (available at http://immunization.acponline.org/app/) that provides the latest ACIP immunization recommendations, searchable by patient age and underlying medical condition.

Vaccinations with multiple doses should not be given at shorter-than-recommended intervals; conversely, administering doses at longer-than-recommended intervals does not typically reduce final immunologic response at series completion. If a vaccination series is interrupted, the schedule should be resumed at the point of interruption. Multiple vaccinations can usually be given simultaneously to improve vaccination rates.

Vaccine administration should be deferred when there is a history of anaphylaxis to vaccine components or if the patient is experiencing a moderate to severe illness; however, vaccines can be administered with several minor conditions, including diarrhea, minor upper respiratory tract infections (with or without fever), otitis media, current antimicrobial therapy, convalescent phase of acute illness, and mild to moderate local reactions to a previous vaccine dose. Contraindications to live vaccines are listed in **Table 12**.

TABLE 11. Summary of Vaccination Recommendations for Adults

Disease	Vaccine Type	ACIP Recommendation
Influenza	Inactivated, live attenuated, recombinant	One dose annually for all persons ≥6 months of age; indications vary by vaccine type (see text)
Tetanus, diphtheria, and pertussis	Inactivated	Primary series for unvaccinated adults; Td booster every 10 y for all adults; one-time pertussis booster with Tdap in adults; all pregnant women between 27 and 36 weeks' gestation during each pregnancy
Varicella	Live attenuated	Two doses given at interval of ≥4 weeks for all persons lacking evidence of VZV immunity[a]
Herpes zoster	Live attenuated	All nonimmunocompromised persons age ≥60 y
Pneumococcal	Inactivated	All adults age ≥65 y; adults ages 19-64 y with risk factors (see Figure 3 and Table 13)
Human papillomavirus	Inactivated	Females at age 11-12 y, or age 13-26 y for unvaccinated females; males at age 11-12 y, or age 13-21 y for unvaccinated males (permitted age 21-26 y); immunocompromised persons (including those infected with HIV) and MSM through age 26 y
Measles, mumps, and rubella	Live attenuated	Adults born in 1957 or later without documented evidence of vaccination or immunity. One dose usually sufficient; second dose recommended for college students, international travelers, and HCWs
Meningococcal	Inactivated	One dose indicated for first-year college students residing in dormitories (unless vaccinated at age ≥16 y), travelers to endemic areas, microbiologists exposed to *Neisseria meningitidis*, military recruits, and exposed persons; two doses indicated for persons with asplenia or complement deficiencies. Revaccination recommended every 5 y for those with persistent risk
Hepatitis A	Inactivated	Any adult requesting immunization and those at high risk (see text)
Hepatitis B	Inactivated	Any adult requesting immunization and those at high risk (see text)

ACIP = Advisory Committee on Immunization Practices; HCW = health care worker; MSM = men who have sex with men; Td = tetanus and diphtheria toxoids; Tdap = tetanus toxoid, reduced diphtheria toxoid, and acellular pertussis; VZV = varicella zoster virus.

[a]Evidence of immunity includes either 1) documentation of receiving two doses of varicella vaccine ≥4 weeks apart, 2) U.S.-born before 1980 except health care providers and pregnant women, 3) varicella or herpes zoster diagnosed by health care provider, or 4) laboratory evidence of immunity.

TABLE 12. Contraindications to Live Vaccines

Pregnancy

HIV or AIDS with a CD4 cell count ≤200/µL or ≤15% of total lymphocytes

Immunosuppressant therapy, including high-dose glucocorticoids (≥20 mg/d of prednisone or equivalent)

Leukemia, lymphoma, or other bone marrow and lymphatic system malignancies

Cellular immunodeficiency

Solid-organ transplant recipient

Current hematopoietic stem cell transplantation

Vaccinations Recommended for All Adults

Influenza

Due to ongoing genetic mutations (antigenic drift), influenza vaccination is necessary each year. Adults who are considered to be at high risk for contracting severe disease and complications include those persons aged 50 years and older, women who may potentially become pregnant during the influenza season, residents of chronic care facilities, immunocompromised individuals, and those who have diabetes mellitus or pulmonary, cardiac (excluding hypertension), liver, or kidney conditions.

Influenza vaccination is recommended for all persons aged 6 months and older unless specifically contraindicated. Vaccination should be offered as soon as the vaccine becomes available and should continue until influenza season has ended.

There are currently three different types of influenza vaccine available in the United States: inactivated influenza vaccine (IIV), live attenuated influenza vaccine (LAIV), and recombinant trivalent influenza vaccine (RIV). IIV is approved for use in all adults, including immunosuppressed persons and pregnant women. Four types of IIV are currently available: standard-dose, egg-based trivalent; standard-dose, egg-based quadrivalent; standard-dose, cell culture–based trivalent; and high-dose trivalent. The quadrivalent vaccine contains two influenza A virus antigens and two influenza B virus antigens, whereas the trivalent vaccines contain two influenza A virus antigens and one influenza B virus antigen. The ACIP has no stated preference for administering the quadrivalent formulation over the trivalent counterparts. The standard-dose, egg-based trivalent and quadrivalent IIVs are approved for all adults of any age, whereas the standard-dose, cell culture–based trivalent IIV is approved for use in adults 18 years of age and older. The intradermally administered standard-dose trivalent IIV may be administered to persons aged 18 to 64 years. The high-dose trivalent vaccine is only approved for use in adults age 65 years and older; it has been shown to be modestly more effective than the standard-dose IIVs in this patient population. All types of IIV can be administered to immunocompromised individuals.

Intranasal LAIV is approved for use in healthy, nonpregnant individuals aged 2 to 49 years. LAIV should be avoided in immunosuppressed individuals and in those with any egg allergies. RIV is also available and is approved for persons aged 18 years and older. RIV does not contain any egg components and can be safely used in individuals with egg allergies. All vaccine formulations should be avoided in persons who previously developed Guillain-Barré syndrome within 6 weeks of receiving the influenza vaccine.

Clinicians frequently encounter patients with a reported history of egg allergy. The ACIP has developed an algorithm for the administration of the influenza vaccine for this group of patients (**Figure 2**).

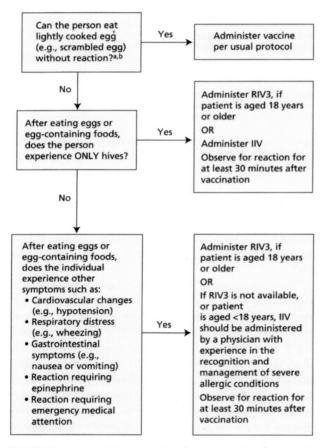

FIGURE 2. Recommendations regarding influenza vaccination of persons who report allergy to eggs.

IIV = inactivated influenza vaccine; RIV3 = recombinant influenza vaccine, trivalent.

[a]Persons with egg allergy might tolerate egg in baked products (for example, bread or cake). Tolerance to egg-containing foods does not exclude the possibility of egg allergy.

[b]For persons who have no known history of exposure to egg, but who are suspected of being egg-allergic on the basis of previously performed allergy testing, consultation with a physician with expertise in the management of allergic conditions should be obtained before vaccination. Alternatively, RIV3 may be administered if the recipient is aged 18 years or older.

Adapted from Grohskopf LA, Olsen SJ, Sokolow LZ, et al; Centers for Disease Control and Prevention. Prevention and control of seasonal influenza with vaccines: recommendations of the Advisory Committee on Immunization Practices (ACIP) – United States, 2014-15 influenza season. MMWR Morb Mortal Wkly Rep. 2014 Aug 15;63(32):691-7. [PMID: 25121712]

Tetanus, Diphtheria, and Pertussis

Although tetanus and diphtheria infections are extremely uncommon, the incidence of pertussis has recently increased, presumably due to waning immunity with age. Primary vaccination against tetanus, diphtheria, and pertussis is recommended during childhood and consists of five doses of the diphtheria and tetanus toxoids and acellular pertussis (DTaP) vaccine administered at 2 months, 4 months, 6 months, 15 through 18 months, and 4 to 6 years of age. A single booster dose of the tetanus toxoid, reduced diphtheria toxoid, and acellular pertussis (Tdap) vaccine is also recommended for children between the ages of 11 and 12 years. Adults who did not receive primary vaccination or who did not complete the primary series, defined as receiving fewer than 3 doses, should begin or complete the primary vaccination series with three doses of tetanus and diphtheria–containing vaccines, one of which should be a Tdap dose. The ACIP makes no recommendations regarding testing of serum antibody levels to confirm immunity. All persons aged 11 years and older who completed the primary series should receive a single booster dose of Tdap, followed by a tetanus and diphtheria toxoids (Td) booster every 10 years thereafter. Tdap can be administered regardless of the interval since the most recent tetanus or diphtheria toxoid–containing vaccine. For pregnant women, one dose of the Tdap vaccine should be administered during each pregnancy between 27 weeks' and 36 weeks' gestation, regardless of when the last dose of Td or Tdap was given.

Vaccinations Recommended for Some Adults
Varicella and Herpes Zoster

Primary infection with varicella zoster virus (VZV) causes varicella (chickenpox). Birth in the United States before 1980 is considered to serve as evidence of immunity against varicella, except in health care professionals, pregnant women, and immunocompromised individuals, all of whom require serologic confirmation. For persons born after 1980, evidence of immunity to varicella includes written documentation of age-appropriate vaccination, serologic confirmation of immunity, or verification of either varicella or herpes zoster diagnosis made by a physician. All individuals who lack evidence of VZV immunity by serologic testing should receive two doses of varicella vaccine, given at least 4 to 8 weeks apart. Women should be assessed for varicella immunity during pregnancy, and if not immune, they should be vaccinated following pregnancy. Vaccination is contraindicated during pregnancy. Revaccination is not currently recommended in patients who received the two-dose vaccination series for primary prevention either as a child, adolescent, or adult.

The herpes zoster vaccine is similar to the varicella vaccine but is significantly more potent. It is recommended for individuals aged 60 years and older regardless of whether they have had a previous zoster episode, but vaccination should be avoided in immunocompromised patients. Vaccination is effective for reducing the occurrence of both herpes zoster and postherpetic neuralgia.

Pneumococcal Disease

Pneumococcal vaccination is indicated for all adults aged 65 years and older and for high-risk persons younger than 65 years (**Table 13**). Two vaccines are currently available: pneumococcal polysaccharide vaccine (PPSV23) is composed of polysaccharide capsular material from 23 pneumococcal subtypes, whereas pneumococcal conjugate vaccine (PCV13) contains capsular material from 13 subtypes conjugated to a nontoxic protein, which increases its immunogenicity. PCV13 is more than 90% effective in preventing invasive pneumococcal disease and is also effective in reducing pneumonia and acute otitis media to a lesser extent, whereas PPSV23 is only 60% to 70% effective in preventing invasive pneumococcal disease and does not reduce the risk of pneumococcal pneumonia.

For pneumococcal vaccine–naïve adults between the ages of 19 and 65 years with certain immunocompromising conditions or who are otherwise at high risk (see Table 13), a single dose of PCV13 should be given, followed by a dose of PPSV23 at least 8 weeks later. For adults between the ages of 19 and 65 years who previously received the PPSV23 vaccine, a single dose of PCV13 should be given at least 1 year after receiving

TABLE 13. Pneumococcal Vaccination Recommendations for Adults Aged 19 Years and Older with Underlying Medical Conditions

Risk Group	Underlying Medical Condition	PCV13 Recommended	PPSV23 Recommended	Revaccination at 5 Years After First Dose
Immunocompetent persons	Chronic heart disease[a]		X	
	Chronic lung disease[b]		X	
	Diabetes mellitus		X	
	CSF leaks	X	X	
	Cochlear implants	X	X	
	Alcoholism		X	
	Chronic liver disease		X	
	Cigarette smoking		X	
Persons with functional or anatomic asplenia	Sickle cell disease/other hemoglobinopathies	X	X	X
	Congenital or acquired asplenia	X	X	X
Immunocompromised persons	Congenital or acquired immunodeficiencies[c]	X	X	X
	HIV infection	X	X	X
	Chronic kidney failure	X	X	X
	The nephrotic syndrome	X	X	X
	Leukemia	X	X	X
	Lymphoma	X	X	X
	Hodgkin lymphoma	X	X	X
	Generalized malignancy	X	X	X
	Iatrogenic immunosuppression[d]	X	X	X
	Solid-organ transplant	X	X	X
	Multiple myeloma	X	X	X

CSF = cerebrospinal fluid; PCV13 = 13-valent pneumococcal conjugate vaccine; PPSV23 = 23-valent pneumococcal polysaccharide vaccine.

[a]Including heart failure and cardiomyopathies.

[b]Including COPD, emphysema, and asthma.

[c]Including B- (humoral) or T-lymphocyte deficiency, complement deficiencies (particularly C1, C2, C3, and C4 deficiencies), and phagocytic disorders (excluding chronic granulomatous disease).

[d]Diseases requiring treatment with immunosuppressive drugs, including long-term systemic glucocorticoids and radiation therapy.

Adapted from Centers for Disease Control and Prevention (CDC). Use of 13-valent pneumococcal conjugate vaccine and 23-valent pneumococcal polysaccharide vaccine for adults with immunocompromising conditions: recommendations of the Advisory Committee on Immunization Practices (ACIP). MMWR Morb Mortal Wkly Rep. 2012 Oct 12;61(40):816-9. [PMID: 23051612]

PPSV23. Giving the PCV13 vaccine sooner than 1 year after administration of PPSV23 appears to reduce the immunogenicity of PCV13. In contrast, PPSV23 can be given as soon as 8 weeks after the administration of PCV13 without concern for reduced immunogenicity.

The ACIP recommends administering PPSV23 alone to selected immunocompetent patients between the ages of 19 and 64 years (see Table 13).

For immunocompetent persons aged 65 years and older who have not received any pneumococcal vaccine, the ACIP recommends administering a single dose of PCV13, followed by a single dose of PPSV23 at least 1 year later. For immunocompetent adults aged 65 years and older who previously received one or more doses of PPSV23, a single dose of PCV13 should be given at least 1 year after the most recent PPSV23 dose (**Figure 3**).

Human Papillomavirus

Human papillomavirus (HPV) is the most common STI in the United States. Genotypes 16 and 18 are responsible for causing most cases of cervical cancer and a large number of cases of vulvar, vaginal, anal, penile, and oropharyngeal cancers. HPV genotypes 6 and 11 cause most cases of genital warts.

Three inactivated vaccines are available: a bivalent vaccine (HPV2), a quadrivalent vaccine (HPV4), and a new nine-valent vaccine (HPV9). All vaccines target genotypes 16 and 18, and the quadrivalent vaccine also targets genotypes 6 and 11. The nine-valent vaccine protects against five additional genotypes that cause cervical cancer, resulting in the potential prevention of 90% of cervical, vulvar, vaginal, and anal cancers.

All vaccines are approved for use in females as a three-dose series at ages 11 to 12 years and between the ages of 13 and 26 years for previously unvaccinated persons. HPV4 and HPV9 are approved for use in males as a three-dose series at ages 11 to 12 years and

between the ages of 13 and 21 years for previously unvaccinated males, although males aged 22 to 26 years can be vaccinated. For immunocompromised persons (including those infected with HIV) and MSM, vaccination is recommended through age 26 years. Vaccination is not recommended during pregnancy.

Measles, Mumps, and Rubella

Adults born before 1957, excluding health care workers, are considered to be immune to measles, mumps, and rubella and do not require vaccination. Adults born in 1957 or later who lack documentation of receiving the measles, mumps, and rubella (MMR) vaccine or who lack serologic evidence of immunity should receive at least one MMR dose. A second dose should be administered to students in postsecondary education, health care workers, and international travelers. The MMR vaccine should be avoided in pregnant women and immunocompromised individuals.

Meningococcal Disease

Individuals with asplenia or persistent complement deficiencies should be given two doses of the meningococcal vaccine, separated by at least 2 months. First-year college students living in a dormitory should be vaccinated, unless they were vaccinated at age 16 years or older. A single dose should be administered to individuals traveling to endemic areas, microbiologists exposed to *Neisseria meningitidis*, military recruits, and at-risk individuals who are exposed to a serogroup contained in the vaccine. Revaccination is recommended every 5 years for individuals who remain at increased risk.

Hepatitis A

Hepatitis A virus (HAV) vaccination is recommended for any adult seeking protection against HAV and for those at risk for infection, including MSM, travelers to endemic regions, users of illicit drugs, those with occupational risk such as health care

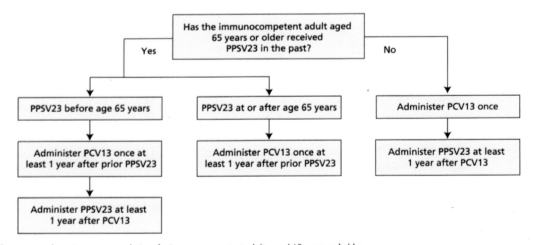

FIGURE 3. Pneumococcal vaccine recommendations for immunocompetent adults aged 65 years and older.

PCV13 = 13-valent pneumococcal conjugate vaccine; PPSV23 = 23-valent pneumococcal polysaccharide vaccine.

NOTE: For adults aged 65 years or older with immunocompromising conditions, functional or anatomic asplenia, cerebrospinal fluid leaks, or cochlear implants, the recommended interval between sequential administration of PCV13 and PPSV23 is at least 8 weeks. For those who previously received PPSV23 before age 65 years and for whom an additional dose of PPSV23 is indicated when aged 65 years or older, this subsequent PPSV23 dose should be given at least 1 year after PCV13 and at least 5 years after the most recent dose of PPSV23.

Recommendations from Kobayashi M, Bennett NM, Gierke R, et al. Intervals between PCV13 and PPSV23 vaccines: Recommendations of the Advisory Committee on Immunization Practices (ACIP). MMWR Morb Mortal Wkly Rep. 2015 Sep 4;64(34):944-7. [PMID: 26334788]

workers, and persons with chronic liver disease or clotting disorders. HAV vaccination of patients infected with either hepatitis B or C is only necessary with evidence of chronic liver disease. The vaccine is typically given as a two-dose regimen.

Hepatitis B

Hepatitis B virus (HBV) vaccination is recommended for any adult seeking protection against HBV and for those at risk due to sexual exposures (MSM, individuals with STIs, individuals not in monogamous relationships, partners of HBsAg-positive individuals) or blood exposures (injection drug users, household contacts of HBsAg-positive persons, health care workers, patients on dialysis). Persons with end-stage kidney disease, HIV-positive persons, persons with chronic liver disease, travelers to endemic areas, persons with diabetes who are younger than age 60 years, and high-risk persons with diabetes who are older than 60 years should also be vaccinated. The vaccine is given as a three-dose regimen.

KEY POINTS

- Even though vaccines are one of the most cost-effective preventive health measures available, immunization rates remain unacceptably low; providing age- and risk-appropriate immunization to patients is essential to the practice of high value care.

- Influenza vaccination is recommended for all persons aged 6 months and older unless specifically contraindicated.

- Pneumococcal vaccination with the 23-valent pneumococcal polysaccharide vaccine (PPSV23) and 13-valent pneumococcal conjugate vaccine (PCV13) is indicated for all adults aged 65 years and older and for certain high-risk persons younger than 65 years.

- Bivalent, quadrivalent, and nine-valent vaccines for human papillomavirus are approved for use in females and quadrivalent and nine-valent vaccines for males between the ages of 11 and 26 years.

- Vaccination with herpes zoster vaccine is recommended for individuals aged 60 years and older, including patients with a previous episode of zoster.

Immunization Recommendations for Specific Populations

Health care workers are at increased risk for both contracting and transmitting influenza, pertussis, varicella, measles, mumps, rubella, and HBV. Annual vaccination against influenza and one-time vaccination against pertussis with Tdap is recommended for all personnel. Written documentation of vaccination or serologic evidence of immunity against varicella, measles, mumps, rubella, and HBV should be obtained for all health care workers. Annual screening to assess exposure to tuberculosis in health care workers is also indicated.

Persons with functional or anatomic asplenia are susceptible to infections with encapsulated organisms and therefore should be vaccinated against pneumococcus, *Haemophilus influenzae* type b, and meningococcus.

Smokers should receive a pneumococcal vaccination and annual influenza vaccination.

International travelers should be appropriately counseled and vaccinated to reduce risk of injury and illness (see MKSAP 17 Infectious Disease, Travel Medicine).

KEY POINTS

- Annual vaccination against influenza and one-time vaccination against pertussis with the tetanus toxoid, reduced diphtheria toxoid, and acellular pertussis (Tdap) vaccine is recommended for all health care workers. **HVC**

- Smokers should receive pneumococcal vaccination and annual influenza vaccination. **HVC**

Healthy Lifestyle Counseling

For adults, the five most common causes of death are heart disease, cancer, chronic lower respiratory diseases, stroke, and accidents. Healthy lifestyle counseling is aimed at preventing these most common causes of death.

Healthy lifestyle counseling for the prevention of cardiovascular and cerebrovascular diseases includes behavioral counseling to encourage healthful diet and exercise, stress reduction and management, and tobacco cessation. The risk of cancers that are associated with tobacco use (such as bladder, lung, and upper airway) can be reduced by encouraging patients to avoid tobacco, quit smoking, or avoid second-hand smoke. Smoking cessation is one of the most important interventions health care providers can encourage to help patients achieve improved short- and long-term health. Cancer prevention counseling may also include guidance on avoiding ultraviolet radiation exposure, appropriate sunscreen use, avoiding alcohol excess, choosing foods wisely, and achieving and maintaining an ideal body weight.

Healthy lifestyle counseling for the prevention of accidents includes counseling on routine seatbelt use, helmet use (for bicycles, motorcycles, and all-terrain vehicles), smoke detectors, weapon safety, and setting water heaters to lower than 49° C (120° F). Best practices to mitigate the risk of firearms in the home include storing firearms and ammunition separately in secure and locked safes, using trigger locks, and encouraging firearm owners to obtain expert training on their use and safety. In households with children, adolescents, persons with mental illness, and others at greater risk for firearm-related accidents, violence, or suicide, the physician may recommend that the patient consider not keeping firearms in the home.

Physicians should provide appropriate brief behavioral counseling to reduce alcohol misuse, including education on avoiding driving, swimming, operating machinery, or boating while using alcohol. Screening for domestic violence, especially in women of childbearing age, and home safety is also recommended. For the aging population, screening for polypharmacy, visual and hearing loss, and elder abuse may also be of value. For persons at risk for falls, exercise or physical therapy and vitamin D supplementation is recommended.

Behavioral Counseling

Behavioral counseling in the health care setting has long been recognized as an integral part of optimizing healthful lifestyle choices and habits. Although moderate- (31-360 minutes) and high-intensity interventions (>360 minutes) have shown better results than brief interventions (1-30 minutes), even 1- to 5-minute interventions have proved effective in curbing tobacco and alcohol misuse. The USPSTF recommends using the 5 A's for clinical counseling regarding tobacco use. With this behavioral framework, the physician Asks about tobacco use; Advises the patient to quit through clear, personalized messages; Assesses willingness to quit; Assists the patient to quit; and Arranges for follow-up and support.

Healthful dietary choices and regular physical activity have been strongly linked with decreased incidence of cardiovascular disease. However, the effect of behavioral counseling in promoting healthful diet and physical activity in adults without known cardiovascular disease, hypertension, hyperlipidemia, or diabetes is small. Moderate-intensity behavioral counseling has shown beneficial effects on intermediate outcomes (blood pressure and laboratory values) but not in patient-important outcomes (cardiovascular events or mortality).

Given small potential effect, time limitations, and opportunity costs, the USPSTF recommends offering dietary and exercise behavioral counseling based only on individual patient circumstances (grade C). Physicians may choose to selectively counsel patients, which may depend on the patients' level of readiness for change, how far they deviate from ideal health habits, and their risk for cardiovascular disease. Tools such as the ASCVD calculator (http://tools.cardiosource.org/ASCVD-Risk-Estimator/) can be used to stratify risk. For those who have hyperlipidemia or other known risk factors for cardiovascular disease, the USPSTF recommends intensive behavioral dietary counseling (grade B recommendation), which can be delivered by internists or by referral to specialists. Additionally, the 2013 joint guideline from the AHA, ACC, and The Obesity Society recommends advising overweight and obese individuals of the increased risk of cardiovascular disease, type 2 diabetes, and mortality with increasing BMI. Overweight and obese adults with cardiovascular disease risk factors should also be counseled that even 3% to 5% weight loss could yield clinically meaningful benefits.

Diet and Physical Activity

Most adults, particularly those with a BMI over 25, can benefit from improving dietary habits and increasing physical activity. The U.S. Department of Health and Human Services (USDHHS) and the AHA have similar recommendations on diet and physical activity. Both organizations recommend limiting the intake of red meat, sugary foods and beverages, saturated fats, sodium, and alcohol (no more than one drink per day for women and two drinks per day for men), while encouraging the intake of fruits, vegetables, whole grains, fiber, low-fat dairy products, poultry, fish, and nuts. The USDHHS and AHA also emphasize that the patient should know his or her daily caloric needs and should not eat more calories than can be expended on a daily basis. The AHA provides a calculator for daily calorie needs at www.myfatstranslator.com/. It is recommended that physical activity be performed for at least 150 minutes per week, usually 30 minutes a day; however, shorter intervals are also encouraged. Muscle-strengthening exercises should be performed at least twice per week.

KEY POINTS

- Moderate- (31-360 minutes) and high-intensity behavioral counseling (>360 minutes) have shown better results than brief behavioral counseling (1-30 minutes); however, even 1- to 5-minute counseling interventions have proved effective in reducing tobacco and alcohol misuse.
- Given small potential effect, time limitations, and opportunity costs, the U.S. Preventive Services Task Force recommends offering dietary and exercise behavioral counseling based only on individual patient circumstances (grade C).
- The U.S. Preventive Services Task Force recommends intensive behavioral dietary counseling for persons who have hyperlipidemia or other known risk factors for cardiovascular disease.

Supplements and Herbal Therapies

The Dietary Supplement Health and Education Act of 1994 defines a dietary supplement as any product (other than tobacco) intended to supplement the diet. This broad definition includes products that contain amino acids, botanicals (including herbals), metabolites, vitamins, and minerals. All products marketed as dietary supplements must be clearly labeled as dietary supplements. Although manufacturers are not allowed to make specific medical claims, they can describe the product's effect on body structure or function. There is no requirement to demonstrate a supplement's efficacy or safety prior to market introduction. Additionally, in order for a supplement to be removed from the market, the FDA must demonstrate that it is unsafe. In contrast, over-the-counter and prescription medications must be proved safe by the manufacturer prior to being introduced on the market. Furthermore, there is not necessarily standardization between supplement preparations in purity, formulation, or dosage.

Recent estimates suggest that nearly half of all adults use dietary supplements for alleviation of chronic disease symptoms and health promotion. Despite widespread usage, patients frequently fail to report supplement use to their health care providers. Because the use of supplements can be associated with adverse effects and can also have interactions with other medications, it is essential that all providers attempt to elicit dietary supplement use in a nonjudgmental manner.

Vitamin supplementation (**Table 14**) is used to treat known deficiencies and to address dietary deficiencies such

TABLE 14. Common Vitamin Supplements

Vitamin	Function	Sources	Deficiency	Toxicity
Water-Soluble Vitamins				
Vitamin B_1 (thiamine)	Cofactor for amino acid and carbohydrate metabolism	Cereals, rice, legumes, pork, yeast	Dry beriberi (peripheral neuropathy), wet beriberi (peripheral neuropathy and cardiomyopathy), Wernicke-Korsakoff syndrome	None
Vitamin B_2 (riboflavin)	Cofactor for multiple pathways, including energy production	Meats, fish, eggs, milk, green vegetables, yeast	Cheilitis, stomatitis, glossitis, pharyngitis	None
Vitamin B_3 (niacin)	Involved in synthesis of carbohydrates, fats, and proteins	Cereals, meats, legumes, seeds, yeast	Pellagra (hyperpigmented rash on sun-exposed skin, confusion, insomnia, vomiting, diarrhea)	Flushing, elevation of serum uric acid levels, nausea, vomiting, pruritus
Vitamin B_5 (pantothenic acid)	Active form is coenzyme A; involved in synthesis of vitamins A and D, cholesterol, steroids, fatty acids, amino acids, proteins, heme A	Broccoli, egg yolk, liver, milk	Anemia, paresthesias, intestinal distress	None
Vitamin B_6 (pyridoxine)	Amino acid metabolism, gluconeogenesis, immune function	Meats, whole grains, nuts, vegetables	Stomatitis, glossitis, cheilitis	Neuropathy, photosensitivity, dermatoses
Vitamin B_9 (folate)	Synthesizes, repairs, and methylates DNA; cofactor	Dark green leafy vegetables	Macrocytic anemia	None
Vitamin B_{12}	Involved in DNA synthesis and regulation; fatty acid and amino acid metabolism	Eggs, meat, milk	Peripheral neuropathy, macrocytic anemia	None
Vitamin C (ascorbic acid)	Antioxidant, cofactor	Citrus fruits, tomatoes, potatoes, broccoli, spinach	Scurvy (bleeding gums, petechiae, hyperkeratosis, arthralgia)	Abdominal bloating and diarrhea with large doses; large doses have not been shown to prevent illness
Biotin	Involved in carbohydrate and lipid metabolism	Egg yolk, liver, soybeans, yeast	Dermatitis, alopecia	None
Fat-Soluble Vitamins				
Vitamin A (retinoic acids)	β-carotene is precursor; vision	Liver, kidney, egg yolk, butter, green leafy vegetables, carrots, sweet potatoes	Xerophthalmia, night blindness (early), complete blindness	Teratogenic; acute toxicity (nausea, vomiting, vertigo, blurred vision); chronic toxicity (hepatotoxicity, visual impairment, ataxia)
Vitamin D	Bone and calcium/phosphorus metabolism	Fortified milk, fish, cod liver oil, eggs, fortified cereals	Hypocalcemia, hypophosphatemia, osteomalacia	Hypercalcemia
Vitamin E	Free radical scavenger	Eggs, meat, leafy vegetables, oil	Neuromuscular disorders, hemolysis	Increased all-cause mortality with ≥400 U/d, hemorrhagic strokes
Vitamin K	Coagulation	Green leafy vegetables	Easy bruising, mucosal bleeding, other bleeding	None

as may occur in patients who follow a restricted diet (vegetarians or vegans). Supplementation in the absence of deficiency is employed by some individuals to prevent disease. Although many patients take multivitamins, evidence is lacking on the benefits of this practice. Additionally, in the Iowa Women's Health Study, use of multivitamins was associated with an increased risk of overall mortality compared with nonuse. The USPSTF recently concluded that there is insufficient evidence to recommend either for or against the use of vitamin A, vitamin C, folic acid, and antioxidant combinations in the prevention of cardiovascular disease and cancer, and the USPSTF recommends against the use of vitamin E and β-carotene for these purposes. The USPSTF also determined that there is insufficient evidence for calcium and vitamin D supplementation to prevent fractures, though the Institute of Medicine recommends intake of 1000 to 1200 mg of calcium daily and 600 to 800 U of vitamin D daily for adult men and women. The USPSTF does recommend that all women who are either planning to become pregnant or capable of becoming pregnant take 400 to 800 µg of folic acid on a daily basis. For patients with age-related macular degeneration, a multivitamin containing copper, zinc, β-carotene (or vitamin A), and vitamins C and E has been shown to slow progression. For smokers with age-related macular degeneration, health care providers should use an alternative formulation that does not contain β-carotene or vitamin A, as high doses have been shown to increase the risk of lung cancer in smokers.

Herbal (botanical) supplements refer to dietary supplements that are plant derived. Despite their long history of use, the efficacy of these substances has only recently been studied. Definitive evidence on the effectiveness of herbal supplements is still either lacking or conflicting. Additionally, many herbals can interact with both prescription and over-the-counter medications, leading to adverse effects and reduced medication efficacy. Some natural products can exert deleterious effects independent of interactions with medications. It is the responsibility of health care providers to be aware of the reasons for use and also of the potential harms (**Table 15**). The National Institute of Health's MedlinePlus directory of herbs and supplements (www.nlm.nih.gov/medlineplus/druginfo/herb_All.html) is a useful resource.

TABLE 15. Common Herbal Supplements

Name	Function	Adverse Effects	Drug Interactions	Effectiveness
Black cohosh	Treatment of menopausal hot flashes	Headaches, stomach discomfort	None	Does not appear to be more effective than placebo
Cranberry	Prevention of urinary tract infections	Heartburn (rare), increased glucose intake	None	Does not appear to be effective
Echinacea	Treatment and prevention of upper respiratory tract infections	Dyspepsia, diarrhea, unpleasant taste	None	Does not appear to be effective in prevention or treatment
Garlic	Reduction in serum cholesterol levels	Bad breath, heartburn, increased risk of bleeding	Isoniazid, saquinavir, nonnucleoside reverse transcriptase inhibitors, warfarin	Does not significantly lower cholesterol levels
Ginkgo biloba	Treatment and prevention of cognitive dysfunction, treatment of peripheral arterial disease	Allergic skin reactions, increased risk of bleeding and bruising	Alprazolam, buspirone, efavirenz, fluoxetine, warfarin	Data appear conflicting, of questionable benefit
Ginseng	Immune system enhancement, stress reduction, general health	Diarrhea, pruritus, insomnia, elevated blood pressure	Warfarin, monoamine oxidase inhibitors	May lower postmeal serum glucose levels and prevent viral upper respiratory tract infections
Milk thistle	Reduction in liver inflammation	Nausea, indigestion, diarrhea	May interact with medications metabolized by CYP2C9 and CYP3A4 enzymes	Does not appear to be effective
Red yeast rice	Treatment of hyperlipidemia	Myalgia, abnormal liver chemistry tests	May interact with medications metabolized by CYP3A4 enzymes	Appears to lower LDL and total cholesterol levels
Saw palmetto	Treatment of benign prostatic hyperplasia-related symptoms	Headache, nausea, dizziness	Oral contraceptives, hormone therapy	Does not appear to be more effective than placebo
St. John's wort	Treatment of depression	Insomnia, vivid dreams, anxiety, restlessness	Many interactions; do not use with antidepressants	Appears effective for mild to moderate depression

Patient Safety and Quality Improvement

Introduction

Patient safety is defined conceptually as prevention of harm to patients, and patient safety practices are those that reduce the risk of adverse events related to exposure to medical care. The Institute of Medicine (IOM) considers patient safety to be indistinguishable from the delivery of high quality health care. However, the process by which patient safety is integrated into daily medical practice and systems of patient care is complex. Not only are individual clinicians required to engage in safe patient practices, but systems of care should ideally be built on a culture of safety, be structured to prevent errors, and be open to change based on errors that do occur.

Quality improvement (QI) consists of systematic and continuous actions that lead to measurable improvement in the quality and safety of patient care. Internists are increasingly becoming involved in QI efforts individually and as a part of interprofessional teams; therefore, it is important to understand QI methods and models of implementation. QI at the health care systems level involves efforts by an organization to understand its own care delivery mechanisms and make changes that lead to improvement in patient safety and the quality of services provided.

Although patient safety and quality are dependent both on the individuals providing care and the systems in which that care takes place, it is often helpful to consider potential issues arising at the direct patient care level and those at the health care systems level.

Direct Patient Care-Related Safety and Quality Issues

Diagnostic Errors

A diagnostic error (a missed, delayed, or incorrect diagnosis) may or may not result in harm to the patient. Despite the fact that diagnostic errors are less common than medication errors, there are twice as many tort claims for diagnostic errors.

Several types of diagnostic errors are common. Cognitive errors involve biases or failed heuristics (shortcuts in reasoning) during medical decision-making. Common examples of cognitive errors include premature closure, anchoring, triage cueing, confirmation bias, and gender bias. Premature closure is concluding the decision-making process before a diagnosis is fully confirmed (for example, when a patient with shortness of breath is diagnosed with a heart failure exacerbation without fully considering other causes such as asthma or pulmonary embolism). Anchoring involves locking into features of a patient's initial presentation despite new information. Triage cueing occurs when a patient's specialist selection or specialty team admission affects the workup and diagnosis (for example, when a patient with chest pain is admitted to a cardiology service and receives an extensive myocardial infarction

workup rather than an evaluation for esophageal reflux). Confirmation bias is the tendency to look for evidence to confirm a suspected diagnosis rather than considering evidence to refute it. Gender bias is the incorrect belief that gender is a factor in the probability of a patient having a certain disease. Suggestions to help avoid diagnostic errors and other examples of heuristics are provided in **Table 16**.

Medication Errors

Between 500,000 and 1.5 million preventable adverse events from medication errors occur each year in the United States, with an estimated 1 medication error daily for each hospitalized patient. The IOM reports that medication errors cause 1 of 131 outpatient deaths and 1 of 854 inpatient deaths. A medication error has been defined as a failure in the treatment process that leads to, or has the potential to lead to, harm to the patient. A medication error can result from prescribing faults of the physician (irrational, inappropriate, or ineffective prescribing; underprescribing; and overprescribing) or from prescription errors (incorrect recipient, drug, formulation, dose, route, timing, frequency, and duration of administration). Medication errors differ from adverse drug effects, which are defined as unintended or harmful reactions to a medication and can occur due to a medication being given appropriately or as a result of a medication error.

Medications with similar names or a low therapeutic index may be more likely to be associated with errors. Polypharmacy, advanced patient age, and kidney or hepatic impairment may also make medication errors more likely. The use of abbreviations and illegible handwriting are easily modifiable factors that can lead to medication errors. Other methods to prevent medication errors include improved drug labeling for sound-alike medications, computerized physician order entry (CPOE), medication reconciliation, and barcode-assisted medication administration.

The Institute for Healthcare Improvement (IHI) has published several tools and how-to guides to decrease harms related to medications. The how-to guides describe key evidence-based care components to prevent adverse drug events and harms from high-alert medications and how to implement these interventions and gauge improvement (available at www.ihi.org). Additionally, the Institute for Safe Medication Practices has published a best practices statement on medication safety issues that cause fatal and harmful errors in patients (available at www.ismp.org/Tools/BestPractices/default.aspX).

Transitions of Care

Transitions between care settings (inpatient and outpatient) provide challenges to patient safety. At discharge, 28% of patients can state all of their medications, and 42% of patients can state their diagnoses, affecting their adherence to discharge instructions. Forty percent of discharged patients have pending laboratory or radiology results of which the ambulatory care physician is unaware, even though roughly 10% of the results are potentially actionable. One in five patients

TABLE 16.	Twelve Tips for Avoiding Diagnostic Errors
Technique	**Comments**
(1) Understand heuristics[a]	*Availability heuristic:* Diagnosing based upon what is most easily available in the physician's memory (e.g., because of a patient recently seen) rather than what is most probable
	Anchoring heuristic: Settling on a diagnosis early in the diagnostic process despite data that refute the diagnosis or support another diagnosis (premature closure)
	Representativeness heuristic: Application of pattern recognition (a patient's presentation fits a "typical" case; therefore, it must be that case)
(2) Utilize "diagnostic timeouts"	Taking time to periodically review a case based on data but without assuming that the diagnosis is that which was previously reached
(3) Practice "worst-case scenario medicine"	Consider the most life-threatening diagnoses first: • Lessens chance of missing these diagnoses • Does not mandate testing for them, however
(4) Use systematic approach to common problems	For example, anatomic approach to abdominal pain beginning from exterior to interior
(5) Ask why	For example, when a patient presents with diabetic ketoacidosis or a COPD exacerbation, ask what prompted this acute exacerbation of a chronic condition
(6) Utilize the clinical examination	Decreases reliance on a single test and decreases chance of premature closure
(7) Use Bayes theorem	Utilize pre- and posttest probabilities • Helps avert premature closure based on a single test result
(8) Acknowledge the effect of the patient	How does the patient make the physician feel? • Physicians may avoid making unfavorable diagnoses in patients with whom they identify • Physicians may discount important data in patients with whom they have difficult encounters
(9) Look for clinical findings that do not fit the diagnosis	Encourages a comprehensive approach and incorporates healthy skepticism
(10) Consider "zebras"	Resist temptation to lock onto common diagnoses at risk of missing the uncommon
(11) Slow down and reflect	Difficult to do in most health care systems, which stress the economy of "getting it right the first time"
(12) Admit mistakes	Awareness of one's own fallibility may lead to fewer diagnostic errors later

[a]Heuristics are shortcuts in reasoning used in discovery, learning, or problem solving.

Based on Trowbridge RL. Twelve tips for teaching avoidance of diagnostic errors. Med Teach. 2008 Jun;30(5):496-500. [PMID: 18576188]

H CONT.

discharged from the hospital will experience an adverse event within 3 weeks of discharge.

To improve patient safety at transitions of care, hospital-to-primary provider communication at discharge, predischarge patient education, medication reconciliation, and timely posthospitalization follow-up are all necessary. Discharge summaries are an important tool for the hospital provider to communicate with the primary provider. Components of a standardized discharge summary are provided in **Table 17**. Timely follow-up with a primary care physician after discharge is also important to prevent rehospitalization.

Medication reconciliation is the process of developing an accurate and comprehensive list of a patient's prescribed and nonprescribed medications and comparing the list to medication orders to rectify any discrepancies. Medication reconciliation is a dynamic process that needs to be completed frequently and at all transitions of care to prevent medication errors, including omissions, duplications, dosing errors, or drug interactions. Despite the recent focus on medication reconciliation, systematic reviews show mixed results on its ability to improve morbidity and mortality.

The IHI has published a how-to guide that summarizes strategies for transitioning patients from the hospital to the next setting of care, with the goal of reducing avoidable readmissions (available at www.ihi.org/resources/Pages/Tools/HowtoGuideImprovingTransitionstoReduceAvoidableRehospitalizations.aspx). **H**

KEY POINT

- Hospital-to-primary provider communication at discharge, predischarge patient education, medication reconciliation, and timely post-hospitalization follow-up are all necessary to improve patient safety during transitions of care.

TABLE 17.	Suggested Content of a Standardized Discharge Summary
Dates of admission and discharge	
Reason for hospitalization	
Discharge diagnosis	
Significant findings from admission workup:	
• History and physical examination	
• Laboratory studies	
• Imaging studies	
• Other tests	
Procedures performed	
Results of procedures and significant testing	
Condition at discharge	
Discharge medications and reasons for any changes from admission medications	
Follow-up issues	
Pending studies and laboratory tests	
Counseling provided to patient and family	
Follow-up appointments/plans	

Systems Patient Care-Related Safety and Quality Issues

Quality Improvement Models

A number of quality improvement models are in use by health care systems; some of these models were developed by the manufacturing industry but are applicable to health care delivery systems. These models apply rigorous processes to identify, measure, and correct areas in need of improvement. The Model for Improvement, Lean, and Six Sigma quality improvement models are compared in **Table 18**.

Model for Improvement

The Model for Improvement involves defining the goal of the project (aim), measuring the baseline to see if interventions lead to improvement (measures), determining what changes can be made to improve quality (ideas), and implementing and testing the change in a process called a Plan-Do-Study-Act (PDSA) cycle (**Figure 4**). For example, the aim of a quality improvement project may be to improve the accuracy of medication lists in patients discharged from the hospital. After study, a quality improvement team may decide to implement

TABLE 18.	Models for Quality Improvement			
Approach	**Goal**	**Methods**	**Sample Use**	
Model for Improvement	Achieve a measurable change in care delivery for a specific patient population	Aim statement, project charter, iterative experiments, PDSA cycle	Improve medication list accuracy at hospital discharge	
Lean	Improve efficiency and eliminate waste in a process	Value stream mapping	Reduce patient waiting times	
Six Sigma	Decrease variability and defects in a process	DMAIC, PDSA cycle	Decrease line-associated infections in an ICU	

DMAIC = Define, Measure, Analyze, Improve, Control; PDSA = Plan, Do, Study, Act.

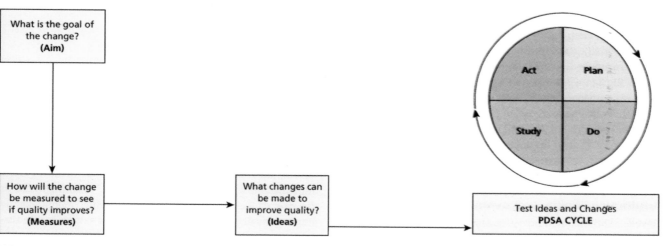

FIGURE 4. Plan-Do-Study-Act (PDSA) Model for Improvement.

CONT.

an intervention whereby a pharmacist will review the list of medications with the patient prior to discharge. A PDSA cycle could be done for a short period to test if the intervention was successful. If problems were encountered, changes in the intervention could be made and additional PDSA cycles completed until the desired improvements were reached. PDSA cycles are rapid tests of change.

Lean

The Lean model, developed by the Toyota Corporation, focuses on closely examining a system's processes and eliminating non-value-added activities, or waste, within that system. Using a tool called value stream mapping that graphically displays the steps of a process (and the time required for each step) from beginning to end, inefficient areas (waste) in a process can be identified and addressed. Lean also uses a 5S strategy (Sort, Shine, Straighten, Systemize, and Sustain). Lean relies on establishing a culture of continuous improvement, in which processes are constantly being refined. Although cost effectiveness is not the focus of the Lean model, cost savings are realized when all process steps add value and waste is eliminated. In the context of health care, the most common type of waste for patients is waiting time; Lean methods could be useful is reducing patient waiting times for various services.

Six Sigma

Six Sigma is a quality improvement model developed by the Motorola Corporation. The name Six Sigma is derived from measures used in industrial manufacturing to indicate the percentage of defect-free products that are created; a Six Sigma measure indicates almost perfect production quality. There are several Six Sigma methodologies, with a stepwise process called DMAIC used primarily to attempt to improve existing processes. DMAIC represents five separate steps: Define, Measure, Analyze, Improve, and Control. The define phase involves developing the aims of the project. In the measure phase, baseline data on the number and types of defects within the system are collected. The analyze step uses the data collected to determine the magnitude of the defects. In the fourth step, solutions are implemented to improve the process. Finally, the control phase works to sustain the gains and disseminate the improvements to other areas. Overall, the goal of Six Sigma is to reduce cost, variation, or defects within a process to make the process more effective. An example of a problem in health care where Six Sigma methods could be employed is a project focusing on decreasing line-associated infections in an ICU. In this case, the defect is the infection, and the goal would be to implement changes so that no future infections were encountered.

Additional Quality Improvement Tools

Several additional methods exist that are helpful in analyzing health care systems for quality improvement. Root cause analysis is a method used to discover the factors that contributed to an error and involves talking to all stakeholders involved in the error. A technique used in root cause analysis is the Five Whys, which involves asking the question "Why?" successively to drill down to the real root of a problem. To organize the root causes, a cause-and-effect diagram (also known as a fishbone diagram or Ishikawa diagram) can be used. The problem, or error, forms the backbone of the diagram and root causes are branched off like ribs. As an example, a quality team may complete a root cause analysis to determine why routine immunizations are not being given in the outpatient setting. After interviewing the physicians, nurses, desk staff, and patients, potential root causes identified might include physician failure to recognize immunization needs or failure to offer immunizations, patient refusal due to lack of insurance coverage or lack of appropriate informed consent, lack of immediate nursing availability, or lack of available immunization supplies.

Another commonly used quality improvement tool is the control chart. Control charts are used to graphically display variation in a process over time and can help determine if variation is from a predictable or unpredictable cause. Additionally, control charts can be used to determine if an intervention has had a positive change. For example, the rate of medication errors could be tracked before and after the initiation of a CPOE system to determine if it has had an impact on reducing errors. **H**

> **KEY POINTS**
>
> - The Model for Improvement involves defining the goal of the project (aim), measuring the baseline to see if interventions lead to improvement (measures), determining what changes can be made to improve quality (ideas), and implementing and testing the change in a process called a Plan-Do-Study-Act cycle.
> - The Lean model focuses on closely examining a system's processes and eliminating non-value-added activities, or waste, within that system.
> - The Six Sigma model has an emphasis on reducing cost, variation, or defects within a process to make the process more effective.

Measurement of Quality Improvement

The measurement of quality improvement is a focus of the Joint Commission, and since 2004, the Joint Commission has required collection of data on core measure sets, such as myocardial infarction, heart failure, pneumonia, and pregnancy. Additionally, the Centers for Medicare and Medicaid have implemented a policy of "meaningful use." Meaningful use is the use of electronic health record (EHR) technology to improve quality, safety, and efficiency, and reduce health disparities; engage patients and family members; improve care coordination; and maintain privacy and security of patient health information. The intended outcomes for meaningful use compliance are better clinical and population health outcomes, increased efficiency, empowered patients, and more robust research data on health outcomes. The meaningful use program is to be implemented in three stages from 2011 to 2016. Eligible professionals and hospitals must achieve specific objectives to qualify for reimbursement and incentive programs; financial penalties took effect in 2015 for providers who did not transition to EHR technology. **ℍ**

Patient-Centered Medical Home

The patient-centered medical home (PCMH) is a health care model in which a patient's comprehensive care is coordinated by a primary provider in a team-based medical practice (**Table 19**). The goal of the PCMH is to improve quality of care, access to services, cost effectiveness, and patient understanding. Studies are ongoing to measure the effectiveness of the PCMH, and the quality core measures have been recommended to ensure standardized and effective care. Programs are also being developed that offer financial incentives to health care providers if they implement the PCMH and meet specific quality measures.

Health Information Technology and Patient Safety

Health information technology has been used as a tool to mitigate medical errors. Three such forms of technology are CPOE, the EHR, and clinical decision support.

CPOE is a system in which the health care provider directly enters patient orders, such as orders for medications or laboratory tests, into a computer interface. The goals of CPOE are to reduce errors due to illegible handwriting, to eliminate confusing abbreviations, and improve order timeliness. Additionally, CPOE systems can use protocols or order sets to standardize care, create one place for medication lists, and employ drug-drug interaction software to reduce medication errors.

An EHR is a collection of all clinical data on a patient in an electronic format. An advantage of an EHR is that it serves as a central repository for patient information for multiple users, including the primary physician, specialists, and nurses. EHRs can also allow for systematic review of indicators, such as preventive service compliance, for a population of patients.

Clinical decision support (CDS) systems use technology to supplement a provider's clinical reasoning, allowing the provider to make an informed decision quickly. The systems are designed to provide relevant and filtered information specific to the patient at an appropriate time. A CDS system may display clinical guidelines and references, provide diagnostic support, house documentation templates, and issue medication interaction warnings. CDS technology can be integrated with CPOE and EHR systems to enhance care delivery.

Health information technology is not without limitations. Systems can be expensive to implement and maintain, and the potential for error is not eliminated with their use. For example, using a CPOE system, a physician may still enter prescriptions for the wrong patient.

National Patient Safety Goals

Since 2002, the Joint Commission has established annual National Patient Safety Goals (NPSGs) to address emerging patient safety issues (www.jointcommission.org/standards_information/npsgs.aspx). The NPSGs apply to multiple patient care settings, including hospitals, ambulatory clinics, behavioral health care centers, nursing care centers, and office-based surgery clinics. Objectives and metrics provided for each NPSG guide the implementation of the goal. For example, a new hospital NPSG introduced in 2014 focuses on clinical alarm systems, which can compromise patient safety if not managed

TABLE 19.	Five Functions and Attributes of the Patient-Centered Medical Home
Comprehensive care	Meets the majority of each patient's physical and mental health care needs, including prevention and wellness, acute care, and chronic care, with a team that may include physicians, advanced practice nurses, physician assistants, nurses, pharmacists, nutritionists, social workers, educators, and care coordinators
Patient-centered	Provides primary health care that is relationship-based with an orientation toward the whole person; ensures that patients are fully informed partners in establishing care plans
Coordinated care	Coordinates care across all elements of the broader health care system, including specialty care, hospitals, home health care, and community services; builds clear and open communication among patients and families, the medical home, and members of the broader care team
Accessible services	Delivers accessible services with shorter waiting times for urgent needs, enhanced in-person hours, around-the-clock telephone or electronic access to a member of the care team, and alternative methods of communication such as e-mail and telephone care
Quality and safety	Demonstrates a commitment to quality and quality improvement by ongoing engagement in activities, such as using evidence-based medicine and clinical decision-support tools to guide shared decision-making with patients and families, engaging in performance measurement and improvement, measuring and responding to patient experiences and patient satisfaction, and practicing population health management

Adapted from U.S. Department of Health and Human Services. Defining the PCMH. Agency for Healthcare Research and Quality Web site. http://pcmh.ahrq.gov/page/defining-pcmh. Accessed May 20, 2015.

properly. With a multi-phase implementation in 2014 and 2016, this NPSG has an initial performance metric of identifying the critical alarm systems to manage based on staff input, risk to patient if alarm is unanswered, alarm necessity, and published guidelines. These safety goals can provide a framework for interprofessional collaboration to achieve quality and safety in health care.

Professionalism and Ethics

Professionalism

A profession is a calling that requires mastery and continuous maintenance of a specialized body of knowledge and skills, commitment to a code of ethics, and self-regulation of its responsibilities to society. Adherence to the principles, responsibilities, and behaviors that characterize a profession constitute professionalism. In exchange for the authority to maintain its unique autonomous role in society, the medical profession must ensure that its members maintain clinical competence and adhere to professional responsibilities and the principles of medical ethics.

The Physician Charter on Medical Professionalism developed by the American Board of Internal Medicine Foundation, the American College of Physicians Foundation, and the European Federation of Internal Medicine focuses on three fundamental principles and ten professional commitments that characterize medical professionalism (**Table 20**). The three fundamental principles in the Charter include primacy of patient welfare, patient autonomy, and social justice. These

TABLE 20. Principles and Commitments of Professionalism

Principle or Commitment	Comment
Fundamental Principle	
Primacy of patient welfare	Altruism is a central trust factor in the physician-patient relationship. Market forces, societal pressures, and administrative exigencies must not compromise this principle.
Patient autonomy	Patients' decisions about their care must be paramount, as long as those decisions are in keeping with ethical practice and do not lead to demands for inappropriate care.
Social justice	Physicians should work actively to eliminate discrimination in health care, whether based on race, gender, socioeconomic status, ethnicity, religion, or any other social category.
Professional Commitment	
Competence	Physicians must be committed to lifelong learning and to maintaining the medical knowledge and clinical and team skills necessary for the provision of quality care.
Honesty with patients	Obtain informed consent for treatment or research. Report and analyze medical errors in order to maintain trust, improve care, and provide appropriate compensation to injured parties.
Patient confidentiality	Privacy of information is essential to patient trust and even more pressing with electronic health records.
Appropriate patient relations	Given the inherent vulnerability and dependency of patients, physicians should never exploit patients for any sexual advantage, personal financial gain, or other private purpose.
Improve quality of care	Work collaboratively with other professionals to reduce medical errors, increase patient safety, minimize overuse of health care resources, and optimize the outcomes of care.
Improve access to care	Work to eliminate barriers to access based on education, laws, finances, geography, and social discrimination. Equity requires the promotion of public health and preventive medicine, as well as public advocacy, without concern for the self-interest of the physician or the profession.
Just distribution of resources	Work with other physicians, hospitals, and payers to develop guidelines for cost-effective care. Providing unnecessary services not only exposes one's patients to avoidable harm and expense but also diminishes the resources available for others.
Scientific knowledge	Uphold scientific standards, promote research, create new knowledge, and ensure its appropriate use.
Manage conflicts of interest	Medical professionals and their organizations have many opportunities to compromise their professional responsibilities by pursuing private gain or personal advantage. Such compromises are especially threatening with for-profit industries, including medical equipment manufacturers, insurance companies, and pharmaceutical firms. Physicians have an obligation to recognize, disclose to the general public, and deal with conflicts of interest that arise.
Professional responsibilities	Undergo self-assessment and external scrutiny of all aspects of one's performance. Participate in the processes of self-regulation, including remediation and discipline of members who have failed to meet professional standards.

Adapted with permission from ABIM Foundation. American Board of Internal Medicine; ACP-ASIM Foundation. American College of Physicians-American Society of Internal Medicine; European Federation of Internal Medicine. Medical professionalism in the new millennium: a physician charter. Ann Intern Med. 2002 Feb 5;136(3):243-6. [PMID: 11827500] Copyrigt 2002, American College of Physicians.

principles embody four basic concepts of medical ethics: beneficence (duty to promote patients' welfare and the health of society), nonmaleficence (duty to avoid harming patients), patient autonomy (duty to respect patients' values, goals, and preferences), and justice (duty to treat patients fairly).

In addition to guiding the patient-physician relationship, professionalism encompasses a wide range of additional responsibilities, including self-assessment and maintaining the highest possible degree of clinical competency, the use of the best available evidence in making diagnostic and treatment decisions, maintaining collaborative relationships with trainees and other health care workers, and participation in activities that seek to advance the public good.

In clinical practice, the principles expressed in the Charter may sometimes be at odds with each other, such as when a physician's desire to promote a patient's welfare conflicts with the patient's health care values, goals, and preferences. Clinical ethics is the identification, analysis, and manner of resolution of these conflicts as they occur.

Primacy of Patient Welfare

Maximizing patient welfare is the primary aim of medicine. There is an expectation that the physician will act on behalf of a patient's best interests (beneficence) while attempting to prevent or minimize harms (nonmaleficence). Patients inherently are vulnerable and dependent due to illness or lack of medical knowledge; they may also have poor health literacy, strained social circumstances, and lack financial and other supportive resources. Therefore, patients must trust that physicians are acting in their best interests and protecting them from harm; in many instances, the physician may effectively be a patient's sole advocate. The ten professional commitments in the Charter are the means by which physicians maximize patient welfare.

Appropriate Physician-Patient Relationships

Patient welfare should be promoted regardless of patient characteristics (age, sex, religion, decision-making capacity, insurance status) or health care setting. Once a physician-patient relationship has been established, the physician has made a commitment to care for the patient regardless of these factors.

Accordingly, the imbalance of power between the physician and the patient should not be exploited to serve the interests of the physician or anyone else (for example, researchers). It is unethical for physicians to become sexually involved with current patients or former patients because vulnerability and transference issues may persist after the professional relationship has ended.

Physicians should maintain appropriate boundaries during the medical history, physical examination, and other health care activities. To avoid patient misperceptions, physicians should describe what they are doing during examinations (for example, "I am going to lift your left breast in order to examine your heart."). At times, a chaperone should be offered (for example, during gynecologic examinations).

Under most circumstances, physicians should avoid caring for family members and close friends. In these situations, the physician's objectivity may be compromised, and patients may receive inferior care, undergo inadequate or inappropriate assessment, or not receive counseling on sensitive issues. Medical records also may not be updated properly.

Online communication and social media can bring substantial benefits to patients and physicians (for example, education and community building); however, they also pose ethical challenges. The American College of Physicians and the Federation of State Medical Boards recently released a policy statement regarding online professionalism. First, online communication with patients should be held to the same standards as in-person contact. Second, online media can blur professional and social boundaries between physicians and patients. Physicians should keep their social and professional online presences separate and conduct themselves professionally in both spheres. Physicians should never post content that might impair relationships with patients or erode public trust in the profession. Online postings are often permanent. Finally, electronic communication should be used only for established physician-patient relationships and with patients' consent. Such communications should be secure and documented in the patients' records.

Challenging Physician-Patient Relationships

Relationships with patients can be challenging or "difficult" for physicians at times. For instance, a patient may reject a physician's recommendations. Under these circumstances, the physician should seek to understand the patient's reasons for the rejection (for example, cultural or religious reasons) and to formulate a mutually agreeable plan. If the patient agrees to, but is nonadherent with, the physician's recommendations, the physician should discern the reasons for the patient's behavior (for example, low health literacy, chaotic home environment, poor transportation, lack of insurance) and address the reasons, if possible, with the assistance of a public health nurse or case worker, social worker, or other professional colleague.

The physician is not obliged to carry out a patient's request for an intervention or treatment that violates the physician's personal values and conscience, standards of medical care and ethical practice, or the law. Again, the physician should attempt to understand the patient's request and seek a mutually agreeable plan. If the matter cannot be resolved, the physician and patient should discuss the option of transferring care of the patient to another physician.

Similarly, circumstances may develop in which there is a lack of trust between the patient and physician, the relationship has become nontherapeutic, and the physician no longer believes he or she can continue to care for the patient. Under these circumstances, physicians may pursue termination of the physician-patient relationship as long as the patient's health is not jeopardized and care can be provided by an

CONT.

alternative provider. The alternative provider must agree to the transfer of care, and the physician should notify the patient in writing of the termination and transfer of care. Physicians should not abandon patients; abandonment is unethical and can be cause for legal action.

Conflicts of Interest

Conflicts of interest, either real or perceived, have the potential to disrupt the trust relationship between the patient, public, and physician. The possibility that medical decisions may be influenced or based on factors other than the patient's best interests may be damaging to the process of providing medical care. Activities that may be viewed as potential conflicts of interest, such as accepting drug samples or gifts or participating in consulting agreements, should be avoided. The Institute of Medicine provides recommendations for controlling conflicts of interest (**Table 21**). In the United States, the Physician Payments Sunshine Act requires pharmaceutical and device companies that participate in federal health care programs to report payments and gifts to physicians and teaching hospitals. **H**

KEY POINTS

- Physicians may pursue termination of the physician-patient relationship as long as the patient's health is not jeopardized and care can be provided by an alternative provider; however, abandonment is unethical and can be cause for legal action.

H Respecting Patient Autonomy
Confidentiality

The principle of patient autonomy requires that physicians maintain patient confidentiality. For a patient to be autonomous,

---

TABLE 21. A Selection of Institute of Medicine Recommendations for Individual Physicians to Control Conflicts of Interest

Forego all gifts or items of material value from pharmaceutical, medical device, and biotechnology companies, accepting only payment at fair market value for a legitimate service in specified situations.

Do not make educational presentations or publish scientific articles that are controlled by industry or contain substantial portions written by someone who is not identified as an author or who is not properly acknowledged.

Do not meet with pharmaceutical and medical device sales representatives except by documented appointment and at the physician's express invitation.

Do not accept drug samples except in certain situations for patients who lack financial access to medications.

Until institutions change their policies, physicians and trainees should voluntarily adopt these recommendations as standards for their own conduct.

Reprinted with permission from Steinbrook R. Controlling conflict of interest—proposals from the Institute of Medicine. N Engl J Med. 2009 May 21;360(21):2160-3. [PMID: 19403898] Copyright 2009, Massachusetts Medical Society.

---

the patient must have control of his or her personal information. Also, maintaining confidentiality is necessary for the proper assessment and treatment of the patient; the patient must trust that his or her personal and medical information will be kept confidential. Release of such information should be done only with the explicit permission of the patient.

Circumstances exist, however, when physicians may be obliged to breach patient confidentiality. Depending on the jurisdiction, physicians may be required to report suspected child abuse, infectious diseases, patients who are a threat to themselves or others, and patients who are hazardous drivers (for example, those with dementia). In these cases, the physician's duty to protect the public's health overrides the duty to maintain patient confidentiality.

Online communication and social media pose substantial challenges to patient confidentiality. Physicians should ensure that electronic communications with patients have adequate security precautions. Physicians should not disseminate patient information using social media.

Another unique challenge to patient confidentiality is genetic testing. If genetic testing is performed, the patient should be informed of the implications of a "positive" test result—not only for the patient, but also for the patient's family. The physician and patient should agree on a plan for disclosing genetic test results to potentially affected family members. Inappropriate disclosure of genetic test results can negatively affect patients and their family members (for example, in regard to insurability and employment). For more information on genetic testing, refer to Routine Care of the Healthy Patient.

Informed Consent

Informed consent includes a discussion of the information that a reasonable patient would want to know about his or her illness (proposed diagnostic and treatment plans, the risks and benefits of the proposed plans, and any alternatives), an assessment of patient understanding, and the acceptance or refusal of the treatment. The patient must have decision-making capacity and make each decision of his or her own free will for consent to be considered valid. Importantly, obtaining a signed consent form is not equivalent to obtaining informed consent; physicians should engage patients in meaningful conversations about their diagnoses and treatment options and document these conversations.

Decision-Making Capacity

Competence is a determination made by the legal system, whereas physicians determine decision-making capacity in the clinical setting. The essential elements of decision-making capacity are an understanding of the risks and benefits of the proposed intervention and the ability to communicate a decision. A diagnosis of dementia or mental illness does not signify that the patient is incapable of making decisions; the physician should ensure such decisions are consistent with the patient's health care values, goals, and preferences. A patient's decision-making capacity should be questioned if the patient does not understand the situation; the patient does not understand the risks, benefits, and alternatives to the decision to be made; or the patient's decision is inconsistent with his or her previously expressed values, goals, and preferences.

A patient with decision-making capacity has the right to refuse a proposed diagnostic or therapeutic intervention, including those that prolong life. Although the physician may regard a given refusal as the wrong decision, the physician must recognize that the refusal is not necessarily irrational. In these instances, the physician should not abandon the patient and should determine the patient's rationale for the refusal (and whether it is informed) and correct misinformation if necessary. If the patient's refusal remains steadfast, the physician should respect the patient's decision and work with the patient to formulate an alternative diagnostic or therapeutic plan.

Advance Care Planning

Advance care planning is a process in which the patient articulates and documents his or her values, goals, and preferences for future health care. Advance care planning includes completion of an advance directive, which contains written instructions for health care that are used in the event that the patient loses decision-making capacity.

Advance directives include the living will and the durable health care power of attorney (or health care proxy). In a living will, the patient outlines preferences regarding specific treatments (for example, mechanical ventilation, hemodialysis, and artificial hydration and nutrition) and management preferences to direct care when he or she is no longer able to make medical decisions. The durable health care power of attorney designates a surrogate who will serve as the legal decision maker in the event the patient is no longer able to make health care decisions.

Ethically and legally, physicians and surrogates are required to adhere to the preferences expressed by patients in their advance directives (assuming that doing so is reasonable and legal). However, in the United States, laws governing advance directives vary by state; an advance directive executed in one state may not fulfill the legal requirements of another state. Physicians should be familiar with these requirements in their jurisdictions.

Unfortunately, only about 20% of U.S. adults have advance directives. Patients, especially those with chronic illnesses and limited longevity, should be encouraged to engage in advance care planning.

Surrogate Decision-Making

For the patient who lacks decision-making capacity, a surrogate must make decisions. If the patient has an advance directive, the person named in that advance directive is the most appropriate (and legal) surrogate. This choice is protected by U.S. federal law and must be respected. If the patient's advance directive does not name a surrogate, or the patient does not have an advance directive, the best surrogate is the person who best knows the patient's health care preferences. This person may not be the next of kin or a family member. Many U.S. states stipulate a hierarchy of surrogate decision-makers in the absence of an advance directive (for example, spouse, followed by adult child). In states that do not stipulate a hierarchy, the surrogate is identified by the patient's loved ones and care team.

Respect for patient autonomy requires that the surrogate adhere to instructions in the patient's advance directive. If the patient does not have an advance directive, the surrogate should make decisions based on substituted judgment (decisions the patient would make if capable). The physician can facilitate the surrogate's substituted judgment with the following question, "If [your loved one] could wake up for 15 minutes and understand his or her condition fully, and then had to return to it, what would he or she tell you to do?" If the surrogate is unable to answer this question or does not know the patient's values, the surrogate should make decisions in the best interest of the patient.

Withholding or Withdrawing Treatment

Patients have the right to refuse or request the withdrawal of any treatment, even those that are life prolonging. In these circumstances, the physician's duty is to understand the reasons for the request and to ensure that the request is informed. If a physician begins or continues a treatment that a patient has refused, the physician, regardless of his or her intent, is committing battery. Notably, patients who lack decision-making capacity also have the right to refuse or request the withdrawal of treatments through advance care planning and surrogate decision makers.

Carrying out a request to withhold or withdraw a life-prolonging treatment is not equivalent to physician-assisted death. The intent of carrying out a request to withhold or withdraw a life-prolonging treatment is to allow for a natural death and to free the patient from the burdens of treatment that he or she perceives as outweighing the benefits. After carrying out such a request, the cause of death is the underlying disease.

Depending on the circumstances, a physician may conscientiously object to a patient's request to withhold or withdraw life-prolonging treatments. In this situation, the physician should arrange for transferring the patient's care to another physician if carrying out the request would violate the physician's conscience.

Physician-Assisted Death

In contrast to carrying out a request to withhold or withdraw a life-prolonging treatment, the intent of physician-assisted death is termination of the patient's life. In physician-assisted suicide, death occurs when the physician provides a means for the patient to terminate his or her life (lethal prescription). In euthanasia, the physician directly terminates the patient's life (for example, by lethal injection). In both physician-assisted suicide and euthanasia, a new pathology is introduced, which is the cause of death. In the United States, physician-assisted death, in the form of lethal prescriptions but not euthanasia, is legal in only a few states. The American College of Physicians does not support the legalization of physician-assisted death, as it may damage the trust established between physician and patient and divert attention from end-of-life care reform.

In caring for patients at the end of life, there may be circumstances in which an intervention may hasten death (for example, intravenous narcotic analgesics). Using such interventions is ethical if doing so satisfies the doctrine of *double effect*: (1) the action itself is good or indifferent (for example, pain control); (2) the good effect (pain control), not the bad effect (death), is intended; (3) the good effect is not achieved by means of the bad effect; and (4) there is a proportionally serious reason (refractory pain due to widely metastatic cancer) for risking the bad effect.

Requests for Interventions

Physicians often encounter patients or surrogates who request specific tests and treatments. However, physicians are not obliged to grant requests for ineffective tests and treatments (for example, antibiotics for viral infection). Physicians should advise patients that using an ineffective intervention does not promote patient well-being, may cause harm, and violates the profession's commitment to stewardship of health care resources.

Patients may also request tests and treatments of questionable efficacy (certain complementary medicine practices) that support uncontroversial ends (improved health and well-being). In these situations, the physician should discern the patient's reasons for the request; inform the patient of the risks, benefits, and alternatives to the requested intervention; and formulate a mutually agreeable care plan. There are instances in which patients and surrogates request tests and treatments that are effective but support controversial ends, which may be best illustrated by requests to sustain the critically ill patient with technologically advanced treatments (mechanical ventilation, hemodialysis, mechanical circulatory support). Such requests reflect a gap between a patient's (or a surrogate's) values and the physician's values regarding goals of care. For example, a physician may regard life-sustaining interventions in the patient in a persistent vegetative state as futile, as the interventions will not restore the patient to health. However, the interventions may be fulfilling what the family desires—keeping the patient alive. For situations in which the physician and patient (or surrogate) cannot agree on how to move forward, a multidisciplinary care conference, consultation with an experienced colleague, and ethics consultation can be helpful. Sometimes, transferring the care of the patient to a colleague who is willing to work with and accommodate the patient's (or surrogate's) preferences resolves the matter. Rarely, resorting to court intervention is necessary. H

- Physicians may be required to breach patient confidentiality to report suspected child abuse, infectious diseases, patients who are a threat to themselves or others, and patients who are hazardous drivers.

- Informed consent includes a discussion of the information that a reasonable patient would want to know about his or her illness, an assessment of patient understanding, and the voluntary acceptance or refusal of the intervention.

- Patients have the right to refuse or request the withdrawal of any treatment, even those that prolong life.

- Physicians are not ethically obliged to grant patient requests for ineffective tests and treatments; they should advise patients that using an ineffective intervention does not promote patient well-being, may cause harm, and violates the profession's commitment to stewardship of health care resources.

Justice

Justice requires that physicians treat patients fairly and that all health care decisions be based on medical need. Unfortunately, evidence suggests that there are disparities in the allocation of health care resources related to sex, race, and socioeconomic status. Physicians should work to eliminate these allocation inequalities and to reduce barriers to care.

Medical Error Disclosure

Medical errors are unintended acts or omissions that harm or have the potential to harm the patient. Research has shown that patients want to be apprised of all medical errors regardless of whether there was an adverse outcome, and the ethics principles of beneficence, patient autonomy, and justice obligate physicians to disclose these errors. A medical error does not necessarily constitute negligent behavior; however, failure to disclose an error may.

Error disclosure has a number of potential benefits. For patients, disclosing errors optimizes informed decision-making and promotes trust. For physicians, disclosing errors may reduce stress and risk for litigation. Although physicians may feel uneasy in disclosing errors to patients, the following approach can mitigate this burden. First, disclosure should be done in private with the patient's loved ones and essential health care team members present. Interruptions should be minimized. Before disclosing the error, the physician should determine the patient's knowledge of the problem and then correct any misinformation. When disclosing the error, the physician should speak clearly (without jargon) and check for comprehension. After disclosing the error, the physician should apologize and advise the patient how the physician and institution will act to prevent similar errors; the physician should not blame others for the error. The physician should also empathetically acknowledge the patient's emotional responses to the disclosure. Finally, the physician should formulate a patient-centered follow-up plan and document the discussion. **H**

> **KEY POINTS**
>
> - Patients want to be apprised of all medical errors regardless of whether there was an adverse outcome; doing so optimizes informed decision-making, promotes trust, and may reduce stress and risk for litigation.

Colleague Responsibility

Physicians have a shared responsibility with other health care professionals in maintaining competence, reducing medical errors, increasing patient safety, minimizing overuse of health care resources, and optimizing outcomes. Physicians should "speak up" about impaired and disruptive colleagues; such colleagues should be confronted directly or reported to appropriate authorities. Physicians should strive to promote a culture of speaking up, and institutions should encourage speaking up and provide relevant training if necessary. In addition to providing direct feedback (confronting an impaired colleague), other means should be available for speaking up (division or department chair, anonymous hotline, quality committee). Institutions should have non-retaliation policies in place for those who make a report. Physicians should also report practices and systems issues that result in suboptimal outcomes and compromise patient safety and quality of care.

Approaching Ethical Dilemmas

When faced with a clinical ethical dilemma, the physician should approach the situation with a review of (1) the medical indications (the patient's medical problems, treatments, and treatment goals), (2) patient preferences (and identifying a surrogate if the patient lacks capacity to make decisions), (3) patient quality of life (including the prospects of restoring the patient–with or without treatment–to normal life, the deficits the patient will experience if treatment is successful, and the patient's and physician's definitions of quality of life), and (4) contextual features (financial, family, legal, religious, and other issues that might affect decision-making). This approach allows for discernment and analysis of the ethically relevant information and usually defines the ethical dilemma. In so doing, it also often suggests a solution to the dilemma.

Nevertheless, physicians may encounter ethical dilemmas that are difficult to resolve. In these situations, ethics consultation should be obtained. The Joint Commission requires that health care institutions have established processes for addressing ethical concerns that arise in clinical practice. **H**

Palliative Care

Introduction

Palliative medicine maximizes quality of life for patients with serious, life-limiting illness. Palliative medicine accomplishes this through meticulous symptom management–whether those symptoms are physical, emotional, spiritual, or social– and by aligning comprehensive care to meet the patients' goals as much as possible. All physicians practice some degree of palliative care; that is, all physicians provide basic symptom management, prognostication, and advance care planning. Although subspecialty palliative care consultation may be appropriate for patients with complex symptoms or fractious communication scenarios, all internists should possess selected palliative medicine skills. It is important to note that subspecialty palliative care consultation neither precludes nor replaces existing care providers; rather, subspecialty palliative care consultation provides an added layer of support, supplementing the care of existing providers rather than supplanting it.

Historically, palliative care was equated only with end-of-life care or hospice; however, palliative care may be accessed at any time during a patient's illness, from diagnosis to death. Palliative care may be provided concurrently with life-prolonging therapies or with therapies with curative intent. Hospice, on the other hand, is a specialized type of palliative care that is reserved for patients in the terminal phase of their disease, arbitrarily defined as the last 6 months of life (**Table 22**). Ideally, palliative care is initiated early and integrated throughout the disease trajectory. Evidence suggests that patients with metastatic non–small cell lung cancer who have palliative care consultation at the time of diagnosis have decreased depression and prolonged life by 2.7 months.

Any patient with a limited life expectancy who has significant symptom burden, who needs assistance determining goals of care or with medical decision-making, or who requires help with advance care planning is appropriate for palliative care. This includes not only those with advanced cancer but also critically ill patients in the ICU and patients with noncancer diagnoses. **H**

TABLE 22. Comparison of Palliative Care and Hospice

Palliative Care	Hospice
Maximize quality of life through meticulous symptom management, clarification of goals of care, and advance care planning	
Can access at any point during life-limiting illness, from diagnosis to death	Can access during terminal phase of disease (life expectancy of less than 6 months)
Can occur concurrently with life-prolonging or curative treatments	Must forego life-prolonging treatments
No limitation on treatment or hospitalization	Goal of avoiding further hospitalization, unless there is no alternative to adequately manage symptoms

HVC • Palliative medicine maximizes quality of life for patients with serious illness through meticulous symptom management and by aligning comprehensive care to meet the patients' goals as much as possible.

HVC • Palliative care may be provided concurrently with life-prolonging therapies or with therapies with curative intent; hospice is palliative care that is reserved for patients in the terminal phase of their disease.

Communication

Outstanding communication skills are necessary for all physicians, especially when negotiating the rocky course of advanced illness. Breaking bad news is particularly difficult for both the patient and provider. Most patients want to be told the truth, but many physicians fear that bad news will diminish patient hope or leave the patient emotionally inconsolable. In fact, physicians can convey bad news and still maintain patient hope. When bad news is communicated in a skillful and empathic manner, patient satisfaction increases, and depression and anxiety decrease.

One strategy for breaking bad news involves communication steps summarized by the SPIKES mnemonic (Setting, Perception, Invitation, Knowledge, Empathy, Strategize) **(Table 23)**. Physicians can balance the medical facts and hope by being sensitive to what patients are ready to hear and how the information is affecting them (S, P, I, K, and E in SPIKES), and emphasizing what can be done (the last S in SPIKES). The key to maintaining hope is to compassionately support the patient through his or her grief and then to reorient the patient's goals toward those that are more achievable. Identifying what is most important to or most feared by the patient within this new medical reality helps to define what the patient hopes to achieve and what the patient hopes to avoid. New goals are set, and with new goals comes the hope to achieve them.

An important aspect of communication with patients is advance care planning, the process of elucidating the patient's future goals of care as disease progresses and identifying a surrogate decision maker. The outcomes of these discussions are recorded in an advance directive. See Professionalism and Ethics for a discussion of advance care planning and advance directives.

• When bad news is communicated in a skillful and empathic manner, patient satisfaction is increased, and depression and anxiety are decreased.

Symptom Management

Meticulous symptom control is one of the cornerstones of palliative medicine. The most common symptoms encountered in patients receiving palliative care include pain, dyspnea, nausea, depression, anorexia, and delirium.

Pain

Pain is common in patients with serious illness. Pain adversely affects functional status and quality of life, and unfortunately, it is often inadequately treated. Patients with serious illness should be routinely assessed for the presence of pain using a pain rating scale. Providers should remain vigilant in addressing emotional, social, and existential distress, which increase suffering related to pain.

	Step	Actions	Comments
TABLE 23.	SPIKES Protocol for Breaking Bad News		
S	Setting	Plan ahead and have the appropriate personnel and family members present. Anticipate and plan for possible patient reactions.	
P	Perception	Ask the patient what he or she has been told about the disease and/or the purpose of the meeting. Correct any misconceptions.	Gauge the patient's understanding of the situation. During this step, avoid the temptation to discuss the medical reality with the patient. Rather, let the patient tell you what he or she has heard.
I	Invitation	Find out how much the patient wants to know and how he or she would prefer to hear information.	If the patient does not want information, ask to whom you should speak on the patient's behalf.
K	Knowledge	Give the patient the news. Use short declarative sentences without jargon. Pause after giving the news to address any emotion.	Provide a "warning shot" that bad news is coming. Do not "sugarcoat" the truth. You cannot change bad news into good news. More words just create confusion.
E	Empathy	Use empathic statements to address emotion. Resist the temptation to rush in and "fix" the situation.	This is a critical step. Empathic statements demonstrate an understanding and continued commitment to the patient despite the bad news, letting the patient know that you are "in this together."
S	Strategize	Emphasize what can be done. Shift hope to achievable goals.	

Based on Baile WF, Buckman R, Lenzi R, Glober G, Beale EA, Kudelka AP. SPIKES-A six-step protocol for delivering bad news: application to the patient with cancer. Oncologist. 2000;5(4):302-11. [PMID: 10964998]

Pharmacologic management of pain progresses in a stepwise manner. The World Health Organization pain ladder has proved efficacious in managing pain (**Figure 5**). Mild pain is treated with nonopioid analgesics such as acetaminophen, NSAIDs, salicylates, or topical agents (lidocaine patches, topical NSAIDs). For moderate pain, a weak opioid such as hydrocodone is added. For severe pain, strong opioids such as morphine, oxycodone, hydromorphone, or fentanyl are used. Additionally, if indicated, adjuvants such as antidepressants or anticonvulsants can be added to the analgesic agents at any step. Dosing of various opioids is delineated in **Table 24**.

Certain opioids should be used with caution or avoided altogether. Fentanyl should only be used in opioid-tolerant patients. Transdermal fentanyl requires adequate subcutaneous fat stores for reliable absorption, and absorption rates are increased by temperature elevations, such as with fever or external heat sources, which can cause overdose. The use of buccal formulations of fentanyl can be especially complicated, as the different buccal formulations are not interchangeable; dosing regimen, escalation, and frequency of use differ between brands. Buccal formulations of fentanyl should only be initiated by experts. Codeine has relatively poor analgesic effect and significant side effects, and as a result, it is not routinely recommended. Meperidine is not recommended for pain due to the accumulation of metabolites with repeated doses, which increases the risk of seizure. Morphine, codeine, and meperidine are all contraindicated in patients with kidney failure (glomerular filtration rate <30 mL/min/1.73 m²). Opioid partial agonists or agonist–antagonist medications, such as

buprenorphine, nalbuphine, and butorphanol, have less incremental analgesic effect when used alone and are therefore used only under limited circumstances. Tramadol and tapentadol are complex drugs that have weak opioid activity and other pharmacologic effects, such as inhibition of serotonin or norepinephrine reuptake, that may result in significant drug interactions. Therefore, tramadol and tapentadol should be used with caution in chronically ill patients for long-term control of pain. Methadone is an excellent and inexpensive pain medication, but complex pharmacokinetics increase the risk for inadvertent overdose. Methadone should only be initiated and titrated by experts.

In the administration of opioids, oral routes are preferred. Use of long-acting formulations is based on patient preference, as there is no evidence of improved pain control with long-acting formulations when compared with short-acting formulations. Intramuscular administration is discouraged because of the associated pain at the injection site. Subcutaneous administration is well tolerated and effective for patients unable to use an oral route. Continuous subcutaneous infusion may be used to achieve a steady state of analgesia in selected patients.

Opioid medications are accompanied by predictable side effects. Constipation is nearly universal, and tolerance to constipation does not develop over time. All patients on scheduled opioids should be on a scheduled stimulant laxative, such as senna or bisacodyl, in combination with docusate. These laxatives should be titrated to effect. If the maximal dose is still ineffective, osmotic laxatives, such as polyethylene glycol powder, sorbitol, or lactulose, can be added. When maximal laxative therapy has failed, methylnaltrexone can be considered. Methylnaltrexone, an injectable peripheral opioid antagonist that does not cross the blood-brain barrier, is very effective in treating opioid-induced constipation without adversely affecting analgesia. Bowel obstruction is an absolute contraindication to methylnaltrexone. Stool softeners are inadequate to manage opioid-induced constipation when given alone.

Nausea related to opioids is not uncommon. No one opioid is known to be less emetogenic than another. Opioid-induced nausea is usually transient, and tolerance generally develops over 2 to 7 days; therefore, opioids should not be switched too quickly in patients with opioid-induced nausea. Antidopaminergic agents, such as metoclopramide or prochlorperazine, are the preferred agents to treat opioid-induced nausea.

Adjunctive medications can be effective for specific pain syndromes. Neuropathic pain is characterized by burning, tingling, or lancinating pain. Tricyclic antidepressants (amitriptyline, nortriptyline), serotonin–norepinephrine reuptake inhibitors (venlafaxine, duloxetine), and antiepileptic medications (gabapentin, pregabalin, carbamazepine) have been shown to be beneficial in neuropathic pain syndromes. Visceral pain is caused by injury to internal organs, most typically malignancy. Visceral pain is often vague, dull, and difficult to localize. In opioid-refractory visceral pain,

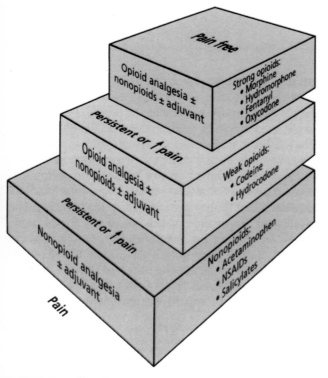

FIGURE 5. World Health Organization analgesic ladder.

TABLE 24. Dosing and Conversion Chart for Opioid Analgesics

| Medication | Usual Starting Dose[a,b] | | Equianalgesic Dosing[c] | |
	Oral	Parenteral	Oral	Parenteral
Hydrocodone	5 mg every 3-4 h	Not available	30 mg	Not available
Oxycodone	5-10 mg every 3-4 h (immediate release or oral solution)	Not available	20 mg	Not available
Morphine[d]	5-15 mg every 3-4 h (immediate release or oral solution)	2.5-5 mg SQ/IV every 3-4 h	30 mg	10 mg
Oxymorphone[e]	10 mg every 4-6 h (immediate release)	1-1.5 mg SQ/IM every 4-6 h	10 mg	1 mg
Hydromorphone	1-2 mg every 3-4 h	0.2-0.6 mg SQ/IV every 2-3 h	7.5 mg	1.5 mg
Fentanyl		25-50 µg IM/IV every 1-3 h	Sublingual tablets, lozenges, films, and buccal formulations available; consultation is advised for dosing of these agents	100 µg (single dose)

Initial transdermal patch dose based on 24-h oral morphine dose

30-59 mg	12 µg/h
60-134 mg	25 µg/h
135-224 mg	50 µg/h
225-314 mg	75 µg/h
315-404 mg	100 µg/h

IM = intramuscularly; IV = intravenously; SQ = subcutaneously.

[a]Adult, opioid-naïve patients with body weight greater than 50 kg (110 lb).

[b]Dose should be reduced by half in older patients or those with liver or kidney disease.

[c]Estimated dose offering equivalent analgesia as other medications.

[d]Morphine should be avoided in patients with kidney failure.

[e]Oxymorphone should be avoided in patients with moderate to severe liver disease.

glucocorticoids can be helpful in decreasing tumor-related swelling and/or peritoneal irritation. Additionally, nerve blocks for the appropriate abdominal plexus can be helpful. Bony metastatic pain is typically complex, involving somatic, neuropathic, and inflammatory components; it is classically worse at night. Anti-inflammatory medications, such as NSAIDs or glucocorticoids, can be particularly helpful. Bisphosphonates can significantly reduce the pain of bony metastases.

Dyspnea

Dyspnea is the subjective sense of breathlessness. Although dyspnea is often related to advanced cardiopulmonary pathology, dyspnea is also common in many chronic progressive diseases near the end of life. In advanced disease, dyspnea may occur with normal oxygen saturations and normal oxyhemoglobin measurements. Reversible causes of dyspnea, such as pleural effusions, infection, and anemia, should be investigated and treated. Any cardiopulmonary pathology, such as heart failure or COPD, should be maximally medically managed.

Oxygen supplementation is helpful if the patient is hypoxic but has not been shown to be effective in the absence of hypoxia. There is mixed evidence regarding the benefit of nonpharmacologic interventions in relieving dyspnea. Mindfulness practices, relaxation, acupuncture, chest wall vibration, or electrical stimulation may be reasonable in selected patients. Systemic opioids are the standard of care for refractory dyspnea in advanced disease. Substantial evidence supports a consensus statement issued by the American College of Chest Physicians that suggests that systemic opioids, dosed and titrated appropriately, are effective and safe for dyspnea in the setting of advanced disease. Conversely, meta-analysis has shown no benefit of nebulized opioids over nebulized saline in the treatment of dyspnea. Benzodiazepines may have a role in the treatment of patients with both dyspnea and anxiety.

Nausea

Nausea and vomiting are a major source of distress for patients. Many patients rate unrelieved nausea as more distressing than unrelieved pain. Management of nausea is based on expert opinion and small case series studies. Most experts recommend attempting to identify the cause of the nausea first. Knowledge of the purported pathophysiologic mechanism of the nausea allows the provider to therapeutically target specific neurotransmitter pathways (**Table 25**). In severely ill patients, more than one mechanism may be at play. For persistent nausea, adding a second medication that targets a different neurotransmitter is appropriate. Glucocorticoids can be adjuvant to all antiemetic therapy and are particularly useful in patients with increased intracranial pressure. **H**

Depression

Anticipatory grief and demoralization are common at the end of life, whereas pathologic depression is never normal. Diagnosing depression in the terminally ill, however, is challenging. Most screening tools for depression rely heavily on the presence of symptoms associated with functions necessary to maintain life (historically termed "vegetative symptoms") such as changes in appetite, sleep, and energy level, which are frequent and anticipated in advanced illness. Helplessness, hopelessness, worthlessness, guilt, and anhedonia are signs of depression rather than normal grief. Suicidal intent is abnormal and should be addressed promptly and aggressively. **Table 26** compares the signs and symptoms of grief to those of depression.

Depression in terminally ill patients responds well to both pharmacologic and nonpharmacologic treatment. Tricyclic antidepressants, selective serotonin reuptake inhibitors, serotonin-norepinephrine reuptake inhibitors, and mirtazapine are all effective agents. Prognosis should be taken into account since these medications take weeks to reach peak effect. If prognosis is less than 6 weeks, a psychostimulant with a faster onset, such as methylphenidate, may be considered.

Anorexia

Anorexia, weight loss, and cachexia reflect a final common pathway during the terminal phase of most disease processes.

Assuming potentially reversible conditions (nausea, altered taste, medication side effects, bowel obstruction, dysphagia, psychological comorbidities) have been ruled out, disease-related cachexia is caused by an altered neurohormonal, inflammatory milieu that results in a profoundly deranged metabolism. The deranged metabolism decreases appetite but also decreases the body's ability to use caloric intake in a productive way. As such, cachexia cannot be fully reversed by conventional nutritional support. Artificial nutrition in cachexia of advanced disease does not improve morbidity or mortality. Medications used to stimulate appetite (progestins, dronabinol, glucocorticoids) do not improve morbidity or mortality, are only effective in 20% to 30% of patients, and are associated with side effects. Head-to-head studies have shown that dronabinol is less effective than progestins or glucocorticoids. Educating patients and families on the etiology and pathophysiology of cachexia is the primary intervention and may help them to better accept the expected course of the disease.

Delirium

H

Delirium is common in terminally ill patients. Potentially reversible causes include medication side effects, inadequately treated pain, urinary obstruction, or bowel impaction. Often, no reversible cause is found. Nonpharmacologic interventions, such as maintaining a calm and quiet environment, reorienting and reassuring the patient, and attempting to normalize sleep-wake cycles, may be helpful in controlling delirium. If these measures fail and the delirium is distressing to the patient or family, pharmacologic therapy may be considered. First-generation antipsychotics, such as haloperidol or chlorpromazine, are usually effective and can be uptitrated as necessary. There is little evidence to support the use of newer-generation antipsychotics over older-generation antipsychotics. Benzodiazepines are less effective than first-generation antipsychotics, are associated with occasional paradoxical reactions, and are only recommended in refractory terminal delirium. **H**

TABLE 25. Treatment of Nausea in the Palliative Care Patient

Cause of Nausea	Mediating Receptor Pathway	Treatment
Gut wall stretching or dilatation (constipation, bowel obstruction, ileus)	Dopamine type 2 (D_2) receptors in the gastrointestinal tract	Antidopaminergic antiemetics (metoclopramide, prochlorperazine, haloperidol)
Gut mucosal injury (radiation, chemotherapy, infection, inflammation, direct tumor invasion)	Serotonin (5-hydroxytryptamine-3 [$5\text{-}HT_3$]) receptors in the gastrointestinal tract	Serotonin antagonists (ondansetron, granisetron)
Drugs, metabolic by-products, bacterial toxins	D_2 receptors, $5\text{-}HT_3$ receptors, and neurokinin type 1 receptors in the chemoreceptor trigger zone	Antidopaminergic antiemetics and serotonin antagonists
Motion sickness, labyrinthine disorders	Histamine type 1 (H_1) receptors and muscarinic acetylcholine receptors in the vestibular system	Anticholinergic antiemetics (scopolamine, diphenhydramine, promethazine)
Anticipatory nausea	Unknown, presumed cerebral cortex	Benzodiazepines
Increased intracranial pressure	Unknown	Glucocorticoids

TABLE 26. Grief Compared with Depression in Terminally Ill Patients

Characteristics of Grief	Characteristics of Depression
Patients experience feelings, emotions, and behaviors that result from a particular loss.	Patients experience feelings, emotions, and behaviors that fulfill criteria for a major psychiatric disorder; distress is usually generalized to all facets of life.
Almost all terminally ill patients experience grief, but only a minority of patients develop full-blown affective disorders requiring treatment.	Major depression occurs in 1%-53% of terminally ill patients.
Patients usually cope with distress on their own.	Medical or psychiatric intervention is usually necessary.
Patients experience somatic distress, loss of usual patterns of behavior, agitation, sleep and appetite disturbances, decreased concentration, and social withdrawal.	Patients experience similar symptoms, plus hopelessness, helplessness, worthlessness, guilt, and suicidal ideation.
Grief is associated with disease progression.	Depression has an increased prevalence (up to 77%) in patients with advanced disease; pain is a major risk factor.
Patients retain the capacity for pleasure.	Patients enjoy nothing.
Grief comes in waves.	Depression is constant and unremitting.
Patients express passive wishes for death to come quickly.	Patients express intense and persistent suicidal ideation.
Patients are able to look forward to the future.	Patients have no sense of a positive future.

Reproduced with permission from Block SD. Assessing and managing depression in the terminally ill patient. ACP-ASIM End-of-Life Care Consensus Panel. American College of Physicians - American Society of Internal Medicine. Ann Intern Med. 2000 Feb 1;132(3):209-18. [PMID: 10651602]

KEY POINTS

- Use of long-acting opioids for pain control is based on patient preference, as there is no evidence of improved pain control with long-acting opioids when compared with short-acting opioids.

- All patients on scheduled opioids should be on a scheduled stimulant laxative, such as senna or bisacodyl, in combination with docusate.

- Systemic opioids are the standard of care for refractory dyspnea in advanced disease.

- Terminally ill patients with depression respond well to tricyclic antidepressants, selective serotonin reuptake inhibitors, serotonin-norepinephrine reuptake inhibitors, and mirtazapine.

Common Symptoms

Introduction

Internists are tasked with diagnosing and treating a wide range of symptoms in adults. Specific symptom complaints account for nearly half of all outpatient visits, with half of these complaints being related to pain, and one third of all symptom complaints ultimately remaining unexplained. However, nearly 75% of symptoms, regardless of type, resolve in 2 weeks.

In evaluating common complaints, clinicians must determine the significance of these symptoms and the need for any further diagnostic testing. Given the array of available diagnostic tests (many of which have high associated costs), it is imperative that each physician approach these symptoms in a systematic manner that utilizes diagnostic testing rationally and cost effectively. This approach forms the basis for the American College of Physicians' High Value Care initiative.

Despite the many advances that have occurred in the field of medicine over the past century, studies indicate that approximately 85% of diagnoses are correctly made simply by performing a detailed history and physical examination. Each question and examination maneuver can be regarded as an independent diagnostic test to help arrive at the correct diagnosis. Therefore, the diagnostic process involves establishing a pretest probability of disease, with sequential application of diagnostic tests, including the history, physical examination, and selected laboratory and/or imaging studies, until a threshold is reached where the physician can be comfortable in either excluding or treating a disorder.

Diagnostic testing beyond the history and physical examination should not be avoided; rather, testing should be used when indicated by the information obtained during patient interactions. A "shotgun" approach to diagnosis, in which the physician orders a barrage of diagnostic tests, is rarely indicated. Studies have shown that nearly 30% of all health care costs in the United States (a total of more than $750 billion each year) are spent unnecessarily on diagnostic testing. Instead, a logical, intentional, and stepwise approach to testing should be used.

It has also been shown that ordering additional diagnostic testing does not alleviate patient fears and concerns. As such, it is important that physicians develop strong relationships with their patients and that physicians explain the rationale for their diagnostic approach while allowing patients to ask questions. Patients should always be made an active partner in their health care.

Given this information, appropriate evaluation of common symptom complexes becomes paramount in order to avoid unnecessary testing, manage costs, and prevent escalation of health-related anxiety. This chapter presents the recommended approaches to managing many symptoms encountered by the general internist, including chronic pain, medically unexplained symptoms, cough, fatigue, dizziness, insomnia, syncope, and edema.

Chronic Noncancer Pain

Chronic pain not caused by cancer is discussed here; see Palliative Care for a discussion of cancer pain. In this context, chronic pain can be defined as pain, with or without a clear precipitant, that has persisted beyond 3 months. Chronic pain results in varying degrees of debility in patients.

The approach to the patient with chronic pain is guided by the type of pain the patient experiences. Pain may be classified by biologic mechanism as neuropathic, nociceptive, or central; however, the physician should keep in mind that once pain becomes chronic, considerable overlap develops. Medication choice is generally based on this classification.

Neuropathic pain is caused by injury or dysfunction of the nervous system. Neuropathic pain is usually described as burning, stinging, tingling, or shooting pain. It typically follows the distribution of the nerve (or nerve root) that is damaged, but it can be bilateral and more diffuse, as in peripheral neuropathies. Pain may be localized, such as in postherpetic neuralgia, or more widespread, such as in diabetic peripheral neuropathy. Physical findings typically reveal pain, numbness, or allodynia (sensitivity to non-noxious stimuli) in the nerve distribution.

Nociceptive pain is pain that is detected by specialized sensory nerves called nociceptors. These nerves are located throughout the soft tissues, such as in muscles and skin, as well as the internal organs. Two types of nociceptive pain exist: somatic pain (pain from the joints, bones, muscles, and other soft tissues) and visceral pain (pain from the internal organs). Nociceptors located in somatic structures provide a wide range of sensory experience, including touch, tickle, pressure, or pain. Somatic pain is usually characterized by more localized, dull, aching, throbbing, or squeezing pain. In contrast, nociceptors in the viscera either transmit no sensation or a poorly localized sensation of fullness, pressure, or pain. Nociceptive pain may have an inflammatory component in some disease states.

Central pain is caused by damage to or dysfunction of the central nervous system, which includes the brain, brainstem, and spinal cord. Central pain syndrome typically occurs shortly after the causative injury or damage, but it may be delayed by months or even years, especially if it is related to stroke. In addition to stroke, this syndrome can be caused by multiple sclerosis, tumors, epilepsy, brain or spinal cord trauma, or Parkinson disease. The character of the pain varies widely and may affect a specific area of the body or occur more diffusely. The pain is usually constant, with bursts of more severe pain, often exacerbated by cough, temperature changes, movement, or emotions. Central pain is often associated with allodynia and/or hyperalgesia (oversensitivity to noxious stimuli). Patients usually describe one or more types of pain sensation, the most prominent being burning. In addition to burning, sensations of numbness, pressure, lacerating pain, aching pain, "pins and needles," and episodic brief bursts of sharp pain have been described. Central pain syndromes can also evolve out of unrelenting chronic pain when persistent stimulation of peripheral pain receptors results in the upregulation of central pain modulators. When such upregulation occurs, the pain generator shifts, becoming more central than peripheral over time. Fibromyalgia is thought to be one example of this type of central pain process.

Assessment

Patients who present with reports of chronic pain should undergo a thorough history and physical examination in an attempt to determine the cause. Specific diagnoses or syndromes should be evaluated and managed accordingly. "Red flag" symptoms, such as nocturnal worsening of pain (often seen in cancer), fever, or weight loss, should spur further investigation. In the absence of red flag symptoms or abnormalities on physical examination, there is little evidence to support additional extensive testing.

The physician should also conduct a thorough assessment to determine all aspects of the patient's life that pain is affecting. A psychosocial history should assess impact of pain on sleep, work function, and family relationships. Functional impairment secondary to pain should be elicited in a detailed and specific way. Psychological screening for depression, anxiety, and somatization is also important. Depression, in particular, very commonly coexists with chronic pain.

Management

When pain becomes chronic, it inevitably affects many aspects of the patient's life. Interventions to improve chronic pain should be multifaceted and individualized. Medications may be part of the treatment plan, but care should be taken to avoid situations in which medications are overemphasized or become the sole management strategy. Patients should be educated early regarding the pathophysiologic mechanisms of chronic pain, the rationale behind a multimodal treatment approach, and reasonable expectations for improvement with the emphasis on functional improvement.

Nonpharmacologic Therapy

Nearly all pain management guidelines recommend introducing an exercise program in patients with chronic pain as a way to both improve pain and function. There is high-quality evidence that shows low-magnitude but significant improvements in both pain and function in certain pain populations. A recent Cochrane review showed an absolute improvement of 8% in pain and 7% in function for adults with osteoarthritis of the hip who exercised. A similar review that focused on patients with nonspecific chronic low back pain showed absolute improvements of 13% and 7% for pain and function, respectively. The type of exercise program will vary from patient to patient, depending on patient needs, preferences, and resources in the community. There is no evidence that one form of exercise is better than another. Options might include formal physical therapy, muscle strengthening, muscle stretching, low-impact aerobic exercise, water-based exercise, or tai chi.

Other nonpharmacologic modalities often employed as part of a multimodal approach to pain management include ice and heat therapy, transcutaneous electric nerve stimulation (TENS), massage, acupuncture, and chiropractic manipulation. Only massage and acupuncture are supported by low-quality evidence, with modest improvements compared with conventional therapy. Optimal duration of treatment for these interventions is unknown.

Chronic pain is often associated with psychological issues. The presence of psychological difficulties should in no way invalidate the patient's report of pain. Identified psychological issues should be specifically addressed as part of the treatment plan. Patients who meet the criteria for diagnosis of a psychological comorbidity, such as depression or anxiety, should be treated accordingly (see Mental and Behavioral Health). Cognitive-behavioral therapy (CBT) is consistently recommended in pain management guidelines to treat chronic pain, and there are data supporting its use but little information to guide pairing a specific technique to a specific type of patient. As such, the supporting data are difficult to interpret. CBT helps replace maladaptive coping skills with more valuable ones. CBT techniques, which may include cognitive restructuring, problem solving, relaxation techniques, and mindfulness-based stress reduction, help mitigate maladaptive behavior patterns, such as catastrophizing, fear avoidance, and overgeneralizing. How individual physicians incorporate CBT techniques into the multimodal management of their patients with chronic pain will depend on local resource availability.

Pharmacologic Therapy

Medications have a role in the management of chronic pain but are more valuable as part of a multimodal approach than as the sole treatment solution.

For neuropathic pain, localized symptoms can be treated with topical agents, such as capsaicin cream or a lidocaine patch or cream. Both topical capsaicin and lidocaine have been shown to be effective for diabetic neuropathy and postherpetic neuralgia. The anticonvulsant drugs gabapentin and pregabalin are considered first-line agents for systemic therapy, are well tolerated, and have the fewest side effects and drug interactions. Carbamazepine has demonstrated efficacy for trigeminal neuralgia, but evidence for effectiveness in other neuropathic syndromes is lacking. Newer anticonvulsants, such as topiramate and lamotrigine, are under investigation for this use. Tricyclic antidepressants, such as amitriptyline and nortriptyline, are effective for neuropathic pain independent of their effect on depression, but they have increased drug interactions, poor side effect profile, and potential cardiac toxicities, especially in the elderly. The serotonin-norepinephrine reuptake inhibitors duloxetine and venlafaxine have demonstrated efficacy in treating diabetic neuropathy. Tramadol and opioids also have demonstrated efficacy in treating neuropathic pain. However, because of the complex risk-benefit ratio associated with these medications, their use should be limited to selected low-risk patients who have failed to respond to more traditional neuromodulators.

For nociceptive pain, acetaminophen is usually the first-line agent owing to its safety and tolerability. NSAIDs can be considered if there is an inflammatory component to the pain and the patient does not have contraindications to oral NSAID use. Ideally, NSAIDs would be used for periodic flares and not on a continuous basis. Topical NSAIDs have improved tolerability, fewer side effects, and demonstrated efficacy in osteoarthritis of the knees.

Central pain syndromes, in particular, benefit from the multimodal approach to pain management. From a pharmacologic standpoint, neuromodulators seem to be the most efficacious medications. Tricyclic antidepressants, serotonin-norepinephrine reuptake inhibitors, gabapentin, and pregabalin are all reasonable options.

Opioid Therapy

Opioid use has increased dramatically in the United States over the past decade. The sales of opioid analgesics quadrupled between 1999 and 2010, and the estimated number of opioid prescriptions filled in the United States exceeded 256 million in 2010. Prescription opioid-related deaths increased from 4000 in 1999 to 14,000 in 2006. Half of fatal overdoses involved concomitant use of sedative-hypnotic medications. In 2012, 60% of prescription opioid overdoses occurred in patients taking opioids as prescribed and within accepted guidelines of prescribing; most of these patients were on high doses of opioids exceeding the equivalent of 100 mg of oral morphine per day.

There is no evidence to support the efficacy of long-term opioids in managing chronic pain. In one study, patients on long-term opioids for chronic pain had more pain, poorer quality of life, and poorer function than a population of patients with chronic pain who were not taking opioids. Any decision to use opioids for the management of chronic non-cancer pain should be entered into carefully and with thorough assessment of risk relative to any potential benefit.

Although the evidence that shows improved outcomes with various risk mitigation strategies is low, the numerous guidelines currently available are in general agreement in their recommendations. Once medical need for opioid analgesia has been established, risk assessment is the next step. The physician should assess the patient for risk of opioid misuse (diversion or addiction) but also for risk of unintended and potentially lethal adverse events. This should include a review of chemical dependency and mental health history. Most guidelines strongly recommend employing a risk assessment tool, such as a DIRE (Diagnosis, Intractability, Risk, and Efficacy) score (**Table 27**). Despite the lack of evidence, written treatment agreements and adherence monitoring, including baseline and periodic urine drug screens and surveillance using prescription monitoring programs, are recommended by most guidelines. Additionally, most guidelines recommend

TABLE 27. DIRE Score: Patient Selection for Chronic Opioid Analgesia

Factor[a]	Explanation
Diagnosis	1 = Benign chronic condition with minimal objective findings or no definite medical diagnosis. Examples: fibromyalgia, migraine, nonspecific back pain
	2 = Slowly progressive condition concordant with moderate pain, or fixed condition with moderate objective findings. Examples: failed back surgery syndrome, back pain with moderate degenerative changes, neuropathic pain
	3 = Advanced condition concordant with severe pain with objective findings. Examples: severe ischemic vascular disease, advanced neuropathy, severe spinal stenosis
Intractability	1 = Few therapies have been tried and the patient takes a passive role in his/her pain management process.
	2 = Most customary treatments have been tried, but the patient is not fully engaged in the pain management process or barriers are present (insurance, transportation, medical illness).
	3 = Patient is fully engaged in a spectrum of appropriate treatments but with inadequate response.
Risk	(R = Total of P + C + R + S below)
Psychological:	1 = Serious personality dysfunction or mental illness interfering with care. Example: personality disorder, severe affective disorder, significant personality issues
	2 = Personality or mental health interferes moderately. Example: depression or anxiety disorder
	3 = Good communication with clinic. No significant personality dysfunction or mental illness
Chemical health:	1 = Active or very recent use of illicit drugs, excessive alcohol, or prescription drug abuse
	2 = Chemical coper (uses medications to cope with stress) or history of chemical dependency in remission
	3 = No chemical dependency history. Not drug-focused or chemically reliant
Reliability:	1 = History of numerous problems: medication misuse, missed appointments, rarely follows through
	2 = Occasional difficulties with compliance but generally reliable
	3 = Highly reliable patient with medications, appointments, and treatments
Social support:	1 = Life in chaos. Little family support and few close relationships. Loss of most normal life roles
	2 = Reduction in some relationships and life roles
	3 = Supportive family/close relationships. Involved in work or school and no social isolation
Efficacy	1 = Poor function or minimal pain relief despite moderate to high doses
	2 = Moderate benefit with function improved in a number of ways (or insufficient information [hasn't tried opioid yet or very low doses or too short of a trial])
	3 = Good improvement in pain and function and quality of life with stable doses over time

[a]For each factor, rate the patient's score from 1 to 3 based on the explanations in the right-hand column. Total score = D + I + R + E. Score of 7-13: Not a suitable candidate for long-term opioid analgesia. Score of 14-21: Good candidate for long-term opioid analgesia.[b]

[b]Score cutoffs were not included on the physician rater's score sheet.

Reprinted with permission from Belgrade MJ, Schamber CD, Lindgren BR. The DIRE score: predicting outcomes of opioid prescribing for chronic pain. J Pain. 2006 Sep;7(9): 671-81. [PMID: 16942953] Copyright 2006, Elsevier.

against concurrently prescribing both opioids and sedative-hypnotics and recommend referral for patients requiring doses of opioids greater than 100-mg oral morphine equivalents per day to physicians or clinics where this level of opioid use may be more closely managed. Furthermore, given the lack of evidence to support chronic opioid therapy, the continued use of opioids for chronic pain should be justified at every follow-up visit by documenting the patient's sustained functional improvement due to effective opioid therapy, lack of adverse events such as opioid-induced side effects (cognitive impairment, sedation, constipation, falls), and lack of aberrant behavior (lost prescriptions, early refill requests, multiple concurrent opioid providers or "doctor shopping," consistently missed appointments, or erratic follow-up).

Physicians must have the fortitude to avoid prescribing opioids to those at significant risk or those who demonstrate adverse events or consistent aberrant behavior.

KEY POINTS

- Studies indicate that approximately 85% of diagnoses are correctly made simply by performing a detailed history and physical examination. **HVC**

- Diagnostic testing beyond the history and physical examination should be used in an intentional, logical, and stepwise fashion; nearly 30% of all health care costs are spent on unnecessary tests and treatments. **HVC**

(Continued)

KEY POINTS (continued)

HVC
- Reasonable quality evidence refutes the commonly held belief that ordering additional, unnecessary diagnostic testing alleviates patient fears and concerns.

HVC
- Nonpharmacologic modalities that can be effective when part of a multimodal approach to pain management include exercise, ice and heat therapy, transcutaneous electric nerve stimulation, massage, acupuncture, and chiropractic manipulation.

- Pharmacologic management of chronic pain may include topical agents, anticonvulsant drugs, tricyclic antidepressants, serotonin-norepinephrine reuptake inhibitors, acetaminophen, NSAIDs, and opioids.

HVC
- There is no evidence to support the efficacy of long-term opioids in managing chronic pain.

Medically Unexplained Symptoms

Many primary care and subspecialty physicians frequently encounter patients with medically unexplained symptoms (MUS), symptoms that cannot be attributed to a known medical cause after examination and testing. In the literature, patients with MUS frequently are described as "challenging," "time consuming," "frustrating," "discouraging," and "puzzling." These symptoms have a higher prevalence in women and in those with lower formal education and lower self-reported quality of life. Patients with MUS also have higher rates of unemployment. Care of patients with MUS and the uncertainty of definitive diagnosis may lead to increased utilization of health care resources, excessive diagnostic testing, and a strained physician-patient relationship. Additionally, family dynamics may be adversely affected.

Some patients with MUS may meet diagnostic criteria for somatic symptom disorder or illness anxiety disorder (replacing the previous diagnostic terms hypochondriasis, conversion disorder, or functional disorder) (Table 28). However, most patients with MUS do not have a clear psychiatric illness. Although psychological factors often play a role in the development of unexplained physical symptoms, there is little evidence to support the premise that psychological distress alone is the cause of the symptoms. Therefore, MUS is the preferred terminology, as this does not imply any sense of psychological causation. Additionally, the presence of symptoms without a medical explanation almost always affects the patient's thoughts, feelings, and actions, and assessing the impact and significance of the symptoms in an individual patient is an essential component of management of MUS.

Clinical Presentation and Evaluation

The most common symptoms in patients presenting with MUS are chest pain, fatigue, dizziness, headache, swelling, back pain, shortness of breath, insomnia, abdominal pain, and numbness. Frequently, patients have seen many primary care

TABLE 28. Diagnostic Criteria for Somatic Symptom Disorder and Illness Anxiety Disorder

Somatic Symptom Disorder	Illness Anxiety Disorder
At least 1 somatic symptom causing distress or interference with daily life	Preoccupation with having or acquiring an illness
Excessive thoughts, behaviors, and feelings related to the somatic symptom(s): Disproportionate or persistent concern about seriousness of symptoms Persistent high level of anxiety about health Excessive focus of time and energy on health concerns	Somatic symptoms are not present or, if present, are only mild in intensity
Persistent somatic symptoms for at least 6 months (the same somatic symptom does not have to persist for 6 months)	

and subspecialty physicians over the course of many years; have undergone extensive laboratory testing, imaging studies, and procedures; and have availed themselves of medical literature in an attempt at self-diagnosis. Because patients with MUS present on a continuum of physical and mental health, a comprehensive, holistic approach is essential. Each presenting symptom merits the relevant history and physical examination. In most cases, a review of prior records should occur before repeating or extending the evaluation unless there is a significant change in the patient's condition. Physicians must possess excellent patient-centered communication skills and listen carefully to the patient, validating concerns and responding to emotions. Additionally, the initial assessment should include specific questions to elicit the patient's concerns, underlying psychological status, and degree of distress and disability attributable to the symptoms (Table 29).

When the history, physical examination, and diagnostic evaluation fail to delineate a precise anatomic or physiologic cause of continued symptoms, patients may request or even demand additional testing. Physicians may comply with these requests, as they feel that a negative result will reassure the patient and themselves. Physicians may also find it challenging to limit further testing, prescribing, or referral because they fear missing an elusive diagnosis. The evidence that more testing helps reassure patients with MUS or improves outcomes is limited. Negative test results may, in fact, increase patient anxiety over a potentially missed diagnosis. In a randomized controlled trial of 150 patients with chronic daily headaches, those randomized to receive MRI had a similar level of symptoms at 1 year compared with those who did not undergo testing; however, physicians made fewer referrals to specialists in the tested patients.

TABLE 29. Elements of a Thorough Assessment of the Patient with Medically Unexplained Symptoms

Why now and what's the agenda? (Questions for the patient)

What is your main concern about this symptom?

What made you come today?

Is there something particular that you hoped I could do for you or your symptoms?

Assess the presentation.

What are the symptoms?

Take a full history of the onset of all symptoms, exacerbating factors, and relieving factors.

How much impairment do the symptoms cause? Do they cause disability? What is a typical day like?

Are there any signs of disease on physical examination?

Encourage discussion of psychosocial difficulties.

Is there associated pathology?

Gather old notes and investigations. Review these first before ordering more investigations.

Balance the iatrogenic risks of further investigation or treatment against the probability of finding associated pathology.

Does the patient have an anxiety or depressive disorder?

Does the patient have any mood symptoms or anxiety symptoms?

Consider using a screening questionnaire, depression scale, the general health questionnaire, or the patient health questionnaire.

Is this some other emotional distress presenting as physical distress?

What is the patient's model of illness?

Who are the patient's supporters?

Reproduced from Hatcher S, Arroll B. Assessment and management of medically unexplained symptoms. BMJ. 2008 May 17;336(7653):1124-8. [PMID: 18483055] with permission from BMJ Publishing Group, Ltd.

Management

Long-term management of the patient with MUS is challenging. A therapeutic alliance and a mutually respectful physician-patient relationship are key features in the successful management of the patient with MUS. In keeping with a patient-centered approach, the patient should be engaged fully in the plan, focusing on physical, psychological, and social aspects of health. The physician and patient should work together to create and maintain an atmosphere of mutual trust.

In addition to physical symptoms, the patient with MUS may manifest primary or secondary signs and symptoms of significant underlying psychological distress, including depression or anxiety. These underlying mental health problems can be overlooked by physicians during the unsuccessful quest for a unifying or previously undiagnosed organic illness. Rather than pursuing further costly, low-value, and potentially risky diagnostic workups and therapies, it may be more beneficial and value driven to assess and treat any potential underlying psychological symptoms and to educate patients with MUS on successful coping skills based on the personal impact of their symptoms. The point of aborting further diagnostic testing and unsuccessful therapy and shifting primary attention toward mental health care requires clinical judgment on an individualized basis and patient engagement in the conversation. Discussions that address the patient's concerns without invalidating their experiences are most likely to be of help to patients who have these difficult and complex problems.

Participation in well-paced exercise programs with gradual increase in activity level, especially in patients with back pain, fatigue, and fibromyalgia, may be more helpful than rest. Patients with MUS have also demonstrated improvement in symptoms with antidepressant therapy. A recent randomized controlled trial documented a clinically significant improvement in the Mental Component Summary of the Short Form (36) Health Survey among patients who participated in a multidimensional protocol, which consisted of 12 monthly visits with trained nurse practitioners and CBT, pharmacologic therapy (antidepressants), and other programs. Patients with lower mental health scores at baseline, severe body pain, nonsevere physical dysfunction, and at least 16 years of education were more likely to show improvement. A follow-up randomized controlled trial of 206 patients found no significant difference in total costs for the group that received the 12-month intervention (emphasizing provider-patient relationship, CBT, and pharmacologic management) than for the control group. However, the intervention group used less medical care outside of the main treatment site and missed 1 less work day per month.

Regularly scheduled follow-up visits and continuity of care are important when treating patients with MUS. Studies suggest that regularly scheduled appointments with targeted physical examination increase physical functioning. In a single-site study, substituting telephone contact for selected face-to-face visits reduced unscheduled clinic visits, medication use, and hospital days and improved function. The overall approach to the patient with MUS on each follow-up visit is outlined in **Table 30** and **Table 31**. Although CBT is generally performed by trained therapists, the internist can reinforce the basic principles at each follow-up visit. The four components of CBT include (1) educating the patient so that he or she understands the plan of care and its purpose, (2) obtaining and reinforcing a commitment from the patient for the chosen plan of care, (3) setting and reviewing mutually chosen patient goals, and (4) negotiating new plans and therapy as needed.

There are minimal data on the long-term prognosis of patients with MUS. In one primary care study, more than 25% of patients had persistent symptoms after 12 months. In a study of patients with MUS who were seen by neurologists, 58% of patients had persistent symptoms at 12 years. The

TABLE 30. Follow-up Evaluation of the Patient with Medically Unexplained Symptoms

Category	Issue	How?	How Often?	Notes
History	Adherence and response to negotiated treatment plan	Ask about level of old symptoms and progress with stated goals	Every week initially until patient is stable, then progressively lengthen interval of visits to 4-12 weeks as tolerated by patient	Help the patient to develop new short-term goals to achieve long-term goals as he or she achieves current goals
	New comorbid organic disease	Monitor for any change in patient's symptoms	Each visit	
	Exploration of nonsomatic symptoms	Show preferential interest in the psychosocial aspects of the patient's story	Each visit	Most will change from a physical symptom focus to a psychosocial focus after 3-4 months
Physical examination	Physical status	Perform a brief physical examination focused on patient's old symptoms	Each visit	
	New comorbid organic disease	Perform a brief physical examination to assess for organic disease pertinent to any change in patient's history, focusing on new signs rather than new symptoms	Each visit	
Laboratory tests	New comorbid organic disease	Order laboratory tests only as needed for new signs	As needed	Recognize that most symptoms will not require laboratory investigations

Adapted with permission from Dwamena FC, Fortin AH, Smith RC. Medically unexplained symptoms. http://smartmedicine.acponline.org/content.aspx?gbosId=24. In ACP Smart Medicine (online database). Philadelphia: American College of Physicians, 2015. Accessed June 25, 2015.

patient should be counseled that treatment may likely improve function and reduce symptoms but is unlikely to produce a cure.

KEY POINTS

HVC • Evidence that further diagnostic testing helps reassure patients with medically unexplained symptoms or improves outcomes is limited; negative test results may, in fact, increase patient anxiety over a potentially missed diagnosis.

HVC • In patients with medically unexplained symptoms, the point of aborting diagnostic testing and unsuccessful therapy and shifting primary attention toward symptom management (and if indicated, mental health care) requires clinical judgment on an individualized basis and patient engagement in the conversation.

Cough

Cough accounts for approximately 30 million physician visits annually, and billions of dollars are spent on prescription and over-the-counter medications as well as homeopathic remedies to relieve this symptom.

An initial approach to the patient is based on duration of cough. Acute cough is present for less than 3 weeks, subacute cough for 3 to 8 weeks, and chronic cough for greater than 8 weeks.

Acute Cough

Acute cough is most commonly caused by viral upper respiratory tract infections (URIs) (rhinosinusitis, pharyngitis) and acute bronchitis. Other causes include pneumonia, COPD, asthma, allergic rhinitis, left ventricular failure, medications, or aspiration.

Rhinosinusitis and acute bronchitis are most commonly caused by influenza types A and B, parainfluenza, coronavirus, rhinovirus, and respiratory syncytial virus. Nonviral causes include *Streptococcus pneumoniae*, *Moraxella catarrhalis*, *Mycoplasma pneumoniae*, *Chlamydophila pneumoniae*, and, more recently, *Bordetella pertussis* (whooping cough). Purulent sputum does not reliably differentiate between viral or bacterial causes. In acute bronchitis, cough may persist for up to 8 weeks due to bronchial hyperreactivity.

Cough that is accompanied by fever, constitutional symptoms, and abnormalities on physical examination is generally indicative of lower respiratory tract infection. A chest radiograph should be obtained in patients who present with these

TABLE 31. Follow-up Management of the Patient with Medically Unexplained Symptoms

Category	Issue	How?	How Often?	Notes
Nonpharmacologic therapy	Maintaining an effective relationship with the patient	Elicit and address the patient's emotional concerns; use a negotiated rather than a prescriptive approach; tailor care to patient's personality; address your own negative reactions to the patient.	Each visit	Monitor the provider-patient relationship regularly as you would, for example, monitor blood pressure in a patient with hypertension. Ask, "So how is all this going; how are you and I working together?" Examples of indicators of an effective relationship are adherence to the treatment plan, friendliness, improved eye contact, positive statements about the provider and the treatment.
	Dissociating treatment regimen from symptoms	Schedule regular, consistent, time-contingent visits rather than ad-hoc (as-needed) visits; give all medications on a scheduled rather than on an as-needed basis.	Each visit	Titrate number of scheduled visits and dosages of different aspects of treatment to patient's needs and progress.
Pharmacologic therapy	MUS symptoms	Consider lowest effective dose of antidepressant and nonnarcotic drugs.	Each visit	Minimize or avoid use of narcotics and tranquilizers.
	Comorbid depression and anxiety	Use full doses of SSRIs or other related antidepressants. If depression has not fully remitted after 6-8 weeks, add a second antidepressant from a different class and titrate to full dose (consider drug interactions). If this is not effective, mental health consultation should be obtained.	As needed	
Patient education	Overall management	Review patient's diary and facilitate understanding of how his or her thoughts, emotions, and behaviors are related to symptoms.	Ongoing	
	Education and treatment plan	Educate the patient so that the patient understands the plan of care and its purpose.	Each visit	
	Reinforcing patient commitment to treatment	Give appropriate praise for commitment behavior such as completing homework; address noncommittal behavior, such as not keeping appointments or visiting an acute care facility without prior discussion.	Each visit	
	Reviewing and revising patient goals	Reinforce previous short-term goals or negotiate new ones to operationalize patient's long-term goals.	Each visit	Help patient to identify solutions to roadblocks.
	Negotiating new plans	Negotiate plans to adjust physical activity; recommend relaxation techniques; refer for physical therapy.	Each visit	Continuously encourage the patient to add new healthy behaviors and to progress in what he or she is already doing.

MUS = medically unexplained symptoms; SSRI = selective serotonin reuptake inhibitor.

Adapted with permission from Dwamena FC, Fortin AH, Smith RC. Medically unexplained symptoms. http://smartmedicine.acponline.org/content.aspx?gbosId=24. In ACP Smart Medicine (online database). Philadelphia: American College of Physicians, 2015. Accessed June 25, 2015.

findings. Influenza should be considered in any patient who presents with cough, fever, myalgia, and headache during the appropriate season (fall to early spring).

Approximately 15% of patients on an ACE inhibitor develop a nonproductive cough. The cough usually begins within 1 week of starting therapy, although it may appear later. If cough is overly troublesome, the medication should be discontinued. It may take up to 4 weeks to subside. Rechallenge with a different ACE inhibitor is not recommended, as there is a high rate of recurrent cough. Angiotensin receptor blockers generally do not cause cough and can be substituted for ACE inhibitors in this instance.

Treatment of acute cough is based on the primary diagnosis and is largely symptomatic. Routine antibiotic treatment of uncomplicated URIs and acute bronchitis in the nonelderly immunocompetent patient is not indicated, a recommendation supported by the Centers for Disease Control and Prevention (CDC) and the Choosing Wisely initiative. Despite efforts to curb inappropriate prescribing of antibiotics, recent evidence has shown that the overall rate of antibiotic prescribing has increased to 71% for patients presenting with symptoms of acute bronchitis. Antibiotic use is costly and potentially harmful, and it should be emphasized that patient satisfaction depends primarily on physician-patient communication rather than on antibiotic prescription.

For patients with the common cold, inhaled ipratropium, cromolyn sodium, first-generation antihistamine-decongestant preparations, and naproxen are helpful in decreasing sneezing and rhinorrhea. First-generation antihistamines and decongestants, however, should be used with caution in older adults. For treatment of cough accompanying the common cold, the American College of Chest Physicians recommends first-generation antihistamine-decongestant preparations (brompheniramine, sustained-release pseudoephedrine). Newer-generation nonsedating antihistamines are ineffective. A review of 17 trials concluded that centrally acting (codeine, dextromethorphan) or peripherally acting (moguisteine) antitussive therapy results in little improvement in cough. β_2-agonists should not be used unless cough is accompanied by wheezing.

Subacute and Chronic Cough

Subacute cough most commonly develops after an infection, including B. pertussis infection. In endemic or sporadic cases of pertussis, patients present with a cough lasting at least 2 weeks plus at least one other clinical finding: paroxysms of coughing, inspiratory "whoop," or post-tussive emesis with no other apparent cause. If infection is unlikely, consideration of the common causes of chronic cough should ensue. Inhaled ipratropium may be beneficial in treating subacute cough if there is no airway hyperreactivity.

Chronic cough has four common causes: upper airway cough syndrome (UACS), asthma, nonasthmatic eosinophilic bronchitis (NAEB), and gastroesophageal reflux disease (GERD). UACS, asthma, and GERD account for approximately 90% of chronic cough cases, excluding cases resulting from smoking or use of ACE inhibitors. Less frequently, chronic cough may be caused by chronic bronchitis, bronchiectasis, lung cancer, aspiration, irritation of the external auditory canal, and psychogenic causes.

Patients with chronic cough, especially smokers, should undergo chest radiography. If the chest radiograph does not reveal a potential cause of cough, the physician should consider UACS, asthma, NAEB, and GERD and begin a stepwise approach for evaluation and treatment. The definitive diagnosis may be suggested by history and physical examination and confirmed by successful empiric treatment.

An algorithmic approach can be used in the immunocompetent patient with chronic cough (excluding the patient who is taking an ACE inhibitor or smoking), leading to successful outcomes in more than 90% of patients (**Figure 6**). In general, if the chest radiograph is unrevealing for a cause of cough, empiric therapy for UACS is begun for 2 to 3 weeks. If the patient does not respond to empiric therapy, appropriate evaluation and treatment for asthma, NAEB, and GERD should follow. All patients with chronic cough who smoke should be offered cessation counseling.

The patient should receive optimized therapy for each diagnosis. For UACS due to allergic rhinitis, intranasal glucocorticoids are effective. For UACS due to nonallergic rhinitis, first-generation antihistamines (for example, chlorpheniramine, brompheniramine, diphenhydramine) and decongestants (pseudoephedrine) remain the therapy of choice. A 2-week trial should be used. Patients with cough-variant asthma may demonstrate reversible airflow obstruction or airway hyperreactivity with bronchoprovocation testing. However, since false-positive results may occur, the diagnosis of asthma should only be given if symptoms abate after 2 to 4 weeks of treatment with an inhaled bronchodilator and inhaled glucocorticoids. In patients in whom UACS and GERD are unlikely by clinical history or who have failed to respond to empiric therapy and in whom pulmonary function tests are normal, sputum testing for eosinophils is a reasonable next evaluation, especially if there is a history of atopy. In patients without airway hyperreactivity but with sputum eosinophilia, NAEB can be diagnosed and subsequently treated with inhaled glucocorticoids. The diagnosis of GERD can be made in patients with typical reflux symptoms (present in 60% of patients) or in those who fit a typical profile and in whom near-complete or complete resolution of symptoms with antireflux treatment occurs. Although 24-hour esophageal pH monitoring may be helpful in the evaluation of suspected GERD, empiric treatment (lifestyle modification and proton pump inhibitor therapy for 1 to 3 months) can be initiated before testing.

In addition to disease-based therapy, symptomatic treatment may be helpful. Broad categories of medications used to treat chronic cough include antitussives (opioids, anesthetics) and protussives (expectorants, mucolytics). Unlike in the treatment of acute cough, studies suggest that opioids may be effective in the treatment of chronic cough. In a recent systematic

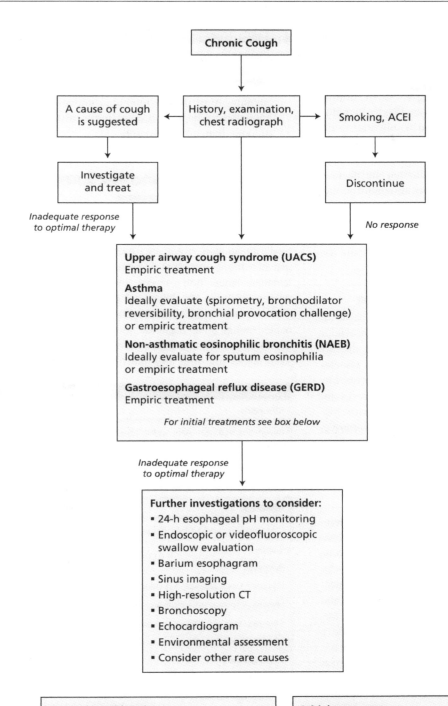

FIGURE 6. Evaluation of chronic cough.

ACEI = ACE inhibitor; LTRA = leukotriene receptor antagonist.

review, opioids were more effective than placebo in decreasing cough frequency and severity and improving quality of life. No one opioid consistently outperformed another in efficacy. There was neither superiority nor inferiority in performance when comparing opioids to peripherally acting anesthetic antitussives (benzonatate). Dextromethorphan was effective in reducing cough severity and/or frequency, but conflicting results were reported in the comparison of dextromethorphan and opioids. Protussives, such as guaifenesin, improve mucus clearance in patients with copious sputum production and decrease irritation of cough reflexes. Protussives may also reduce cough intensity. In patients with refractory chronic cough, gabapentin may be considered. In a randomized, double-blind, placebo-controlled trial, gabapentin significantly improved cough-specific quality of life (number needed to treat = 3.58). The onset of action of gabapentin was within 4 weeks.

Cough in the Immunocompromised Patient

Special consideration must be given to infectious causes of cough in the immunocompromised patient, who is at risk for the common community-acquired infections but also for tuberculosis, *Pneumocystis jirovecii*, *Aspergillus* species, *Cryptococcus* species, cytomegalovirus, varicella, herpes simplex, and, less commonly, parasitic infections. The severity and duration of the immunosuppression, and whether the primary impairment is in humoral or cell-mediated immunity, can help focus the differential diagnosis. The patient should be started on empiric therapy for suspected infectious causes while diagnostic testing is performed.

Hemoptysis

Hemoptysis, the coughing up of blood from the lower respiratory tract, must be distinguished from nasopharyngeal bleeding or hematemesis, which involves vomiting of blood from the gastrointestinal tract. Sources of hemoptysis include the tracheobronchial tree (bronchitis, bronchiectasis, tumor), pulmonary parenchyma (abscess, pneumonia, tuberculosis, Goodpasture syndrome, granulomatosis with polyangiitis [formerly known as Wegener granulomatosis]), and pulmonary vasculature (arteriovenous malformations, pulmonary embolism, mitral stenosis, left-sided heart failure). Hemoptysis most commonly results from infection or malignancy. All patients with hemoptysis should receive chest radiography and, if indicated, chest CT and/or bronchoscopy.

> **KEY POINTS**
> - A chest radiograph should be obtained in patients who present with cough that is accompanied by fever, constitutional symptoms, and abnormalities on physical examination.
>
> HVC
> - Routine antibiotic treatment of uncomplicated upper respiratory infections and acute bronchitis in the nonelderly immunocompetent patient is not indicated.
>
> *(Continued)*

> **KEY POINTS** *(continued)*
> - Upper airway cough syndrome, asthma, and gastroesophageal reflux disease account for approximately 90% of chronic cough cases, excluding cases resulting from smoking or use of ACE inhibitors, and an algorithmic approach can be used, leading to successful outcomes in more than 90% of patients.

Fatigue and Systemic Exertion Intolerance Disease

Fatigue is an exceedingly common symptom, affecting up to one third of patients in primary care. Fatigue can be caused by a medical condition, psychiatric disorder, or lifestyle factors. The patient's history and physical examination should be used to differentiate fatigue from excessive somnolence, dyspnea, and true muscle weakness. The differential diagnosis is large; more common causes are listed in **Table 32**. The history and physical examination should guide diagnostic testing. If the history (including depression screen, medication reconciliation, and assessment of sleep habits and drug use) and physical examination do not

TABLE 32. Common Causes of Fatigue

Lifestyle
Sleep deprivation; poor sleep habits
Alcohol
Extremes of activity
Drug dependency (overuse and withdrawal)
Medical
Chronic liver and kidney disease
Cancer
Anemia
Chronic lung disease; hypoxemia
Hyperglycemia; uncontrolled diabetes mellitus
Thyroid disorder (hyper- and hypothyroidism)
Medication side effects
β-blockers
Antihistamines
Antidepressants
Benzodiazepines
Antipsychotics
Obesity
Heart failure
HIV/AIDS
Psychological
Depression
Anxiety
Stress

suggest a particular etiology, reasonable initial laboratory tests for evaluating fatigue include a complete blood count, thyroid-stimulating hormone level, electrolyte panel, fasting glucose, serum creatinine, and liver chemistry tests. Further diagnostic testing is likely to be unrevealing.

Systemic exertion intolerance disease (SEID), formerly known as chronic fatigue syndrome, is a complex and disabling condition without known causation or curative treatment. SEID affects between 800,000 and 2.5 million people in the United States and is more prevalent in women than in men. In February 2015, the Institute of Medicine defined the diagnostic criteria for SEID, which include (1) reduction or impairment in the ability to carry out normal daily activities, accompanied by profound fatigue that is not relieved by rest; (2) post-exertional malaise (worsening of symptoms after physical, cognitive, or emotional effort); and (3) unrefreshing sleep. In addition to the three major criteria, the patient must also demonstrate either cognitive impairment or orthostatic intolerance (symptoms that worsen when a person stands upright and improve when the person lies back down). Symptoms should be present for more than 6 months; however, they may persist for years, and many patients never regain their previous level of health or function. Other associated symptoms include pain, failure to recover from a prior infection, sore throat, painful or tender axillary or cervical lymph nodes, sensitivity to external stimuli (food, chemicals, drugs), and abnormal immune function; fibromyalgia and irritable bowel syndrome are common comorbidities.

Evaluation

The initial approach to the patient presenting with SEID includes obtaining a detailed history and performing a thorough physical examination. The assessment should incorporate a complete review of over-the-counter medications and appropriate screening for depression, sleep disorders, and alcohol or other substance abuse.

There is no specific objective laboratory test to diagnose SEID, and since the presenting symptoms are nonspecific, it remains a diagnosis of exclusion. Recommended value-based screening tests include complete blood count, glucose levels, and thyroid function tests. If indicated by the history and physical examination, electrolytes, calcium, serum creatinine, liver enzyme levels, albumin, INR, total bilirubin, and antinuclear antibodies may be obtained. Viral titers are not recommended. Gender and age-appropriate evidence-based screening should be up to date.

Management

There is no curative treatment for SEID, and no specific medications are approved by the FDA for the treatment of SEID. Management strategies are limited and should be tailored to address the most bothersome symptoms and those that disrupt the patient's daily activities. A team approach to care, utilizing the internist, psychologists trained in CBT, psychiatrists, physical therapists, exercise physiologists, physiatrists, and support groups, may be beneficial.

In the most recent systematic review with meta-analysis evaluating treatment modalities in patients with SEID, two studies reported that severely debilitated patients receiving rintatolimod, an immune modulator and antiviral agent, demonstrated a slight improvement in performance compared with placebo. This drug is not currently available in the United States. Other prescription drugs (galantamine, hydrocortisone, IgG, and fluoxetine) or complementary and alternative approaches, including diets, supplements, and phototherapy, provided no benefit. Although there were inconsistencies among studies included in the review, some found that counseling and CBT improved fatigue, physical function, quality of life, and work impairment. Graded exercise training was also found to improve function, fatigue, and work impairment. Graded exercise training gradually and consistently increases baseline activity level, avoiding extremes in exercise or periods of inactivity and deconditioning.

One 4-week randomized placebo-controlled trial with methylphenidate demonstrated clinically significant (>33% increase) improvement in fatigue and concentration in approximately 20% of patients. Opioids are not indicated for long-term management of pain.

Adequate restorative sleep is essential, and sleep hygiene techniques should be reviewed with the patient. Although strong evidence is lacking for relaxation and stress-reduction programs (biofeedback, massage, meditation, yoga, tai chi), some patients may experience improvement in symptoms with these modalities. Coexisting medical conditions should be appropriately treated.

Approximately 70% of patients with SEID meet criteria for the diagnosis of depression, anxiety, or dysthymia. These diagnoses should be recognized, and the patients should be treated appropriately.

The long-term prognosis for the patient with SEID is variable, which may frustrate both the patient and the physician. In one of the largest follow-up cohorts, functional impairment persisted at 2 to 4 years in 33% of patients. Identified factors for symptom persistence at 2.5 years are more than eight medically unexplained symptoms not included in the SEID case definition, lifetime history of dysthymia, duration of SEID greater than 1.5 years, less than 16 years of formal education, and age greater than 38 years.

To ensure ongoing monitoring and stability of symptoms, and to support the patient with SEID, regular follow-up is recommended. Polypharmacy, excessive testing, and multiple referrals should be avoided.

KEY POINTS

- Treatment strategies that have been shown to have meaningful benefit for patients with systemic exertion intolerance disease are cognitive-behavioral therapy and graded exercise training.

- No pharmacologic agent is FDA approved for the treatment of systemic exertion intolerance disease.

Dizziness

Approach to the Patient with Dizziness

Dizziness is a common nonspecific symptom that is especially prevalent in the elderly. Although dizziness is sometimes challenging to classify, the physician should attempt to place the symptom into one of four categories based on history and physical examination: (1) vertigo, (2) presyncope, (3) disequilibrium, or (4) nonspecific dizziness. Studies conducted in primary care settings, emergency departments, or dizziness clinics report that approximately 50% of patients with dizziness have vertigo, 4% to 14% of patients have presyncope, and 1% to 16% of patients have disequilibrium. The remaining patients have a psychiatric disorder, hyperventilation, multiple causes, or an unknown cause. In patients presenting to the emergency department, dizziness is the most common symptom linked to a missed diagnosis of stroke.

Acute vestibular syndrome (AVS) is defined as rapid-onset dizziness that is continuous for more than 24 hours and is associated with nystagmus, unsteadiness of gait, nausea, vomiting, and intolerance to head movement. Hemiparesis, hemisensory loss, gaze palsy, and other focal neurologic events are not present. Several common, benign conditions may cause AVS, including vestibular neuronitis and labyrinthitis. However, AVS may also result from brainstem or cerebellar infarction or hemorrhage. Therefore, it is important to consider these diagnoses when evaluating patients with AVS. The continuous and prolonged nature of symptoms in AVS tends to exclude transient and intermittent conditions, such as benign paroxysmal positional vertigo, vestibular migraine, Meniere disease, and transient ischemic attack.

Vertigo

Vertigo is the illusion of either personal or environmental movement. It is frequently associated with nausea and made worse with head movement. Although classically described as a spinning sensation, patients may report swaying, tilting, or other less abrupt movement. Once vertigo is suspected, the next important step is to distinguish central from peripheral causes. The Dix-Hallpike maneuver (**Figure 7**) can help with this task. The latency (time of onset of nystagmus after positioning the patient), direction, and duration of nystagmus should be observed, and habituation (less severe or shorter duration vertigo with repeated assumption of the triggering position), fatigability (decrease in the intensity and duration of nystagmus with repeated maneuvers), and severity of symptoms should be determined. **Table 33** outlines how to interpret the different findings in the Dix-Hallpike maneuver.

Peripheral Vertigo

The most common cause of vertigo is benign paroxysmal positional vertigo (BPPV), which is attributed to debris (canalithiasis), usually in the posterior semicircular canal, perturbing labyrinthine sensory receptors and resulting in the erroneous perception of angular head acceleration. The vertiginous sensation in patients with BPPV is brief (10-30 seconds) and is precipitated by abrupt head movement. Nausea is a common accompaniment. Recurrence rates are high.

Vestibular neuronitis (or labyrinthitis, if hearing is affected), another cause of peripheral vertigo, may follow a viral syndrome that has affected the vestibular portion of cranial nerve VIII. Symptoms are generally more severe and of longer duration than in BPPV and may take longer to resolve. The physical examination findings for both BPPV and labyrinthitis are similar; mixed upbeat-torsional nystagmus may occur, but no focal neurologic findings are present.

Less common causes of peripheral vertigo are Meniere disease (classic triad of vertigo, hearing loss, tinnitus), perilymphatic fistula (vertigo and hearing loss with history of straining or trauma), vestibular schwannoma (acoustic neuroma), aminoglycoside toxicity, herpes zoster, and migraine.

For patients with BPPV, the Epley maneuver (**Figure 8**), also known as the canalith repositioning procedure, is an effective and safe treatment. The American Academy of Neurology and American Academy of Otolaryngology recommend using the Epley maneuver for BPPV involving the posterior canal. Pharmacologic therapy for BPPV generally is ineffective for cure but, as with other causes of peripheral vertigo, may be used for symptom relief. These medications include centrally acting antihistamines (meclizine), vestibular suppressants (benzodiazepines), and antiemetic drugs (**Table 34**, on page 55). It is recommended that these medications be used only for short periods of time, as more prolonged use may suppress vestibular feedback and central compensation mechanisms. Data supporting the use of glucocorticoids, calcium channel blockers, betahistine, and other complementary approaches are weak. Vestibular rehabilitation therapy, delivered by trained physical or occupational therapists, is effective for patients with peripheral vertigo, especially if referred early. Treatment modalities center on desensitization exercises and improving balance.

Central Vertigo

Approximately 20% of cerebrovascular accidents are located in the posterior fossa, and the predominant symptom is dizziness in up to 70% of these strokes. Although disorders of the peripheral vestibular system may cause debilitating symptoms, diseases associated with central vertigo, resulting in ischemia, infarction, or hemorrhage of the cerebellum or brainstem, may be life threatening. Patients at high risk include those with hypertension, diabetes, hyperlipidemia, or advanced age. These patients may have recurrent episodes over the preceding weeks or months, so it is important to elicit a history of similar events. Vertebrobasilar stroke is usually, but not always, accompanied by dysarthria, dysphagia, diplopia, weakness, or numbness. In a systematic review, focal neurologic signs were present in 80% of patients with stroke who presented with dizziness. Cerebellar infarct may present with gait or truncal ataxia or with vertigo alone. In one study, gait unsteadiness was reported in 55% of patients with central vertigo.

Demyelinating conditions, such as multiple sclerosis, can present with vertigo, although a history of other relapsing and

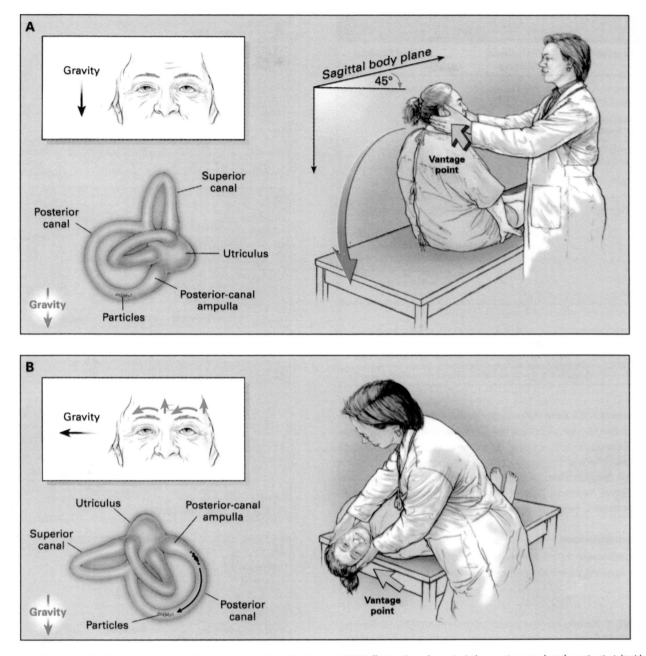

FIGURE 7. The Dix-Hallpike test of a patient with benign paroxysmal positional vertigo (BPPV) affecting the right ear. In *A*, the examiner stands at the patient's right side and rotates the patient's head 45 degrees to the right to align the right posterior semicircular canal with the sagittal plane of the body. In *B*, the examiner moves the patient, whose eyes are open, from the seated to the supine right-ear-down position and then extends the patient's neck slightly so that the chin is pointed slightly upward. The latency, duration, and direction of nystagmus, if present, and the latency and duration of vertigo, if present, should be noted. The red arrows in the inset depict the direction of nystagmus in patients with typical BPPV. The presumed location in the labyrinth of the free-floating debris thought to cause the disorder is also shown.

Reprinted with permission of the Massachusetts Medical Society from Furman JM, Cass SP. Benign paroxysmal positional vertigo. N Engl J Med. 1999;341:1590-6. [PMID: 10564690] Copyright ©1999 Massachusetts Medical Society.

remitting neurologic abnormalities, including optic neuritis, is usually present. Other rarer causes of central vertigo include Wernicke syndrome, brainstem encephalitis, and migraine.

In the patient presenting with a suspected central cause of vertigo, MRI is more sensitive than CT for detecting ischemia and is the preferred diagnostic study for nonhemorrhagic stroke. Noncontrast CT can detect hemorrhagic stroke with

high sensitivity; however, hemorrhage accounts for only about 4% of cases of central vertigo.

Presyncope

Presyncope is near loss of consciousness without loss of postural tone. Classic vertigo is absent, but patients may have difficulty distinguishing "lightheadedness" from true vertigo.

TABLE 33. Interpretation of Dix-Hallpike Maneuver Findings in Evaluation of Vertigo		
Characteristic	**Peripheral Disease**	**Central Disease**
Latency of nystagmus[a]	2-40 s	No latency
Duration of nystagmus	<1 min	>1 min
Severity of symptoms	Severe	Less severe
Fatigability[b]	Yes	No
Direction of nystagmus	Unidirectional, mixed upbeat and torsional with a small horizontal component[c]	Direction of nystagmus may depend on direction of gaze; may be purely vertical or horizontal without a torsional component

[a]Time to onset of nystagmus after positioning the patient.

[b]Decrease in the intensity and duration of nystagmus with repeated maneuvers.

[c]In benign paroxysmal positional vertigo, this pattern of nystagmus is provoked with the affected ear positioned downward when the posterior semicircular canal is involved (most common); when the anterior semicircular canal is involved, nystagmus is mixed downbeat and torsional with the affected ear positioned upward.

The absence of loss of consciousness distinguishes presyncope from true syncope, although the pathophysiology may be similar. Presyncope is the result of a decrease in global cerebral perfusion, tachyarrhythmias, bradyarrhythmias, valvular heart disease, hypotension, or vasovagal reaction (see Syncope). In addition to dizziness, patients with presyncope may also experience nausea, warmth, or tunnel vision.

Disequilibrium

Disequilibrium is an unsteadiness, or sense of imbalance, with standing or walking. The elderly are primarily at risk for

FIGURE 8. The Epley maneuver (canalith or particle repositioning maneuver) for the treatment of a patient with benign paroxysmal positional vertigo (BPPV) affecting the right ear. The presumed position of the debris within the labyrinth during the maneuver is shown in each panel. The maneuver is a three-step procedure. First, a Dix-Hallpike test is done with the patient's head rotated 45 degrees toward the right ear and the neck slightly extended with the chin pointed slightly upward. This position results in the patient's head hanging to the right (A). Once the vertigo and nystagmus provoked by the Dix-Hallpike test cease, the patient's head is rotated about the rostral-caudal body axis until the left ear is down (B). Then the head and body are further rotated until the head is face down (C). The vertex of the head is kept tilted downward throughout the rotation. The maneuver usually provokes brief vertigo. The patient should be kept in the final, facedown position for about 10 to 15 seconds. With the head kept turned toward the left shoulder, the patient is brought into the seated position (D). Once the patient is upright, the head is tilted so that the chin is pointed slightly downward.

Reprinted with permission of the Massachusetts Medical Society from Furman JM, Cass SP. Benign paroxysmal positional vertigo. N Engl J Med. 1999;341:1590-6. [PMID: 10564690] Copyright ©1999 Massachusetts Medical Society.

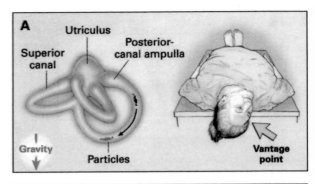

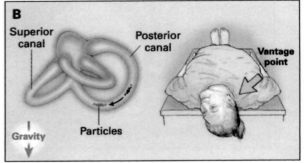

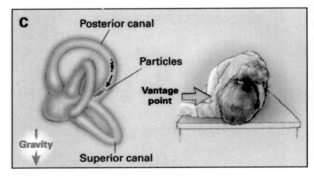

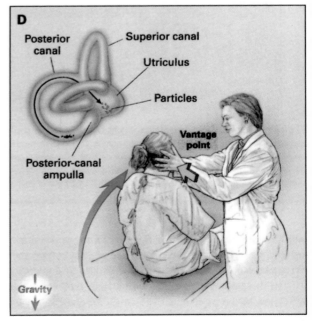

TABLE 34. Symptomatic Drug Therapy for Benign Paroxysmal Positional Vertigo

Drug	Drug Class	Dosage	Side Effects	Precautions	Clinical Use
Clonazepam	Benzodiazepine	0.25 mg PO BID	Drowsiness, confusion, respiratory depression, tolerance, dependence, anterograde amnesia, hepatotoxicity, myasthenia	Avoid with pregnancy, closed-angle glaucoma, severe liver disease. Caution with depression, psychosis. Use low dose with mild to moderate liver disease, elderly, CKD. Metabolized by CYP3A4.	Anxiety associated with dizziness
Diazepam	Benzodiazepine	1 mg PO BID	Same as with clonazepam	Same as with clonazepam. Metabolized by CYP2C19 and CYP3A4.	Anxiety associated with dizziness
Meclizine	Centrally acting antihistamine	25 mg PO four times daily	Drowsiness, fatigue, confusion, headache, xerostomia	Avoid with closed-angle glaucoma, MAOI therapy. Caution with elderly, pulmonary disease, diabetes mellitus, seizure disorder, cardiovascular disease, liver disease.	Mild dizziness and nausea
Prochlorperazine	Antiemetic	5-10 mg PO three or four times daily	Agitation, lethargy, dystonia, extrapyramidal symptoms, anticholinergic effects, cardiac conduction disturbances	Avoid with elderly, dementia, liver or kidney impairment, Parkinson disease, seizure disorder. Multiple drug interactions.	Dizziness and nausea

BID = twice daily; CKD = chronic kidney disease; CYP = cytochrome P450 isoenzyme; MAOI = monoamine oxidase inhibitor; PO = orally.

---

disequilibrium. Causes include impaired visual or auditory acuity, impaired proprioception, motor weakness, joint pain, psychiatric disease, orthostasis, or neuropathic and cerebellar diseases affecting balance and gait. Patients may also experience disequilibrium as a side effect of medication use. Frequently, more than one cause can be identified. Although patients with disequilibrium have difficulty standing or walking, they do not experience true vertigo; sitting or lying down relieves the sensation. Physical therapy, visual and auditory screening followed by correction of impairment, and mobility aids that stabilize ambulation can be beneficial in reducing severity of symptoms and fall risk.

Nonspecific Dizziness and Chronic Subjective Dizziness

Some patients may complain of other dizzy sensations, such as lightheadedness, floating, swimming, heavy-headedness, and feeling "spaced out," that do not fit into a specific diagnostic category. Although nonspecific dizziness may be associated with a wide variety of other medical and psychological conditions,

it may also occur in otherwise healthy individuals. Appropriate evaluation includes a patient-specific assessment for possible associated conditions by history and physical examination and selected diagnostic testing as indicated.

In patients with dizziness or disequilibrium that is present for most days over a period of at least 3 months that cannot be explained by an identifiable underlying cause, chronic subjective dizziness (CSD) should be considered. Symptom severity may fluctuate, but symptoms are usually more severe when walking or standing and less severe when lying down. Symptoms are often worsened with motion, highly stimulating or moving visual environments, and settings with indistinct visual orientation clues (for example, a dimly lit room). CSD can be precipitated by an acute disorder affecting the vestibular system and is often accompanied by the presence of medical and/or psychiatric problems, such as depression, anxiety, or obsessive-compulsive traits. Physical examination findings are normal, as are vestibular testing results. Treatment is multimodal: pharmacologic therapy, vestibular and balance rehabilitation therapy (VBRT), and CBT. Selective serotonin reuptake inhibitors are effective in treating CSD, even in patients without psychiatric comorbidity; they are usually effective in the low therapeutic range. Vestibular suppressants (for example, meclizine) are not effective in treating CSD. VBRT is a program of habituation/desensitization exercises that can be integrated with medication and psychotherapy. All patients with CSD should undergo VBRT. Additionally, CBT may be beneficial if there is a coexisting psychiatric disorder in patients with CSD, although it appears to be less effective for improving the physical symptoms of dizziness.

KEY POINTS

- Dizziness is the most common symptom linked to a missed diagnosis of stroke in patients presenting to the emergency department.

HVC
- The Dix-Hallpike maneuver can be used to distinguish central from peripheral causes of vertigo; for peripheral causes, the Epley maneuver is an effective and safe treatment; neuroimaging is not necessary in patients with peripheral vertigo.

- In the patient presenting with a suspected central cause of vertigo, MRI is more sensitive than CT for detecting ischemia and is the preferred diagnostic study for non-hemorrhagic stroke.

- Vertebrobasilar stroke as a cause of vertigo is usually accompanied by dysarthria, dysphagia, diplopia, weakness, or numbness.

Insomnia

Insomnia is defined as the inability to initiate or maintain adequate sleep and is a common disorder. Its prevalence is higher in women; older adults (in whom it is estimated to occur in up to 34%); patients with depression, stress, or altered sleep cycles; and patients who engage in long-distance traveling. Insomnia can lead to daytime somnolence, work absenteeism, motor vehicle accidents, poor general health, functional impairment, and impaired quality of life.

Evaluation

The initial comprehensive assessment of the patient with insomnia should include a history and physical examination, along with a psychological and psychiatric assessment. The history should elicit past and current symptoms of sleep apnea, restless legs syndrome, hypothyroidism, arthritis, cardiopulmonary disease, neurologic disease, and depression. Obtaining a history of medication and other substance use, including caffeine and other stimulants, alcohol, and over-the-counter medications, and a detailed description of sleep behavior and sleep environment is essential. A 2-week diary, documenting all activities from bedtime to final arising time, can be helpful. The patient should be encouraged to include all activities related to the use of electronic devices at night as well. Studies suggest that mobile device usage while in bed

before going to sleep is positively associated with insomnia. A targeted physical examination, with appropriate laboratory testing, to uncover medical conditions associated with sleep disturbance is indicated in most patients.

Additional selected diagnostic testing is useful for patients in whom the history is consistent with sleep-disordered breathing (sleep apnea), periodic limb movement disorders, or narcolepsy, or who fail to respond to initial therapeutic measures for insomnia. These specialized testing modalities, such as polysomnography and multiple sleep latency tests, require referral to sleep specialists and sleep laboratories.

Management
Nonpharmacologic Therapy

The initial treatment of insomnia focuses on implementing good sleep hygiene, which refers to the optimization of the environmental and behavioral factors associated with sleep. Key instructional information to discuss with the patient is outlined in **Table 35**.

CBT for insomnia is brief, multicomponent therapy that includes both cognitive components (to provide sleep education and address maladaptive beliefs and expectations about sleep) and behavioral components (including sleep restriction therapy, stimulus-control therapy, and relaxation techniques). Sleep restriction may be helpful in the motivated patient if the techniques of sleep hygiene are inadequate. Sleep restriction limits and then gradually increases the time in bed for sleep, and utilizes the concept of sleep efficiency (total sleep time divided by total time in bed). The patient is instructed to keep

TABLE 35.	Techniques for Good Sleep Hygiene
During the Day	
Ensure adequate exposure to natural light	
Avoid napping	
Avoid the following close to bedtime:	
Substances that may fragment sleep (caffeine, nicotine, alcohol, pseudoephedrine)	
Vigorous exercise	
Large meals	
Emotionally upsetting activities or conversations	
At Bedtime	
Establish a regular relaxing bedtime routine (30 minutes)	
Associate the bed and the bedroom with sleep	
Keep the bedroom quiet and dark	
Keep stable bedtime and arising time	
Spend no more than 20 minutes awake in bed	
Spend no more than 8 hours in bed	
Avoid use of television, radio, computer, or phone (texting) in bed	

Based on Masters PA. In the clinic. Insomnia. Ann Intern Med. 2014 Oct 7;161(7): ITC1-15; quiz ITC16. [PMID: 25285559]

a sleep diary for 2 weeks and to calculate the average total sleep time per day. The patient then spends that amount of time in bed, keeping the arising time constant. The time in bed gradually increases by 15 minutes as long as the sleep efficiency is greater than 85%. Stimulus-control therapy reinforces the connection between the bedroom and sleep by setting bedtimes and awaking times, removing stimuli that may keep the patient awake (electronic devices), and restricting the use of the bedroom to sleep. Relaxation techniques such as diaphragmatic breathing, visualization, and progressive muscle relaxation, sometimes coupled with biofeedback, are also effective behavioral treatments for insomnia.

CBT for insomnia is highly effective and is generally recommended as initial treatment. Unfortunately, not all clinicians are skilled at providing all of the elements of CBT, and referral for specific components to trained therapists may be needed.

Pharmacologic Therapy
The role of over-the-counter and prescription sleep aids is limited in chronic insomnia due to the potential for adverse effects and dependency. Pharmacologic therapy should generally be considered only after behavioral therapy has been insufficient in controlling insomnia symptoms.

Over-the-Counter Medications
Sedating antihistamines, such as diphenhydramine, are commonly used to treat insomnia. Although they may induce sedation, the resultant anticholinergic side effects, daytime somnolence, and cognitive impairment limit their overall safety and benefit, especially in the elderly, and they are generally not recommended. Antihistamines are also contraindicated in patients with glaucoma and men with benign prostatic hyperplasia. Melatonin may be effective for short-term insomnia due to travel or shift work. The efficacy and safety for melatonin's long-term use, as well as for other marketed natural remedies, are unknown. Alcohol, though sedating, is not recommended as it disrupts continuous sleep.

Prescription Medications
Approximately 9 million Americans take prescription medication for poor sleep, and 59 million sleeping pills were prescribed in the United States in 2012. The prevalence of use is higher in women and increases with age and level of education. Although targeted use can be effective in improving sleep, prescription sleep agents are approved only for short-term (1-month) continuous use; however, there are less data regarding using these medications on an as-needed basis. The two most commonly prescribed categories of medication are benzodiazepines, which are nonselective γ-aminobutyric acid (GABA)-receptor agonists, and nonbenzodiazepines, which are chemically unrelated to benzodiazepines and are more selective GABA-receptor agonists. Prescription drugs that are FDA approved for the treatment of insomnia are compared in **Table 36**. The American Geriatrics Society recommends that benzodiazepines of any type be avoided for the treatment of insomnia in the elderly, as an increased sensitivity to these medications coupled with decreased metabolism raise the risk of delirium, falls, fractures, cognitive impairment, and motor vehicle accidents in this population.

Although effective for short-term therapy, the use of benzodiazepines (flurazepam, triazolam, temazepam) is limited by tolerance; the side effects of daytime somnolence, falls, cognitive impairment, anterograde amnesia; and the potential for dependence. Rebound insomnia may occur upon discontinuation, especially if discontinuation is abrupt. The selective nature and shorter half-life of nonbenzodiazepines (zolpidem, zaleplon, eszopiclone) leads to fewer side effects (including rebound insomnia), making these drugs better initial choices if pharmacotherapy is warranted. However, sedation, disorientation, and agitation may occur as well as, rarely, sleep driving, sleep walking, and sleep eating.

Some antidepressants are sedating and may improve sleep. Doxepin, in low doses, is the only antidepressant approved for the treatment of insomnia. Most expert opinion recommends against using antidepressants for treating insomnia in patients without depression; however, doxepin, trazodone, and mirtazapine can be useful if a sedating antidepressant is indicated.

In patients with restless legs syndrome, dopaminergic agonists have been effective in reducing involuntary leg movement and, hence, improving sleep. Pramipexole or ropinirole are the drugs of choice.

Referral
Referral to a sleep specialist and/or psychiatrist is indicated if the diagnosis remains uncertain or if the initial treatments are ineffective. Additionally, referral to the appropriate specialist may be indicated to assist in the management of the underlying cause of the insomnia.

KEY POINTS
- The initial treatment of insomnia is nonpharmacologic and focuses on implementing good sleep hygiene via patient education or brief cognitive-behavioral therapy. **HVC**
- Although effective for short-term treatment of insomnia, the use of benzodiazepines is limited by dependence, tolerance, and the side effects of daytime somnolence, falls, cognitive impairment, and anterograde amnesia. **HVC**

Syncope
Syncope is nontraumatic, complete transient loss of consciousness and loss of postural tone. Onset is abrupt and recovery is spontaneous, rapid, and complete. Syncope accounts for 6% of hospital admissions each year, and syncope-related hospital admissions cost $2.4 billion annually in the United States.

Syncope is caused by global cerebral hypoperfusion secondary to a decrease in cardiac output and/or a decrease in

TABLE 36. FDA-Approved Prescription Drug Treatment for Insomnia

Agent[a]	Usual Dosage	Onset of Action[b]	Duration of Action[c]	Notes
Benzodiazepines (oral)				
Estazolam	1-2 mg	Slow	Intermediate	
Flurazepam	15-30 mg	Rapid	Long	
Quazepam	7.5-15 mg	Slow	Long	
Temazepam	7.5-30 mg	Slow	Intermediate	
Triazolam	0.125–0.5 mg	Rapid	Short	Short-acting benzodiazepines have been associated with an increased risk of anterograde amnesia
Nonbenzodiazepines				
Zolpidem				
Oral tablet	5-10 mg	Rapid	Short	
Extended-release oral tablet	6.25-12.5 mg	Rapid	Intermediate	
Sublingual				
Intermezzo (Transcept Pharmaceuticals)	1.75-3.5 mg	Rapid	Short	Indicated for as-needed use for treatment of middle-of-the-night insomnia with ≥4 h of sleep time remaining
Edluar (Meda Pharmaceuticals)	10 mg	Rapid	Short	
Oral spray	10 mg	Rapid	Short	
Eszopiclone	1-3 mg	Rapid	Intermediate	The recommended initial dose was reduced to 1 mg because of prolonged impaired driving skills, memory, and coordination at the previously recommended 3-mg dose
Zaleplon	10-20 mg	Rapid	Short	
Orexin-Receptor Antagonist				
Suvorexant	5-20 mg	Slow	Long	The recommended initial dose is 10 mg; the daily dose should not exceed 20 mg
Antidepressant				
Doxepin	3-6 mg	Rapid	Intermediate	
Melatonin Agonist				
Ramelteon	8 mg	Rapid	Short	

[a]All agents classified as schedule C-IV by the Drug Enforcement Agency (DEA) except doxepin and ramelteon, which are not scheduled.

[b]Onset of action: rapid = 15 to 30 minutes; slow = 30 to 60 minutes.

[c]Based on elimination half-life and preparation: short = 1 to 5 hours; intermediate = 5 to 12 hours; long = greater than 12 hours.

Reprinted with permission from Masters PA. In the clinic. Insomnia. Ann Intern Med. 2014 Oct 7;161(7):ITC1-15; quiz ITC16. [PMID: 25285559]

systemic resistance. Specific etiology is based on underlying pathophysiologic mechanisms (**Table 37**). Neurally mediated syncope, the most common cause of syncope, generally occurs with standing and is associated with a prodrome of nausea, lightheadedness, and warmth. It may follow cough, urination, defecation, pain, or laughing. Orthostatic syncope is associated with a decline of 20 mm Hg or more in systolic blood pressure (SBP) (or ≥10 mm Hg drop in diastolic blood pressure) within 3 minutes of standing. Orthostatic syncope occurs as a result of primary autonomic failure, secondary autonomic failure (diabetes, amyloidosis, spinal cord injuries, Parkinson disease), hypovolemia, medications (vasodilators, diuretics), or age-associated changes in blood pressure regulation. Cardiac syncope, most commonly caused by an arrhythmia, is typically abrupt and without prodrome. A history of coronary artery or valvular heart disease may not be present. Patients may report palpitations, which may occur in the seated or recumbent position, immediately before syncope. Cerebrovascular disease is a rare cause of syncope. With cerebrovascular disease of the anterior circulation, global cerebral hypoperfusion is rare;

TABLE 37. Classification of Syncope

Neurally Mediated Syncope (Reflex Syncope)
Vasovagal
Situational
Carotid sinus syndrome

Orthostatic Syncope
Primary
Secondary
Drug-induced
Volume depletion

Cardiac Syncope
Tachyarrhythmia or bradyarrhythmia
Atrioventricular block
Structural heart disease
Valvular heart disease (aortic stenosis)
Cardiomyopathy
Hypertrophic cardiomyopathy
Atrial myxoma
Ischemia
Other (saddle pulmonary embolism, aortic dissection, pulmonary hypertension)

Cerebrovascular Syncope
Vertebrobasilar transient ischemic attack
Subclavian steal

Psychiatric Disease (Pseudosyncope)

Unknown

dizziness and vertigo are the hallmark symptoms of posterior circulation disease. With either severe anterior or posterior cerebrovascular disease, other neurologic symptoms would be expected to precede or accompany syncope.

Diagnosis and Evaluation

The purpose of the initial evaluation of the patient with syncope is to substantiate true syncope, identify patients at risk for subsequent life-threatening events or sudden death, and identify specific etiology. The first step in the approach is to distinguish true syncope from nonsyncope. Although dizziness, vertigo, and seizures may be confused with syncope, a careful history can usually distinguish between these conditions. Dizziness and vertigo do not lead to loss of consciousness, and seizures generally are accompanied by aura, rhythmic involuntary movements, postictal confusion, and, occasionally, urinary and fecal incontinence; a history of tongue biting is helpful for ruling in, but not ruling out, a seizure diagnosis.

The physical examination should include orthostatic blood pressure measurements and a careful cardiovascular examination, including auscultation for valvular heart disease

(aortic stenosis) and the murmur of hypertrophic cardiomyopathy, especially with syncope related to exertion. In the appropriate patient, carotid sinus massage can detect carotid sinus hypersensitivity (ventricular pause >3 seconds and/or decrease in SBP >50 mm Hg). This response may predict subsequent spontaneous asystole. Carotid massage, however, should not be performed in patients with a transient ischemic attack or stroke within the past 3 months or in those with known carotid stenosis.

In addition to a history and physical examination with orthostatic blood pressure measurements, the European Society of Cardiology and National Institute for Health and Care Excellence recommend 12-lead electrocardiography (ECG). If structural heart disease is suspected, echocardiography is recommended. The cause of syncope can be identified in up to 50% of patients by utilizing this approach.

The subsequent evaluation should include only tests that are most likely to inform the diagnosis, management, and prognosis. In a study of 1920 hospitalized patients, the most commonly ordered tests, in addition to ECGs, were telemetry (95%), cardiac enzymes (95%), and CT of the head (63%). These tests, along with echocardiography, carotid ultrasonography, and electroencephalography, aided diagnosis in less than 2% of patients and altered management decisions in less than 5% of patients. The most valuable diagnostic and management test was postural blood pressure. The American College of Physicians does not recommend brain imaging, either with CT or MRI, in the evaluation of a patient with simple syncope and with a normal neurologic examination.

The diagnostic yield of 24- to 48-hour electrocardiographic monitoring is low (1%-2%), unless there are frequent episodes over a short period of time. More prolonged rhythm monitoring with external loop event recorders (ELRs) improves yield if the patient has clinical or ECG features of arrhythmia-related syncope and an intersymptom interval of less than 4 weeks. Implantable loop recorders (ILRs) may be beneficial in patients with unexplained recurrent syncope when the intersymptom interval is more than 4 weeks. In pooled data, the average yield of ILRs in diagnosing syncope was 32% over 18 months and 50% at 2 years. In two randomized controlled trials of recurrent unexplained syncope, ILRs were twice as effective as ELRs, tilt-table testing, and electrophysiologic studies. Electrophysiologic studies are useful in unexplained syncope in patients suspected to have arrhythmias and structural or ischemic heart disease. Diagnostic testing for cardiac arrhythmias is further discussed in MKSAP 17 Cardiovascular Medicine.

Tilt-table testing may be helpful in patients with reflex syncope triggered by standing, patients in high-risk settings (for example, construction workers, surgeons) with a single unexplained episode of syncope, patients with recurrent episodes in the absence of organic heart disease, or patients with recurrent episodes in the presence of heart disease when cardiac causes of syncope are excluded. The low sensitivity, specificity, and reproducibility of tilt-table testing limit its diagnostic potential.

CONT.

Recently, specialized syncope centers have been established. Although studies report increased diagnostic yield and reduction in hospital admissions and testing, long-term outcomes are unknown.

Risk Stratification and Decision for Hospital Admission

Forty percent of patients who present to emergency departments with syncope are admitted to the hospital. Many of these admissions are unnecessary, as only 5% to 6% of these patients have severe physical injuries that require hospital care. The goal of the physician is to identify patients who are at high short-term risk for adverse cardiovascular outcomes (**Table 38**). When the criteria for high risk are absent, a life-threatening event is rare.

The recently validated ROSE (Risk stratification Of Syncope in the Emergency department) rule identifies independent clinical predictors for short-term (1-month) risk of acute myocardial infarction, life-threatening arrhythmia, pacemaker implantation, pulmonary embolism, stroke, intracranial or subarachnoid hemorrhage, need for blood transfusion, or acute surgical procedure. These predictors are elevated B-type natriuretic peptide concentration (≥300 pg/mL), bradycardia (≤50 beats/minute), fecal occult blood in patients with suspected gastrointestinal bleeding, anemia (hemoglobin ≤9 g/dL [90 g/L]), chest pain with syncope, ECG with Q waves (not in lead III), and oxygen saturation less than or equal to 94% on ambient air. If any of these indicators are present in the patient with syncope, the patient should be considered high risk and should be admitted for evaluation and monitoring.

Management

Therapy is guided by the underlying etiology. The treatment for neurally mediated syncope is reassurance, education, and avoidance of hypotensive agents. Orthostatic syncope resulting from hypovolemia may be treated with volume expansion and correction of any other potential contributing factors, such as medications that may cause hypovolemia or hypotension. In patients with persistent orthostatic changes following optimization of volume and other possible contributing factors, other medications are often used, although data on these agents for treating orthostatic syncope are limited. Fludrocortisone, β-blockers, and selective serotonin reuptake inhibitors have not been shown to be uniformly beneficial. Midodrine, an α-agonist, may be effective; however, its use is limited by the side effects of hypertension and urinary retention. Pacemakers are only recommended for patients with symptomatic bradycardia or asystolic pauses. Most patients with cardiac syncope are referred to cardiologists.

Prognosis

Prognosis, like treatment, depends upon the cause of the syncope. Patients with neurally mediated syncope have the same mortality rate as that of comparably aged healthy individuals. Cardiac syncope is associated with 1-year mortality rate of 18% to 33%, and the mortality rate with syncope due to cerebrovascular disease is less than 10%. In addition to clinical predictors of adverse outcomes in the ROSE rule, age greater than 65 years, abnormal ECG, history of heart failure, ischemic heart disease, ventricular arrhythmias, and lack of warning signs or symptoms have been shown to adversely affect outcomes. Gender, tilt-test response, and severity of presentation have low predictive value for adverse outcomes. Quality of life is adversely affected in patients with recurrent syncope, especially the elderly. Driving restrictions may also be imposed on patients with recurrent syncope, and physicians should be familiar with the state laws that govern these restrictions.

KEY POINTS

- The physical examination of the patient with syncope should include orthostatic blood pressure measurements and a careful cardiovascular examination, including auscultation for valvular heart disease (aortic stenosis) and the murmur of hypertrophic cardiomyopathy, especially with syncope related to exertion.

- The most valuable diagnostic and management test in patients with syncope is postural blood pressure measurement; extensive additional testing, including telemetry, cardiac enzyme testing, CT of the head, echocardiography, carotid ultrasonography, and electroencephalography, aided diagnosis in less than 2% of patients and altered management decisions in less than 5% of patients.

- The American College of Physicians does not recommend brain imaging, either with CT or MRI, in the evaluation of a patient with simple syncope and a normal neurologic examination.

(Continued)

TABLE 38.	High-Risk Criteria for the Patient with Syncope

Features suggesting arrhythmic syncope

    Clinical: syncope during exertion, palpitations at time of syncope, family history of sudden death

    Electrocardiography: nonsustained ventricular tachycardia, bifascicular block, sinus bradycardia (<50 beats/min or sinoatrial block), prolonged QT interval

Severe structural or coronary artery disease

    Heart failure

    Low ejection fraction

    Previous myocardial infarction

Comorbidities

    Severe anemia

    Electrolyte disturbances

- The majority of patients with syncope can be safely managed as outpatients; indications for hospital admission for patients with syncope include presence of severe traumatic injuries or a high short-term risk for adverse cardiovascular outcomes.

- High short-term risks for adverse cardiovascular outcomes for patients with syncope include history suggestive of arrhythmic syncope (syncope during exertion, palpitations at the time of syncope, family history of sudden death, abnormal electrocardiographic findings), severe structural or coronary heart disease (heart failure, low ejection fraction, previous myocardial infarction), and comorbidities (severe anemia, electrolyte disturbances).

Lower Extremity Edema

Lower extremity edema results from increased movement of fluid from the intravascular to the interstitial space or decreased movement of fluid from the interstitium into the capillaries or lymphatic vessels. The mechanism involves one or more of the following: increased capillary hydrostatic pressure, decreased plasma oncotic pressure, increased capillary permeability, or obstruction of the lymphatic system.

Lower extremity edema can usually be subdivided into systemic and more localized causes. Systemic causes such as heart failure, cirrhosis, the nephrotic syndrome, chronic kidney disease, and obstructive sleep apnea typically cause bilateral fluid accumulation in gravity-dependent areas. Bilateral leg edema may also be caused by certain medications (**Table 39**). Unilateral leg edema is most commonly due to venous thromboembolism or cellulitis, but it can also be caused by lymph obstruction from significant joint swelling or prior surgery or other processes that disturb lymphatic drainage in the leg or pelvis.

TABLE 39. Drugs Commonly Associated with Edema

Androgens
Aromatase inhibitors
Calcium channel blockers
Clonidine
Estrogens
Gabapentin and pregabalin
Glucocorticoids
Hydralazine
Insulin
Minoxidil
NSAIDs
Progestins
Tamoxifen
Thiazolidinediones

Although the differential diagnosis for the cause of lower extremity edema is broad, a careful history and physical examination are central to establishing a correct diagnosis and to guiding diagnostic testing. In patients with generalized edema, obtaining a complete blood count, electrolytes, blood urea nitrogen level, serum creatinine level, liver chemistry tests, serum albumin level, and urinalysis is a reasonable initial step. For patients with acute unilateral leg pain and swelling, venous ultrasonography to evaluate for thromboembolism should be considered. Subsequent testing should be based on the likelihood of the potential causes of edema that may be present in a specific patient; treatment is based on managing the underlying cause.

Chronic Venous Insufficiency

Leg edema is frequently caused by chronic venous insufficiency, which can result from various conditions that damage the leg veins and their valves. Risk factors associated with the development of chronic venous insufficiency include tobacco use, obesity, increasing age, family history of venous disease, history of venous thromboembolism and/or lower extremity trauma, and pregnancy. Postthrombotic syndrome is the development of chronic venous insufficiency following an acute deep venous thrombosis.

The edema associated with chronic venous insufficiency typically is insidious in onset. It worsens with prolonged standing and is improved with elevating the legs and with walking. Leg discomfort is another common manifestation of chronic venous insufficiency. The pain is often gradual in onset and is described as a tired or heavy sensation in the legs. Pain is also worsened with prolonged standing and improves with walking and leg elevation. Other symptoms can include pruritus, skin discoloration, and ulceration. On examination, there is leg edema, and skin findings can include a shiny, atrophic appearance to the skin in addition to varicose veins and telangiectasias. In severe cases, there may be ulceration overlying the medial malleolus. The ulceration is often surrounded by skin that is erythematous, scaled, and weeping. The pain associated with venous ulcers is variable, ranging from mild to severe. Additional diagnostic testing is not usually necessary to correctly diagnose chronic venous insufficiency; however, venous duplex ultrasonography can help to determine severity and document valvular incompetence.

For patients with chronic venous insufficiency, first-line therapy includes compression, leg elevation, and exercise. Addressing reversible risk factors, such as weight loss in obese patients, is also advisable. Diuretics should generally be avoided in these patients. Ablation therapy (chemical, surgical, and thermal) should be reserved for patients who have failed to respond to conservative therapy for at least 6 months and who have documented retrograde valvular flow on duplex ultrasonography (>0.5 seconds in duration). Compression stockings are frequently used to prevent postthrombotic syndrome following venous thromboembolism, although a recent randomized controlled trial did not find any benefit. Dry skin, itching, and eczematous changes are treated with moisturizers. Venous ulcers are discussed within MKSAP 17 Dermatology.

Musculoskeletal Pain

Low Back Pain

Diagnosis and Evaluation

Low back pain may be acute (lasting <4 weeks), subacute (lasting 4-12 weeks), or chronic (lasting >12 weeks). Most episodes are self-limited, and 90% of patients recover fully within 6 weeks. Recommendations from the American College of Physicians for diagnosing and treating patients with low back pain are provided in **Table 40**.

History and Physical Examination

Patients with low back pain can be grouped into one of three broad categories: those having nonspecific pain (about 85%); those having pain with radiculopathy or spinal stenosis (about 7%); and those having pain possibly associated with another specific spine disorder, such as cancer (0.7%), compression fracture (4%), infection (0.01%), or ankylosing spondylitis

(0.3%). Low back pain my also stem from problems outside of the back (such as pancreatitis, aortic aneurysm, systemic illness, nephrolithiasis), but these conditions are unlikely to present with an isolated symptom of low back pain. Prevalence of various causes of back pain should be considered when assessing a patient, and testing to rule out uncommon causes in patients without risk factors or supportive history should not be performed. The history and physical examination should focus on determining the likelihood of a specific underlying condition causing the back pain and identifying neurologic involvement.

Although most patients with low back pain have nonspecific findings, features of the history associated with specific underlying disorders are presented in **Table 41**. A stepwise approach to the initial evaluation (**Figure 9**) and management

---

TABLE 40. Recommendations for Managing Low Back Pain

Perform a focused history and physical examination, including assessment of psychosocial risk factors, to classify patients into one of three broad categories:

- Nonspecific low back pain
- Back pain potentially associated with radiculopathy or spinal stenosis
- Back pain potentially associated with another specific spinal cause

Do not routinely obtain imaging or other diagnostic tests in patients with nonspecific low back pain.

Perform diagnostic imaging and testing when severe or progressive neurologic deficits are present or when serious underlying conditions are suspected.

Evaluate patients with persistent low back pain and signs or symptoms of radiculopathy or spinal stenosis with MRI (preferred) or CT only if they are potential candidates for surgery or epidural glucocorticoid injection for suspected radiculopathy.

Provide patients with evidence-based information on low back pain with regard to their expected course, advise patients to remain active, and provide information about effective self-care options.

Consider the use of medications with proven benefits in conjunction with back care information and self-care. For most patients, first-line medication options are acetaminophen or NSAIDs.

For patients who do not improve with self-care options, consider the addition of nonpharmacologic therapy with proven benefits, such as spinal manipulation, exercise therapy, and massage therapy.

Adapted with permission from Chou R, Qaseem A, Snow V, et al; Clinical Efficacy Assessment Subcommittee of the American College of Physicians; American College of Physicians; American Pain Society Low Back Pain Guidelines Panel. Diagnosis and treatment of low back pain: a joint clinical practice guideline from the American College of Physicians and the American Pain Society. Ann Intern Med. 2007 Oct 2;147(7):478-91. Erratum in: Ann Intern Med. 2008 Feb 5;148(3):247-8. [PMID: 17909209]

TABLE 41. History Features and Suggested Diagnoses in Low Back Pain

Suggested Diagnosis	History Feature
Cancer	Unexplained weight loss
	Failure to improve after 1 month
	No relief with bed rest
Infection	Fever
	Injection drug abuse
	Urinary tract infection
	Skin infection
Inflammatory/ rheumatologic condition	Presence of morning stiffness
	Pain not relieved when supine
	Pain persisting for >3 months
	Gradual onset
	Involvement of other joints
Nerve root irritation (radiculopathy)	Sciatica
	Increased pain with cough, sneeze, or Valsalva maneuver
Spinal stenosis	Severe leg pain
	No pain when seated
	Pseudoclaudication[a]
Compression fracture	Trauma
	Glucocorticoid use
	Osteoporosis
Cauda equina syndrome[b]	Bowel or bladder dysfunction
	Saddle sensory loss
	Rapidly progressive neurologic deficits

[a]Lower extremity symptoms caused by lumbar spinal stenosis mimicking vascular ischemia, including worsened pain with walking or standing and relief with sitting; also termed neurogenic claudication.

[b]Compression of the lumbar and sacral nerves below the termination of the spinal cord (conus medullaris). Characterized by back pain; sensory changes in the S3 to S5 dermatomes (saddle anesthesia); bowel, bladder, and sexual dysfunction; and absent Achilles tendon reflexes bilaterally.

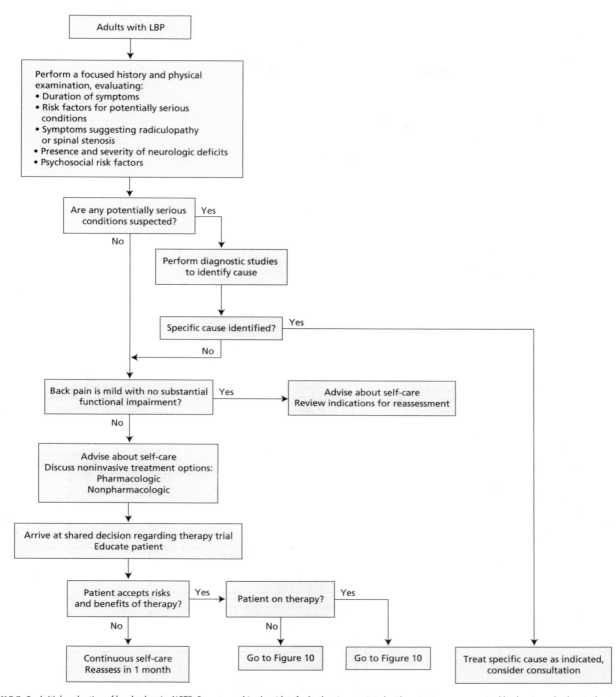

FIGURE 9. Initial evaluation of low back pain. NOTE: Do not use this algorithm for back pain associated with major trauma, nonspinal back pain, or back pain due to systemic illness.

LBP = low back pain.

Adapted with permission from Chou R, Qaseem A, Snow V, et al; Clinical Efficacy Assessment Subcommittee of the American College of Physicians; American College of Physicians; American Pain Society Low Back Pain Guidelines Panel. Diagnosis and treatment of low back pain: a joint clinical practice guideline from the American College of Physicians and the American Pain Society. Ann Intern Med. 2007 Oct 2;147(7):478-91. [PMID: 17909209] Copyright 2007, American College of Physicians.

(**Figure 10**) of low back pain is provided. Age is a useful predictor to help differentiate causes of low back pain, as the risk for concerning diagnoses, cancer, compression fractures, and spinal stenosis are significantly more likely in patients older than 50 years.

Physical examination findings may help determine whether the patient has nonspecific low back pain, radiculopathy or spinal stenosis, or a specific spinal pathology. Skin findings such as erythema or psoriasis may suggest infection or an inflammatory arthritis. Percussion over the spinal processes

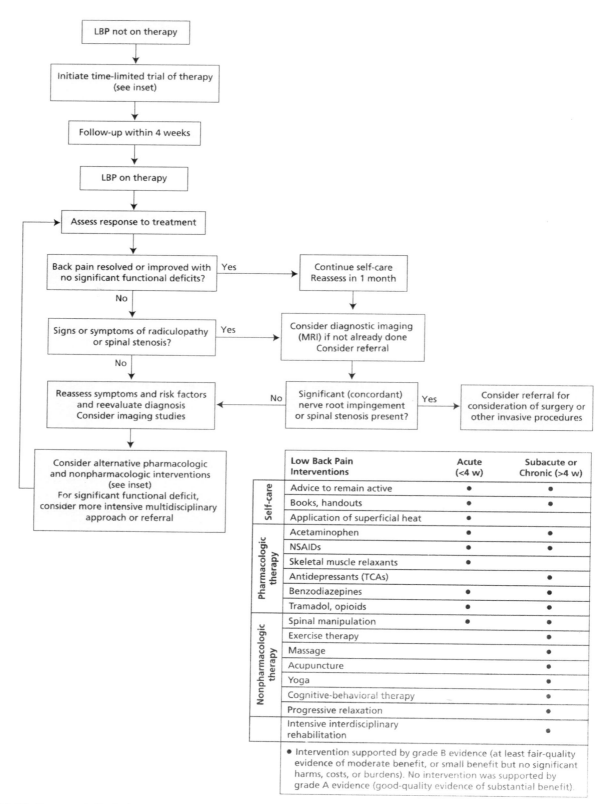

FIGURE 10. Management of low back pain.

LBP = low back pain; TCAs = tricyclic antidepressants.

Adapted with permission from Chou R, Qaseem A, Snow V, et al; Clinical Efficacy Assessment Subcommittee of the American College of Physicians; American College of Physicians; American Pain Society Low Back Pain Guidelines Panel. Diagnosis and treatment of low back pain: a joint clinical practice guideline from the American College of Physicians and the American Pain Society. Ann Intern Med. 2007 Oct 2;147(7):478-91. [PMID: 17909209] Copyright 2007, American College of Physicians.

that induces pain may indicate compression fracture or disk space infection. Reproduction of pain with palpation over the paraspinus muscles or the posterior superior iliac spine is more consistent with nonspecific (musculoskeletal) pain. Reproduction of the pain with back range of motion can also be helpful in determining etiology.

Physical examination findings for patients with possible lumbar disk herniation and nerve root impingement are provided in **Table 42**. The straight-leg raise test has a sensitivity of 91% for diagnosing disk herniation. This maneuver involves raising the patient's leg 30 to 70 degrees off the table with the patient in the supine position. A positive test is defined as development of a shooting or electric shock sensation from the hip to the ankle when the leg is raised.

KEY POINT

- In patients with low back pain, the history and physical examination should focus on determining the likelihood of a specific underlying condition causing the pain and identifying neurologic involvement.

Further Diagnostic Testing

Most patients who present with back pain do not require additional imaging or testing and will recover with supportive measures. Diagnostic studies should not be routinely obtained in patients with nonspecific low back pain; such testing should be reserved for patients with severe or progressive neurologic deficits, patients for whom a serious underlying condition is suspected, or patients who do not have symptom improvement after 4 to 6 weeks of conservative management.

In patients with radiculopathy or spinal stenosis, routine imaging has not been shown to improve outcomes. For those patients in whom a trial of conservative therapy fails, further testing might be considered. The American College of Physicians recommends MRI (preferred) or CT for radiculopathy or spinal stenosis only for those patients who are candidates for epidural glucocorticoid injection or surgery. If cancer or vertebral infection is suspected, a plain radiograph, MRI, or

erythrocyte sedimentation rate may be helpful. MRI or electromyography should be considered in patients with suspected spinal stenosis, cauda equina syndrome, or severe and progressive neurologic deficits. A vertebral fracture can usually be diagnosed by plain radiography. If features of ankylosing spondylitis are present, plain radiography of the sacroiliac joints and erythrocyte sedimentation rate may help determine the cause of pain.

When to Refer

Indications for surgical referral include features of cauda equina syndrome (a surgical emergency), presence of severe neurologic deficits, suspected spinal cord compression, neuromotor deficits, or significant pain that persists after 6 weeks of conservative therapy. **H**

KEY POINTS

- Most patients who present with low back pain do not require additional imaging or testing. **HVC**

- Diagnostic testing for low back pain should be reserved for patients with severe or progressive neurologic deficits, patients for whom a serious underlying condition is suspected, or patients who do not have symptom improvement after 4 to 6 weeks of conservative management. **HVC**

Treatment

Most patients with acute low back pain recover quickly no matter what therapeutic intervention is used. Because the overall prognosis for acute musculoskeletal low back pain is excellent, therapeutic interventions should focus on symptom management and maintaining function (see Figure 10). Follow-up should occur within 4 weeks to determine response to therapy and whether additional treatment or evaluation is needed. If there is no response to treatment, additional workup for spinal stenosis or radiculopathy should be considered if suggestive symptoms are present. If no symptoms of spinal stenosis are present, alternative pharmacologic and nonpharmacologic interventions should be considered.

TABLE 42. Physical Examination Findings for Lumbar Disk and Nerve Root Impingement

Disk	Nerve Root	Affected Reflex	Involved Muscles	Location of Altered Sensation
L3-L4	L4	Patellar reflex	Anterior tibialis (dorsiflexion and inversion of foot at ankle)	Medial leg, medial foot, medial aspect of great toe
L4-L5	L5	None	Extensor hallucis longus, anterior tibialis, deep peroneal (extension of great toe and dorsiflexion of foot at ankle); extensor digitorum longus and brevis (dorsiflexion of toes 2, 3, 4); gluteus medius and minimus (hip and pelvic abduction)	Lateral leg; dorsum of foot; toes 2, 3, 4
L5-S1	S1	Achilles tendon reflex	Gastrocnemius and soleus (plantar flexion of foot at ankle); peroneus longus and brevis (foot plantar flexion and eversion); gluteus maximus (hip extension)	Posterior aspect of the leg, lateral aspect of foot, lateral aspect of little toe

Nonpharmacologic Treatment

An important part of treatment of acute low back pain is educating patients that recovery is generally quick regardless of the intervention used. Whenever possible, maintaining daily activities should be encouraged. Application of heat may also be beneficial for acute back pain. Bed rest for patients with and without sciatica should generally be avoided, as bed rest is associated with decrease in functional recovery and increase in pain. Spinal manipulation is associated with modest benefits in treating acute low back pain, comparable to conventional therapy. Physical therapy is not typically recommended for treatment of acute low back pain.

For subacute and chronic low back pain, interdisciplinary rehabilitation (physician coordination of psychological, physical, and vocational therapy) has been shown to improve pain. A systematic review concluded that massage for low back pain may be beneficial for patients with subacute and chronic pain without neurologic symptoms. Lumbar supports are unlikely to be better than no intervention at all. Acupuncture, yoga, cognitive-behavioral therapy, and intensive rehabilitation should be reserved for patients with chronic low back pain.

Pharmacologic Treatment

Acetaminophen or NSAIDs are first-line pharmacotherapy for low back pain. NSAIDs should be used with caution in patients at increased risk for nephrotoxicity or for gastrointestinal ulcer. All NSAIDs are equally effective for treatment of low back pain. Opioid analgesics may be helpful when acetaminophen or NSAIDs are not adequate. Medications should be given at the lowest possible dose and for the shortest possible time. Muscle relaxants and benzodiazepines may be modestly beneficial for pain relief; however, side effects of dizziness and sedation limit their usefulness. Systemic glucocorticoids have not been shown to be effective in the treatment of low back pain.

Interventional and Surgical Treatment

Epidural glucocorticoid injections may provide short-term relief for patients with radiculopathy caused by disk herniation; however, the FDA issued a warning in 2014 regarding injection of glucocorticoids into the epidural space. The warning states that these injections may result in rare, but serious, adverse events, such as vision loss, stroke, paralysis, and death. Furthermore, the FDA states that the effectiveness and safety have not been established and glucocorticoids are not approved for this use.

Surgery has been shown to have definite benefits only for patients with disk herniation causing persistent radiculopathy, patients with painful spinal stenosis, and those with cauda equina syndrome. For patients with radiculopathy, diskectomy is associated with improved outcomes at 6 to 12 weeks compared with nonsurgical therapy. In patients with spinal stenosis, decompressive laminectomy has been shown to provide moderate benefit compared with nonsurgical therapy for the

first 1 to 2 years postoperatively. However, effects diminish over time.

Treatment of cauda equina syndrome typically involves prompt surgical decompression of the affected area of the spinal cord.

KEY POINTS

- Most patients with acute musculoskeletal low back pain have an excellent prognosis no matter what therapeutic intervention is used; therapeutic interventions should focus on symptom management and maintaining function.

- Most patients with acute low back pain should try to maintain daily activities and avoid bed rest whenever possible.

- Acetaminophen or NSAIDs is first-line pharmacotherapy for treatment of low back pain.

- Surgery has been shown to have definite benefits only for patients with low back pain due to disk herniation causing persistent radiculopathy, patients with painful spinal stenosis, and those with cauda equina syndrome.

Neck Pain

Diagnosis and Evaluation

Neck pain may be broadly grouped into three categories (Table 43). Mechanical pain arises from the muscles, soft tissues, and joints. Neurogenic pain originates from cervical nerve roots or the spinal cord. Systemic diseases induce neck pain because of inflammation or mass effect.

Onset, character, and location of neck pain should be determined, along with precipitating and mitigating factors and any associated symptoms. Physical examination should focus on reproducing the pain by palpation, assessing range of motion, and testing strength and reflexes, as well as identifying any upper motoneuron signs.

Mechanical neck pain is usually an aching sensation that is isolated to the neck but can radiate to the posterior head or shoulders. History often reveals an antecedent injury, such as a fall or motor vehicle accident. Mechanical neck pain can also be exacerbated by an unaccustomed activity or overuse. Physical examination findings usually show decreased range of motion, tenderness to palpation, and reproduction of the pain with flexion or extension.

Neurogenic neck pain is usually described as a burning or tingling sensation that may radiate down the arms. Dermatomal numbness or muscle weakness may be present (Table 44). On physical examination, maneuvers to compress the spinal nerves may reproduce the pain or cause radiation down the arms. Examples include worsening of symptoms with extension and rotation of the patient's neck toward the symptomatic side when an axial load is placed on the patient's head (Spurling test), and improvement when the symptomatic arm is lifted above the head with resting of the hand on the top

TABLE 43. Evaluation of Neck Pain

Category	History	Physical Examination Findings
Mechanical neck pain (muscle, ligament, facet, intervertebral disk, soft tissue)	Pain (usually episodic, deep, dull, and aching) and stiffness	Decrease in active and passive range of motion
	Pain may be precipitated or aggravated by excessive or unaccustomed activity or sustaining an awkward posture without a specific injury	Superficial tenderness indicates soft-tissue pain; deep tenderness indicates muscle or bone pain
	Ligament, muscle, and facet pain are localized and asymmetric	Pain on extension or ipsilateral lateral flexion usually indicates facet pain; pain on flexion or contralateral lateral flexion usually indicates soft-tissue pain
	Pain from upper cervical segments is referred toward the head; pain from lower segments is referred to the upper limb girdle	
Neurogenic neck pain (cervical nerve root and/or spinal cord)	Significant root pain; sharp, intense, often described as a burning sensation; may radiate to the trapezial and periscapular regions or down the arm	Neurologic examination may show motor weakness, usually involving several cervical levels and often asymmetric, affecting one or both arms
	Numbness in a dermatomal distribution and motor weakness in a myotomal distribution	Look for plantar extensor response, gait disorder, and spasticity in patients with spinal cord involvement
	Symptoms often more severe with certain movement	Bilateral or multilevel involvement indicates more severe pathology
Neck pain associated with systemic disease	Fever, malaise, or pain in areas in addition to the neck	Complete physical examination may show underlying systemic disease, such as inflammatory joint disease, organ infection, or neoplastic process
	Pain is usually severe, relentless, and progressive	
	Symptoms or signs may be progressive despite treatment	

Adapted with permission from Huang S, Tsang IK. Neck pain. http://smartmedicine.acponline.org/content.aspx?gbosId=88. In ACP Smart Medicine (online database). Philadelphia: American College of Physicians, 2015. Accessed May 5, 2015.

TABLE 44. Physical Examination Findings for Cervical Disk and Nerve Root Impingement

Disk	Nerve Root	Affected Reflex	Involved Muscles	Location of Altered Sensation
C4-C5	C5	Biceps reflex	Deltoid, biceps, and rhomboid (arm abduction and flexion at the shoulder)	Lateral arm
C5-C6	C6	Brachioradialis reflex	Biceps and brachioradialis (wrist extensors and elbow flexors)	Anterior lateral forearm, palm, thumb, and second digit
C6-C7	C7	Triceps reflex	Triceps and finger extensors (elbow and finger extensors)	Middle of the palm and third digit
C7-T1	C8	None	Finger flexors	Anterior and medial hand and forearm, fourth and fifth digits
T1-T2	T1	None	Hand intrinsics (abduction and adduction)	Anterior medial arm (distal aspect of arm to proximal aspect of forearm)

of the head (shoulder abduction relief test). Both of these tests have low to moderate sensitivity but relatively high specificity for cervical nerve root compression. Upper motoneuron findings such as spasticity or hyperreflexia may indicate spinal cord involvement.

Features in the history that indicate a possible systemic origin of neck pain include fever, weight loss, polyarthritis, and changes in vision, as well as a history of immunosuppression, cancer, or injection drug use.

Imaging studies are not needed for most patients with neck pain. When mechanical pain is present, imaging is primarily indicated after trauma to rule out fracture. Plain cervical radiography may be helpful for evaluating older patients with examination findings suggestive of malignancy or degenerative osteoarthritic changes. MRI or CT myelography is indicated for patients with neurologic signs of weakness or spinal cord involvement. Imaging may also be indicated if tumor, abscess, or pathologic fracture is suspected.

Laboratory testing is also not needed for most patients with neck pain. However, if a systemic illness such as an infectious, malignant, or rheumatologic disorder is suspected, targeted blood tests (such as erythrocyte sedimentation rate, C-reactive protein measurement, and complete blood count) may aid in establishing the diagnosis.

KEY POINT

HVC
- Imaging studies and laboratory testing are not needed for most patients with neck pain; patients with a history of trauma, presence of neurologic signs or symptoms, fever, weight loss, or immunosuppression may require additional testing.

Treatment

The mainstays of treatment for neck pain are mobilization, exercise, and analgesic agents. Most patients with neck pain recover with conservative therapy. Mechanical neck pain is treated with mobilization and physical therapy that focuses on improving range of motion and posture; systematic reviews have shown that these interventions improve neck pain over the short and intermediate terms. Over-the-counter acetaminophen and NSAIDs often provide acute pain relief. Opioid analgesic agents and skeletal muscle relaxants should only be used if over-the-counter agents are ineffective in treating moderate to severe neck pain. Neurogenic neck pain may respond to agents such as gabapentin and tricyclic antidepressants. Therapy for neck pain associated with systemic illness should focus on treating the underlying condition.

Acupuncture has been studied in the treatment of chronic neck pain and may provide short-term improvement in symptoms. Glucocorticoid injections have been used for patients with cervical radiculopathy that does not respond to pharmacotherapy; however, the FDA does not approve glucocorticoids for this use. Systemic glucocorticoids are not indicated for the treatment of neck pain. Surgery may be beneficial for patients with progressive neurologic symptoms that are caused by a defined anatomic abnormality. Surgical management of chronic neck pain is controversial and is usually limited to patients with neurologic symptoms.

KEY POINT

HVC
- Most patients with neck pain recover with conservative therapy, including mobilization, exercise, analgesic agents, and physical therapy.

Upper Extremity Disorders
Thoracic Outlet Syndrome

Thoracic outlet syndrome is caused by compression of the brachial plexus, subclavian artery, and subclavian vein as these structures pass through the thoracic outlet. There are three main clinical subtypes of thoracic outlet syndrome, defined by the primary structure involved.

Neurogenic thoracic outlet syndrome is the most common subtype and is caused by compression of the brachial plexus nerve roots as they exit the triangle formed by the first rib and the scalenus anticus and medius muscles. Symptoms include paresthesias and pain that typically worsen with activities that involve continued use of the arm or hand, especially those that include elevation of the arm. First-line therapy consists of physical therapy, rest, avoiding aggravating activities, and ergonomic modifications. Surgical intervention consists of resection of the first rib and anterior scalenectomy; surgery can be considered in patients who fail to respond to conservative measures.

Venous thoracic outlet syndrome is usually caused by thrombosis of the subclavian and/or axillary veins as they pass through the triangle formed by the clavicle, first rib, and subclavius and scalenus anticus muscles. Common symptoms include pain, swelling, and cyanosis, which occur with repeated activities involving the arms, especially when such activities involve using the arm above the plane of the shoulder. Dilated collateral veins may be seen on the chest wall, neck, and shoulder. First-line therapy consists of timely catheter-directed thrombolysis, followed by surgical decompression shortly thereafter.

Arterial thoracic outlet syndrome refers to compression of the subclavian artery usually by a cervical rib or anomalous bone, with or without distal thromboembolism. It is the least common form of thoracic outlet syndrome but is potentially dangerous as it can result in significant morbidity. This compression leads to ischemic symptoms such as exertional pain, easy fatigability, pallor, and paresthesias in the involved arm. Surgical repair or resection alleviates the compression of the affected structure. For patients with associated thrombosis, treatment consists of catheter-directed thrombolysis for patients with mild symptoms and surgical embolectomy for patients with more severe symptoms.

Shoulder Pain
Diagnosis and Evaluation

The initial diagnostic step is to determine whether the pain is originating in the shoulder or referred from a distant site. Pain with shoulder movement accompanied by stiffness and limited range of motion favors an intrinsic disorder, whereas a normal shoulder examination suggests referred pain. Neck pain and stiffness, decreased neck range of motion, and pain extending below the elbow all support pain being referred from the cervical spine.

Shoulder examination includes inspection, palpation, range-of-motion testing, and specific test maneuvers (**Table 45**). Both shoulders should be fully exposed to detect asymmetry. All important structures should be palpated in a systematic manner. Both active and passive range of motion should be tested. Articular disorders are characterized by limited active and passive movements, whereas extra-articular disorders are associated only with limited active movements.

TABLE 45. Shoulder Examination Maneuvers

Test	Description
Cross-arm	Patient abducts arm to 90 degrees and then actively adducts arm across body. Positive test: Pain in the acromioclavicular joint region (suggests acromioclavicular joint disorder)
Drop-arm	Patient's arm is passively abducted to 90 degrees; patient is then asked to slowly lower arm to waist. Positive test: Patient's arm will drop down (indicates supraspinatus tear)
External rotation lag	Patient's arm is abducted to 20 degrees. Examiner passively externally rotates arm. Positive test: Patient is unable to maintain a position of full external rotation (suggests possible tear of supraspinatus and infraspinatus muscles)
External rotation resistance	Patient's arm is placed at side with elbow flexed 90 degrees. Examiner stabilizes elbow and applies force proximal to wrist while patient attempts external rotation. Positive test: Pain or weakness (suggests infraspinatus tear or tendinopathy)
Hawkins	Patient's shoulder is flexed to 90 degrees, elbow is flexed to 90 degrees, and forearm is placed in neutral rotation. Then, while supporting the arm, the humerus is rotated internally. Positive test: Pain (suggests subacromial impingement)
Internal rotation lag	Patient internally rotates arm behind back. Examiner lifts hand off patient's back and patient is asked to maintain position while examiner applies a counteracting force. Positive test: Patient is unable to maintain position (suggests subscapularis tear)
Neer	Patient's scapula is stabilized and shoulder is flexed with arm fully pronated. Positive test: Pain (suggests subacromial impingement or rotator cuff tendinitis)
Painful arc	Patient actively abducts arm. Positive test: Pain between 60 and 120 degrees of abduction (suggests subacromial impingement)
Yergason	Patient's elbow is flexed to 90 degrees with thumb pointing up. Examiner grasps wrist and attempts to resist active supination and elbow flexion by patient. Positive test: Pain (suggests bicipital tendinitis)
"Empty can"	Patient's shoulder is passively abducted to 90 degrees in forward flexion and then is maximally internally rotated with thumb pointing down. Examiner applies downward pressure at wrist or elbow while patient resists. Positive test: Weakness (suggests supraspinatus tendon tear)

KEY POINT

- When evaluating patients with shoulder pain, pain with shoulder movement accompanied by stiffness and limited range of motion favors an intrinsic disorder, whereas a normal shoulder examination suggests referred pain.

Rotator Cuff Disorders

Rotator cuff disorders include rotator cuff tendinitis, rotator cuff tears, and subacromial bursitis. The subacromial impingement syndrome results from altered mechanics of the shoulder that lead to compression of the soft tissues of the shoulder complex between the humeral head and the undersurface of the acromion, acromioclavicular joint, or the coracoacromial arch, leading to rotator cuff tendinitis and subacromial bursitis. Pain is often described as dull and worsened with overhead activities and at night. The site of pain varies but is frequently located in the deltoid region. Decreased range of motion, weakness, and stiffness may also be reported.

On examination, posterior inspection may reveal supraspinatus and infraspinatus muscle atrophy. Tenderness associated with bicipital tendinitis may be elicited on palpating the insertion of the long head of the biceps tendon. Active range of motion is usually limited, whereas passive range of motion is preserved. Strength is usually preserved in the absence of a full-thickness rotator cuff tear. Specific maneuvers for diagnosis can generally be divided into those that attempt to provoke pain, such as the painful arc test (**Figure 11**), and those that assess strength, such as the drop-arm test (**Figure 12**; see Table 45). Only limited and largely suboptimal quality data exist concerning the usefulness of each of these maneuvers. Imaging of the shoulder is typically not needed but should be considered if a full-thickness rotator cuff tear is suspected or if there is diagnostic uncertainty. MRI is the preferred imaging modality.

Conservative therapy is indicated for patients with suspected rotator cuff tendinitis and subacromial bursitis. Patients should be instructed to avoid repetitive overhead activities and to refrain from lifting heavy objects. Performing exercises that strengthen the rotator cuff muscles and improve flexibility has also been shown to be effective in improving pain, as has the use of NSAIDs. Although data are limited, acetaminophen can be used as a safe alternative to NSAIDs. The effectiveness of

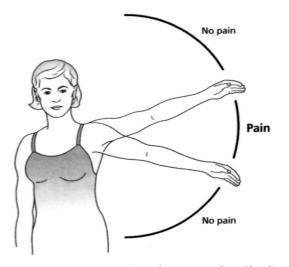

FIGURE 11. The painful arc test. The painful arc test is performed by asking the patient to actively abduct the affected arm and is considered to be positive when pain is present between 60 degrees and 120 degrees of active abduction. A positive test result suggests the presence of subacromial impingement syndrome due to subacromial bursitis or rotator cuff tendinitis.

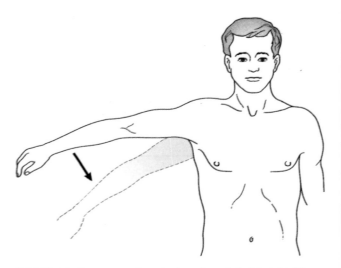
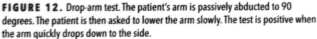

FIGURE 12. Drop-arm test. The patient's arm is passively abducted to 90 degrees. The patient is then asked to lower the arm slowly. The test is positive when the arm quickly drops down to the side.

subacromial glucocorticoid injections appears to be short-lived, although the available evidence is conflicting. Given the conflicting evidence, it is reasonable to offer a single glucocorticoid injection to patients who fail to respond to 4 to 6 weeks of the aforementioned measures or initially in patients whose pain is so severe that they are unable to participate in therapy.

Initial management of partial rotator cuff tears is identical to that for rotator cuff tendinitis and subacromial bursitis. Immediate surgery is indicated for an acute full-thickness tear in younger patients, although full-thickness tears are frequently managed conservatively in older patients. Surgery may also be considered for patients with partial tears who fail to respond to conservative therapy.

- Although most rotator cuff tears can be managed conservatively, immediate surgery is indicated for younger patients with an acute full-thickness tear, and surgery may be indicated for patients with partial tears who do not respond to conservative therapy.

Adhesive Capsulitis

Adhesive capsulitis ("frozen shoulder") is a poorly understood condition associated with development of glenohumeral joint capsule thickening and fibrosis. It most frequently occurs in patients aged 40 to 70 years and is more common in women than in men. Adhesive capsulitis may be idiopathic but may also occur following shoulder injury or surgery. Other associated conditions include diabetes mellitus, hypothyroidism, Parkinson disease, stroke, and prolonged immobility. Patients report loss of shoulder movement accompanied by pain. Examination discloses tenderness at the deltoid insertion site and significant loss of both active and passive range of motion. Plain radiographs are typically normal.

Injection of glucocorticoids into the glenohumeral joint appears to be beneficial, particularly when it is performed early in the course of the disease. Benefits are likely due to the effect of the glucocorticoid on reducing intra-articular inflammation. A systematic review supports giving up to three intra-articular glucocorticoid injections. Physical therapy appears to be less beneficial than intra-articular glucocorticoid injection, although there may be a role for physical therapy following glucocorticoid injection. NSAIDs and acetaminophen can be used for pain control. Surgery is generally reserved for patients who do not improve with 6 to 12 weeks of conservative measures. Patients should be informed that improvement in range of motion and pain may not occur for several years postoperatively.

- Glucocorticoid injections into the glenohumeral joint appear to be beneficial in the treatment of adhesive capsulitis.

Acromioclavicular Joint Degeneration

Acromioclavicular joint degeneration typically presents as pain located on the superior aspect of the shoulder, although pain may be poorly localized. The acromioclavicular joint is often tender to palpation. Pain is frequently elicited on physical examination with the arm on the affected side adducted across the body (see cross-arm test in Table 45) and with abduction beyond 120 degrees. Plain radiographs reveal degenerative changes. Treatment includes NSAIDs and activity modification. Glucocorticoid injection may also provide short-term pain relief. Surgery is rarely indicated.

Elbow Pain
Diagnosis and Evaluation

Elbow pain may originate from disease in the elbow joint, its adjacent tissues, or proximate nerves. Neck, shoulder, and wrist pathology may also cause pain referred to the elbow. Thorough examination of the neck and affected arm is required.

Epicondylosis

Epicondylosis and epicondylitis are terms used interchangeably to refer to noninflammatory pathology of the major tendons traversing the elbow joint. Lateral and medial epicondylosis are considered to be overload injuries, which occur after minor, often unrecognized, trauma to the proximal insertion of the extensor (tennis elbow) or flexor (golfer's elbow) muscles of the forearm. Lateral epicondylosis is induced by activities requiring repetitive wrist extension, such as prolonged computer use or racquet sports. Pain is located over the lateral elbow but may also radiate to the dorsal forearm. Tenderness over the lateral elbow and pain with resisted wrist extension are characteristic examination findings. Medial epicondylosis is caused by repetitive wrist flexion. Pain and tenderness are located over the medial elbow and ventral forearm and worsen with resisted wrist flexion.

Imaging studies are not indicated for patients with clinical findings consistent with epicondylosis. Initial management includes NSAIDs and avoidance of activities that cause pain. A brace may be useful when exacerbating activities cannot be avoided. Both oral and topical NSAIDs may provide short-term pain relief. Gentle physical therapy (stretching and strengthening exercises) can begin after the acute pain has improved. Glucocorticoid injections may improve symptoms in the short-term, but data are conflicting on long-term benefit. Surgery is indicated only for patients with intractable pain.

KEY POINT

- Imaging studies are not indicated for patients with clinical findings consistent with epicondylosis.

Olecranon Bursitis

Trauma, gout, rheumatoid arthritis, and infection may cause inflammation of the olecranon bursa. Examination reveals swelling and tenderness over the posterior elbow but normal range of motion (**Figure 13**). Most cases are of benign cause (painless swelling) and are self-limited with conservative management including ice, compression elbow sleeve, and avoiding trauma by protective padding over the elbow. Aspiration with fluid culture, cell count, and crystal analysis should be performed in patients with severe pain, fever, or other suspicion of infection. The cornerstone of therapy is patient education regarding joint protection, such as avoiding impact and pressure on the elbow. Noninfectious olecranon bursitis may be treated with NSAIDs. Glucocorticoid injections have questionable efficacy and considerable side effects (for example, hyperglycemia, infection); therefore, they should be reserved for refractory cases. Infectious or refractory bursitis may require surgery.

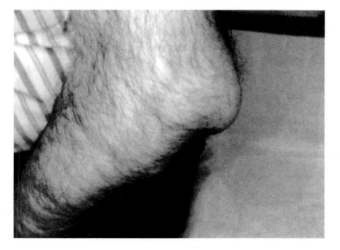

FIGURE 13. Olecranon bursitis with swelling restricted to the posterior elbow.

Ulnar Nerve Entrapment

Ulnar nerve entrapment, sometimes referred to as cubital tunnel syndrome, may occur at the level of the elbow and may be caused by bone spurs, ganglion cysts, ulnar nerve subluxation, or constriction from fibrous tissue. Repetitive elbow flexion and extension can further exacerbate the syndrome. Symptoms and signs range from elbow pain that worsens with flexion of the elbow to paresthesias and numbness of the fourth and fifth fingers and weakness of the interosseous muscles. Diagnosis may be made clinically in patients with characteristic manifestations, although electromyography may be helpful in some patients. Plain radiography is useful to identify potential bony causes, although MRI and ultrasound are usually reserved for unclear cases. Initial treatment consists of activity modification, NSAIDs, splinting the elbow at night to prevent prolonged elbow flexion, and use of an elbow pad during the day to avoid direct trauma. Surgery is reserved for patients who fail to respond to conservative measures.

Wrist and Hand Pain

Carpal Tunnel Syndrome

Carpal tunnel syndrome is caused by median nerve compression within the carpal tunnel. Pain and paresthesias are typically present in a median nerve distribution (**Figure 14**) but may radiate into the arm and involve all five fingers. Pain frequently worsens at night and with repetitive actions. Bilateral symptoms are common (>50% of patients). Known risk factors include obesity, female gender, pregnancy, hypothyroidism, diabetes mellitus, and connective tissue disorders.

Common findings on physical examination include hypalgesia of the median nerve distribution and weakness of thumb abduction. Thenar muscle atrophy suggests severe disease. The presence of Phalen and Tinel signs has minimal diagnostic utility. Hand diagrams are useful diagnostic instruments for identifying symptom patterns associated with carpal tunnel syndrome. When diagnostic uncertainty exists, nerve conduction studies can be obtained.

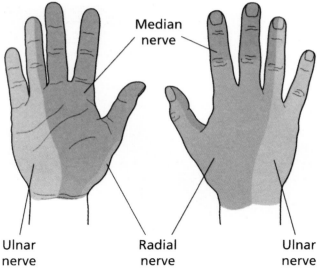

Median nerve

Ulnar nerve

Radial nerve

Ulnar nerve

FIGURE 14. Innervation of the hand.

For patients with mild to moderate symptoms, initial therapy consists of avoiding repetitive hand and wrist motions. Neutral-position wrist splinting appears to be more effective when used full time rather than only at night. Local glucocorticoid injection can provide short-term symptomatic improvement (up to 10 weeks), and a 2-week course of an oral glucocorticoid can result in short-term symptom improvement lasting for up to 1 month. Data are lacking for use of NSAIDs and vitamin B$_6$. Surgery is considered first-line therapy for those who have severe disease on nerve conduction testing and in those who have muscle wasting on examination. Additional indications for surgery include failure to respond to conservative therapy, intolerable pain, and progressive numbness or weakness.

KEY POINT

HVC
- Surgery in carpal tunnel syndrome is reserved for patients who do not respond to conservative measures, have intolerable pain, have severe disease on nerve conduction testing, or have evidence of muscle wasting on examination.

Other Causes of Wrist and Hand Pain

Hamate fractures may be due to trauma or to repetitive forces such as swinging a baseball bat. Initial treatment usually consists of a short-arm cast, although surgical intervention should be considered in patients with displaced fractures.

A history of falling on an outstretched hand accompanied by pain in the anatomic snuffbox should raise suspicion for a scaphoid fracture. If plain radiographs are initially normal but clinical suspicion for a scaphoid fracture remains high, management includes immobilization with a thumb splint and repeating radiographs in 10 to 14 days. MRI is both highly sensitive and specific for diagnosing scaphoid fractures and can be useful when plain radiographs are inconclusive and a high degree of clinical suspicion remains.

Subacute pain at the thumb base that radiates to the distal radius is characteristic of de Quervain tenosynovitis (inflammation of the dorsal thumb tendons). Examination reveals distal radial styloid tenderness and pain with resisted thumb abduction and extension. Pain is also caused when the patient makes a fist over the thumb with ulnar deviation (Finkelstein test). Initial treatment consists of applying ice, using NSAIDs, and splinting. For patients with persistent symptoms who fail to improve after 4 to 6 weeks of initial therapy, local glucocorticoid injection should be offered. Glucocorticoid injection can be repeated 4 to 6 weeks later if there is no significant improvement. Surgery is reserved for patients who fail to respond to two glucocorticoid injections.

Osteoarthritis of the first carpometacarpal and proximal and distal interphalangeal joints is common. Pain is usually insidious in onset, worsens with activity, and improves with rest. Management of osteoarthritis is addressed in MKSAP 17 Rheumatology.

Ganglion cysts are cystic swellings overlying tendon sheaths or joints that are thought to be caused by herniated synovial tissue. Asymptomatic ganglion cysts do not require treatment, as they frequently regress in size. When painful, cysts can be aspirated and injected with either a crystalline glucocorticoid or hyaluronidase. For ganglion cysts that are symptomatic and fail to respond to aspiration and injection, surgical resection is a highly effective treatment option.

Ulnar nerve entrapment at the wrist may cause sensory and motor abnormalities; however, this is seen infrequently compared with carpal tunnel syndrome.

Lower Extremity Disorders
Hip Pain
Diagnosis and Evaluation

Hip pain can arise from the hip joint or from surrounding structures, including the pelvis, abdomen, or retroperitoneum. Therefore, patients reporting hip pain should be asked to identify the specific location of the pain and characterize the associated discomfort. History should focus on what activities make the pain worse or better, trauma, prior surgeries, prior cancer, occupational activities, and a review of the gastrointestinal, gynecologic, and genitourinary systems.

Physical examination should include observation of gait, inspection and palpation of the affected and unaffected hips, examination of the sacroiliac and knee joints, and hip range-of-motion testing. Having the patient isolate the most painful area by pointing with one finger may also be helpful. The FABER test assesses the ability to Flex, ABduct, and Externally Rotate the hip (**Figure 15**). If the sacroiliac joint is painful with the FABER test and there is no pain on passive range of motion, sacroiliac joint disease is likely.

The American College of Rheumatology appropriateness criteria endorse plain radiographs of the hip and pelvis as initial testing in patients with acute or chronic hip pain. Advanced imaging techniques are usually not needed and should be

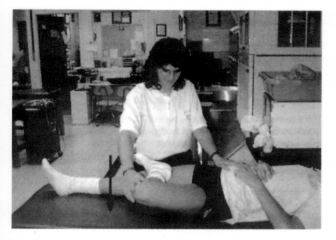

FIGURE 15. The FABER test assesses Flexion, ABduction, and External Rotation of the hip. With the leg in a figure-four position, the normal leg should attain a parallel plane with the table. Gentle downward pressure on the knee in this position simultaneously places stress on the ipsilateral sacroiliac joint.

Reprinted with permission from Davis MF, Davis PF, Ross DS. ACP Expert Guide to Sports Medicine. Philadelphia, PA: American College of Physicians; 2005:360. Copyright 2005, American College of Physicians.

reserved for patients in whom osteonecrosis, occult fracture, or tumor is suspected, or in those in whom the diagnosis remains unclear or other specific diagnoses are being considered.

Specific Causes of Hip Pain

Degenerative hip disease is common and usually presents with pain radiating to the groin that often becomes worse with weight bearing. On physical examination, internal and external rotation at the hip will be limited or painful. Plain radiographs can confirm the diagnosis; changes include superolateral joint space narrowing with subchondral sclerosis. Cystic changes can also occur, and the femoral head can appear to be irregular. Oral analgesic agents are the initial treatment (see MKSAP 17 Rheumatology).

Patients with trochanteric bursitis describe an aching sensation over the greater trochanteric bursa (lateral hip) that may radiate to the buttock or knee and is often worse when lying on the affected side. It can be differentiated from hip joint pain in that it does not usually radiate to the groin or limit hip range of motion on examination. Diagnosis is made by history and by eliciting pain with palpation over the greater trochanter or reproduction of the pain when the patient takes a step up. Oral analgesic agents and physical therapy to improve gait, strength, and range of motion are first-line treatments. If these therapies are not effective, consideration of glucocorticoid injection is warranted.

Meralgia paresthetica is caused by entrapment of the lateral femoral cutaneous nerve. Patients often present with paresthesias over the anterolateral thighs. Risk factors include obesity, pregnancy, diabetes mellitus, and tight clothing or belts around the waist. Treatment should focus on mechanisms to relieve the entrapment (for example, avoiding tight clothing, weight loss). Oral analgesic agents can also provide symptomatic relief. Additionally, more aggressive management of diabetes may be indicated in appropriate patients.

Piriformis syndrome is caused by compression of the sciatic nerve by the piriformis muscle. Patients describe chronic posterior pain in the buttock. Risk factors include prolonged sitting, such as in truck drivers. Analgesic agents and physical therapy focusing on stretching exercises are the mainstays of therapy.

Osteonecrosis (avascular necrosis) of the femoral head is caused by a loss of blood supply and subsequent death and collapse of the bone. Risk factors include glucocorticoid use, prior fracture or radiation exposure, excessive alcohol use, and sickle cell anemia. Patients may initially report pain with weight bearing, but the pain can progress significantly to occur at rest and can be associated with significant decrease in joint function. Imaging with MRI (early-stage disease) or plain radiographs (later-stage disease) is necessary to establish the diagnosis. Initial treatment includes therapies to control pain (such as NSAIDs), reduced weight bearing, and range of motion exercises. Most patients with osteonecrosis will eventually need surgical intervention with hip replacement.

KEY POINT

- If the FABER (Flex, ABduct, and Externally Rotate) test demonstrates limited range of motion or hip pain, hip pathology is likely.

Knee Pain
Diagnosis and Evaluation

Pain location, circumstances of onset (including antecedent trauma), and duration can help to narrow the differential diagnosis of knee pain. Other signs and symptoms, including joint stiffness, locking, instability, and constitutional symptoms, may provide additional diagnostic clues.

Examination should be performed with both knees fully exposed. Both knees should be inspected for asymmetry, swelling, or erythema and palpated to detect focal tenderness, joint effusion, or warmth. Active and passive range of motion should then be assessed, followed by maneuvers that test the integrity of the knee ligaments and menisci (**Table 46**). Referred pain to the knee should always be considered, especially when the knee examination is normal.

Arthrocentesis is indicated for patients presenting with acute-onset knee pain accompanied by an effusion, overlying erythema, warmth, and marked tenderness. Plain radiographs are generally needed for evaluation of acute pain only if a fracture due to trauma is suspected.

Degenerative disease of the knee is discussed in MKSAP 17 Rheumatology.

KEY POINT

- In patients with acute knee pain, plain radiographs are generally needed only if a traumatic fracture is suspected.

HVC

TABLE 46. Knee Examination Maneuvers

Test	Purpose	Description
Anterior drawer	ACL integrity	Patient is supine with hip flexed to 45 degrees and knee flexed to 90 degrees. Examiner sits on dorsum of foot and places hands on proximal calf and then pulls anteriorly while assessing movement of tibia relative to femur.
		Positive test: Increased laxity with lack of firm end point (suggests ACL tear)
Lachman	ACL integrity	Patient is supine with leg in slight external rotation and knee flexed 20 degrees to 30 degrees at examiner's side. Examiner stabilizes femur with one hand and grasps proximal calf with other. Calf is pulled forward while assessing movement of tibia relative to femur.
		Positive test: Increased laxity with lack of firm end point (suggests ACL tear)
Posterior drawer	PCL integrity	Patient is supine with hip flexed to 45 degrees and knee flexed to 90 degrees. Examiner sits on dorsum of foot and places hands on proximal calf, and then pushes posteriorly while assessing movement of tibia relative to femur.
		Positive test: Increased laxity with lack of firm end point (suggests PCL tear)
Valgus stress	MCL integrity	Patient is supine with knee flexed to 30 degrees and leg slightly abducted. Examiner places one hand on lateral knee and other hand on medial distal tibia and applies valgus force.
		Positive test: Increased laxity and pain (suggests MCL tear)
Varus stress	LCL integrity	Patient is supine with knee flexed to 30 degrees and leg slightly abducted. Examiner places one hand on medial knee and other hand on lateral distal tibia and applies varus force.
		Positive test: Increased laxity and pain (suggests LCL tear)
Thessaly	Meniscal integrity	Examiner holds patient's outstretched hands while patient stands on one leg with knee flexed to 5 degrees and with other knee flexed to 90 degrees with foot off of floor. Patient rotates body internally and externally three times. Repeat with knee flexed 20 degrees. Always perform on uninvolved knee first.
		Positive test: Medial or lateral joint line pain (suggests meniscal tear)
Medial-lateral grind	Meniscal integrity	With patient supine, examiner places calf in one hand and thumb and index finger of opposite hand over joint line and applies varus and valgus stress to tibia during extension and flexion.
		Positive test: Grinding sensation palpable over joint line (suggests meniscal injury)
Noble	Iliotibial band integrity	With patient supine, examiner repeatedly flexes and extends knee with examiner's thumb placed on lateral femoral epicondyle.
		Positive test: Reproduces patient's pain (suggests iliotibial band syndrome)

ACL = anterior cruciate ligament; LCL = lateral collateral ligament; MCL = medial collateral ligament; PCL = posterior cruciate ligament.

Ligament and Meniscal Tears

Anterior cruciate ligament injury usually occurs when a person rapidly decelerates and pivots but may also develop following direct trauma resulting in knee hyperextension. A complete tear should be suspected when a popping sound is reported and the patient reports pain and knee instability. Knee swelling that begins within 2 hours is also common. The characteristic examination finding is a large effusion with increased laxity seen on both the anterior drawer and Lachman tests. Acute posterior cruciate ligament tears result from posteriorly directed forces on the knee, such as in car accidents when the knee is flexed and strikes the dashboard or when an athlete falls on a knee that is flexed. On examination, increased laxity is seen with the posterior drawer test.

A complete medial collateral ligament tear results from a direct valgus (medially directed) force and typically presents as joint instability accompanied by medial knee pain and swelling. Examination discloses medial joint line tenderness and increased laxity and pain with valgus stress. A lateral collateral ligament tear results from a direct varus (laterally directed) force and is associated with lateral knee pain and swelling. On examination, there is lateral joint line tenderness and increased laxity and pain with varus stress.

Acute meniscal tears occur from a twisting of the knee when the foot is planted and the knee is flexed. Patients with acute meniscal tears are typically able to continue participating in the activity that resulted in the injury. Chronic degenerative meniscal tears are becoming increasingly common and occur in older adults in the absence of significant twisting. Locking and catching are common symptoms of meniscal injuries. Patients with meniscal injuries frequently have positive Thessaly and medial-lateral grind tests on examination. Initial therapy for acute meniscal tears includes rest, ice, and physical therapy to strengthen the quadriceps and hamstring muscles. Consideration for surgical intervention for acute meniscal tears is typically limited to patients who have significant mechanical symptoms that persist beyond 4 weeks. MRI is reserved for patients in whom surgery is being considered and in patients with persistent locking and catching despite appropriate initial management. First-line therapy for chronic degenerative meniscal tears is physical therapy. Surgery for chronic degenerative meniscal tears is usually limited to patients with persistent mechanical symptoms or effusions.

Patellofemoral Pain Syndrome

Patellofemoral pain syndrome is characterized by anterior knee pain that is usually gradual in onset and worsens with running, prolonged sitting, and climbing stairs. The exact cause is not clear but appears to be due to multiple factors that affect the load distribution underneath the patella including deconditioning and patellofemoral malalignment. On physical examination, patellar tracking should be assessed by medially and laterally displacing the patella. Applying direct pressure to the patella with the knee extended may reproduce the pain. Imaging studies are usually not needed.

Treatment is challenging because of the varied causes but generally includes addressing the underlying disorder, activity modification, and physical therapy. NSAIDs, acetaminophen, bracing, and patellar taping all have limited efficacy.

Bursitis

Prepatellar bursitis is caused by inflammation of the prepatellar bursa that overlies the patella. Patients present with acute anterior knee pain and swelling. Possible causes include trauma, infection, and gout. Physical examination reveals a palpable fluid collection with preserved active and passive range of motion of the knee. Aspiration is indicated for both diagnostic and therapeutic purposes. After aspiration, a compression dressing should be applied and patients should be advised to avoid kneeling.

Pes anserine bursitis is caused by inflammation of the pes anserine bursa located at the proximal anteromedial tibia. It usually develops as a result of overuse or constant friction and stress on the bursa. Pes anserine bursitis is common in athletes, particularly runners. Persons with osteoarthritis of the knee are also susceptible. Tenderness on the anteromedial aspect of the knee 5 to 8 cm below the joint line is reproduced by palpation or by having the patient take a step up. Treatment consists of anti-inflammatory medications and application of ice as well as avoidance of direct pressure, squatting, and overuse. If conservative measures are ineffective, glucocorticoid injection may be considered.

Iliotibial Band Syndrome

Iliotibial band syndrome is caused by inflammation of the distal iliotibial band as it slides over the lateral femoral epicondyle during knee movement. It can occur from overuse or from alterations in anatomic alignment or biomechanical function. It is a common cause of lateral knee pain in runners and can also occur in patients with significant leg length difference, excessively pronated foot, genu varum, or gluteal muscle weakness. Pain initially may be present only at completion of an activity but can progress to occur earlier during the activity and even at rest. Physical examination reveals tenderness to palpation approximately 2 cm proximal to the lateral knee joint line accompanied by weakness of hip abductors, knee flexors and extensors, and a positive Noble test (see Table 46). Initial treatment consists of activity modification, ice application, and NSAIDs to reduce inflammation. Once inflammation subsides, stretching and then strengthening exercises are indicated.

Popliteal Cyst

Popliteal (Baker) cysts in adults are synovial fluid–containing extensions of the knee joint space and generally occur as the result of osteoarthritis or trauma of the knee. The cyst is usually asymptomatic but may become painful as it enlarges. Swelling is seen in the popliteal fossa on physical examination. The knee should be examined for signs of meniscal pathology, effusion, or mechanical signs that indicate an intra-articular irritant causing excessive joint fluid. Treatment is usually directed at the underlying cause of the increased synovial fluid (such as repair of a torn meniscus or knee replacement). The cyst is often not diagnosed until it ruptures, which may result in significant pain and swelling of the calf, mimicking thrombophlebitis.

Ankle and Foot Pain

Ankle Sprains

Most ankle sprains result from inversion injuries that damage the lateral ankle ligaments. Characteristic findings include pain, swelling, and decreased proprioception. Physical examination reveals swelling, ecchymosis, and lateral ankle tenderness. Immediate inability to bear weight may indicate a more serious injury.

High ankle sprains result from excessive dorsiflexion or eversion that causes injury to the tibiofibular syndesmotic ligaments connecting the distal tibia and fibula. Pain can be elicited by compressing the leg at midcalf (squeeze test) or by having the patient cross the legs with the midcalf of the injured leg resting on the other knee (crossed-leg test).

The Ottawa ankle and foot rules (**Figure 16**) are useful in excluding ankle fractures, with an extremely high sensitivity (>95%). According to these validated rules, radiographs should be obtained when a patient is unable to walk four steps both immediately after the injury and during evaluation and when focal tenderness is present at the posterior aspect of either malleolus, the navicular bone, or the fifth metatarsal base. If these criteria are not met, obtaining radiographs is not necessary, as the probability of an ankle fracture is exceedingly low.

Initial therapy includes Rest, Ice, Compression, and Elevation (RICE). NSAIDs are useful for pain control. Early mobilization appears to be superior to prolonged rest. Once pain and swelling subside, proprioception training along with range-of-motion and strengthening exercises should be initiated to prevent chronic instability and predisposition to reinjury. Surgery is indicated only for patients with complete tears and those with chronic instability in whom conservative interventions are ineffective.

KEY POINT

HVC
- The Ottawa ankle and foot rules are useful in excluding ankle fractures, with an extremely high sensitivity (>95%); if these rules are not met, obtaining radiographs is not necessary, as the probability of an ankle fracture is exceedingly low.

Hindfoot Pain

Achilles tendinopathy commonly occurs in persons who begin exercising or increase exercise too rapidly. The usual presentation is of posterior heel pain, stiffness, and tenderness approximately 2 to 6 cm proximal to the Achilles tendon insertion. Pain is generally burning, worsens with activity, and improves with rest. Treatment consists of rest, activity modification, and application of ice. NSAIDs can be used for pain control.

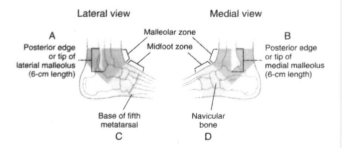

FIGURE 16. Ottawa ankle and foot rules. An ankle radiographic series is indicated if a patient has pain in the malleolar zone and any of the following findings: bone tenderness at *A*, bone tenderness at *B*, or inability to bear weight immediately and in the emergency department (or physician's office). A foot radiographic series is indicated if a patient has pain in the midfoot zone and any of the following findings: bone tenderness at *C*, bone tenderness at *D*, or inability to bear weight immediately and in the emergency department (or physician's office).

Achilles tendon rupture should be suspected when a person participating in a strenuous activity such as basketball hears a popping sound in the heel. Rarely, fluoroquinolone antibiotics are associated with Achilles tendinopathy or rupture. Sudden posterior heel pain is common but not always present. Plantar flexion may be preserved. Patients usually have a positive Thompson test (sensitivity, 96%; specificity 93%) (**Figure 17**). A palpable tendon defect may be present. Treatment is controversial. Patients treated with either surgery or immobilization of the ankle in plantar flexion accompanied by an early range-of-motion protocol appear to have a similar risk of rerupture, although surgery is associated with a high risk of complications, including infection.

Plantar fasciitis is characterized by pain and tenderness near the medial plantar heel surface. Pain typically occurs upon awakening and after prolonged rest. Risk factors include obesity, improper footwear, overpronation, pes cavus, pes planus, and leg-length discrepancies. Management should be individualized to address specific historical and examination findings and reevaluated at regular intervals. Initial treatment is multimodal and consists of patient education, activity modification, application of ice, correcting improper mechanics (for example, using arch supports for pes planus), and heel stretches. Acetaminophen or NSAIDs can be used to control pain, although neither is thought to alter the underlying pathologic process. For patients who fail to respond to the aforementioned therapies, ultrasound therapy and glucocorticoid injections may be beneficial, although some experts do not recommend glucocorticoid injections because of the risk of fat atrophy in the heel pad. Plantar fascia release is reserved for patients in whom other therapies are ineffective.

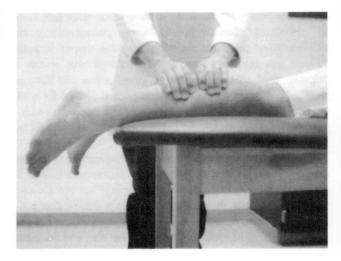

FIGURE 17. Thompson test. The patient is positioned in the prone position. The examiner squeezes mid-calf and observes for plantar flexion of the foot. When the patient has an intact Achilles tendon, plantar flexion will occur. When there is a complete Achilles tendon rupture, no plantar flexion is observed.

- Achilles tendon rupture should be suspected when a person participating in a strenuous activity such as basketball hears a popping sound in the heel.

- Plantar fasciitis is characterized by pain and tenderness near the medial plantar heel surface; the pain typically occurs upon awakening and after prolonged rest.

- Initial treatment of plantar faciitis is multimodal and consists of patient education, activity modification, application of ice, correcting improper mechanics, and heel stretches.

Midfoot Pain

Tarsal tunnel syndrome is usually caused by posterior tibial nerve compression within the tarsal tunnel below the medial malleolus. It most commonly arises in the setting of a calcaneous, medial malleolus, or talus fracture, but it can also be associated with rheumatoid arthritis, diabetes mellitus, thyroid disorders, pregnancy, and wearing tight-fitting shoes. Patients commonly present with pain and paresthesias in the medial ankle extending into the foot that worsen with standing, walking, and running. Pain can be reproduced by tapping on the posterior tibial nerve along its course. Treatment includes activity modification, orthotics, anti-inflammatory agents, and occasionally glucocorticoid injections. Surgical decompression is reserved for patients who do not benefit from conservative measures.

Forefoot Pain

Hallux valgus deformity (bunion) is characterized by lateral great toe deviation with bony deformity on the medial aspect of the first metatarsal phalangeal joint. Osteoarthritis can develop in this joint, and bursitis can occur overlying the bony deformity. Treatment includes NSAIDs, orthotic devices, and possibly surgery.

Morton neuroma refers to common digital nerve entrapment that usually occurs between the third and fourth toes. Patients describe a "walking on a pebble" sensation and burning pain with weight bearing that radiates distally into the toes. Treatment consists of using metatarsal padding, wearing broad-toed footwear, and avoiding high-heeled shoes. For patients who fail to respond to these conservative measures, a single combination lidocaine and glucocorticoid injection often provides significant pain relief. Surgical intervention is reserved for patients who fail to respond to at least 12 months of conservative therapy.

Dyslipidemia
Evaluation of Lipid Levels

Screening for lipid disorders is discussed in Routine Care of the Healthy Patient.

In a marked change from previous guidelines, the 2013 American College of Cardiology/American Heart Association (ACC/AHA) cholesterol treatment guideline does not focus on LDL cholesterol treatment targets, but rather on a person's overall risk of developing atherosclerotic cardiovascular disease (ASCVD). Furthermore, although non-HDL cholesterol (total cholesterol minus HDL cholesterol) represents the sum of all potentially atherogenic cholesterol, non-HDL cholesterol treatment targets are no longer included in the current ACC/AHA management guidelines. Therefore, the primary utility of measuring specific lipid levels is for ASCVD risk assessment.

LDL Cholesterol

LDL cholesterol is the most atherogenic of the lipoproteins. Elevated LDL cholesterol is strongly associated with increased risk of cardiovascular disease. Although statin therapy lowers LDL cholesterol levels and reduces the risk of cardiovascular events, no randomized trials have demonstrated the value of treating to specific LDL cholesterol goals, which is the basis for the change in guideline recommendations. The utility of LDL cholesterol measurement is therefore limited to determining the need for treatment and monitoring the response to therapy. Patients with an LDL cholesterol level of 190 mg/dL (4.92 mmol/L) or higher should be evaluated for familial hypercholesterolemia and secondary causes of hyperlipidemia, including hypothyroidism, diabetes mellitus, and glucocorticoid use.

Triglycerides

Prevailing literature suggests that elevated triglyceride levels more likely represent a marker of metabolic syndrome and cardiovascular disease than a cause. Therefore, they are not measured routinely as part of assessing risk for ASCVD. However, severe fasting hypertriglyceridemia (≥500 mg/dL [5.65 mmol/L]), which is associated with familial combined hyperlipidemia, excessive alcohol use, hypothyroidism, exogenous estrogens, chronic kidney disease, and use of protease inhibitors, can trigger pancreatitis with postprandial triglyceride level increases (to >1000 mg/dL [11.30 mmol/L]). Measurement of triglyceride levels is indicated in these clinical situations as well as before initiation of drug therapy.

HDL Cholesterol

HDL cholesterol levels have a strong inverse correlation with cardiovascular risk. However, the pathophysiologic link between low HDL cholesterol and ASCVD is uncertain, especially as studies have yet to clearly demonstrate a reduction in cardiovascular risk with HDL cholesterol–raising medications. Subsequently, the ACC/AHA cholesterol treatment guideline provides no recommendation for treatment of low HDL cholesterol levels. However, HDL cholesterol level is a factor used in 10-year ASCVD risk estimation.

Nonstandard Lipid Risk Factors

Currently, there is insufficient evidence to support the routine measurement of lipoprotein(a), apolipoprotein B, and LDL particles in the evaluation or management of dyslipidemia. Several other biomarkers and cardiovascular tests have been shown to correlate with increased cardiovascular risk (**Table 47**). The ACC/AHA guideline does not include them as primary factors to be considered in treatment decisions, although these risk factors may be used to guide the decision to initiate statin

therapy in patients who do not clearly meet treatment criteria. Carotid artery intima-media thickness measurement is not recommended for ASCVD risk assessment in primary prevention.

KEY POINTS

- The 2013 American College of Cardiology/American Heart Association cholesterol treatment guideline does not focus on LDL cholesterol treatment targets, but rather on a person's overall risk of developing atherosclerotic cardiovascular disease.

- Patients with an LDL cholesterol level of 190 mg/dL (4.92 mmol/L) or higher should be evaluated for familial hypercholesterolemia and secondary causes of hyperlipidemia, including hypothyroidism, diabetes mellitus, and glucocorticoid use.

- There is insufficient evidence to support the routine measurement of lipoprotein(a), apolipoprotein B, and LDL particles in the evaluation or management of dyslipidemia.

TABLE 47. Additional Risk Factors for Atherosclerotic Cardiovascular Disease

African-American ancestry

Family history of premature cardiovascular disease (onset before age 55 y in first-degree male relative or before age 65 y in first-degree female relative)

Elevated lifetime risk (>50% for men, >40% for women) of cardiovascular disease (as determined from the ASCVD Risk Estimator based on the Pooled Cohort Equations [available at http://tools.cardiosource.org/ASCVD-Risk-Estimator/])

LDL cholesterol ≥160 mg/dL (4.14 mmol/L)

High-sensitivity C-reactive protein ≥2 mg/L

Coronary artery calcium score ≥300 or ≥75th percentile for age

Ankle-brachial index <0.90

ASCVD = atherosclerotic cardiovascular disease.

Data from Stone NJ, Robinson JG, Lichtenstein AH, et al; American College of Cardiology/American Heart Association Task Force on Practice Guidelines. 2013 ACC/AHA guideline on the treatment of blood cholesterol to reduce atherosclerotic cardiovascular risk in adults: a report of the American College of Cardiology/American Heart Association Task Force on Practice Guidelines. J Am Coll Cardiol. 2014 Jul 1;63 (25 Pt B):2889-934. Erratum in: J Am Coll Cardiol. 2014 Jul 1;63(25 Pt B):3024-3025. [PMID: 24239923]

Management of Dyslipidemias

Therapeutic Lifestyle Changes

The AHA and ACC advise counseling all adult patients on healthy lifestyle modifications prior to, and in addition to, pharmacologic therapy for dyslipidemia. Habits that should be encouraged include avoiding tobacco, maintaining a healthy weight, and regularly engaging in physical exercise.

A heart-healthy diet emphasizing the intake of vegetables, fruits, whole grains, and low-fat dairy products, while limiting the intake of red meats and simple carbohydrates, reduces LDL cholesterol levels. The DASH (Dietary Approaches to Stop Hypertension) eating plan (**Table 48**) has been shown to lower

TABLE 48. Dietary Approaches to Stop Hypertension (DASH) Eating Plan

Food	Number of Servings[a]	Serving Examples
Fats and simple carbohydrates	Limited	Sugar (1 tbsp)
Lean meats (including fish and poultry)	2 or fewer	Fish or poultry (3 oz)
Legumes, nuts, seeds	4-5 per week	Nuts (1/3 cup), seeds (2 tbsp), peanut butter (2 tbsp), beans (1/2 cup)
Low-fat or non-fat dairy products	2-3	Skim milk (1 cup), yogurt (1 cup), low-fat cheese (1 oz)
Fruits	4-5	Fresh fruit (size of a baseball), fruit juice (1/2 cup), dried fruit (1/4 cup)
Vegetables	4-5	Raw lettuce or spinach (1 cup), cooked carrots or broccoli (1/2 cup), vegetable juice (1/2 cup)
Grains	7-8 (at least 3 whole-grain foods due to higher fiber and nutrient content)	Bread (1 slice); cooked rice, cereal, or pasta (1/2 cup); dry cereal (1 oz)

oz = ounce; tbsp = tablespoon.

[a]For a daily 2000-calorie diet.

Adapted from National Heart, Lung, and Blood Institute. Following the DASH eating plan. www.nhlbi.nih.gov/health/health-topics/topics/dash/followdash. Updated June 6, 2014. Accessed June 24, 2015.

LDL cholesterol levels more than 10 mg/dL (0.26 mmol/L) while also lowering HDL cholesterol levels 4 mg/dL (0.10 mmol/L). Adjusting the DASH eating plan to replace 10% of calories from carbohydrates with 10% of calories from protein provides a small additional reduction in LDL cholesterol levels, HDL cholesterol levels, and triglyceride levels (reduction of 16 mg/dL [0.18 mmol/L]); replacing 10% of calories from carbohydrates with 10% of calories from unsaturated fat slightly increases HDL cholesterol levels and lowers LDL cholesterol and triglycerides levels. Reducing the intake of saturated fatty acids to 5% to 6% of calories and reducing the intake of *trans* fatty acids also provides slight improvements in lipid profiles. Limitation of dietary cholesterol has no clear impact on dyslipidemia.

The ACC/AHA guideline on lifestyle management to reduce cardiovascular risk recommends that adults engage in aerobic physical activity (3-4 sessions per week, with an average of 40 minutes per session, and involving moderate- to vigorous-intensity physical activity) to lower LDL cholesterol levels, non-HDL cholesterol levels, and blood pressure. Aerobic exercise reduces LDL cholesterol levels by 3 to 6 mg/dL (0.08-0.16 mmol/L) and non-HDL cholesterol levels by 6 mg/dL (0.16 mmol/L). Data on the impact of exercise on triglyceride or HDL cholesterol levels have been more inconsistent.

Drug Therapy

Strong evidence indicates that statins are effective in both primary and secondary prevention of ASCVD. The ACC/AHA cholesterol treatment guideline identifies four patient groups for which there is evidence that treatment of hyperlipidemia with statin therapy is beneficial: (1) established clinical ASCVD, (2) LDL cholesterol level of 190 mg/dL (4.92 mmol/L) or higher, (3) diabetes and age 40 to 75 years with an LDL cholesterol level of 70 to 189 mg/dL (1.81-4.90 mmol/L) and no ASCVD, and (4) no ASCVD or diabetes and estimated 10-year ASCVD risk greater than or equal to 7.5% as estimated by the Pooled Cohort Equations. When statin therapy is indicated, either high- or moderate-intensity therapy is utilized based upon the clinical scenario (**Figure 18**).

In patients with clinical ASCVD (coronary artery disease, peripheral arterial disease, cerebrovascular disease), the decision to give high- or moderate- intensity statin dosing is based upon the patient's age and tolerance to the statin dose. High-intensity therapy, defined as statin doses with expected LDL cholesterol reduction of 50% or more, is recommended for all patients aged 75 years and younger who can tolerate it. Atorvastatin and rosuvastatin are the only high-intensity statins recommended by the ACC/AHA cholesterol treatment guideline. Simvastatin, 80 mg/d, has been studied in trials, but this dosage is not recommended by the FDA because of an increased risk of rhabdomyolysis. Moderate-intensity therapy is recommended for patients with risk factors for statin-related adverse effects, including age older than 75 years, impaired kidney or liver function, muscle disorders, and use of drugs affecting statin metabolism (calcium channel blockers, fibrates, protease inhibitors, amiodarone, macrolide antibiotics). Moderate-intensity statin treatment provides an expected reduction in LDL cholesterol of 30% to 49% (**Table 49**).

Patients over the age of 20 years with an LDL cholesterol level of 190 mg/dL (4.92 mmol/L) or higher should receive a high-intensity statin unless they have risk factors for statin-associated side effects.

For patients 40 to 75 years of age with diabetes and an LDL cholesterol level of 70 to 189 mg/dL (1.81-4.90 mmol/L), intensity of statin therapy is dictated by the estimated 10-year risk for ASCVD. High-intensity statin therapy should be used in these patients with a 10-year ASCVD risk of 7.5% or higher, whereas moderate-intensity therapy should be used if the risk is below 7.5%.

Patients with no history of ASCVD or diabetes and an LDL cholesterol level of 70 to 189 mg/dL (1.81-4.90 mmol/L) are candidates for either high- or moderate-intensity statin therapy if their 10-year ASCVD risk is greater than or equal to 7.5%. Thorough discussion of the benefits and risks of statin therapy of either potency is necessary before starting treatment. In select patients who do not qualify for one of the indication groups, statin therapy may be considered based on additional factors (see Table 47).

Clinical judgment and patient preference must be taken into account when selecting a statin dose. Furthermore, adjustment of statin therapy after failure to achieve the expected LDL cholesterol reduction requires individualized decision-making. Alteration of a well-tolerated statin regimen that was started before the release of the updated guideline is not necessarily indicated.

Before initiating statin treatment, a fasting lipid panel and alanine aminotransferase (ALT) level should be obtained. Baseline creatine kinase (CK) measurement is not routinely indicated before starting statin therapy. During statin treatment, monitoring of ALT and CK is only required if a patient develops symptoms of liver or muscle disease. To determine medication adherence and response to therapy, repeat lipid panels should be obtained 1 to 3 months after initiation of statin treatment and then every 3 to 12 months as clinically indicated.

Statins may cause myopathy and liver aminotransferase elevations and are associated with an increased risk of diabetes and, possibly, cognitive dysfunction. The incidence of these adverse effects ranges from 1% to 10%, but permanent disability related to statin intolerance is rare. For patients with signs or symptoms of statin intolerance, the benefits and risks of continued statin therapy should be discussed with the patient. Often, switching to a different statin or decreasing the dosage eliminates side effects. In those patients unable or unwilling to take statins, alternative cholesterol-lowering therapy should be considered.

Combination and Nonstatin Drug Therapy

Nonstatin drugs, such as ezetimibe, fibrates, niacin, bile acid sequestrants, and omega-3 fatty acids, favorably affect lipid profiles, and some reduce cardiovascular events compared with placebo. However, there are minimal data supporting the

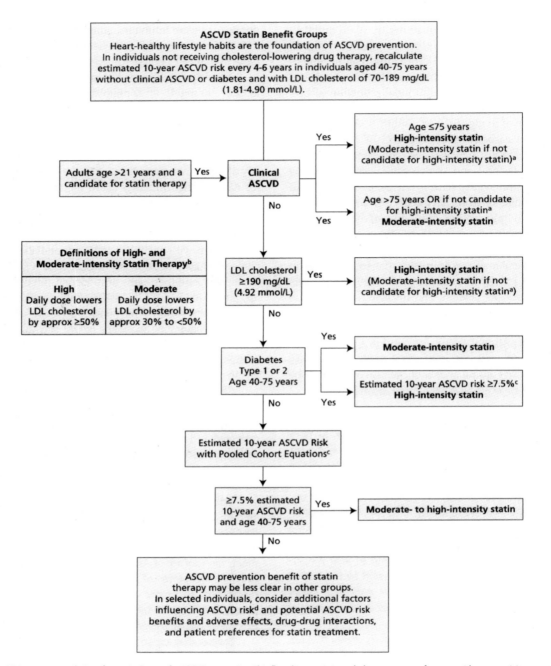

FIGURE 18. Major recommendations for statin therapy for ASCVD prevention. This flow diagram is intended to serve as a reference guide summarizing recommendations for ASCVD risk assessment and treatment. Assessment of the potential for benefit and risk from statin therapy for ASCVD prevention provides the framework for clinical decision-making incorporating patient preferences.

ASCVD = atherosclerotic cardiovascular disease.

[a]Moderate-intensity statin therapy should be used in individuals in whom high-intensity statin therapy would otherwise be recommended when high-intensity statin therapy is contraindicated or when characteristics predisposing them to statin-associated adverse effects are present.

Characteristics predisposing individuals to statin adverse effects include, but are not limited to:

• Multiple or serious comorbidities, including impaired kidney or liver function
• History of previous statin intolerance or muscle disorders
• Unexplained alanine aminotransferase elevations >3 times upper limit of normal
• Patient characteristics or concomitant use of drugs affecting statin metabolism
• >75 years of age

Additional characteristics that may modify the decision to use higher statin intensities may include, but are not limited to:

• History of hemorrhagic stroke
• Asian ancestry

[b]Percent reduction in LDL cholesterol can be used as an indication of response and adherence to therapy but is not in itself a treatment goal.

[c]The Pooled Cohort Equations can be used to estimate 10-year ASCVD risk in individuals with and without diabetes. A downloadable spreadsheet enabling estimation of 10-year and lifetime risk for ASCVD and a web-based calculator are available at http://my.americanheart.org/cvriskcalculator and www.cardiosource.org/science-and-quality/practice-guidelines-and-quality-standards/2013-prevention-guideline-toold.aspx.

[d]Primary LDL cholesterol level ≥160 mg/dL (4.14 mmol/L) or other evidence of genetic hyperlipidemias; family history of premature ASCVD with onset <55 years of age in a first-degree male relative or <65 years of age in a first-degree female relative; high sensitivity C-reactive protein ≥2 mg/L; coronary artery calcium score ≥300 or ≥75th percentile for age, sex, and ethnicity; ankle-brachial index <0.90; or elevated lifetime risk of ASCVD.

Reprinted with permission from Stone NJ, Robinson JG, Lichtenstein AH, et al; American College of Cardiology/American Heart Association Task Force on Practice Guidelines. 2013 ACC/AHA guideline on the treatment of blood cholesterol to reduce atherosclerotic cardiovascular risk in adults: a report of the American College of Cardiology/American Heart Association Task Force on Practice Guidelines. Circulation. 2013; Epub 2013 Nov 12. Copyright 2013, American Heart Association, Inc.

TABLE 49. High- and Moderate-Intensity Statin Therapy

High-Intensity (≥50% LDL Cholesterol Reduction with Daily Dose)	Moderate-Intensity (30% to <50% LDL Cholesterol Reduction with Daily Dose)
Atorvastatin 40-80 mg	Atorvastatin 10-20 mg
	Rosuvastatin 5-10 mg
	Simvastatin 20-40 mg
Rosuvastatin 20-40 mg	Pravastatin 40-80 mg
	Lovastatin 40 mg
	Fluvastatin 40 mg twice daily

Adapted with permission from Stone NJ, Robinson JG, Lichtenstein AH, et al; American College of Cardiology/American Heart Association Task Force on Practice Guidelines. 2013 ACC/AHA guideline on the treatment of blood cholesterol to reduce atherosclerotic cardiovascular risk in adults: a report of the American College of Cardiology/American Heart Association Task Force on Practice Guidelines. J Am Coll Cardiol. 2014 Jul 1;63(25 Pt B):2889-934. Erratum in: J Am Coll Cardiol. 2014 Jul 1;63(25 Pt B):3024-3025. [PMID: 24239923] Copyright 2014, Elsevier.

use of nonstatin drugs combined with statin therapy to further reduce ASCVD events. Nonstatin drugs are also associated with many significant side effects (**Table 50**). Therefore, the ACC/AHA cholesterol treatment guideline recommends consideration of these drugs only in high-risk patients (those with known ASCVD, diabetes, or LDL cholesterol level ≥190 mg/dL [4.92 mmol/L]) who fail to respond as expected to the recommended intensity of a statin or have poor tolerance to statins.

Management of Hypertriglyceridemia

Patients with elevated triglyceride levels should be counseled on weight loss (if appropriate), regular aerobic exercise, abstinence from alcoholic beverages, avoidance of *trans* fatty acids, and limitation of saturated fats and added sugars. Polyunsaturated omega-3 fatty acids should be included in the diet due to their favorable impact on triglyceride levels.

In patients with a fasting triglyceride level of 500 mg/dL (5.65 mmol/L) or higher, triglyceride-lowering drug therapy (alone or in combination with therapy to reduce LDL cholesterol if a concurrent indication for treatment exists) is useful to prevent pancreatitis. Fibrates are the most potent triglyceride-lowering agents, causing an average reduction in triglyceride levels of 30% to 50%. Niacin, statins, and omega-3 fatty acid supplements also provide significant reduction in triglyceride levels (see Table 50).

KEY POINTS

- Strong evidence indicates that statins are effective in both primary and secondary prevention of atherosclerotic cardiovascular disease.

- In patients with clinical atherosclerotic cardiovascular disease, high-intensity therapy (statin doses with expected LDL cholesterol reduction of 50% or more) is recommended for all patients aged 75 years and younger who can tolerate it.

- In patients with clinical atherosclerotic cardiovascular disease who have risk factors for statin-related adverse effects, including age older than 75 years, impaired kidney or liver function, muscle disorders, and use of drugs affecting statin metabolism, moderate-intensity statin treatment should be used.

- Patients over the age of 20 years with an LDL cholesterol level of 190 mg/dL (4.92 mmol/L) or higher should receive a high-intensity statin unless they have risk factors for statin-associated adverse effects.

- For patients 40 to 75 years of age with diabetes mellitus and an LDL cholesterol level of 70 to 189 mg/dL (1.81-4.90 mmol/L), intensity of statin therapy is dictated by the estimated 10-year risk for atherosclerotic cardiovascular disease (ASCVD); patients with a 10-year ASCVD risk of 7.5% or higher should receive high-intensity statin therapy, and patients with a 10-year ASCVD risk below 7.5% should receive moderate-intensity therapy.

(Continued)

TABLE 50. Characteristics of Nonstatin Drugs

Medication	Effects on Lipids			Adverse Effects
	LDL Cholesterol	HDL Cholesterol	Triglycerides	
Ezetimibe	↓↓	—	—	Abdominal pain, fatigue, myositis, elevated liver aminotransferases (especially when combined with statins)
Bile acid sequestrants	↓↓	—	↑[a]	Constipation, nausea, bloating, elevated liver aminotransferases, interference with medication/vitamin absorption
Fibrates	↓	↑	↓↓↓	Nausea, abdominal pain, myositis (particularly when combined with statins)
Niacin	↓	↑↑	↓↓	Flushing, nausea, diarrhea, gout, hyperglycemia, myositis
Omega-3 fatty acids	—	↑	↓↓↓	Bloating, fishy taste

[a]Bile acid sequestrants increase triglyceride levels only if baseline triglycerides are elevated.

- Patients with no history of atherosclerotic cardiovascular disease (ASCVD) or diabetes mellitus and an LDL cholesterol level of 70 to 189 mg/dL (1.81-4.90 mmol/L) are candidates for either high- or moderate-intensity statin therapy if their 10-year ASCVD risk is greater than or equal to 7.5%.

HVC
- Baseline creatine kinase measurement is not routinely indicated before starting statin therapy or for monitoring therapy in the absence of symptoms of muscle disease.

Dyslipidemia Management in Unique Populations

Evidence suggests that it is safe to continue statin therapy in a patient older than 75 years if the patient is already taking and tolerating statin drugs. Moderate-intensity statin therapy is effective for the secondary prevention of ASCVD in this population. The use of statins for primary prevention or at high intensity in patients older than 75 years is not well supported.

Due to a paucity of evidence, the ACC/AHA guidelines provide no recommendations for statin therapy in patients who require hemodialysis or patients with New York Heart Association functional class II to IV heart failure.

Metabolic Syndrome
Epidemiology and Pathophysiology

The concurrence of type 2 diabetes and multiple cardiovascular disease risk factors, including abdominal obesity, dyslipidemia, hypertension, and hyperglycemia, is known as the metabolic syndrome. Diagnosis of metabolic syndrome is made by the presence of three of the five diagnostic criteria used by the International Diabetes Federation and the AHA (Table 51).

Metabolic syndrome may be present in over 25% of the world population, with even higher rates in Mexican Americans and black women. Metabolic syndrome is associated with a 5- to 10-fold increase in the risk of developing diabetes and a 1.5- to 2-fold increase in ASCVD risk.

There is still much debate on whether the metabolic syndrome is a truly unique entity with its own pathophysiologic basis. The insulin resistance, hyperinsulinemia, and increased adipocyte cytokines seen in this condition induce vascular endothelial changes that promote atherosclerosis. Additionally, metabolic syndrome is associated with several other pathologic changes, including hepatic steatosis, kidney impairment, sleep apnea, and polycystic ovary syndrome.

Management

The AHA recommends weight loss with a goal BMI of less than 25, exercise for at least 30 minutes per day five times weekly, and a heart-healthy diet (as described previously).

TABLE 51. Criteria for Clinical Diagnosis of the Metabolic Syndrome

Measure	Categorical Cut Points
Elevated waist circumference[a]	Population- and country-specific definitions
Elevated triglycerides (drug treatment for elevated triglycerides is an alternate indicator)[b]	≥150 mg/dL (1.7 mmol/L)
Reduced HDL cholesterol level (drug treatment for reduced HDL cholesterol is an alternate indicator)[b]	<40 mg/dL (1.0 mmol/L) in men; <50 mg/dL (1.30 mmol/L) in women
Elevated blood pressure (antihypertensive drug treatment in a patient with a history of hypertension is an alternate indicator)	Systolic ≥130 and/or diastolic ≥85 mm Hg
Elevated fasting glucose[c] (drug treatment of elevated glucose level is an alternate indicator)	≥100 mg/dL (5.6 mmol/L)

[a]It is recommended that the International Diabetes Federation (IDF) cut points (waist circumference ≥94 cm [37 in] in men or ≥80 cm [31.5 in] in women) be used for non-Europeans and either the IDF or American Heart Association/National Heart, Lung, and Blood Institute cut points (waist circumference ≥102 cm [40.2 in] in men or ≥88 cm [34.6 in] in women) be used for people of European origin until more data are available.

[b]The most commonly used drugs for elevated triglycerides and reduced HDL cholesterol are fibrates and nicotinic acid. A patient taking one of these drugs can be presumed to have high triglycerides and low HDL cholesterol. High-dose omega-3 fatty acids presumes high triglycerides.

[c]Most patients with type 2 diabetes mellitus will have the metabolic syndrome by the proposed criteria.

Reprinted with permission from Alberti KG, Eckel RH, Grundy SM, et al. Harmonizing the metabolic syndrome: a joint interim statement of the International Diabetes Federation Task Force on Epidemiology and Prevention; National Heart, Lung, and Blood Institute; American Heart Association; World Heart Federation; International Atherosclerosis Society; and International Association for the Study of Obesity. Circulation. 2009 Oct 20; 120(16):1640-5. [PMID: 19805654] Copyright 2013, American Heart Association, Inc.

Patients with hypertension should be treated aggressively to achieve the blood pressure goals outlined in the report from the panel members appointed to the Eighth Joint National Committee (see MKSAP 17 Nephrology). Similarly, dyslipidemia should be treated as detailed previously, and hyperglycemia should be managed per guidelines from the American Diabetes Association. In some studies, metformin has been shown to reduce the risk of developing metabolic syndrome; however, therapeutic lifestyle interventions are as effective or superior to metformin.

The AHA recommends low-dose aspirin for patients with metabolic syndrome and a 10-year cardiovascular risk of 10% or higher.

- The American Heart Association recommends low-dose aspirin for patients with metabolic syndrome and a 10-year cardiovascular risk of 10% or higher.

Obesity

Definition and Epidemiology

Obesity is currently defined as a BMI greater than or equal to 30, whereas overweight is defined as a BMI between 25 and 29.9 (**Table 52**). Online BMI calculators are widely available (https://www.nhlbi.nih.gov/guidelines/obesity/BMI/bmicalc.htm).

The prevalence of obesity has increased dramatically in recent decades. Currently, one third of U.S. adults are obese. Obesity is a leading cause of preventable death and is associated with increased risk for dyslipidemia, type 2 diabetes mellitus, hypertension, cardiovascular disease (CVD), stroke, cancer (breast, colon, and endometrial), osteoarthritis, obstructive sleep apnea, and other diseases. These risks increase with rising BMI. Obesity is also associated with reduced quality of life, impaired physical functioning, and increased health care costs.

Screening and Evaluation

Although current guidelines and recommendations urge physicians to identify and counsel overweight or obese patients, obesity is often not diagnosed or addressed as a medical issue in affected adults. Patients who report being told they are obese by physicians are more likely to have realistic self-perceptions of weight, greater desire to lose weight, and to have made attempts to lose weight.

The U.S. Preventive Services Task Force (USPSTF) recommends screening all adults for obesity by calculating BMI but concludes that there is no evidence regarding an appropriate interval for obesity screening. The American Heart Association (AHA), American College of Cardiology (ACC), and The Obesity Society (TOS) recommend screening for overweight and obesity annually (or more frequently depending on the patient) by calculating BMI and measuring waist circumference at the level of the iliac crest. Central adiposity (waist circumference >102 cm [40 in] in men and >88 cm [35 in] in women) is associated with increased cardiovascular risk independent of BMI.

TABLE 52. Classification of Overweight and Obesity by BMI

Category	BMI	Obesity Class
Underweight	<18.5	
Normal	18.5-24.9	
Overweight	25.0-29.9	
Obesity	30.0-34.0	I
	35.0-39.9	II
Extreme obesity	≥40	III

Reprinted from National Heart, Lung, and Blood Institute. Aim for a Healthy Weight. www.nhlbi.nih.gov/health/educational/lose_wt/BMI/bmi_dis.htm. Accessed June 24, 2015.

In evaluating the obese patient, the chronology of weight gain, prior weight loss attempts, eating and exercise patterns, family history of obesity, and use of medications that promote weight gain (**Table 53**) should be elicited. A history of risk factors for and symptoms of obesity-associated comorbidities, including insulin resistance and type 2 diabetes, dyslipidemia, hypertension, CVD, stroke, sleep apnea, gallstones, hyperuricemia and gout, and osteoarthritis, should also be obtained. During the history, obese patients should be asked about their perceptions of healthy weight and their own weight.

Evaluation should include a thorough physical examination. Additionally, the AHA/ACC/TOS Guideline for the Management of Overweight and Obesity in Adults recommends obtaining a fasting glucose level and fasting lipid profile in obese patients. Further testing should be guided by the history and physical examination.

KEY POINT

- The U.S. Preventive Services Task Force recommends screening all adults for obesity by calculating BMI.

Treatment

Treatment of overweight and obese patients should begin with establishing a weight loss goal and individualized treatment plan. A reasonable goal is weight loss of 0.5 kg to 1.0 kg (1.1-2.2 lb) per week to achieve a total weight loss of 10%. The mainstay of obesity treatment is lifestyle modification that includes diet for weight loss, increased physical activity, and behavioral therapy. A strategy that combines all three elements is likely to be more successful than any one element alone. Involving dieticians, exercise therapists, and behavioral therapists in the process increases the chances of success. Some patients may also be candidates for pharmacologic treatments and bariatric surgery. The overall management of the obese patient is presented in **Figure 19**.

TABLE 53. Medications That Promote Weight Gain

Drug Category	Example Medications
α-Blockers	Clonidine, prazosin, terazosin
Antidiabetic drugs	Insulin, sulfonylureas (especially glyburide and glipizide), thiazolidinediones
Anticonvulsant drugs	Carbamazepine, gabapentin, valproic acid
Antidepressant drugs	Amitriptyline, imipramine, doxepin, paroxetine, mirtazapine
Antihistamines	Cyproheptadine
Atypical antipsychotic drugs	Clozapine, olanzapine, quetiapine, risperidone
β-blockers	Atenolol, metoprolol, propranolol
Glucocorticoids	Prednisone
Hormonal contraceptives	Progestins (especially depot injections)

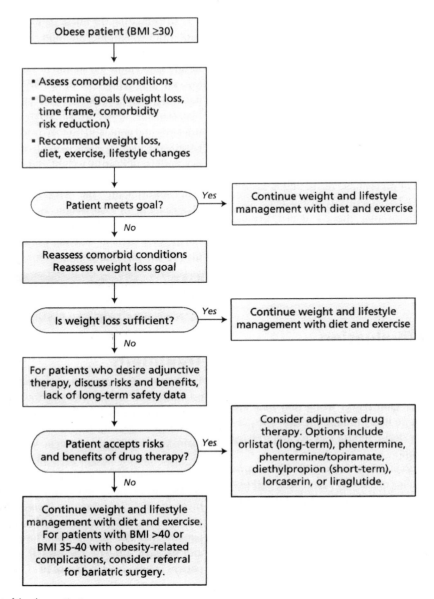

FIGURE 19. Management of the obese patient.

Adapted with permission from Snow V, Barry P, Fitterman N, Qaseem A, Weiss K; Clinical Efficacy Assessment Subcommittee of the American College of Physicians. Pharmacologic and surgical management of obesity in primary care: a clinical practice guideline from the American College of Physicians. Ann Intern Med. 2005;142(7):526. [PMID: 15809464] Copyright 2005, American College of Physicians.

Lifestyle Modification

According to the USPSTF and the AHA/ACC/TOS obesity guideline, all obese patients should be offered a comprehensive lifestyle intervention (comprised of diet, physical activity, and behavioral treatments) for weight loss. Additionally, the USPSTF recommends offering overweight or obese adults who have cardiovascular risk factors intensive behavioral counseling interventions to promote a healthful diet and physical activity for CVD prevention. In overweight and obese adults with cardiovascular risk factors such as hypertension, hyperglycemia, and hyperlipidemia, lifestyle changes that result in modest and sustained weight loss (3% to 5%) produce clinically meaningful health benefits (reduced triglycerides, blood glucose, hemoglobin A_{1c}, and risk for type 2 diabetes). Greater weight loss results in greater benefits (reduced blood pressure and improved LDL and HDL cholesterol levels).

Reduced Dietary Energy Intake

Maintaining a continuous negative energy balance (that is, energy intake less than expenditure) of 500 kcal/d results in a weight loss of about 0.5 kg (1.1 lb) per week. Calorie restriction can be further guided by estimating a patient's basal energy requirement using the Harris-Benedict equation; calculators are available online (http://www-users.med.cornell.edu/~spon/picu/calc/beecalc.htm). Based on the result, a specific daily calorie limit should be prescribed (typically, 1500-1800 kcal/d for men and 1200-1500 kcal/d for women).

All diets, when effective, maintain negative energy balance. There are numerous diet options available, including very-low-fat diets, high-protein and low-carbohydrate diets, pattern diets (for example, the Mediterranean diet), and meal replacement diets. After diet implementation, the average total weight loss in obese adults is maximal at 6 months (typical range, 4-12 kg [8.8-26.5 lb]); thereafter, weight regain usually occurs (typical range of total weight loss at 1 year, 4-10 kg [8.8-22 lb]; at 2 years, 3-4 kg [6.6-8.8 lb]).

In a recent meta-analysis, investigators compared weight loss outcomes for various popular diets. All diets were superior to no diet at 6 months (median difference in weight loss, 8.7 kg [19.2 lb]); however, weight loss differences between individual diets were nonexistent or minimal. These results suggest that clinicians should prescribe a diet with which the patient will adhere (that is, a diet that is palatable and affordable) and that maintains negative energy balance in order to achieve weight loss. Inadequate exercise and sleep compromise the success of dietary interventions.

Exercise

Most studies have shown little or no weight loss with exercise programs alone; however, regular exercise improves fitness and maintains weight after weight loss. Overweight and obese patients should be advised to engage in physical activities, such as brisk walking, for 30 minutes or longer per day, at least 5 days per week.

Overweight and obese patients should also be encouraged to engage in activities that increase nonexercise activity thermogenesis (NEAT), which is defined as all of the energy expended except during sleeping, eating, and exercising. NEAT has dramatically declined during the past 100 years due to the sedentary aspects of modern life (reliance on automobiles and appliances). People who engage in activities that increase NEAT (for example, parking farther from workplaces, climbing stairs instead of using elevators, doing desk work while standing) are less likely to gain weight.

Behavioral Therapy

Overweight and obese patients should be provided with strategies to facilitate a shift from personal maladaptive eating patterns toward healthful eating and exercise. Although best conducted by a trained therapist, behavioral therapy can be initiated by internists. Specifically, internists can emphasize the behavioral therapy components of self-monitoring, stimulus control, goal setting, and social support.

Self-monitoring of energy intake and expenditure has been shown to facilitate weight loss and is a key component of behavioral therapy. It frequently involves the use of food and activity diaries and self-weighing.

Stimulus control entails modifying the physical environment by purchasing low-energy-density foods (high-fiber foods) for consumption, keeping unhealthy foods unavailable, and avoiding sugar-sweetened drinks and fast foods. Patients should also be advised to modify their cognitive environment

through avoidance (placing food out of sight), distraction (going for a walk rather than eating), and reframing (shifting focus from the pleasure of eating to the adverse consequences of obesity). Planning for high-risk situations (for example, "If I am tempted by food at the ball game, I will chew gum.") is also essential.

Goal setting involves establishing explicit, reasonable, and proximate weight loss and exercise goals. When a goal is achieved, a new one should be set. If a goal is not achieved, the patient should determine the reason why and then set a new goal.

Patients should be advised to enlist social support to adhere with diet and exercise plans. Including family members and spouses may also lead to increased weight loss.

A recent meta-analysis assessed the effects of behavioral interventions in obese patients. Participants who received behavioral interventions experienced more weight loss (3.0 kg [6.6 lb]) and were less likely to develop diabetes and hypertension than participants in the control group.

If weight plateauing occurs despite these lifestyle interventions, the physician should review the patient's diet and physical activities, recalculate the patient's daily calorie limit, and make new recommendations. These recommendations may include referral to dieticians, nutritionists, and behavioral therapists, whose assistance may facilitate the patient's weight loss.

KEY POINTS

- The mainstay of obesity treatment is lifestyle modification that includes diet for weight loss, increased physical activity, and behavioral therapy; a strategy that combines all three elements is likely to be more successful than any one element alone.

- Patients who maintain a continuous negative energy balance of 500 kcal/d lose about 0.5 kg (1.1 lb) per week.

- Obese patients should be advised to engage in physical activities, such as brisk walking, for 30 minutes or longer per day, at least 5 days per week.

Pharmacologic Therapy

Pharmacologic therapy may be used as an adjunct to diet, physical activity, and behavioral treatments in patients with a BMI of 30 or higher or in patients with a BMI of 27 or higher with overweight- or obesity-associated comorbidities. Drugs used in the treatment of obesity generally produce weight loss by reducing absorption of dietary fat or suppressing appetite.

Orlistat is an inhibitor of gastric and pancreatic lipases that results in malabsorption of approximately 30% of ingested fat. A meta-analysis showed that 12 months of orlistat treatment (120 mg three times daily), compared with placebo, resulted in greater reductions in weight (mean difference, 2.9 kg [6.4 lb]), BMI, waist circumference, blood pressure, blood cholesterol levels, and risk for type 2 diabetes. Diarrhea and oily stools are common side effects but subside over time. Given its mechanism of action, patients taking orlistat should also take a daily multivitamin containing vitamins A, D, and E, although the multivitamin should be taken 2 hours before or 2 hours after orlistat. A reduced-strength form (60 mg) of orlistat is available over the counter; this dose is also effective for weight loss.

Combination low-dose phentermine (a sympathomimetic drug) and low-dose topiramate (an antiepileptic drug) has demonstrated efficacy in reducing weight, possibly by suppressing appetite, altering taste, and increasing metabolism. In a 56-week trial, patients taking placebo achieved weight loss of 1.4 kg (3.1 lb), whereas patients taking 7.5 mg phentermine/46 mg topiramate had weight loss of 8.1 kg (17.9 lb). Patients taking 15 mg phentermine/92 mg topiramate lost 10.6 kg (23.4 lb). Both treatment groups that received phentermine-topiramate experienced improved blood pressure, fasting glucose levels, and lipid levels. Contraindications to phentermine-topiramate include pregnancy, glaucoma, hyperthyroidism, and recent use of monoamine oxidase inhibitors; its long-term safety and efficacy are unknown.

Lorcaserin, a brain serotonin 2C receptor agonist, acts as an appetite suppressant. In a 1-year trial, treatment with lorcaserin was superior to placebo and resulted in an additional weight loss of 3.6 kg (7.9 lb). Lorcaserin also led to significant reductions in BMI, waist circumference, and systolic blood pressure. Lorcaserin should be used with caution in patients taking medications that increase serotonin levels. There are limited data on the long-term safety and efficacy of lorcaserin.

The FDA recently approved combination sustained-release bupropion (a norepinephrine-dopamine reuptake inhibitor) and sustained-release naltrexone (an opioid receptor antagonist) for weight loss. In a 56-week trial, patients who received placebo achieved weight loss of 1.9 kg (4.2 lb), whereas patients taking sustained-release naltrexone (16 mg/d) plus sustained-release bupropion (360 mg/d) had weight loss of 6.5 kg (14.3 lb). Those taking combination sustained-release naltrexone (32 mg/d) and sustained-release bupropion (360 mg/d) lost 8.0 kg (17.6 lb). Combination bupropion-naltrexone is contraindicated in patients with epilepsy or uncontrolled hypertension and in patients taking opioids or opioid agonists.

The FDA also recently approved liraglutide, an injectable long-acting glucagon-like peptide-1 agonist used to improve glycemic control in patients with type 2 diabetes, for use as an adjunct to a reduced-calorie diet and increased physical activity for chronic weight management in adult patients with a BMI of 30 or greater or 27 or greater in the presence of at least one weight-related comorbid condition. The average weight loss with liraglutide is about 5%. If, after 16 weeks of treatment, a patient has not lost at least 4% of baseline weight, the drug should be stopped. Liraglutide is contraindicated in patients with multiple endocrine neoplasia syndrome type 2 and patients with a family or personal history of medullary thyroid carcinoma.

Several sympathomimetic drugs (phentermine, phendimetrazine, diethylpropion, and benzphetamine) are available specifically for short-term use (12 weeks or less) in the treatment of obesity. Hypertension may be experienced as a side effect of these drugs.

KEY POINT

- Pharmacologic therapy may be used as an adjunct to diet, physical activity, and behavioral treatments in patients with a BMI of 30 or higher or in patients with a BMI of 27 or higher with overweight- or obesity-associated comorbidities.

Bariatric Surgery

Bariatric surgery should be considered in all patients with a BMI of 40 or higher and in patients with a BMI of 35 or higher with obesity-related comorbid conditions. Since the bariatric surgery requirement of a BMI of 35 or higher was established, emerging evidence has supported the clinical and cost effectiveness of surgical intervention in patients with a BMI of 30 to 35 who do not achieve substantial weight and comorbidity improvement with nonsurgical methods. However, most guidelines (and third-party payers) still support withholding surgical intervention until the BMI is 35 or higher. Candidates should be evaluated by a multidisciplinary team with medical, surgical, nutritional, and psychiatric expertise. Additional criteria for bariatric surgery are presented in **Table 54**.

TABLE 54. Patient Criteria for Bariatric Surgery

BMI ≥40 or BMI 35-39.9 and obesity-related comorbidities (e.g., type 2 diabetes mellitus, coronary heart disease, obstructive sleep apnea, osteoarthritis)

Unlikeliness to lose weight or maintain weight loss with nonsurgical interventions

Acceptable operative risk

Knowledge of the benefits, risks, and alternatives of the proposed procedure

Commitment to ongoing diet, physical activity, and behavioral treatments after the procedure

Awareness of how life may change as a result of the procedure (e.g., need to chew food thoroughly, inability to eat large meals)

No psychological contraindications to surgery

Commitment to lifelong medical follow-up including monitoring for nutritional deficiencies

Evaluation by a multidisciplinary team with medical, surgical, nutritional, and psychiatric expertise

Adapted from National Institute of Diabetes and Digestive and Kidney Diseases, National Institutes of Health. Bariatric Surgery for Severe Obesity. Bethesda, Md: National Institutes of Health; March 2009, Updated June 2011. NIH Publication No. 08-4006. Available at www.niddk.nih.gov/health-information/health-topics/weight-control/bariatric-surgery-severe-obesity/Pages/bariatric-surgery-for-severe-obesity.aspx. Accessed June 24, 2015; Thompson WG, Cook DA, Clark MM, Bardia A, Levine JA. Treatment of obesity. Mayo Clin Proc. 2007 Jan;82(1):93-101. [PMID: 17285790]; and Vest AR, Heneghan HM, Schauer PR, Young JB. Surgical management of obesity and the relationship to cardiovascular disease. Circulation. 2013 Feb 26;127(8):945-59. [PMID: 23439447]

Bariatric surgical procedures result in reduced stomach capacity (restriction), malabsorption of ingested nutrients, hormone changes that suppress appetite, or a combination of these mechanisms. Mortality risk associated with bariatric surgery is low. Weight loss equal to or greater than 50% of excess body weight (current weight minus ideal body weight) is considered a success.

Commonly performed bariatric procedures include laparoscopic adjustable gastric banding, Roux-en-Y gastric bypass, and sleeve gastrectomy (**Figure 20**). Laparoscopic adjustable gastric banding, a restrictive procedure, involves placement of a soft silicone band below the gastroesophageal junction, which results in a small (approximately 30 mL) gastric pouch. The band is adjusted (via a port) to achieve early satiety without dysphagia. Three to 6 years after gastric banding, excess weight loss is 45% to 72%.

Roux-en-Y gastric bypass, a combination restrictive and malabsorptive procedure, involves creation of a small (30 mL) proximal gastric pouch, which is separated from the distal stomach and connected to a Roux limb of small bowel. Digestion and absorption of nutrients occur in the mid-small intestine. With Roux-en-Y gastric bypass, stomach capacity is reduced, as is absorption of calories. Additionally, delivery of nutrients to the mid-small intestine triggers hormone changes that suppress appetite. Three to 6 years after Roux-en-Y gastric bypass, excess weight loss is 62%.

Sleeve gastrectomy, a restrictive procedure, involves resection of the greater curvature of the stomach; this procedure reduces stomach capacity and suppresses appetite by removing tissue that produces ghrelin, a hunger-stimulating hormone. Excess weight loss 3 to 6 years after sleeve gastrectomy is 53% to 77%.

In a meta-analysis that compared bariatric surgery with nonsurgical treatment (diet, exercise, behavioral modification, and medications), participants randomized to bariatric surgery lost more weight (26.0 kg [57.3 lb]) and were more likely to experience remission of type 2 diabetes and metabolic syndrome, improved quality of life, and reduced medication use. Evidence suggests that bariatric surgery is also associated with reduced mortality and improvement of obstructive sleep apnea, osteoarthritis, and other conditions.

Patients who undergo bariatric surgery should continue dietary, physical activity, and behavioral measures and should receive nutrient replacement therapy (**Table 55**). Complications of bariatric surgery are discussed in MKSAP 17 Gastroenterology and Hepatology.

TABLE 55. Nutrient Deficiencies and Replacement after Bariatric Surgery	
Nutrient Deficiency	**Replacement Therapy**
Iron	MVI with iron, or elemental iron 80-100 mg/d orally
Vitamin B$_{12}$	Vitamin B$_{12}$ 500-1000 µg/d orally, or 1000 µg IM monthly
Folic acid	MVI with folate; for women of childbearing age, folate 1 mg/d orally
Calcium	Calcium citrate 1500 mg/d orally
Vitamin D	Vitamin D 400-800 U/d orally
Thiamine	25-50 mg/d orally
Vitamin A	MVI daily; if deficient, 2500 U/d orally with ongoing monitoring
Vitamin E	MVI daily; if deficient, 10 mg/d orally
IM = intramuscularly; MVI = multivitamin.	

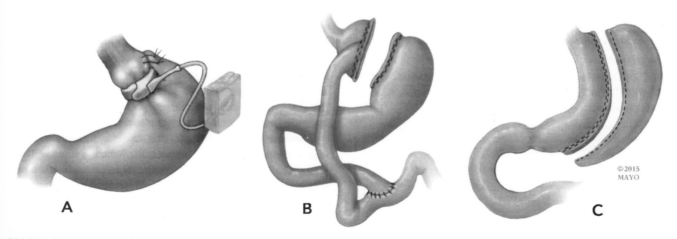

FIGURE 20. Commonly performed surgical procedures for obesity. *A,* gastric banding; *B,* Roux-en-Y gastric bypass; *C,* sleeve gastrectomy.

- Bariatric surgery should be considered in all patients with a BMI of 40 or higher and in patients with a BMI of 35 or higher with obesity-related comorbid conditions.

- Patients who undergo bariatric surgery lose more weight and are more likely to experience remission of type 2 diabetes mellitus and metabolic syndrome, improved quality of life, and reduced medication use than patients who receive nonsurgical treatment alone.

Men's Health

Male Sexual Dysfunction

Erectile Dysfunction

Erectile dysfunction (ED) is the inability to maintain an erection that is adequate for sexual performance. Incidence increases with age; approximately two thirds of men report some degree of ED by the age of 70 years. The most important risk factor is cardiovascular disease (diabetes mellitus, hyperlipidemia, hypertension, smoking, family history). Other risk factors include aging, obesity, sedentary lifestyle, prior genitourinary surgery, substance abuse, and trauma. Neurologic (dementia, multiple sclerosis, stroke, quadriplegia), hormonal (hypogonadism, hypothyroidism, hyperprolactinemia), and psychiatric (depression) conditions are also risk factors for ED. Medications, especially psychiatric and antihypertensive agents, are common causes of ED (**Table 56**).

The history for ED should include an accurate description to verify that patients are not experiencing decreased libido, premature ejaculation, anorgasmia, or an anatomic problem such as penile curvature or pain from Peyronie disease. Determining sudden onset of symptoms and persistence of

TABLE 56. Drugs Commonly Associated with Erectile Dysfunction

Antidepressants: monoamine oxidase inhibitors, selective serotonin reuptake inhibitors, tricyclic antidepressants

Benzodiazepines

Opioids, nicotine, alcohol, amphetamines, barbiturates, cocaine, marijuana, methadone

Anticonvulsants: phenytoin, phenobarbital

Antihypertensives and diuretics: α-blockers, β-blockers, calcium channel blockers, clonidine, spironolactone, thiazide diuretics, loop diuretics, ACE inhibitors

5α-Reductase inhibitors: dutasteride, finasteride

Antihistamines and histamine H_2-receptor antagonists: dimenhydrinate, diphenhydramine, hydroxyzine, meclizine, promethazine, cimetidine, nizatidine, ranitidine

NSAIDs: naproxen, indomethacin

Parkinson disease medications: levodopa, bromocriptine, biperiden, trihexyphenidyl, benztropine, procyclidine

firm nocturnal or morning erections are important indicators of an inorganic (psychological) etiology of ED. Assessment of coinciding medical or psychiatric conditions, relationships (including the partner's condition), and history of surgery or trauma is appropriate.

Physical examination includes vital signs, genital examination, digital rectal examination, lower extremity pulses, secondary sexual characteristics, and a neurologic assessment. The choice of laboratory studies is directed by findings on the history and examination. Based on typical causes of ED, testing may include glucose, lipids, and thyroid-stimulating hormone. The role of routine hormonal testing is less clear, with inconclusive evidence regarding its value in diagnosis and guiding therapy. If pursued, a fasting morning total testosterone level is the most appropriate study.

Treatment should be based on the underlying etiology. First-line therapy includes lifestyle modification (smoking cessation and weight loss), psychotherapy, and/or phosphodiesterase type 5 (PDE-5) inhibitor therapy. Obese patients may experience substantial improvements in erectile function solely from weight loss (BMI <30).

PDE-5 inhibitors increase cyclic guanosine monophosphate (cGMP) levels in the corpus cavernosum of the penis, which leads to vascular smooth muscle relaxation, increased penile blood flow, and erection. Available formulations include sildenafil, vardenafil, and tadalafil, all of which are believed to be equally efficacious. Avanafil is a newer PDE-5 inhibitor medication that was recently approved by the FDA. Because ED shares many risk factors with atherosclerotic disease, it is important to assess cardiovascular risk and safety for sexual activity before initiating a PDE-5 inhibitor (**Table 57**). For all PDE-5 inhibitors, starting with a low dose and increasing the dose based on response and side effects is indicated. Sildenafil should be taken on an empty stomach at least 1 hour before sex; counselling patients on the proper use of PDE-5 inhibitors leads to success in a high proportion of repeat users. PDE-5 inhibitors are generally well tolerated and safe. The most common side effect is headache (10%). Other side effects include dizziness, dyspepsia, flushing, rhinitis, syncope, and blue visual disturbances from inhibition of PDE-6 in the retina. PDE-5 inhibitors are contraindicated in patients taking nitrates and should be used with caution in patients taking α-blockers (such as tamsulosin) due to the risk of profound hypotension. PDE-5 inhibitors also inhibit cytochrome P-450 3A4 and may alter the metabolism of medications metabolized through this pathway (for example, protease inhibitors, erythromycin, ketoconazole).

Second-line treatment for ED includes intraurethral or injected prostaglandin E_1 (alprostadil), which is more efficacious than PDE-5 inhibitors at producing erections but is more inconvenient and less tolerated. Penile pump therapy may also be considered.

The evidence of effectiveness of testosterone replacement therapy for ED in men with low serum levels is conflicting but should not be considered except in men with clinical hypogonadism.

TABLE 57. Third Princeton Consensus Conference Guidelines for Treatment of Erectile Dysfunction in Patients with Cardiovascular Disease or Cardiac Risk Factors

Risk Level	Treatment Recommendation
Low Risk	
Patients who are able to do moderate-intensity exercise without symptoms	Can initiate or resume sexual activity or treat for ED with PDE-5 inhibitor (if not using nitrates)
Successfully revascularized patients (e.g., coronary artery bypass grafting, coronary stenting, or angioplasty)	
Asymptomatic controlled hypertension	
Mild valvular disease	
Mild left ventricular dysfunction (NYHA functional class I and II) who can achieve 5 METS without ischemia as determined by recent exercise testing	
Intermediate/Indeterminate Risk	
Mild to moderate stable angina	Further cardiac evaluation and restratification before resumption of sexual activity or treatment for ED
Recent MI (2-8 weeks) without intervention awaiting exercise ECG	If the patient can complete 4 minutes of the standard Bruce treadmill protocol without symptoms, arrhythmias, or a decrease in blood pressure, treatment for ED can be safely initiated
Heart failure (NYHA functional class III)	
Noncardiac atherosclerotic disease (clinically evident PAD, history of stroke/TIA)	
High Risk	
Unstable or refractory angina	Defer sexual activity or ED treatment until cardiac condition is stabilized and reassessed
Uncontrolled hypertension	
Moderate to severe heart failure (NYHA functional class IV)	
Recent MI (<2 weeks) without intervention	
High-risk arrhythmia (exercise-induced ventricular tachycardia, ICD with frequent shocks, poorly controlled atrial fibrillation)	
Obstructive hypertrophic cardiomyopathy with severe symptoms	
Moderate to severe valvular disease (particularly aortic stenosis)	

ECG = electrocardiography; ED = erectile dysfunction; ICD = implantable cardioverter-defibrillator; METS = metabolic equivalents; MI = myocardial infarction; NYHA = New York Heart Association; PAD = peripheral arterial disease; PDE = phosphodiesterase; TIA = transient ischemic attack.

Recommendations from Nehra A, Jackson G, Miner M, et al. The Princeton III Consensus recommendations for the management of erectile dysfunction and cardiovascular disease. Mayo Clin Proc. 2012 Aug;87(8):766-78. [PMID: 22862865]

Premature Ejaculation

Premature ejaculation is defined as ejaculation that occurs sooner than desired. Treatments are counseling and pharmacologic therapy. Topical medications (lidocaine, prilocaine), which work by reducing tactile stimulation, may be used with or without a condom. Oral medications (fluoxetine, paroxetine, sertraline) work based on their tendency to cause delayed ejaculation as a side effect.

Decreased Libido

Decreased libido is defined as diminished desire for sexual activity. Hypoactive sexual desire disorder is diagnosed when impaired libido causes marked distress and harms interpersonal relationships. Common causes are aging, hypogonadism, hyperprolactinemia, medications, and psychiatric conditions (mainly depression). Treatment is directed at the underlying cause. Many so-called natural supplements have been touted as effective for treating decreased libido and sexual dysfunction; however, none of these supplements has strong evidence to support their efficacy. Furthermore, the FDA has warned that many of the ingredients in these products are potentially harmful.

KEY POINTS

- First-line therapy for erectile dysfunction includes lifestyle modification, psychotherapy, and/or phosphodiesterase type 5 inhibitor therapy.

- Because erectile dysfunction shares many risk factors with atherosclerotic disease (smoking, diabetes, hypertension, hyperlipidemia, and family history of cardiovascular disease), it is important to assess cardiovascular risk and safety for sexual activity before initiating a phosphodiesterase type 5 inhibitor.

- Phosphodiesterase type 5 inhibitors are contraindicated in patients taking nitrates and should be used with caution in patients taking α-blockers due to the risk of profound hypotension.

Androgen Deficiency

The diagnosis of androgen deficiency is based on typical symptoms and documented hypogonadism (**Table 58**). Testing should be performed judiciously because symptoms of hypogonadism overlap with many common conditions. The Endocrine Society guidelines recommend against screening of asymptomatic men in the general population, regardless of age.

History should address conditions that alter testosterone production or metabolism, including systemic illnesses and medications (for example, high-dose systemic glucocorticoids, opioids, marijuana), or conditions that lower testosterone transiently, such as eating disorders and excessive exercise. Diagnosis of hypogonadism can be made by obtaining a fasting morning total testosterone level and confirming abnormal results with at least one repeat test. Before initiating treatment, identifying the cause of hypogonadism is indicated, including whether it is primary or secondary in origin. Treatment goals include inducing and maintaining secondary sex characteristics as well as improving well-being, sexual function, muscle mass/strength, and bone mineral density. Due to potential adverse effects, testosterone therapy is contraindicated in patients with prostate or breast cancer, prostate nodules or induration, a prostate-specific antigen (PSA) level greater than

4 ng/mL (4 µg/L) or greater than 3 ng/mL (3 µg/L) if at high risk for prostate cancer, a hematocrit greater than 50%, severe obstructive sleep apnea, severe lower urinary tract symptoms, or poorly controlled heart failure.

See MKSAP 17 Endocrinology and Metabolism for details on the evaluation of hypogonadism and testosterone treatment.

KEY POINTS

- Current guidelines recommend against screening for androgen deficiency in asymptomatic men, regardless of age.
- Diagnosis of hypogonadism can be made by obtaining a fasting morning total testosterone level and confirming abnormal results with at least one repeat test.

Benign Prostatic Hyperplasia

Benign prostatic hyperplasia (BPH) is a common cause of lower urinary tract symptoms (LUTS) in men. The prostate is about the size of a walnut in men aged 30 years and gradually increases in size. Most men older than 60 years have LUTS. BPH begins in the central transition zone of the prostate and causes obstruction to urine flow, which may ultimately lead to detrusor muscle dysfunction and uninhibited bladder contractions. LUTS may be categorized by the type of symptoms. Obstructive symptoms include decreased stream, urinary retention, incomplete emptying, and incontinence. Irritative symptoms, which are caused by detrusor hyperactivity and may occur later in the course of BPH, include nocturia, frequency, and urgency.

Diagnosing BPH can be challenging because of the many causes of LUTS; furthermore, there is poor correlation between prostate size on examination and urinary symptoms. Nonetheless, a careful history and examination can usually render the diagnosis. Men older than 50 years are likely to have BPH as a cause for LUTS, whereas men younger than 40 years are likely to have other causes for LUTS. Some medications may cause LUTS, including diuretics (urinary frequency), sympathomimetics, and anticholinergics (increased urethral sphincter tone and decreased detrusor muscle contractions); over-the-counter medications (especially sympathomimetic decongestants and anticholinergic antihistamines) may also cause LUTS. Other causes of LUTS are malignancy (prostate, bladder), infection (prostatitis, sexually transmitted infections), neurologic (spinal cord injury, stroke, Parkinson disease), medical conditions (poorly controlled diabetes mellitus, hypercalcemia), and behavior (alcohol or caffeine intake, excessive water consumption).

The American Urological Association (AUA) guidelines recommend obtaining a baseline AUA Symptom Index (AUA-SI) score to determine the severity of and to monitor LUTS. This questionnaire (available at www.hiv.va.gov/provider/manual-primary-care/urology-tool1.asp) assesses urinary frequency, nocturia, weak stream, hesitancy, intermittency, incomplete emptying, and urgency and generates a score reflecting mild,

TABLE 58. Symptoms and Signs Suggestive of Androgen Deficiency in Men

More Specific Symptoms and Signs
Incomplete or delayed sexual development, eunuchoidism
Reduced sexual desire (libido) and activity
Decreased spontaneous erections
Breast discomfort, gynecomastia
Loss of body (axillary and pubic) hair, reduced shaving
Very small (especially <5 mL) or shrinking testes
Inability to father children, low or zero sperm count
Height loss, low-trauma fracture, low bone mineral density
Hot flushes, sweats

Less Specific Symptoms and Signs
Decreased energy, motivation, initiative, and self-confidence
Feeling sad or blue, depressed mood, dysthymia
Poor concentration and memory
Sleep disturbance, increased sleepiness
Mild anemia (normochromic, normocytic, in the female range)
Reduced muscle bulk and strength
Increased body fat, BMI
Diminished physical or work performance

Adapted with permission from Bhasin S, Cunningham GR, Hayes FJ, et al; Task Force, Endocrine Society. Testosterone therapy in men with androgen deficiency syndromes: an Endocrine Society clinical practice guideline. J Clin Endocrinol Metab. 2010 Jun;95(6):2537. [PMID: 20525905] Copyright 2010, The Endocrine Society.

moderate, or severe symptoms. Prostate examination can reveal the characteristic findings of BPH, including symmetric enlargement and a firm consistency (like the tip of nose). Findings of prostate adenocarcinoma include asymmetry, induration, and nodularity. The penile meatus should be inspected to exclude evidence of stricture. The abdomen should be palpated to exclude masses or bladder distention. The examination should also exclude neurologic defects such as decreased anal sphincter tone, absent cremasteric reflex, saddle anesthesia, and lower extremity neurologic abnormalities. The AUA recommends urinalysis to exclude infection and malignancy (hematuria). Because PSA may be elevated in BPH, and increased levels of PSA associated with BPH do not reliably correlate with lower urinary tract symptoms, PSA testing is not required for the diagnosis of BPH and is not routinely followed in patients with BPH. Although not required for diagnosis, uroflow studies are a noninvasive means for evaluating LUTS and may be helpful in some patients in whom the cause is unclear. Accurate interpretation requires a minimum urine volume of 150 mL. Peak flow rates of less than 15 mL/s are often found in BPH, although this finding may also be associated with detrusor muscle dysfunction.

The main goals of treatment of BPH are to reduce symptoms from LUTS and improve quality of life. The AUA suggests a treatment approach based on AUA-SI score severity. Mild LUTS (AUA-SI score <8) can be addressed by conservative measures and observation. The approach to moderate to severe LUTS (AUA-SI score ≥8) may range from conservative measures and observation to medical treatment or invasive interventional therapy such as transurethral resection of the prostate (TURP) or transurethral needle ablation (TUNA). Conservative measures to treat LUTS in men with BPH include reduced fluid intake, timed voiding (every 3 hours while awake), limiting caffeine/alcohol, modifying medications, improving mobility, and avoiding bladder irritants.

First-line pharmacotherapy for LUTS due to BPH that does not respond to conservative measures consists of α-blockers, which act on the dynamic component of bladder outlet obstruction by relaxing smooth muscles in the urethral and bladder neck. Common side effects are headache, dizziness, nasal congestion, hypotension, edema, palpitations, fatigue, and ED. α-Blockers currently FDA approved for treatment of LUTS are alfuzosin, doxazosin, tamsulosin, terazosin, and silodosin. All α-blockers are equally effective but differ with regard to their cardiovascular safety and tolerability. Generally, α-blockers that are efficacious in treating hypertension (doxazosin, terazosin, alfuzosin) are more likely to cause more hypotensive side effects than tamsulosin and silodosin, which have little effect on blood pressure. The PDE-5 inhibitor tadalafil is also available for treatment of BPH, which may be a reasonable option for men with BPH and erectile dysfunction. Combinations of α-blockers and PDE-5 inhibitors can cause significant hypotension and should be initiated with caution.

Pharmacologic agents that inhibit the action of testosterone have also been shown to be efficacious in treating BPH.

5α-reductase inhibitors (5-ARIs) act on the anatomic component of bladder outlet obstruction by reducing the conversion of testosterone to dihydrotestosterone in the prostate, thus reducing prostate size and growth. 5-ARIs are most effective in men with large prostates (>40 mL), moderate to severe symptoms, and elevated PSA. Because 5-ARIs are associated with major reductions in PSA, it is recommended that physicians multiply the value of the PSA by 2 in patients taking 5-ARIs who require PSA testing. 5-ARIs reduce prostate size gradually, so the therapeutic effect may require several months. These medications are well tolerated; side effects include ejaculatory dysfunction and decreased libido. The combination of α-blockers and 5-ARIs is recommended in men with large prostates and elevated PSA levels.

Numerous herbal medications have been used for BPH, including saw palmetto, African star grass, African plum tree bark, rye grass pollen, stinging nettle, and cactus flower; however, recent studies have demonstrated no clear benefit.

Indications for referral to a urologist and possible invasive treatment for BPH include severe symptoms refractory to medical therapy, acute urinary retention, bladder stones, persistent gross hematuria, recurrent urinary tract infections, and obstructive nephropathy.

KEY POINTS

- First-line pharmacotherapy for benign prostatic hyperplasia consists of α-blockers.

- 5α-Reductase inhibitors are most effective in men with benign prostatic hyperplasia who have large prostates, moderate to severe symptoms, and elevated prostate-specific antigen levels.

Acute Testicular and Scrotal Pain

Common causes of acute testicular pain are testicular torsion, epididymitis, orchitis (viral, such as the mumps), and extension of infection from the epididymis or the urinary tract. Other causes are referred pain from abdominal aortic aneurysm, inguinal hernia with strangulation of the bowel/omentum, nephrolithiasis, lumbosacral nerve impingement, and retroperitoneal inflammation.

The causes of testicular and scrotal pain are usually diagnosed by history and examination. Discussion should include onset (sudden or gradual), pain quality and severity, LUTS, trauma, and association of pain with sexual activity. Examination includes scrotal inspection, palpation, transillumination, and the cremasteric reflex (stroking the inner thigh and observing rise in ipsilateral testicle). Testing includes urinalysis with microscopy to exclude infection as well as testicular ultrasonography.

Testicular Torsion

Testicular torsion occurs when the testes twist on the spermatic cord, leading to ischemia; it is considered a surgical emergency. It is most common in boys and men younger than

30 years. Symptoms are sudden and severe, including scrotal pain along with nausea and vomiting. Examination reveals a testis that is high riding, oriented transversely, and edematous. Testicular pain worsens with manual elevation, and the cremasteric reflex may be absent. Assessing blood flow using Doppler ultrasonography is sensitive (82%) and specific (100%) in making the diagnosis. Treatment is surgical decompression to restore blood flow.

Epididymitis

Epididymitis causes pain superolateral to the testicle and results from inflammation of the epididymis. Although symptoms are usually subacute, the pain ranges from acute to chronic and may be accompanied by dysuria, frequency, and urgency. Examination is remarkable for pain that is relieved by testicular elevation.

Epididymitis is most commonly infectious in etiology. Infectious epididymitis is characterized by acute onset, fever, leukocytosis, and possibly concomitant prostatitis. Infectious epididymitis has a bimodal distribution: men younger than 35 years and older than 55 years. In younger patients, sexually transmitted infections (chlamydia and gonorrhea) are most likely. In older patients and those who practice anal intercourse, *Escherichia coli*, Enterobacteriaceae, and *Pseudomonas* species should be considered. In older men and persons who practice anal intercourse, infectious epididymitis should be treated with ceftriaxone and a fluoroquinolone. All other men are treated with ceftriaxone (250-mg intramuscular injection in one dose) plus doxycycline (100 mg by mouth twice daily for 10 days).

Epididymitis can also be due to noninfectious causes (for example, trauma, autoimmune disease, or vasculitis). Treatment includes scrotal support, ice, and NSAIDs.

KEY POINTS

- Testicular torsion occurs when the testes twist on the spermatic cord, leading to ischemia; it is a surgical emergency treated with surgical decompression.

- Infectious epididymitis in older men and persons who practice anal intercourse is treated with ceftriaxone and a fluoroquinolone; all other men are treated with ceftriaxone plus doxycycline.

Hydroceles, Varicoceles, and Epididymal Cysts

Hydroceles

Hydroceles are fluid collections between layers of the tunica vaginalis and occur in approximately 1% of adult men. Communicating hydroceles involve fluid that flows from the peritoneal space into the scrotum through a patent processus vaginalis, whereas simple hydroceles do not have this communication. Most hydroceles are asymptomatic, but larger ones may be painful. Examination typically reveals a tense,

smooth, and transilluminating scrotal mass; this is in contrast to varicoceles, hernias, and solid masses, which do not transilluminate. Ultrasonography is used for confirmation. Treatment is reserved for large, painful hydroceles and communicating hydroceles, which may require surgery or aspiration with sclerotherapy.

Varicoceles

Varicoceles are caused by dilation of the testicular vein and pampiniform plexus. They are common, occurring in 15% of adult men. Varicoceles are believed to be a leading cause of infertility, as 40% of men who are infertile have varicoceles. Examination reveals a left-sided (90%) scrotal mass with a "bag of worms" consistency that increases with standing and decreases while supine. Ultrasonography is used for confirmation. Management is usually conservative. Surgery may be indicated in men with infertility and abnormal sperm counts; however, surgical repair may increase sperm counts without improving fertility.

Epididymal Cysts

Epididymal cysts are fluid-filled structures that contain spermatozoa and occur near the head of the epididymis. When greater than 2 cm in diameter, they are termed spermatoceles. Epididymal cysts and spermatoceles are usually asymptomatic, nontender to palpation, and confirmed by ultrasonography. Surgery is required only in rare cases of chronic pain.

Acute and Chronic Prostatitis and Pelvic Pain

Prostatitis and pelvic pain account for approximately 2 million physician visits annually. Presenting symptoms typically include pain originating from the perineum, testes, penis, or suprapubic region or as LUTS such as dysuria, frequency, and incomplete emptying.

Causes of symptomatic prostatitis may be acute bacterial infection (discussed in further detail in MKSAP 17 Infectious Disease), chronic bacterial infection, or chronic abacterial prostatitis/chronic pelvic pain syndrome. In patients with chronic symptoms, the National Institutes of Health Chronic Prostatitis Symptom Index can be used to aid in the diagnosis and symptom monitoring of prostatitis (www.prostate.net/wp-content/uploads/pdf/chronic-prostatitis-symptom-test.pdf).

Evaluation of symptoms of prostatitis and pelvic pain include the exclusion of identifiable sources of symptoms originating from the urethra, testicles, rectum, or bladder. In acute prostatitis, the prostate is typically very tender and edematous, whereas the degree of prostate tenderness is much more variable with chronic bacterial prostatitis or chronic abacterial prostatitis/chronic pelvic pain syndrome. Laboratory evaluation of suspected prostatitis includes urinalysis with microscopy and gram stain and culture; vigorous prostate massage is not indicated in acute prostatitis due to lack of diagnostic or therapeutic benefit. Imaging is not required for uncomplicated cases of acute prostatitis. **Table 59** provides details on the classification and management of prostatitis.

- Causes of symptomatic prostatitis may be acute bacterial infection, chronic bacterial infection, or chronic abacterial prostatitis/chronic pelvic pain syndrome.

Hernias

Hernias are organs that bulge through an area of muscle or weak connective tissue, which may be congenital or acquired. Most hernias occur in the groin; they may also occur in the abdomen (ventral, umbilical) or at incision sites. Hernias are exacerbated by increased intra-abdominal pressure from straining or coughing. Hernias are more common in men.

Inguinal hernias can be direct or indirect. Direct hernias involve the herniation of intra-abdominal contents through a weak region of the fascia between the rectus abdominis and inguinal ligament. Indirect hernias, which comprise the vast majority, involve the protrusion of contents through the internal inguinal ring. Femoral hernias, which are less common, are due to protrusion of contents through the femoral canal.

Symptoms of inguinal hernias include an asymptomatic bulge, pressure in the groin or abdomen, and severe pain from movement of abdominal contents into the inguinal ring or scrotum. Direct hernias present with a low abdomen bulge, are less painful, and less frequently incarcerate. Diagnosis is made by physical examination, which reveals a visible, palpable bulge in the lower abdomen or within the inguinal canal

TABLE 59. Classification and Management of Prostatitis

Class	Definition	Symptoms	Management
I. Acute bacterial prostatitis (see MKSAP 17 Infectious Disease)	Acute infection of the prostate	Fever, LUTS, prostate tenderness on examination	Empiric antibiotic coverage for gram-negative organisms, usually with a fluoroquinolone or trimethoprim-sulfamethoxazole; narrow antibiotic spectrum based on Gram stain and culture results, if available
II. Chronic bacterial prostatitis	Recurrent infection of the prostate	Pain, LUTS	First-line treatment is an antibiotic with good penetration into prostatic tissue, often with an extended, 1-month course of a fluoroquinolone
III. Chronic abacterial prostatitis/chronic pelvic pain syndrome (CPPS)	No demonstrable infection	Pain, LUTS	Often refractory to treatment; usually treated with a 1-month course of empiric therapy (not supported by evidence and not repeated if ineffective); other treatments are NSAIDs, α-blockers for LUTS, muscle relaxants, finasteride, gabapentin for neuropathic pain and if other drugs are ineffective; efficacy of complementary treatments (e.g., pollen extract, saw palmetto) not determined; in the absence of structural causes for pain, surgery should be avoided
IIIA. Inflammatory CPPS	Leukocytes in semen, expressed prostatic secretions, or post-prostatic massage urine		
IIIB. Noninflammatory CPPS	No leukocytes in semen, expressed prostatic secretions, or post-prostatic massage urine		
IV. Asymptomatic inflammatory prostatitis	Detected either by prostate biopsy, or the presence of leukocytes in semen samples during evaluation for other disorders	No symptoms	

LUTS = lower urinary tract symptoms.

Class and Definition columns reprinted from Litwin MS, McNaughton-Collins M, Fowler FJ Jr., et al. The National Institutes of Health chronic prostatitis symptom index: development and validation of a new outcome measure. Chronic Prostatitis Collaborative Research Network. J Urol. 1999 Aug;162(2)369-375. [PMID: 10411041] with permission from American Urological Association. Copyright 1999, American Urological Association.

or scrotum that increases with standing and the Valsalva maneuver.

Asymptomatic hernias may be monitored, but patients should be educated on symptoms and potential complications such as strangulation and incarceration. Symptomatic hernias require surgical consultation for consideration of repair. The benefit of laparoscopic versus open repair remains controversial. Hernia repair with polypropylene mesh may have lower complication rates. Possible complications of surgery include infection, seroma, hematoma, chronic pain, and recurrence.

KEY POINT

- Asymptomatic hernias may be monitored; symptomatic hernias require surgical consultation for consideration of repair.

Women's Health
Abnormal Uterine Bleeding
Clinical Presentation

Abnormal uterine bleeding can generally be categorized into ovulatory and anovulatory patterns. Ovulatory abnormal uterine bleeding (menorrhagia) occurs at normal, regular intervals but is excessive in volume or duration. Women with ovulatory bleeding have estrogen-mediated endometrial proliferation, produce progesterone, slough the endometrium regularly following progesterone withdrawal, and have a minimal risk of developing uterine cancer. Menorrhagia may be caused by coagulation disorders, anatomic abnormalities such as polyps or fibroids, medications that interfere with hemostasis, and thyroid dysfunction. Approximately 50% of women with menorrhagia have no identifiable cause.

Anovulatory cycles are characterized by unpredictable bleeding of variable flow and duration caused by absence of normal cyclic hormonal flux. Without cyclic progesterone, the estrogen-mediated endometrium proliferates excessively, resulting in endometrial instability, erratic bleeding, and increased risk of uterine cancer. Terms commonly associated with anovulatory bleeding include amenorrhea (absent menses for more than three cycles), oligomenorrhea (abnormally infrequent menses occurring at intervals of more than 35 days), and metrorrhagia (menses at irregular intervals with excessive bleeding or lasting more than 7 days). These terms apply only to women of reproductive age who are menstruating. Approximately 6% to 10% of women with anovulation have polycystic ovary syndrome. Other causes include diabetes mellitus, thyroid disorders, hyperprolactinemia, and medications such as antiseizure and psychotropic agents.

Anovulation increases in perimenopause and can cause abnormal uterine bleeding, including menorrhagia, metrorrhagia, and menometrorrhagia. The perimenopausal transition begins with changes in the interval between menstrual periods and ends 1 year after the last period; it is highly variable, lasting between 4 to 8 years.

Any uterine bleeding is always abnormal in postmenopausal women (absent menses for 1 year) and requires further evaluation.

KEY POINT

- Any uterine bleeding is always abnormal in postmenopausal women and requires further evaluation.

Evaluation

Initial evaluation of abnormal uterine bleeding in premenopausal women includes a detailed history, noting estimated changes in menstrual pattern and severity of bleeding, such as needing increased numbers of pads or tampons, leaking through pads or tampons, and the presence of clots. The history may provide clues to an underlying endocrine or bleeding disorder, liver or kidney disease, or sexually transmitted infection (STI). Physical examination requires a complete pelvic examination. Screening studies for cervical malignancy should be current. Because pregnancy commonly causes changes in the normal bleeding pattern, pregnancy testing must be performed in all women. Other laboratory tests should be based on clinical evaluation.

Abnormal ovulatory bleeding warrants consideration of a possible bleeding disorder or other causes of excessive bleeding, such as a structural uterine abnormality (polyps, fibroids). In women with anovulatory bleeding, exposure to unopposed estrogen increases the risk for endometrial cancer. Additional risk factors for endometrial cancer in premenopausal women include obesity, nulliparity, age 35 years or older, diabetes mellitus, family history of colon cancer, infertility, and treatment with tamoxifen. In women younger than 35 years of age with anovulatory bleeding and no other risk factors for endometrial cancer, no additional evaluation prior to treatment is usually indicated. However, in women younger than 35 years of age with risk factors, or any patient with anovulatory bleeding 35 years of age or older, endometrial biopsy should be performed to exclude significant endometrial pathology. Transvaginal ultrasonography is not helpful in evaluating premenopausal bleeding unless a structural uterine abnormality is suspected as a cause of bleeding.

Perimenopause is frequently characterized by abnormal bleeding patterns and should be approached on an individualized basis. Pelvic examination and transvaginal ultrasound are useful for ruling out common causes of bleeding, such as endometrial hyperplasia, polyps, and STIs, and endometrial sampling is definitive in cases of diagnostic uncertainty or increased risk for endometrial cancer. Unless bleeding is excessive, laboratory studies, including hormone levels, are generally not indicated.

In postmenopausal women, any vaginal bleeding requires assessment to exclude malignancy. Initial evaluation may be with either transvaginal ultrasonography or endometrial biopsy; both studies are not required. When transvaginal ultrasonography is performed as an initial study and an endometrial thickness of less than or equal to 4 mm is found, endometrial sampling is not required. Endometrial thickness of greater than 4 mm should be further evaluated by endometrial sampling.

- Because pregnancy commonly causes changes in the normal bleeding pattern, pregnancy testing must be performed in all women with abnormal uterine bleeding before more extensive testing is ordered.
- Exposure to unopposed estrogen increases the risk for endometrial cancer in women with prolonged anovulation.

Management

Management of abnormal ovulatory bleeding is focused on addressing any underlying causes and reducing flow volume, which may be done with hormonal therapy or other treatments such as NSAIDs. Treatment of anovulatory bleeding is directed toward restoring hormonal balance and stabilizing the endometrium. A progestin such as medroxyprogesterone acetate may be used to promote withdrawal bleeding for women who wish to become pregnant. Hormonal contraceptives may be used to regulate cycles for women not desiring pregnancy. NSAIDs can decrease uterine bleeding by up to 40%, owing to the high concentrations of prostaglandins in the endometrium. Tranexamic acid, an antifibrinolytic agent that stabilizes clot formation, is FDA-approved for treatment of menorrhagia but is expensive. Patients with severe bleeding may require short courses of gonadotropin-releasing hormone (GnRH) agonists or intravenous high-dose estrogens. Endometrial ablation or hysterectomy may be considered for patients who do not respond to medical treatment or in whom anatomic causes are identified.

Breast Mass

Clinical Presentation

A breast mass is characterized by a lesion that persists throughout the menstrual cycle and differs from the surrounding breast tissue and the corresponding area in the contralateral breast. The differential diagnosis of a palpable breast mass includes cyst, abscess, fibroadenoma, fat necrosis, and neoplasm. Distinguishing between benign and malignant breast masses is critical. Although up to 90% of breast masses are benign cysts or fibroadenomas, neither the history nor the physical examination findings can definitively rule out underlying malignancy.

- Although up to 90% of breast masses are benign cysts or fibroadenomas, neither the history nor the physical examination findings can definitively rule out underlying malignancy.

Evaluation

Evaluation of a palpable breast mass varies, based on the patient's age and risk factors and the degree of clinical suspicion. Mammography and ultrasonography are the initial imaging modalities. Ultrasonography is often preferred in women younger than age 35 years because the increased density of breast tissue in younger women limits the usefulness of mammography. Ultrasonography may also be a better choice for pregnant patients in order to avoid radiation exposure. The main utility of ultrasonography is its ability to differentiate cystic from solid lesions. A simple cyst is likely to be benign if it has symmetric, round borders with no internal echoes; aspiration reveals nonbloody fluid and complete resolution of the cyst. Any bloody fluid obtained from cyst aspiration requires cytologic examination. A solid lesion with uniform borders and uniformly sized internal echoes is consistent with a benign fibroadenoma, but it must be evaluated completely with fine needle aspiration or biopsy.

A suspicious mass is solitary, discrete, hard, and sometimes adherent to adjacent tissue. If such a mass is present, mammography is performed before a pathologic diagnosis is attempted. The radiologist should be informed of the area of clinical concern to ensure that any noted mammographic abnormalities correspond to the clinical findings. Which breast is to be imaged, clock face location of the mass, dimension, and distance from the areola must be indicated. On mammography, an irregular mass with microcalcifications or spiculations is suspicious for malignant disease, and biopsy is mandatory.

Mammography results are reported in a standardized format called BI-RADS (Breast Imaging Reporting and Data System) that uses a 0 to 6 scale (**Table 60**). Approximately 10%

TABLE 60.	Breast Imaging Reporting and Data System (BI-RADS) Assessment Categories
Category 0	Mammography: Incomplete—Need additional imaging evaluation and/or prior mammograms for comparison
	Ultrasound and MRI: Incomplete—Need additional imaging evaluation
Category 1	Negative
Category 2	Benign
Category 3	Probably benign
Category 4	Suspicious
	Mammography and ultrasound:
	Category 4A: Low suspicion for malignancy
	Category 4B: Moderate suspicion for malignancy
	Category 4C: High suspicion for malignancy
Category 5	Highly suggestive of malignancy
Category 6	Known biopsy-proven malignancy

Reprinted with permission of the American College of Radiology (ACR) from D'Orsi CJ, Sickles EA, Mendelson EB, et al. ACR BI-RADS® Atlas, Breast Imaging Reporting and Data System. Reston, VA, American College of Radiology; 2013. No other representation of this material is authorized without expressed, written permission from the ACR. Refer to the ACR website at http://www.acr.org/Quality-Safety/Resources/BIRADS for the most current and complete version of the BI-RADS® Atlas.

to 20% of palpable breast cancers are not detected by ultrasonography or mammography. If a mass is present, a nondiagnostic mammogram or ultrasound should not be considered proof of the absence of malignancy, and tissue diagnosis is indicated.

Definitive diagnosis is obtained by tissue sampling using fine needle aspiration, core needle biopsy with or without stereotactic or ultrasound guidance, or excisional biopsy. Fine needle aspiration, generally reserved for ultrasound-confirmed cystic lesions, requires an experienced cytopathologist for interpretation. Core needle biopsy is the test of choice for most solid lesions, as it provides more tissue for histology and tissue markers. Excisional biopsy is used when core needle biopsy findings are nondiagnostic or when biopsy and imaging studies do not concur. Further management of abnormal pathologic findings requires consultation with a breast surgeon and oncologist.

KEY POINTS

- The initial imaging modalities for evaluating a palpable breast mass are mammography and ultrasonography; ultrasonography is often preferred in women younger than age 35 years and pregnant women.
- Any solid mass on imaging must be evaluated completely with fine needle aspiration, core needle biopsy, or excisional biopsy.

Breast Pain

Clinical Presentation

Breast pain (mastalgia) is common and may be cyclic, noncyclic, or extramammary. Generalized mastalgia may be caused by hormonal changes related to pregnancy, hormonal contraception, and medications. Many younger women experience cyclic breast discomfort with the onset of menses. The discomfort is typically bilateral, lasts for several days, and varies in intensity. Noncyclic breast pain is more likely to be unilateral and may be caused by trauma, cysts, duct ectasia, mastitis, ligamentous stretching secondary to large breasts, or a breast mass. Extramammary pain (breast pain referred from other areas) may be caused by musculoskeletal, cardiac, gastrointestinal, or spinal disorders. Chest wall pain, which is a common cause of extramammary pain, typically presents with unilateral, localized, reproducible discomfort.

Evaluation

A thorough history with attention to type of pain, location, and relationship to menses and a careful physical examination are essential to rule out palpable masses or anatomic causes. Women with a palpable breast mass should be referred for diagnostic imaging. Chest wall pain is typically reproduced by palpation or by examination maneuvers that place stress on the painful musculoskeletal structures. All women who are evaluated for mastalgia should be up to date on routine mammographic screening, according to age and personal risk factors for breast cancer.

KEY POINT

- In women with mastalgia, the evaluation focuses on excluding palpable masses or anatomic causes.

Treatment

Because most symptoms of cyclic mastalgia are self-limited, management usually requires only education, reassurance, and appropriate breast support. Studies have not shown that caffeine restriction or vitamin E administration is beneficial. Medical treatment may be considered for women with severe and persistent pain that interferes with quality of life. Danazol is the only therapy that is FDA approved for the treatment of cyclic mastalgia, but side effects limit its use.

KEY POINT

- Because most symptoms of cyclic mastalgia are self-limited, management usually requires only education, reassurance, and appropriate breast support.

Chronic Pelvic Pain

Chronic pelvic pain (CPP) in women is a syndrome of intermittent or constant noncyclic pain of at least 6 months' duration that localizes to the lower abdomen or pelvis and is sufficiently severe to cause functional disability. Prevalence estimates vary, but in one representative study of female patients aged 15 to 73 years, a point prevalence of 3.8% was comparable with that of asthma (3.7%) and chronic back pain (4.1%).

CPP often presents a diagnostic and therapeutic challenge. It is frequently associated with endometriosis, pelvic adhesions, myofascial pain disorders, interstitial cystitis, irritable bowel syndrome, sleep disorders, and depression. Many women have more than one associated disorder. Risk factors for CPP include physical, sexual, and emotional abuse; pelvic inflammatory disease; obstetric or gynecologic disorders; psychological disorders; abdominopelvic surgery; and chronic pain syndromes, such as fibromyalgia.

Evaluation includes screening for gynecologic, gastrointestinal, urologic, and psychological disorders, and a detailed physical examination is warranted. Laboratory studies are based upon clinical indication. Transvaginal ultrasonography is helpful for identifying anatomic pathology, and a normal study aids in providing reassurance. Laparoscopy may be indicated for evaluation of severe symptoms of unclear etiology.

Treatment should be directed toward the specific cause, if identified. In patients without a clearly defined pathophysiologic or anatomic cause, therapy is usually targeted toward general pain management. NSAIDs may be used as first-line short-term therapy for most women with moderate CPP. Other therapeutic interventions include antidepressant agents, biofeedback, cognitive-behavioral therapy, physical therapy, hypnosis, acupuncture, meditation, and stress-reduction techniques.

- NSAIDs may be used as first-line short-term therapy for most women with moderate chronic pelvic pain in patients without a clearly defined pathophysiologic or anatomic cause.

Contraception

Nearly 50% of all pregnancies in the United States are unintended, with higher prevalence among younger women, racial and ethnic minorities, and women at lower socioeconomic levels. Unintended pregnancy is associated with poor maternal and infant outcomes. Strategies to reduce unintended pregnancy require assessing pregnancy risk, counseling patients regarding contraceptive options, and ensuring correct and consistent use of contraceptives. Most women can start most contraceptive methods at any time, and appropriate methods are available for women with serious medical conditions, in whom the risk of pregnancy-related adverse events is high. The U.S. Selected Practice Recommendations for Contraceptive Use are a useful guide to contraceptive use and detail medical eligibility criteria (www.cdc.gov/reproductivehealth/UnintendedPregnancy/USSPR.htm).

Available contraceptive methods include hormonal contraception; long-acting reversible preparations, including intrauterine devices (IUDs); barrier contraceptives; and sterilization (**Table 61**).

- Strategies to reduce unintended pregnancy require assessing for pregnancy risk, counseling patients regarding contraceptive options, and ensuring correct and consistent use of contraceptives.

Hormonal Contraception

Other than a thorough history, blood pressure, and BMI measurements, few examinations or tests, if any, are needed before starting a contraceptive method. A negative pregnancy test should be obtained if more than 7 days have elapsed since the start of normal menses. In healthy women of reproductive age, a pelvic examination is not needed before beginning hormonal contraception. Various types of hormonal contraception include oral contraceptive pills, transdermal patch, vaginal ring, and long-acting reversible contraceptives.

- Healthy women of reproductive age generally do not require a pelvic examination or other studies before beginning hormonal contraception.

Oral Contraceptive Pills

Oral contraceptive pills are the most common form of contraception. These include combination estrogen-progestin and progestin-only pills. Combination preparations differ based on the strength of estrogen and the type of progestin component. All preparations are therapeutically equivalent in preventing pregnancy. The mechanisms of action include inhibition of ovulation, alteration of the cervical mucus to an environment less conducive to sperm migration, and inhibition of endometrial proliferation. Benefits of combined hormonal contraception are summarized in Table 61. Contraindications to combination products include uncontrolled hypertension, breast cancer, venous thromboembolism, liver disease, and migraine with aura. Estrogen-containing preparations are contraindicated in women older than 35 years who smoke more than 15 cigarettes a day. Progestin-only pills, also called the "mini-pill," may be used by women with contraindications to estrogen.

In addition to oral contraceptive pills, other methods of hormonal contraceptive delivery include transdermal patches and vaginal rings.

Medications that induce the cytochrome P-450 3A4 (CYP3A4) class of liver enzymes may reduce the effectiveness of hormonal contraceptives. These may include, but are not limited to, rifampin, griseofulvin, antiseizure agents (see MKSAP 17 Neurology), St. John's wort, and antiretroviral drugs.

- Contraindications to oral combination estrogen-progestin contraceptives include uncontrolled hypertension, breast cancer, venous thromboembolism, liver disease, and migraine with aura.
- Estrogen-containing contraceptive pills are contraindicated in women older than 35 years who smoke more than 15 cigarettes daily.

Long-Acting Reversible Contraceptives

Long-acting reversible contraceptives contain progestin and include depot medroxyprogesterone acetate injections, subcutaneous implants, and progestin-containing IUDs. These preparations are less reliant on user adherence than oral contraceptive pills and are highly effective. Return of fertility may be delayed with these methods, with the median time to conception of 10 months after cessation of use. As with other progestin-only methods, irregular bleeding and amenorrhea are prevalent, and weight gain is a common side effect.

Depot medroxyprogesterone acetate is given by intramuscular or subcutaneous injection every 3 months following a negative pregnancy test. The etonogestrel implant is a single matchstick-sized rod inserted subdermally in the upper inner arm and is effective for 3 years.

IUDs are a long-acting reversible contraceptive method in which a small T-shaped device is placed inside the uterus. The levonorgestrel IUD is available in two dosage formulations, one that releases 14 µg and is effective for 3 years and one that releases 20 µg and is effective for 5 years. The levonorgestrel-containing IUD releases a low dose of progestin, which causes endometrial atrophy and generally leads to

TABLE 61. Comparison of Contraceptive Options

Agent	Percent (%) of Women Experiencing Unintended Pregnancy Within the First Year of Use		Advantages	Disadvantages
	Typical Use	Perfect Use[a]		
Combination estrogen-progestin preparations			Decreased incidence of endometrial and ovarian cancers	Increased risk of myocardial infarction, ischemic stroke, VTE, hypertension
			Decreased dysmenorrhea, menorrhagia, symptomatic ovarian cysts	Increased risk of cancers of the cervix, liver, and breast
			Less iron-deficiency anemia	Breakthrough bleeding
Oral	9	0.3	Easy to use	May exacerbate migraine
			Rapidly reversible	
Patch	9	0.3	Easier adherence	Local skin reaction
				Increased estrogen dose, thus higher VTE risk
Vaginal ring	9	0.3	Easier adherence	Requires self-insertion
			Lowest level of systemic estrogen	
Progestin-only preparations "Mini-pill"			Use when estrogen is contraindicated	Irregular bleeding, breakthrough bleeding
				Must maintain precise daily dosing schedule
Long-acting reversible preparations				Irregular bleeding, amenorrhea, decreased bone mineral density (especially in adolescents)
Depot medroxyprogesterone acetate (IM or SQ)	6	0.2	Administered every 3 months	Delayed return to ovulation (10 months)
			Decreased risk of endometrial cancer, PID	
			Improves endometriosis	
			Decreased menstrual frequency	
Progestin implants	0.05	0.05	Effective up to 3 years	Delayed return to ovulation (6 months)
Intrauterine devices			Least dependence on user	Bleeding, pain, expulsion (rare); no protection from STIs
Copper	0.8	0.6	Nonhormonal	
			Effective up to 10 years	
Levonorgestrel	6	0.2	Decreased blood loss, decreased anemia	
			Effective up to 5 years	
Barrier methods			Only use when needed	Most user-dependent
Cervical cap	16-32	9-26		Requires spermicide
Diaphragm	12	6		Requires spermicide
Male condom	18	2	Protection from STIs	
Female condom	21	5	Protection from STIs	
Vaginal sponge	12-24	9-20		
Sterilization				
Female (tubal ligation)	0.5	0.5	May reduce ovarian cancer risk	Surgical complications
				Regret
				Increased risk of ectopy if pregnancy occurs
Male (vasectomy)	0.15	0.10	Lower costs, fewer complications, and more effective than tubal ligation	Surgical complications

IM = intramuscular; PID = pelvic inflammatory disease; SQ = subcutaneous; STI = sexually transmitted infection; VTE = venous thromboembolism.

[a]Perfect use implies correct and consistent use exactly as directed/intended. Typical use reflects rates in actual practice with patients.

decrease or absence of menstrual flow. A nonhormonal copper IUD is also available. IUDs are extremely effective and provide long-term protection of 3 to 10 years, depending on the type. They may be placed at any time except during pregnancy in an office setting, without need for anesthesia, in both nulliparous and multiparous women. Expulsion of the device occurs in 2% to 10% of women within the first year. IUDs do not increase risk of ectopic pregnancy, pelvic inflammatory disease, or infertility.

KEY POINT

- Long-acting reversible contraceptives contain progestin and include depot medroxyprogesterone acetate injections, subcutaneous implants, and progestin-containing intrauterine devices; they are less reliant on user adherence than oral contraceptive pills and are highly effective.

Barrier Contraceptive Methods

Barrier methods (see Table 61) provide as-needed contraception but are substantially less reliable than hormonal methods. All barrier methods are more effective when used with spermicides; spermicides alone are not a reliable method of contraception. Condoms reduce risk of STIs. Evidence is strongest for prevention of HIV infection when male condoms are used. Combining a barrier method with a hormonal method is always recommended to prevent STIs, as well as to prevent unintended pregnancy.

KEY POINT

- Combining a barrier method with a hormonal method is always recommended to prevent sexually transmitted infections, as well to prevent unintended pregnancy.

Sterilization

Female surgical sterilization is highly successful and safe and has a low risk for complications. The fallopian tubes can be occluded by ligation, occlusive clips or rings, or with cauterization. Tubal occlusion should be considered a permanent end to fertility and should not be performed in women who may desire future pregnancy. The incidence of regret is significantly higher in women under age 30 years and in those who are postabortion or postpartum at the time of the procedure.

Emergency Contraception

Emergency contraception is postcoital hormonal contraception used to prevent pregnancy after inadequately protected coitus. Two methods are FDA approved: over-the-counter levonorgestrel (1.5 mg) and prescription ulipristal (30 mg). Both are taken as a single dose. The primary documented mechanism of action for both levonorgestrel and ulipristal is interference with the process of ovulation. Ulipristal has been shown to prevent ovulation both before and after the luteinizing hormone surge has started, delaying follicular rupture for at least 5 days. Both agents have no effect on an established pregnancy and do not increase rates of miscarriage.

Ulipristal has slightly greater efficacy than levonorgestrel, and efficacy for both products increases the earlier they are used. Both levonorgestrel and ulipristal may be taken up to 5 days (120 hours) after intercourse. Both agents are less effective in obese women.

KEY POINT

- Two methods of emergency contraception are over-the-counter levonorgestrel and prescription ulipristal; both are taken as a single dose and are effective for up to 5 days (120 hours) after intercourse.

Dysmenorrhea

Dysmenorrhea (painful menstruation) occurs in up to 50% of adolescents and young adults and is classified as primary or secondary. Primary dysmenorrhea, which occurs in 90% of patients, is associated with normal ovulatory cycles and no pelvic pathology. The prevalence of primary dysmenorrhea decreases with increasing age and is highest in the 20- to 24-year-old age group. A secondary cause, such as endometriosis, fibroids, or uterine pathology, is found in 10% of patients. Symptoms of dysmenorrhea include severe abdominal cramps, backache, headache, nausea, vomiting, and diarrhea. Symptoms coincide with the onset of menses and last 2 to 3 days.

Dysmenorrhea is sometimes associated with other cyclic symptom complexes such as premenstrual syndrome and premenstrual dysphoric disorder. These disorders include a wide range of physical and psychological symptoms that begin approximately 1 week before menses and typically cease with menstruation (see Mental and Behavioral Health).

Initial evaluation includes a thorough history, with attention to risks for infection and possible physical, sexual, or emotional abuse. It is important to distinguish between pain associated with menstruation and pain that occurs at other times. If pelvic pathology (previous irradiation, trauma, infection, foreign body) is not suspected and a diagnosis of primary dysmenorrhea is made, symptomatic treatment may begin without further testing. Both NSAIDs and cyclooxygenase-2 inhibitors are effective. For patients with incomplete relief of symptoms, use of combined hormonal contraceptive therapy is effective. Extended-cycle combined oral contraceptive pills may be particularly useful for this indication.

KEY POINTS

- In a patient with dysmenorrhea, if pelvic pathology is **HVC** not suspected and a diagnosis of primary dysmenorrhea is made, symptomatic treatment may begin without additional evaluation.

- Both NSAIDs and cyclooxygenase-2 inhibitors are effective initial therapy for primary dysmenorrhea; combined hormonal contraceptive therapy is effective for patients whose symptoms do not resolve completely after initial therapy.

Female Sexual Dysfunction

Female sexual dysfunction describes sexual difficulties that are persistent and personally distressing to the patient. Up to 35% of sexually active women are affected, with a peak occurrence in middle age. Asking an open-ended question about sexual concerns, including pain with intercourse, is appropriate. When indicated, a complete sexual history should be obtained, including a review of medications, medical history, psychiatric disorders, and reproductive surgeries that can contribute to sexual dysfunction. Identifying problems with relationships, desire, arousal, orgasm, or pain may help in determining the cause and potential treatment strategies. Screening for concurrent depression is indicated, as sexual dysfunction and depression often coexist. A pelvic examination is helpful in identifying specific areas of pain or tenderness, menopausal genitourinary symptoms, decreased lubrication, or tissue friability. Laboratory testing is recommended only if an underlying disorder is suspected. If further evaluation is needed, validated self-report questionnaires, such as the Female Sexual Function Index, can supplement the clinical assessment.

KEY POINT

- Women with possible sexual dysfunction should be screened for depression, as both disorders may coexist.

Classification of Female Sexual Disorders

According to the DSM-5, abnormalities in female sexual response fall into three categories: sexual interest/arousal disorder, orgasmic disorder, and genitopelvic pain/penetration disorder. Sexual interest/arousal disorder includes female hypoactive desire dysfunction and female arousal dysfunction; it is diagnosed if a woman reports at least three of the following symptoms: lack of sexual interest, lack of sexual thoughts or fantasies, decreased initiation of sexual activity or decreased responsiveness to partner's initiation attempts, reduced excitement or pleasure during sexual activity, decreased response to sexual cues, or decreased sensations during sexual activity. Female orgasmic disorder is the persistent or recurrent absence, delay, or diminished intensity of orgasm following a normal excitement phase. Genitopelvic pain/penetration disorder is diagnosed when there is difficulty in vaginal penetration, marked vulvovaginal or pelvic pain during penetration, fear of pain or anxiety about pain in anticipation of or during penetration, or tightening or tensing of pelvic floor muscles during attempted penetration. The diagnosis of a sexual disorder requires both significant distress more than 75% of the time and a minimum duration of 6 months.

Treatment

Therapy is aimed at identifying and treating underlying contributing causes, which may include vulvodynia (an idiopathic chronic pain syndrome affecting the vulvovaginal area), vaginitis, interstitial cystitis, pelvic adhesions, infections, or endometriosis. Coexisting genitourinary syndrome of menopause or inadequate lubrication may worsen genitopelvic pain/penetration disorder and generally can be diagnosed on physical examination. Vaginal or systemic hormone therapy frequently improves atrophy and lubrication and helps alleviate dyspareunia.

Successful treatment strategies must address the complex psychological and behavioral changes that accompany these disorders. Cognitive-behavioral therapy is most effective in helping to minimize negative attitudes and decrease anxiety. Individual and couples psychotherapy or sex therapy may be beneficial. Sex therapy is a form of talk therapy comprised of a combination of counseling, cognitive-behavioral interventions, and treatment of concomitant psychiatric conditions such as depression and anxiety disorders. With genitopelvic pain/penetration disorder, sex therapy with systematic desensitization teaches deep muscle relaxation and uses objects of increasing diameter, such as dilators, to achieve gradual vaginal tolerance.

There are currently no FDA-approved pharmacologic agents for treatment of sexual dysfunction in women. Although study results are inconsistent, systemic hormone therapy may improve sexual function. Treatment with low-dose testosterone in women has been shown to increase sexual function scores and the number of satisfying sexual episodes; however, it may be associated with adverse effects and therefore has not been FDA approved for female sexual dysfunction. Phosphodiesterase inhibitors are generally ineffective in women.

Menopause

Menopause describes the cessation of menses and fertility and is definitive once a woman has experienced amenorrhea for 12 months. Menopause may be natural, surgical (induced by bilateral oophorectomy), or medical (induced by chemotherapy or medical treatment). The average age of experiencing natural menopause is 51 years, and 95% of women will experience menopause between ages 40 and 59 years. Menopause occurring before age 40 years is known as premature menopause.

The transitional phase of perimenopause varies in length and may begin as early as 8 years before the final menstrual period. Irregular menstrual cycles, sometimes associated with vasomotor symptoms, are characteristic findings. The length of the menstrual cycles may increase or decrease as episodes of anovulation become more frequent. Follicle-stimulating hormone (FSH) levels begin to rise during perimenopause. However, FSH levels fluctuate depending on the frequency of anovulation. Hormone measurements during perimenopause are imprecise, cannot predict onset of menopause, and are therefore not recommended. Salivary testing of reproductive hormones is inaccurate and never indicated, and measurement of FSH is not routinely needed. The North American Menopause Society suggests measurement of FSH only to evaluate premature menopause. After 1 year of amenorrhea, a woman is considered to be postmenopausal, and elevated serum FSH levels stabilize (>35 mU/mL [35 units/L]).

The hallmark symptoms of menopause vary greatly in severity, duration, and frequency but may include vasomotor symptoms (hot flushes, night sweats) and urogenital symptoms (vaginal dryness, dyspareunia). Symptoms generally resolve spontaneously within a few years, and treatment should be based on symptom severity.

The differential diagnosis of menopausal symptoms associated with amenorrhea includes thyroid disease, elevated serum prolactin levels, and pregnancy, and testing for these conditions may be considered in selected patients.

Contraceptive needs must continue to be addressed during perimenopause. For perimenopausal women without contraindications, the use of combined hormonal oral contraceptive pills is helpful in providing both vasomotor symptom relief and contraception.

KEY POINTS

- Hormone measurements during perimenopause are imprecise, cannot predict onset of menopause, and are therefore not recommended.
- Contraceptive needs should continue to be addressed during perimenopause.

Management of Vasomotor Symptoms

The most effective treatment of moderate to severe vasomotor symptoms is systemic hormone therapy. Multiple formulations and routes of administration are available, and all formulations are equally effective. The lowest dose that alleviates symptoms should be used initially, titrating up if needed. Although supporting data are limited, transdermal estrogen may be associated with less thromboembolic risk than oral estrogen because transdermal delivery avoids the hepatic first-pass effect.

A stepwise approach for initiating hormone therapy in women ages 50 to 59 years who have experienced menopause at the median age is presented in **Table 62**. Effectiveness of treatment is based on relief of symptoms. In light of the risks and benefits, hormone therapy may be used to treat troubling menopausal symptoms in healthy women younger than 60 years and within 10 years of menopause, with consideration of symptom severity and risk factors. The low absolute risk of adverse events supports the option to prescribe hormone therapy for women with moderate to severe vasomotor or urogenital symptoms who are at low risk for coronary heart disease, stroke, thromboembolic disease, and breast cancer.

All women with an intact uterus who are treated with hormone therapy must receive progestin to avoid estrogen-induced endometrial proliferation. Several preparations are available and may be given continuously or cyclically to confer endometrial protection. Limited evidence suggests that micronized progesterone confers less risk of thromboembolism than does medroxyprogesterone acetate. Continuous daily estrogen-progestin does not result in cyclic bleeding, an option

TABLE 62. Initiating Systemic Hormone Therapy in Women Ages 50-59 Years[a]

Step 1: Confirm that hot flushes/night sweats are moderate to severe in intensity and refractory to lifestyle modifications and/or vaginal symptoms have been refractory to local therapies.

Step 2: Assess for contraindications to systemic hormone therapy.

Step 3: Assess the patient's baseline risk for stroke, cardiovascular disease, and breast cancer (consider using the 10-year ASCVD risk calculator, Framingham stroke risk score, Framingham CHD risk score, and Gail model risk score to quantify this risk). If the Framingham stroke or CHD risk score is >10% or Gail model risk score is elevated, consider alternatives to systemic hormone therapy.[b,c]

Step 4: Use the lowest dose of estrogen that relieves menopausal symptoms.

Step 5: Add systemic progesterone therapy to estrogen therapy in women who have an intact uterus.

Step 6: Assess symptoms and side effects after initiating therapy and adjust the dose of estrogen if symptoms are persistent.

Step 7: Reassess symptoms and risk factors for cardiovascular disease, stroke, and breast cancer annually.

Step 8: Discontinue systemic hormone therapy if the risks of treatment outweigh the benefits.

ASCVD = atherosclerotic cardiovascular disease; CHD = coronary heart disease.

[a]According to the North American Menopause Society, systemic hormone therapy should be avoided in women 60 years and older who have experienced menopause at the median age (51 years). If a woman has experienced menopause later than the median age, these guidelines apply within the first 10 years of menopause.

[b]Some experts indicate that systemic hormone therapy is safe in women who have experienced menopause within the last 5 years and have a Framingham CHD risk score of 10% to 20%.

[c]The majority of participants in the Women's Health Initiative had a Gail model risk score of less than 2%.

preferred by most women at midlife. Women treated with cyclic progestin may have withdrawal bleeding and should be counseled regarding this effect. Duration of combined estrogen-progestin use beyond 5 years is associated with increased risk of breast cancer and necessitates individualized risk assessment.

Absolute contraindications to hormone therapy include pregnancy, unexplained vaginal bleeding, prolonged immobilization, coronary heart disease or high risk for cardiovascular disease, or history of stroke, thromboembolic disease, or breast or endometrial cancer. Discontinuation should be individualized based on clinical symptoms and risk-to-benefit ratio. The need for continued treatment should be reevaluated annually as many women will experience diminished symptoms over time.

KEY POINTS

- Systemic hormone therapy is the most effective treatment of moderate to severe vasomotor symptoms during menopause and also provides contraception.

(Continued)

KEY POINTS *(continued)*

- All women with an intact uterus who are treated with estrogen therapy must also receive progestin to avoid estrogen-induced endometrial proliferation.

- Hormone therapy should not be initiated in women 60 years of age and older.

- Duration of combined estrogen-progestin use beyond 5 years is associated with an increased risk of breast cancer and necessitates individualized risk assessment.

Management of Genitourinary Symptoms

Mild to moderate genitourinary symptoms can be effectively treated with vaginal lubricants. Vaginal estrogen therapy is FDA-approved for women who have moderate to severe urogenital symptoms and do not respond to lubricants. Preparations include estrogen creams, vaginal estradiol tablets, and a low-dose estradiol vaginal ring. Low-dose vaginal estradiol tablets (10-25 µg) and the estradiol vaginal ring (8-9 µg) have minimal systemic estrogen absorption. Because estradiol absorption is insufficient to cause endometrial proliferation, concurrent progestin is typically not indicated when low-dose local estrogen is used to treat genitourinary syndrome of menopause.

KEY POINTS

- Vaginal estrogen therapy is indicated for treatment of moderate to severe genitourinary symptoms of menopause that do not respond to initial use of vaginal lubricants.

- Concurrent progestin is typically not indicated when low-dose local estrogen is used to treat genitourinary syndrome of menopause, since estradiol absorption is insufficient to cause endometrial proliferation.

Nonhormonal Therapy

Nonhormonal options for women with contraindications to hormone therapy or who wish to avoid the associated risks include low-dose antidepressant agents and gabapentin, which have been shown to help modulate vasomotor symptoms. Selective serotonin reuptake inhibitors and serotonin-norepinephrine reuptake inhibitors in low doses that have been shown to have efficacy greater than placebo include venlafaxine, desvenlafaxine, paroxetine, citalopram, and escitalopram. Data regarding black cohosh are inconclusive, as are studies of other herbs, soy, and other phytoestrogens.

KEY POINT

- Alternatives to hormone therapy for management of menopausal symptoms include low-dose antidepressant agents and gabapentin.

Preconception Care

Preconception counseling can significantly reduce the risk for preterm birth and birth anomalies. Preconception risk should be assessed, including personal and family medical history and psychosocial risk (**Table 63**). An obstetric history of pregnancy-induced hypertension, preeclampsia, or gestational diabetes is strongly predictive of future risk. Discussion should include maintenance of a healthy lifestyle; weight management; and tobacco, alcohol, and illicit drug cessation. Medications should be reviewed in order to minimize teratogenic exposure (**Table 64**). The pregnancy letter categories that have been used by the FDA to characterize the safety of drugs in pregnancy are provided in **Table 65**. The FDA has published changes in pregnancy and lactation labeling for prescription drugs, effective June 30, 2015 (see www.fda.gov/Drugs/DevelopmentApprovalProcess/DevelopmentResources/Labeling/ucm093307.htm). The pregnancy letter categories will be removed with the new labeling requirements; however, for prescription drugs that were previously approved, these changes will be phased in gradually. Labeling will include information relevant to the use of the drug in pregnant women (such as dosing and potential risks to the developing fetus), information about using the drug while breastfeeding (such as the amount of drug in breast milk and

TABLE 63. Preconception Risk Assessment

Risk Category	Specific Items to Assess
Reproductive awareness	Desire for pregnancy, number and timing of desired pregnancies, age-related changes in fertility, sexuality, contraception
Environmental hazards and toxins	Exposure to radiation, lead, mercury
Nutrition and folic acid consumption	Healthy diet, daily consumption of folic acid, restricting consumption of shark, swordfish, king mackerel, and tilefish to fewer than 2 servings weekly (owing to high mercury content)
Genetics	Family history of inherited genetic disorders
Substance abuse	Use of tobacco, alcohol, illicit drugs
Medical conditions	Seizure disorder, diabetes mellitus, hypertension, thyroid disease, asthma, HIV infection, systemic lupus erythematosus
Obstetric history	Pregnancy-induced hypertension, preeclampsia, gestational diabetes
Medications	Over-the-counter and prescription medications, potential teratogens
Infectious diseases and vaccinations	Immunity to varicella, rubella, pertussis, tetanus; risk for hepatitis B
Psychosocial concerns	Depression, interpersonal/family relationships, risk for abuse (physical, sexual, emotional)

Based on Johnson K, Posner SF, Biermann J, et al; CDC/ATSDR Preconception Care Work Group; Select Panel on Preconception Care. Recommendations to improve preconception health and health care—United States. A report of the CDC/ATSDR Preconception Care Work Group and the Select Panel on Preconception Care. MMWR Recomm Rep. 2006 Apr 21;55(RR-6):1-23. [PMID: 16617292]

TABLE 64.	Teratogenic Medications Commonly Prescribed by Internists
ACE inhibitors	
Androgens, testosterone derivatives	
Carbamazepine	
Folic acid antagonists	
Lithium	
Phenytoin	
Primidone	
Statins	
Tetracycline, doxycycline	
Valproic acid	
Vitamin A derivatives: isotretinoin, retinoids, etretinate	
Warfarin	

TABLE 65.	FDA Classification of Drugs in Pregnancy[a]	
Class	**Fetal Effect of Drug During Pregnancy**	
A	No disclosed fetal effects	
B	Animal studies failed to demonstrate fetal risk	
C	Animal studies suggest adverse fetal effects	
D	Evidence of human fetal risk	
X	Documented fetal abnormalities	

[a]The FDA has published changes in pregnancy and lactation labeling for prescription drugs, effective June 30, 2015. A summary of these changes is available here: www.fda.gov/Drugs/DevelopmentApprovalProcess/DevelopmentResources/Labeling/ucm093307.htm. The pregnancy letter categories will be removed with the new labeling requirements; however, for prescription drugs that were previously approved, these changes will be phased in gradually.

potential effects on the breastfed infant), and information regarding potential risks to females and males of reproductive potential who take the drug.

Measurements of BMI and blood pressure are essential. The pelvic examination may include screening cervical cytology. Testing for STIs and screening for HIV infection are also indicated. All women who are considering pregnancy should be routinely assessed for immunity to varicella and rubella. In nonimmune women, vaccination for rubella and varicella should be administered at least 4 weeks before conception to minimize fetal risk. Other routine immunizations should be current.

Supplementation with folic acid (400 µg/d) reduces the risk of neural tube defects. Because these defects occur very early in gestation, when a woman might not be aware of pregnancy, folic acid supplementation is generally recommended for all women who are of reproductive age. Supplementation with low-dose iron may reduce the risk for maternal anemia. A daily prenatal multivitamin that contains iron and folic acid, while not replacing a healthy diet, is reasonable for all women who are planning pregnancy or who may become pregnant.

- Women considering pregnancy should be routinely assessed for immunity to varicella and rubella, and other routine immunizations should be current.

Vaginitis

Vaginitis describes infectious and noninfectious conditions that cause vulvovaginal symptoms, including abnormal vaginal discharge, vulvar itching, burning, irritation, and malodor. Although vaginal discharge is frequently reported, it may not be due to infection, since normal vaginal secretions vary in color, amount, and consistency throughout the menstrual cycle. When discharge is associated with abnormal findings, the differential diagnosis most commonly includes bacterial vaginosis, vulvovaginal candidiasis, and trichomoniasis (**Table 66**). Vaginal irritation also may be caused by dermatologic conditions or allergic reactions, cervical infections, or genitourinary syndrome of menopause. A woman may have more than one type of infection at a time.

History should include duration of symptoms, relationship to the menstrual cycle, use of douches or other products, sexual activity and risk behavior, dysuria, dyspareunia, and discharge characteristics, including color, consistency, odor, pain, and itching. Risk for STIs should be considered. The vulva and vagina should be inspected for erythema, excoriations, and lesions, and vaginal wall secretions should be collected for pH, amine whiff testing, and saline and 10% potassium hydroxide (KOH) microscopy.

Bacterial Vaginosis

Bacterial vaginosis is the most common cause of vaginal discharge or malodor. It is characterized by an imbalance in the normal vaginal bacterial flora, with a decrease in hydrogen peroxide–producing lactobacilli and an increase in *Gardnerella vaginalis*, *Mycoplasma* species, and other anaerobic bacteria. When vaginal alkalinity increases after intercourse or during menses, the odor becomes stronger and is predictive of bacterial vaginosis. Bacterial vaginosis is associated with increased risk of adverse pregnancy outcomes, including preterm labor and pregnancy loss, and with increased risk for STIs and HIV infection.

Symptomatic patients may report a thin, white or gray homogeneous discharge that has a "fishy" or unpleasant odor. Accepted clinical criteria for diagnosing bacterial vaginosis include the presence of three of four characteristics: vaginal pH greater than 4.5, amine ("fishy") odor on the application of 10% KOH to vaginal secretions (whiff test), the presence of a thin homogeneous vaginal discharge, and the finding of at least 20% clue cells on a microscopic saline wet mount examination. Clue cells are squamous vaginal epithelial cells with a large number of coccobacillary organisms attached to the cell surface, causing stippling and obscuring the cell borders (**Figure 21**). Other point-of-care

TABLE 66. Clinical Presentation, Evaluation, and Management of Vaginitis

Cause of Vaginitis	Clinical Presentation	Evaluation	Management
Bacterial vaginosis	Malodorous or "fishy" vaginal discharge, often most noticeable after intercourse Increased thin white or gray discharge Symptoms other than malodor may be minimal	pH ≥4.5 KOH amine whiff test positive Saline wet mount >20% epithelial clue cells	Metronidazole: 500 mg orally twice daily for 7 days[a] (avoid alcohol during treatment and for 24 hours after last dose); or vaginal gel (0.75%) 5 g into vagina at bedtime for 5 nights Clindamycin: 300 mg orally twice daily for 7 days; or vaginal cream (2%) 5 g into vagina for 7 nights Note: Use oral regimens in pregnancy.
Vulvovaginal candidiasis	Itching, irritation, dysuria, dyspareunia, vulvodynia, excoriation, erythema, fissures Increased thick white discharge (although may be normal)	pH ≤4.5 KOH amine whiff test negative KOH wet mount with hyphae, pseudohyphae, or yeast	**Uncomplicated[b]** Fluconazole: 150 mg orally as a single dose Butoconazole vaginal: (2% cream) 5 g into vagina at bedtime for 3 nights Clotrimazole vaginal: (1% cream) 5 g into vagina at bedtime for 7-14 nights; or 100 mg vaginal tablet into vagina at bedtime for 7 nights; or 200 mg (two vaginal tablets) into vagina once daily at bedtime for 3 nights Miconazole vaginal: (2% cream) 5 g into vagina at bedtime for 7 nights; or 100 mg vaginal suppository into vagina at bedtime for 7 nights; or 200 mg vaginal suppository into vagina at bedtime for 3 nights Note: Single-dose vaginal preparations and non-imidazoles are available but less effective. **Complicated[c]** Longer duration of initial oral or topical treatment, followed by maintenance therapy: Fluconazole 150 mg orally every 3 days for a total of three doses; or topical imidazole therapy for 7-14 nights Following this, maintenance therapy is based on refractory or recurrent symptoms: Fluconazole 150 mg orally weekly for 6 months; or 200 mg orally weekly for 8 weeks; or 200 mg orally twice weekly for 4 months; or 200 mg orally once monthly for 6 months
Trichomoniasis	Increased discolored discharge (yellowish, gray, and/or frothy) Dyspareunia, dysuria, itch, erythema, postcoital bleeding, abdominal pain Punctate cervical hemorrhages ("strawberry" cervix)	pH ≥4.5 KOH amine whiff test negative Saline wet mount with trichomonads, leukocytes NAAT or rapid assay positive	Metronidazole[a]: 2 g orally as a single dose; or 500 mg orally twice daily for 7 days Note: Avoid alcohol during treatment and for 24 hours after last dose.

KOH = potassium hydroxide; NAAT = nucleic acid amplification test.

[a]Safe in pregnancy.

[b]Uncomplicated vulvovaginal candidiasis: *Candida albicans*, mild to moderate symptom severity, healthy nonpregnant women, four or fewer episodes per year.

[c]Complicated vulvovaginal candidiasis: Severe symptoms, suspected or proven non-albicans *Candida*, more than four episodes a year, uncontrolled diabetes mellitus, or immunosuppression.

tests that can aid in diagnosis utilize nucleic acid testing. Because of their low specificity, vaginal cultures are not recommended.

Treatment is with metronidazole or clindamycin, both of which are available in either oral or topical preparations. Both oral treatments are safe in pregnancy; oral metronida- zole is most cost effective. Although the pathogenesis is poorly understood, bacterial vaginosis is associated with high rates of recurrence (30%-60%). Condom use may help prevent recurrence, and douching should be avoided. Data regarding the usefulness of probiotics to increase lactobacilli are inconclusive.

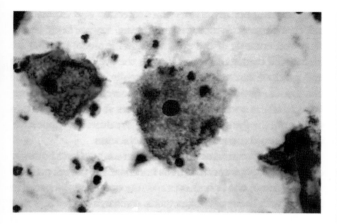

FIGURE 21. Clue cells. Vaginal epithelial cells with bacteria adherent to their surface are termed clue cells and are characteristic of bacterial vaginosis.

KEY POINT

- Clinical criteria for diagnosing bacterial vaginosis include the presence of three of four characteristics: vaginal pH greater than 4.5, positive whiff test, thin homogeneous vaginal discharge, and at least 20% clue cells on saline microscopy.

Vulvovaginal Candidiasis

Vulvovaginal candidiasis (VVC) is a common cause of vaginal symptoms in women and occurs in up to 40% of women who are evaluated for such symptoms in the primary care setting. Uncomplicated VVC develops in immunocompetent women, is sporadic and infrequent, and is likely due to *Candida albicans*. Most healthy women with uncomplicated VVC have no identifiable precipitating factors, although prevalence increases in women who are pregnant, have diabetes mellitus, or require treatment with antibiotics or glucocorticoids. Complicated VVC is recurrent (four or more episodes in 1 year), characterized by more severe symptoms, and may be due to non-albicans *Candida* such as *Candida glabrata*. It may develop in women who have uncontrolled diabetes, are immunosuppressed, or are pregnant.

A diagnosis of VVC is suggested by the presence of external dysuria and vulvar pruritus, pain, irritation, and redness. Signs include vulvar edema; fissures; excoriations; or thick, white, curdy vaginal discharge. The diagnosis can be made when a saline or 10% KOH wet mount of vaginal discharge shows yeast, hyphae, or pseudohyphae. Because VVC is associated with a normal vaginal pH (<4.5), pH testing is not useful.

As the sensitivity of microscopy is low, empiric treatment of VVC can be considered if symptoms are accompanied by characteristic findings. Several therapeutically equivalent topical and oral drugs are available, although among the topically applied drugs, imidazoles (fluconazole, miconazole, clotrimazole) are more effective than nystatin. Short-course over-the-counter intravaginal imidazole therapy may effectively treat uncomplicated VVC, as does prescription fluconazole, 150 mg orally in a single dose. A combined approach is often effective. Severe VVC requires topical therapy, preferably with an imidazole, administered intravaginally daily for 3 to 7 days with or without fluconazole, 150 mg orally every third day for a total of three doses.

Recurrent VVC is common, and retreatment is based on severity and persistence of symptoms. The pathogenesis is poorly understood, and many women have no identifiable predisposing or underlying conditions. Recurrence is treated initially with oral fluconazole every third day for a total of three doses or a 7- to 14-day course of an intravaginal imidazole. Long-term weekly suppressive oral antifungal therapy may be required to control recurrent VVC, and recurrence rates remain high after discontinuation of treatment.

KEY POINTS

- As the sensitivity of microscopy is low, empiric treatment of vulvovaginal candidiasis can be considered if symptoms are accompanied by characteristic findings.
- Short-course, over-the-counter intravaginal imidazole therapy may effectively treat uncomplicated vulvovaginal candidiasis, as does prescription fluconazole, 150 mg orally in a single dose.

Trichomoniasis

Trichomoniasis, which is caused by *Trichomonas vaginalis*, is the most common nonviral STI worldwide. Unlike other STIs that predominate in adolescents and younger adults, rates of trichomoniasis are evenly distributed among women of all age groups.

T. vaginalis is a flagellated protozoan that exclusively infects the urogenital tract, causing inflammatory vaginitis and urethritis. Although the presentation is variable, many women develop a copious, malodorous, pale yellow or gray frothy discharge with vulvar itching, burning, and postcoital bleeding.

The diagnosis has traditionally been made by direct microscopic examination of a wet mount of vaginal fluid to determine the presence of motile trichomonads. Although trichomoniasis is associated with a vaginal pH greater than 4.5, the specificity of an abnormal vaginal pH and the sensitivity of saline microscopy findings are both low. Point-of-care vaginal swab rapid immunoassays and nucleic acid amplification tests (NAATs) for detection of *T. vaginalis* have replaced microscopy or culture as the gold standard for diagnosis. NAATs can be performed on a vaginal (or endocervical) swab, urine sample, or specimens collected for liquid-based Pap tests. Once trichomoniasis is identified, testing for other STIs should be considered. Any patient who tests positive for *T. vaginalis* should be retested 3 months after treatment.

All women with symptoms should be treated with metronidazole, 2 g orally in a single dose, which is associated with high cure rates. In addition, treatment of the sexual partner is essential for preventing reinfection. Metronidazole may be safely given at any stage of pregnancy. Inadequate response to treatment may be caused by reinfection or by diminished responsiveness to metronidazole. If the latter is suspected, a

7-day course of metronidazole, 500 mg twice daily, usually results in clinical resolution.

Eye Disorders

Red Eye

Conjunctivitis

Red eye is the most frequently encountered eye disorder. As a general approach to the patient with red eye, if pain is present, especially in the setting of visual loss, pupillary distortion, or corneal involvement, emergent ophthalmology referral is indicated. In the absence of pain, continuous discharge suggests the presence of conjunctivitis, which is the most common cause of red eye.

Conjunctivitis is categorized as infectious (bacterial or viral) or noninfectious (allergic or nonallergic). History may reveal typical causes, such as allergies, viral or bacterial infections, and contact lens wear. On examination, the conjunctiva (bulbar and tarsal) appears red and vessels may be visible. In general, conjunctivitis is a diagnosis of exclusion; in a patient with red eye and discharge, a diagnosis of conjunctivitis is made only if the vision is normal and there is no evidence of angle closure glaucoma, iritis, or keratitis.

Viral conjunctivitis (**Figure 22**), typically caused by an adenovirus, is often acute, unilateral, and associated with antecedent upper respiratory tract infection and exposure to infected persons. Symptoms are itching, foreign body sensation, and crusting of the eyelids following sleep. Patients are considered contagious for as long as the eye continues to tear and produce discharge, which is usually 3 to 7 days. While contagious, patients should perform careful hand washing. Food handlers and health care providers should not return to work until the eye symptoms subside. Treatment is supportive, including cold compresses and artificial tears.

Bacterial conjunctivitis (**Figure 23**) in adult patients is usually caused by *Staphylococcus aureus* infection. The patient presents with redness in one or both eyes and mucopurulent discharge. In patients with bacterial conjunctivitis, discharge is thick and may be yellow or green in color, whereas discharge appears watery in patients with viral conjunctivitis. Treatment of bacterial conjunctivitis involves broad-spectrum topical antibiotics (erythromycin ophthalmic 0.5% ointment, bacitracin/polymyxin B ophthalmic ointment), which should be used for 5 to 7 days.

Patients with allergic conjunctivitis present with itching, sneezing, and tearing. Inspection may reveal the presence of bilateral redness and chemosis (conjunctival edema). Treatment includes oral antihistamines, topical antihistamines (olopatadine ophthalmic 0.1%, ketotifen ophthalmic), and artificial tears.

Nonallergic conjunctivitis can result from dry eye or insult with a foreign body or chemical. Nonallergic conjunctivitis typically resolves within 24 hours, although topical lubricants may be beneficial.

Episcleritis and Scleritis

Episcleritis (**Figure 24**) is an abrupt inflammation of the superficial vessels of the episclera, a thin membrane that lies just beneath the conjunctiva. The cause is often unclear; rarely, it is associated with systemic rheumatic disease. Patients with episcleritis frequently present without pain or decreased visual acuity. On examination, the inflammation appears

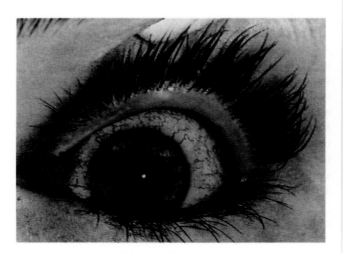

FIGURE 22. Viral conjunctivitis. Diffuse conjunctival injection and erythema, usually with a watery or mucoserous discharge, is characteristic of viral conjunctivitis.

Eye with Viral Conjunctivitis. Digital image. Wikimedia Commons. 1 Feb 2010. Web. 16 May 2012. http://commons.wikimedia.org/wiki/File:An_eye_with_viral_conjunctivitis.jpg.

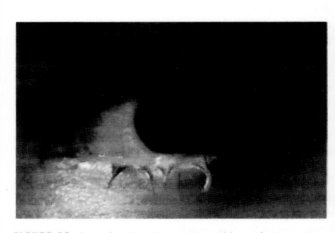

FIGURE 23. Bacterial conjunctivitis. In patients with bacterial conjunctivitis, eye discharge is thick and may be yellow or green in color.

Swollen Eye with Conjunctivitis. Digital image. Wikimedia Commons. 8 Feb 2008. Web. 16 May 2012. http://commons.wikimedia.org/wiki/File:Swollen_eye_with_conjunctivitis.jpg.

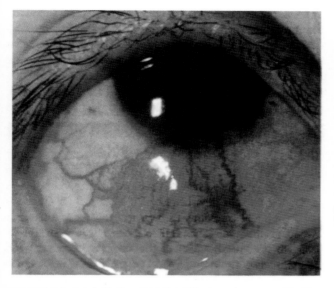

FIGURE 24. Episcleritis. Superficial dilated blood vessels are seen, with white sclera visible between the blood vessels.

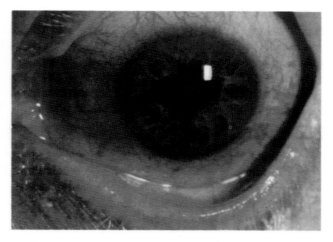

FIGURE 25. Nongranulomatous iritis (anterior uveitis). The conjunctival vessels are most dilated at the corneal edge, resulting in a circumferential redness around the iris, which is termed ciliary flush.

more localized than with conjunctivitis, which is typically diffuse. White sclera can be seen between superficial dilated blood vessels. Episcleritis typically resolves spontaneously.

Scleritis is inflammation of the sclera, the fibrous layers of the eye underlying the episclera and conjunctiva. Anterior scleritis, which is most common, involves the superficial sclera and deep vessels of the episclera. It has several forms, including diffuse, nodular, and necrotizing; the necrotizing form is more often associated with systemic inflammatory disorders. Posterior scleritis involves the deeper structures of the eye. Roughly half of patients with scleritis have an underlying systemic disease, such as an inflammatory connective tissue disorder or infection. Patients may present with severe ocular pain, photophobia, tearing, and vision changes. On examination, the sclera may have a blue or violet coloration and be tender to palpation.

Episcleritis must be distinguished from scleritis, as scleritis can be a sight-threatening condition. Generally, episcleritis is painless and involves no vision changes, whereas scleritis is painful and associated with visual impairment. Patients with scleritis, or any patients in whom the diagnosis is unclear, must be urgently referred to an ophthalmologist.

Uveitis

Uveitis (**Figure 25**) is inflammation of the middle eye, which includes the iris, ciliary body, and choroid (the vascular layer lying between the retina and the sclera). Uveitis can either be idiopathic or occur as part of an underlying systemic condition, such as autoimmune disorders, arthritides associated with HLA-B27 antigen, infection, malignancy, and sarcoidosis. Presenting symptoms of uveal inflammation are eye redness, pain, and photophobia. On examination, the conjunctival vessels are most dilated at the corneal edge, resulting in a circumferential redness around the iris (ciliary flush). The pupil may have an irregular

shape because it has become attached to the anterior surface of the lens or the posterior surface of the cornea. Uveitis requires urgent referral to an ophthalmologist.

Blepharitis

Blepharitis (**Figure 26**) is a diffuse inflammation of the sebaceous glands or lash follicles of the eyelids. Common causes are *Staphylococcus aureus* infection, rosacea, and seborrheic dermatitis. The patient may report a gritty, burning sensation and crusting or matting, especially upon awakening. Treatment includes warm compresses, application of diluted shampoo with a cotton tip applicator, topical antibiotics (for staphylococcal infections), and oral tetracyclines (for infections associated with rosacea).

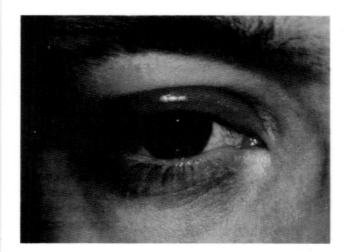

FIGURE 26. Blepharitis. Erythematous, edematous eyelids typically seen in blepharitis.

Blepharitis. Digital image. Wikimedia Commons. 2 May 2012. Web. 13 Nov 2014. https://commons.wikimedia.org/wiki/File:Blepharitis.JPG.

Subconjunctival Hemorrhage

Subconjunctival hemorrhage (**Figure 27**) is extremely common and usually benign in origin. Examination reveals a blotchy redness (from extravascular blood) that is typically confined to one area of the conjunctiva. Subconjunctival hemorrhage is painless but nonetheless alarming to patients. Most cases resolve within several weeks without intervention.

> **KEY POINTS**
>
> HVC
> - Viral conjunctivitis is often acute, unilateral, and associated with antecedent upper respiratory tract infection and exposure to infected persons; treatment is supportive.
> - Patients with bacterial conjunctivitis present with eye discharge that is thick and yellow or green in color.
> - Allergic conjunctivitis presents with itching, sneezing, tearing, bilateral redness, and chemosis (conjunctival edema) and can be treated with oral antihistamines, topical antihistamines, and artificial tears.
> - Episcleritis is painless and involves no vision changes, whereas scleritis is painful and associated with visual impairment.

Corneal Disorders

Corneal abrasions are secondary to trauma from foreign bodies and usually heal within 48 hours. Symptoms are pain, foreign body sensation, photophobia, and tearing. Physical examination requires eversion of the lid for inspection and removal of foreign bodies. The cornea can be examined by applying fluorescein dye and examining with a Wood lamp or slit lamp. Management consists of antibiotic ointments that provide comfort. Acute pain control can be achieved with topical NSAIDs, such as diclofenac and ketorolac. Topical anesthetics should be avoided after the initial examination, as they can retard healing and cause further corneal damage. A follow-up examination in 24 hours should be arranged to ensure that the corneal abrasion has healed. Eye patching is not recommended for corneal abrasions.

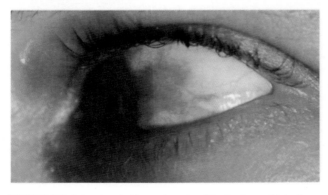

FIGURE 27. Subconjunctival hemorrhage. A well-localized superficial collection of extravasated blood is visible; the sclera and conjunctiva are not involved.

Subconjunctival hemorrhage. Digital image. Wikimedia Commons. 28 Jun 2011. Web. 16 May 2012. http://commons.wikimedia.org/wiki/File:Subconjunctival_hemorrhage_eye.JPG.

Corneal ulcers (**Figure 28**) are caused by trauma, contact lens wear, herpes simplex virus infection, bacterial infection, and connective tissue disorders (ankylosing spondylitis). On inspection, corneal ulcers are visible with fluorescein dye; herpes infections often manifest as a dendritic-appearing defect. Corneal ulcers can cause permanent visual loss and require referral to an ophthalmologist.

> **KEY POINT**
>
> - Corneal abrasions are managed with topical antibiotic ointments and topical NSAIDs; topical anesthetics and eye patching are not indicated.

Cataract

Cataracts are opacifications of the lens. Cataracts are very common and occur in over 50% of people older than 80 years in the United States. They are a leading cause of visual impairment and blindness worldwide. Risk factors include aging, family history, smoking, diabetes mellitus, ultraviolet B radiation exposure, and use of systemic glucocorticoids. Symptoms are decreased visual acuity, impaired night vision, glare, and diplopia. Ophthalmoscopic examination reveals opacification of the lens and diminished or absent light reflex. Surgery is indicated when symptoms interfere with activities of daily living; however, not all patients with cataracts will require surgery.

Glaucoma

Primary Open Angle Glaucoma

Primary open angle glaucoma (POAG), the most common type of glaucoma, is a progressive optic neuropathy associated with increased intraocular pressure (IOP) without obstruction to the normal drainage pathways of the aqueous humor. POAG is a leading cause of permanent blindness worldwide. Risk factors are age older than 40 years, family history, and race (incidence in blacks is approximately four times higher than in whites). POAG presents with bilateral peripheral visual loss

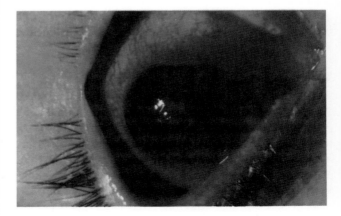

FIGURE 28. Corneal ulcer. Corneal epithelial defect with associated conjunctival injection.

that occurs gradually and painlessly; it may impair central visual acuity in later stages. Because the onset is gradual and asymptomatic, it often goes unnoticed by the patient. The U.S. Preventive Services Task Force has found that there is insufficient evidence to support the practice of screening for glaucoma. Physical examination reveals increased cup:disc ratio (>0.5), vertical extension of the central cup, and disc hemorrhages. The primary treatment is lowering IOP with medications (**Table 67**). Other interventions include laser therapy and surgical therapy, such as iridectomy or trabeculectomy.

Acute Angle Closure Glaucoma

Acute angle closure glaucoma (AACG) is caused by increased IOP resulting from blocked drainage of the aqueous humor. Symptoms are severe eye pain, headache, and decreased visual acuity. Occasionally, patients experience nausea, vomiting, and visual halos. Ophthalmoscopic examination reveals a mid-dilated (4-6 mm), nonreactive pupil and IOP greater than 50 mm Hg. There is an immediate threat of blindness from optic nerve atrophy in patients with AACG, so urgent referral to an ophthalmologist is required. Additionally, patients with chronic angle closure glaucoma should avoid certain medications that cause pupillary dilatation, including decongestants, anticholinergic agents, adrenergic agents, antidepressants, antipsychotic agents, and motion-sickness medications.

> **KEY POINTS**
>
> - Primary open angle glaucoma presents with bilateral peripheral visual loss that occurs gradually and painlessly.
>
> - Acute angle closure glaucoma presents with severe eye pain, headache, decreased visual acuity, a mid-dilated (4-6 mm) nonreactive pupil, and elevated intraocular pressure; urgent referral to an ophthalmologist is required to prevent blindness.

Age-Related Macular Degeneration

Age-related macular degeneration (AMD) is a degenerative disease of the macula. It is a leading cause of visual loss among elderly patients. AMD may be classified as either dry or wet (**Figure 29**). Dry AMD, which accounts for approximately 85% of cases, involves the deposition of extracellular material (drusen) in the macular region of one or both eyes. If the drusen become confluent in the macula, visual acuity will decrease but rarely below 20/40. Patients often report a gradual loss of vision.

A small percentage of patients with dry AMD will progress to develop new vessel growth under the retina (wet AMD). Bleeding and exudation result in sudden (or rapid onset over weeks), painless blurring or warping of central vision. Wet AMD, which often involves only one eye, results in severe visual loss.

Risk factors for developing AMD are advanced age, family history, smoking, and cardiovascular disease. Smoking cessation decreases the risk for developing AMD and should be recommended to all patients who smoke.

Dry AMD cannot be reversed with treatment; however, progression to advanced dry AMD may be slowed with the use of zinc or antioxidants. There is no evidence that antioxidants have a role in AMD prevention. Laser photocoagulation is recommended for wet AMD with extrafoveal lesions. Additionally, intraocular injection of inhibitors of vascular endothelial growth factor (VEGF) has been used to slow neovascularization of wet AMD.

> **KEY POINT**
>
> - Progression to advanced dry age-related macular degeneration may be slowed with smoking cessation and the use of zinc or antioxidants.

TABLE 67. Drug Treatment for Primary Open Angle Glaucoma

Agent	Mechanism of Action	Systemic Side Effects
β-Blockers (timolol)	Decreases inflow	Bradycardia, heart block, bronchospasm, decreased libido, central nervous system depression, mood swings
Nonselective adrenergic agonists (epinephrine)	Decreases inflow and increases outflow	Hypertension, headaches, extrasystole
Selective α₂-adrenergic agonists (brimonidine)	Decreases inflow and increases outflow	Hypotension, vasovagal attack, dry mouth, fatigue, insomnia, depression, syncope, dizziness, anxiety
Parasympathomimetic agents (pilocarpine, echothiophate iodide)	Increases outflow	Increased salivation, increased gastric secretion, abdominal cramps, urinary frequency, shock
Oral carbonic anhydrase inhibitors (acetazolamide)	Decreases inflow	Acidosis, depression, malaise, hirsutism, paresthesias, numbness, blood dyscrasias, diarrhea, weight loss, kidney stones, loss of libido, bone marrow suppression, hypokalemia, bad taste, increased serum urate level
Topical carbonic anhydrase inhibitors (dorzolamide)	Decreases inflow	Lower incidence of systemic effects compared with oral carbonic anhydrase inhibitors
Prostaglandin analogues (latanoprost)	Increases outflow	Flu-like symptoms, joint and muscle pain
Hyperosmotic agents (mannitol)	Reduces vitreous and aqueous volume	Headache, heart failure, expansion of blood volume, nausea, vomiting, diarrhea, electrolyte disturbance, kidney failure

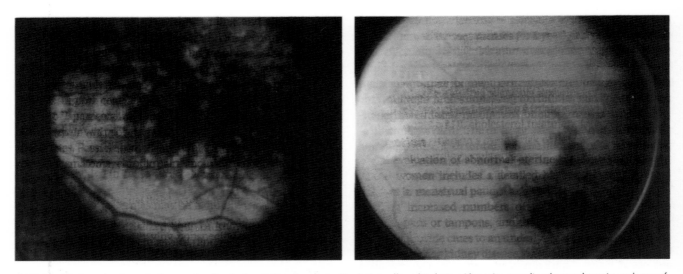

FIGURE 29. Age-related macular degeneration. The dry form (*left*), is characterized by distinct yellow-white lesions (drusen) surrounding the macular region and areas of pigment mottling. The wet form (*right*), is characterized by clumps of hyperpigmentation, hypopigmentation, and evidence of subretinal hemorrhage.

Retinal Detachment

Retinal detachment (**Figure 30**) occurs mainly in patients with myopia. Symptoms are floaters, flashes of light (photopsias), and squiggly lines, followed by a sudden, peripheral visual field defect that resembles a black curtain and progresses across the entire visual field. Emergent ophthalmology referral is crucial, as prognosis depends on the time to surgical treatment.

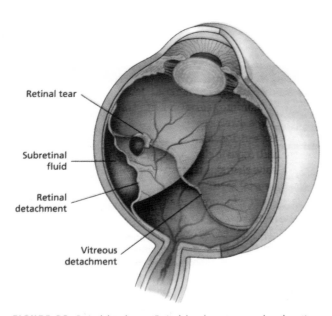

FIGURE 30. Retinal detachment. Retinal detachment occurs when the retina separates from the underlying retinal pigment epithelium and choroid and may be caused by a tear in the retina, leakage or exudation from beneath the retina, or vitreous traction pulling on the retina.

KEY POINT

- Emergent ophthalmology referral is crucial for patients with suspected retinal detachment, as prognosis depends on the time to surgical treatment.

Dry Eye

Dry eye, also called keratoconjunctivitis sicca, includes symptoms of dryness, irritation, and burning that generally worsen throughout the day. Irritants, such as smoke, allergens, and low humidity, may exacerbate symptoms.

The mechanisms of dry eye include disruption of tear secretion and increased tear evaporation. Decreased tear secretion usually results from inflammation of the lacrimal glands and may be related to systemic diseases, such as Sjögren syndrome and rheumatoid arthritis. Increased tear evaporation can be caused by increased size of the palpebral fissure, as seen in Graves ophthalmopathy, or by meibomian gland dysfunction, which reduces the tear film. Sjögren syndrome, Graves disease, and Bell palsy can cause persistent dry eye that results in corneal injury. Other risk factors for dry eye are advanced age, female sex, medications (antihistamines, selective serotonin reuptake inhibitors), diabetes mellitus, or a history of laser-assisted in-situ keratomileusis (LASIK) procedure.

Treatment focuses on reducing inflammation and correcting lid pathology that disrupts the tear film. Common treatments for dry eye are artificial tears and warm compresses. Gentle scrubs with diluted shampoo may be used for meibomianitis. Oral tetracyclines are used to treat lid inflammation. Topical cyclosporine and glucocorticoid drops are reserved for patients with dry eye from systemic illness. Punctal or canalicular plugs, very small devices that are inserted into the tear ducts to decrease tear evaporation, may be used in patients who fail to respond to conservative treatment for dry eye. Temporary or semi-permanent plugs are available.

Retinal Vascular Occlusion

Retinal Artery Occlusion

Central retinal artery occlusion (CRAO) is caused by thrombi or emboli. CRAO is most commonly associated with carotid artery atherosclerosis, although it may result from other vascular disease (carotid artery dissection), hematologic disease, or inflammatory disease (giant cell arteritis). Patients are usually elderly and present with profound and sudden painless vision loss.

Funduscopic examination reveals an afferent pupillary defect and cherry red fovea that is accentuated by a pale retinal background (**Figure 31**). Prognosis is based on visual acuity at presentation. Ischemia that lasts 4 hours or longer tends to result in irreversible vision loss. Treatment may include measures to lower IOP. Emergent ophthalmology consultation is required.

Retinal Vein Occlusion

Central retinal vein occlusion (CRVO) is usually caused by occlusion of the central retinal vein by a thrombus, whereas branch retinal vein occlusion (BRVO) is most commonly caused by arterial compression of the vein. Patients with CRVO present with sudden, painless, unilateral visual loss often mixed with "sparkles"; symptoms may be sudden or evolve over hours to days. BRVO is typically asymptomatic. Risk factors for retinal vein occlusion are advanced age, smoking, diabetes mellitus, hypertension, hyperlipidemia, obesity, glaucoma, retinal arteriolar defects, and hypercoagulable states.

Funduscopic examination may reveal an afferent pupillary defect, congested retinal veins, scattered retinal hemorrhages, and cotton wool spots in the region of occlusion (**Figure 32**). Severe visual impairment at presentation signifies the risk of permanent visual loss. Immediate ophthalmology consultation is necessary.

KEY POINT

- Patients with central retinal artery occlusion, caused by thrombi or emboli, present with profound and sudden vision loss; emergent ophthalmology consultation is required.

Eye Emergencies

Eye emergencies may include causes of acute visual loss (retinal detachment, CRAO, CRVO, temporal arteritis, endophthalmitis, orbital cellulitis, optic neuritis, chemical injury) as well as trauma to the globe, eyelid, nasolacrimal system, or tarsal plate.

Endophthalmitis is inflammation of the aqueous and vitreous humors. It is usually caused by bacterial or fungal infection following surgery. Treatment includes intravitreal antibiotics. Prognosis is dependent on how quickly treatment is started and the virulence of the pathogen.

Orbital cellulitis, another ocular emergency, results from infection of tissues posterior to the orbital septum, a membrane that extends from the orbital rims to the eyelids. Preseptal (periorbital) cellulitis originates from the eyelids and facial tissue that is anterior to the orbital septum. Orbital cellulitis often results from contiguous dental or sinus infections.

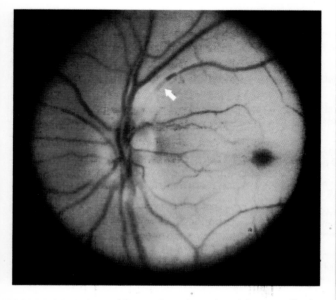

FIGURE 31. Occlusion of the central retinal artery (*arrow*) characterized by the appearance of an opalescent retina, retinal pallor, and "cherry-red spot" defining the fovea.

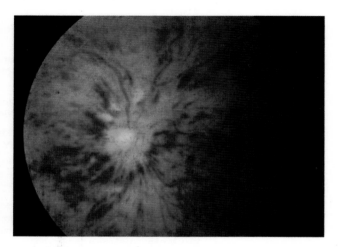

FIGURE 32. Central retinal vein occlusion characterized by optic disk swelling, dilated and tortuous veins, flame-shaped retinal hemorrhages, and cotton-wool spots ("blood and thunder").

Symptoms are eye swelling, erythema, pain, and fever. Orbital cellulitis may be distinguished from preseptal cellulitis by examining pupillary reflexes and function of the extraocular muscles and obtaining a CT scan to exclude deeper infection.

Herpes zoster involving the trigeminal nerve distribution and especially the tip of the nose (Hutchinson sign) correlates with sight-threatening herpes zoster ophthalmicus. Patients who present with Hutchinson sign require ophthalmologic evaluation.

Optic neuritis, inflammation of the optic nerve, can also result in acute visual loss. It occurs most commonly in people who are middle-aged, white, and female and is often associated with multiple sclerosis. Presenting symptoms include eye pain, blurred vision, visual field defects, and changed color perception. Evaluation includes ophthalmologic evaluation and MRI of the brain. Treatment may include systemic glucocorticoids, although optic neuritis usually resolves spontaneously.

In the case of chemical eye injuries, patients may present with severe pain, decreased visual acuity, eye redness, and photophobia and may not be able to open the eyelids. The eye should be treated with at least 30 minutes of eye irrigation while awaiting ophthalmologic evaluation. **H**

Ear, Nose, Mouth, and Throat Disorders

Hearing Loss

Hearing loss affects 28 million U.S. adults, and it is the third most common chronic health problem in the geriatric population. Hearing loss is generally categorized as conductive or sensorineural, although patients can have mixed hearing disorders (**Table 68**). Conductive hearing loss results from a mechanical problem in the ear canal, tympanic membrane, or ossicles that prevents the transmission of sound to the cochlea. Patients with conductive problems will describe general hearing loss, frequently with associated pain or drainage. Sensorineural hearing loss is caused by damage to the cochlea or acoustic nerve. Patients with sensorineural hearing loss will often describe difficulty hearing people speak, especially if there is background noise. Associated symptoms can include tinnitus or vertigo.

The U.S. Preventive Services Task Force concludes that the current evidence is insufficient to assess the balance of benefits and harms of screening for hearing loss in asymptomatic adults

TABLE 68.	Common Causes of Hearing Loss
Disease	**Notes**
Conductive	
Cerumen impaction	Cerumen may completely obstruct ear canal, causing conductive hearing loss. Impacted cerumen can be removed with gentle irrigation or an ear curette. No removal needed if asymptomatic.
Otosclerosis	Bony overgrowth of the stapes footplate with eventual fixation. Family history of otosclerosis is common. Treatment is stapedectomy or stapedotomy. Hearing aid may be helpful.
Tympanic membrane perforation	Often heals without intervention. Ear should be kept dry. Refer for possible repair if associated with significant hearing loss or possible middle ear pathology.
Cholesteatoma	An expanding mass composed of keratinizing squamous epithelial cells that may contain cholesterol crystals. Although histologically benign, it may erode extensively into local structures, including the cochlea, ossicles, tympanic membrane, and facial nerve. Treatment is surgical removal.
Sensorineural	
Presbycusis	Age-related hearing loss; typically symmetric high-frequency hearing loss. Hearing aids are mainstay of treatment.
Sudden sensorineural hearing loss	Unclear etiology; presents as a sudden loss of hearing that is sensorineural in nature. Rapid treatment with glucocorticoids may improve outcome.
Meniere disease	Classically presents as a triad of sensorineural hearing loss, tinnitus, and vertigo, although all three are not necessarily present in each patient. Symptoms may fluctuate, and attacks are often precipitated by high salt intake.
Acoustic neuroma	Benign neoplasm, usually causing sensorineural hearing loss, tinnitus, and sometimes vertigo. A family or personal history of neurofibromatosis type 2 puts patients at high risk for these tumors, often bilaterally.
Noise-induced	History of chronic noise exposure or sudden, short exposure to noise blast. Prevention is mainstay of treatment; hearing aids if condition is already advanced.
Drug-induced	History of ototoxic medication use (aminoglycosides, chemotherapeutic agents [irreversible], aspirin and NSAIDs [partially reversible], antimalarial agents [reversible], loop diuretics [sometimes irreversible]).
Both Conductive and Sensorineural	
Infection	Middle ear infection may impair movement of the tympanic membrane or ossicles, producing reversible conductive hearing loss. Viral cochleitis may cause reversible sensorineural hearing loss. Chronic ear infection may lead to conductive hearing loss.
Head trauma	May produce a conductive hearing loss from ossicular disruption and hemotympanum or a sensorineural hearing loss from cochlear fracture or auditory nerve injury.

aged 50 years or older. If undertaken, screening can be completed by simply asking the patient if he or she has difficulty hearing. Self-reported hearing loss has been shown to have 90% agreement with audiometric assessment in patients older than age 50 years. Validated screening questionnaires, such as the Hearing Handicap Inventory for the Elderly, have been shown to have high positive likelihood ratios for hearing loss. Additionally, asking close contacts about a patient's hearing impairment is important because patients may not self-perceive hearing loss. The whispered voice test is another reliable screening method for hearing loss. The examiner stands at arm's length behind the patient, and the patient occludes the untested ear canal. The examiner whispers six sets of three letter or number combinations to the patient. Failure to repeat at least three of the six sets correctly constitutes a positive result. The finger rub test involves the examiner gently rubbing his or her fingers together 6 inches (15 cm) from the patient's ear. A positive test result occurs when the patient fails to identify the rubbing in three of six attempts.

Physical examination for hearing loss should focus on differentiating between conductive and sensorineural causes using the Weber and Rinne tests (**Table 69**). During physical examination, visualization of the ear canal is important to determine if a mechanical obstruction or tympanic membrane disorder exists. Formal audiometry should be completed in patients when the etiology of the hearing loss is not evident upon examination. Imaging, usually with MRI, is rarely needed and should be reserved for patients with progressive, unilateral, or accompanying neurologic symptoms.

Sudden sensorineural hearing loss, in which the patient has a 30-dB loss over 3 days or less, requires urgent referral to an otolaryngologist and MRI to determine the underlying cause. Approximately 90% of cases are idiopathic; however, viral infection, bacterial meningitis, Lyme disease, migraine, Meniere disease, acoustic neuroma, head injury, drug reactions, and neurosarcoidosis can be causes. Most cases occur unilaterally. Treatment commonly involves glucocorticoids, although systematic reviews have shown limited success compared with placebo. Most patients recover completely within 2 weeks.

Hearing aids, which amplify environmental sounds, may be beneficial in treating conductive or sensorineural hearing loss in appropriate patients. Studies indicate that approximately 25% of patients who would benefit from hearing aids actually acquire them. Cost can create a barrier for some patients, as hearing aids are expensive and are usually not covered by insurance. Hearing aids are available in multiple styles, including behind-the-ear, in-the-canal models, and some newer hearing aids can be adjusted for only those frequencies requiring amplification.

KEY POINTS

- Screening for hearing loss can be accomplished by questioning the patient, as self-reported hearing loss has been shown to have 90% agreement with audiometric assessment in patients older than age 50 years.
- Sudden sensorineural hearing loss, in which the patient has a 30-dB loss over 3 days or less, requires urgent referral to an otolaryngologist and MRI to determine the underlying cause.

Tinnitus

Tinnitus is the perception of sound (for example, whistling, buzzing, ringing) in one or both ears that is not associated with an external stimulus. Tinnitus is most commonly caused by abnormalities within the auditory system but can occasionally have a vascular etiology. Common causes include excessive noise exposure (both acute and chronic), otosclerosis, barotrauma, infection, vascular insufficiency, Meniere disease, and metabolic disorders. Ototoxic medications may also cause tinnitus (**Table 70**). Most medications associated with ototoxicity are only ototoxic at high doses or toxic levels. Tinnitus due to medication exposure is usually reversible, with the exception of platinum-based chemotherapeutic agents and aminoglycosides.

The characteristics of tinnitus can help facilitate diagnosis and treatment. Tinnitus can be classified as pulsatile (coinciding with the patient's heartbeat) or continuous (nonpulsatile). Pulsatile tinnitus suggests a vascular etiology, such as arteriovenous malformation, atherosclerosis, carotid artery disease, aneurysm, or paraganglioma. For nonpulsatile tinnitus, time of onset, laterality, and other associated symptoms are also helpful in determining the etiology. For example, tinnitus developing in the setting of progressive hearing loss in an older

TABLE 69. Distinguishing between Conductive and Sensorineural Hearing Loss with the Weber and Rinne Tests

Condition	Weber Test[a] Result	Rinne Test[b] Result	Differential Diagnoses
Conductive hearing loss	Louder in the affected ear	Decreased in the affected ear (bone conduction > air conduction)	Cerumen impaction, foreign body, otitis media, otosclerosis, perforated tympanic membrane
Sensorineural hearing loss	Louder in the unaffected ear	As loud or louder in the affected ear (air conduction > bone conduction)	Presbycusis, Meniere disease, acoustic neuroma, sudden sensorineural hearing loss

[a]A 256-Hz vibrating tuning fork (although a 512-Hz tuning fork may be used) is applied to the forehead or scalp at the midline, and the patient is asked if the sound is louder in one ear or the other; a normal test shows no lateralization.

[b]A 512-Hz vibrating tuning fork is applied to the mastoid process of the affected ear until it is no longer heard. The fork is then repositioned outside of the external auditory canal, and the patient is asked if he or she can again hear the tuning fork; with a normal test, air conduction is greater than bone conduction, and the tuning fork can be heard.

TABLE 70. Drugs Commonly Associated with Tinnitus

Antibiotics (aminoglycosides, erythromycin, vancomycin, neomycin, polymyxin B)

Antimalarial agents (chloroquine, hydroxychloroquine, quinine)

Benzodiazepines

Chemotherapeutic agents (mechlorethamine, vincristine, carboplatin, cisplatin)

Carbamazepine

Loop diuretics

Quinidine

Salicylates

NSAIDs

Tricyclic antidepressants

patient suggests age-related hearing loss (presbycusis); unilateral tinnitus may be caused by otitis media or cerumen impaction; and tinnitus associated with unilateral sensorineural hearing loss is suggestive of acoustic neuroma.

Physical examination for tinnitus is similar to that for hearing loss. Additionally, cranial nerves should be examined for evidence of brainstem involvement. If pulsatile tinnitus is present, auscultation for bruits over the neck, periauricular area, orbits, and mastoid should be performed.

After initial history and examination, the evaluation of patients with tinnitus should include audiometry. Since various metabolic abnormalities may be associated with tinnitus (hypo- and hyperthyroidism, anemia, hyperlipidemia, zinc and vitamin B_{12} deficiencies), obtaining thyroid studies, a complete blood count, lipid studies, and zinc and vitamin B_{12} levels may be considered if clinically appropriate. Most patients with tinnitus do not require neuroimaging; however, patients with unilateral or pulsatile tinnitus, asymmetric hearing loss, or focal neurologic abnormalities should be considered for additional diagnostic imaging.

Mild tinnitus that is minimally bothersome to the patient may not require treatment. Treatment for bothersome tinnitus is directed toward the underlying disorder. Medications are largely ineffective; neurocognitive interventions (including cognitive-behavioral therapy) to help the patient cope with the problem are usually more successful. Sound-masking noise generators are sometimes employed, although limited data exist to support their effectiveness.

KEY POINT

- Medications are largely ineffective in the treatment of tinnitus; neurocognitive interventions to help the patient cope with the problem are usually more successful.

Otitis Media and Otitis Externa

Acute otitis media is characterized by fluid and inflammation in the middle ear accompanied by symptoms of infection.

Many patients with acute otitis media will first present with viral upper respiratory tract infection symptoms. Eustachian tube dysfunction, which impairs drainage and causes retention of fluid in the middle ear, is a predisposing factor. In acute otitis media, if the tympanic membrane ruptures, purulent drainage from the ear canal may be present. Otitis media with effusion is defined as fluid in the middle ear but without signs of infection. Otitis media with effusion often occurs after a case of acute otitis media or may be associated with allergies. It is also more likely if eustachian tube dysfunction is present. Evidence to guide treatment of acute otitis media in adults is lacking; however, oral antibiotics (for example, amoxicillin), analgesic therapy, and decongestants are the mainstays of treatment. If there is no response to oral antibiotics within 2 to 3 days, consideration of a broader-spectrum antibiotic is appropriate. Complications include hearing loss, tympanic membrane perforation, meningitis, and mastoiditis. Otitis media with effusion may resolve spontaneously; decongestants, antihistamines, or nasal glucocorticoids are frequently used as therapy, although evidence of their effectiveness is limited.

Otitis externa, which ranges from mild inflammation to severe infection of the external ear canal, can manifest acutely or chronically. Acute otitis externa usually has a bacterial cause, accounting for 90% of cases, whereas chronic otitis externa is frequently the result of fungal infection, allergy, or systemic dermatitis. Swimming can contribute to otitis externa (also known as swimmer's ear) when moisture in the ear canal breaks down the canal's tissue, leading to a favorable environment for bacterial growth. Manipulation or trauma to the ear canal is also a predisposing factor for the development of otitis externa. Treatment for both mild and severe cases includes dilute acetic acid solution and ototopical agents containing neomycin, polymyxin B, and hydrocortisone. Oral antibiotics are indicated for patients whose infection extends beyond the external ear canal, for older patients, for those who have not responded to topical treatment, for immunocompromised patients, and for patients with diabetes mellitus. Patients with malignant otitis externa (a necrotizing infection of the ear canal and osteomyelitis of the skull base) or disease involving the temporal or mastoid bones should be hospitalized and treated with intravenous antibiotics.

Cerumen Impaction

Symptoms of impaction can include itching, pain, hearing loss, odor, or tinnitus. Treatment is only indicated in symptomatic patients or if the tympanic membrane needs to be visualized. Treatment options include ceruminolytic agents, manual removal (with plastic or metal loop or spoon), and irrigation. Suction devices are also available that are useful in removing soft cerumen. No ceruminolytic has been shown to be superior to any other. Manual removal does not subject the ear canal to moisture, so it may be associated with lower rates of infection. However, manual removal requires operator skill and a cooperative patient.

Upper Respiratory Tract Infections

Sinusitis

Acute sinusitis can have bacterial or viral causes. In addition to the duration of symptoms, the time course and pattern of disease progression are important in differentiating viral and bacterial rhinosinusitis. Most patients with uncomplicated viral upper respiratory tract infections (URIs) do not have fever. However, if fever is present, it tends to occur early in the illness, often in conjunction with other symptoms, such as myalgia and headache. Fever and constitutional symptoms usually resolve within 24 to 48 hours, after which respiratory tract symptoms become more prominent. In most cases of uncomplicated viral URI, sinus symptoms peak between days 3 and 6 and resolve by day 10. In contrast, patients with acute bacterial sinusitis usually have symptoms (fever, purulent nasal discharge accompanied by nasal obstruction, facial pain/pressure/fullness, tooth pain) that persist without improvement for 10 days from symptom onset. Bacterial sinusitis may also present after a viral URI as a sudden onset of worsening symptoms after typical viral URI symptoms are improving (5-6 days).

Imaging with plain radiographs or CT is rarely needed and does not help in distinguishing bacterial from viral sinusitis. Initial treatment of acute sinusitis (viral and bacterial) is focused on symptom relief. Analgesics, decongestants (systemic or topical), antihistamines, intranasal glucocorticoids, and nasal saline irrigation are frequently prescribed. Although more than 90% of cases of acute sinusitis are viral in origin, antibiotics are frequently prescribed for patients presenting with acute sinusitis symptoms, resulting in inappropriate antibiotic overuse. The Infectious Diseases Society of America (IDSA) recommends initial symptomatic treatment with initiation of antibiotics only in patients with 3 to 4 days of severe symptoms (fever, purulent drainage, and facial pain), worsening of symptoms that were initially improving, or failure to improve with symptomatic treatment after 10 days. Amoxicillin-clavulanate and doxycycline are recommended as first-line antimicrobial therapy. Macrolides, trimethoprim-sulfamethoxazole, and second- and third-generation cephalosporins are no longer recommended because of bacterial resistance. Second-line therapy is higher-dose amoxicillin-clavulanate or doxycycline. Fluoroquinolones should be reserved for those who have failed to respond to initial therapy or those with a history of penicillin allergy, and as second-line therapy for patients at high risk for bacterial resistance. **Figure 33** provides an algorithmic approach for the treatment of acute bacterial rhinosinusitis.

Rhinitis

Allergic rhinitis should be suspected if rhinitis symptoms (sneezing, congestion, rhinorrhea) are associated with a season, environment, or exposure. A thorough history focusing on symptom triggers is necessary for diagnosis. A management algorithm for patients with rhinitis is provided in **Figure 34**. If the history and examination are suggestive of allergic rhinitis, a therapeutic trial for symptom relief is indicated. Pharmacotherapy may include intranasal glucocorticoids, oral antihistamines, intranasal antihistamines, oral leukotriene inhibitors, or intranasal cromolyn. In general, topical agents should be tried before oral agents. Combining therapies may be helpful in patients who have persistent symptoms when using a single agent. If the patient does not respond to these therapies, referral to an allergist-immunologist may be necessary for skin testing, immunotherapy, and medication adjustment.

Nonallergic (vasomotor) rhinitis is defined as chronic rhinitis symptoms without an associated exposure. Patients may describe triggers such as food, odors, or temperature. Treatments include intranasal glucocorticoids, antihistamines, anticholinergics, and nasal saline irrigation. Nasal irrigation can be completed using isotonic saline administered with a specific device (neti pot) that allows the solution to be poured into one nostril with drainage out through the other nostril while keeping the mouth open to breathe. Rhinitis medicamentosa is the syndrome of chronic rhinitis resulting from long-term use of topical nasal decongestants. Treatment involves discontinuing the decongestant; intranasal glucocorticoids may be beneficial.

Pharyngitis

Pharyngitis most frequently has a viral cause (up to 80% of cases). However, group A streptococcal (GAS) pharyngitis, which accounts for approximately 15% of cases, should be detected to prevent potentially serious complications, such as acute rheumatic fever. Diagnosis and treatment of patients with GAS pharyngitis is aided by the four-point Centor criteria: (1) fever, (2) absence of cough, (3) tonsillar exudates, and (4) tender anterior cervical lymphadenopathy. No additional testing or treatment is needed for patients who meet zero or one criterion. Patients who meet two or three criteria should have a confirmatory test (either a rapid antigen detection test for GAS or throat culture) and be treated based on the findings. Rapid antigen detection testing for GAS has a specificity of greater than 95% and a sensitivity of 85% to 95%. Patients with four criteria are at highest risk and can be treated empirically. Penicillin is first-line treatment for GAS pharyngitis, and erythromycin or azithromycin are alternatives in patients who are allergic to penicillin. Complications of GAS pharyngitis include rheumatic fever and peritonsillar abscess.

Pharyngitis can also be caused by group C and group G streptococci. Patients will present with symptoms similar to GAS pharyngitis, although the syndrome is often less severe with groups C and G streptococci. Groups C and G streptococci

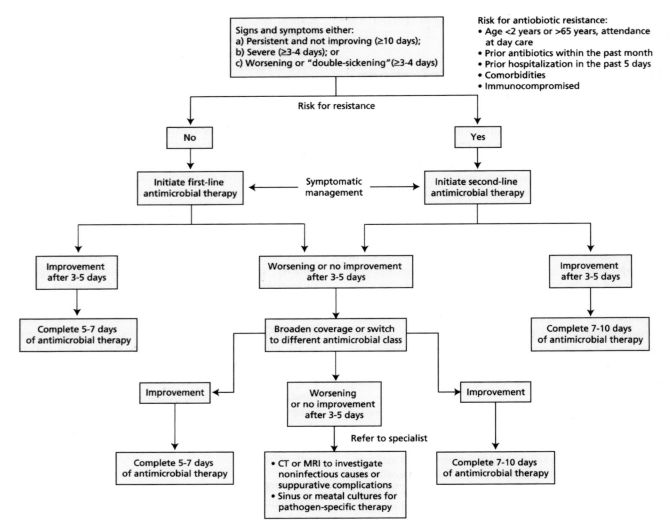

FIGURE 33. Algorithm for the management of acute bacterial rhinosinusitis.

Reprinted from Chow AW, Benninger MS, Brook I, et al; Infectious Diseases Society of America. IDSA clinical practice guideline for acute bacterial rhinosinusitis in children and adults. Clin Infect Dis. 2012 Apr;54(8):e72-e112. [PMID: 22438350] by permission of Oxford University Press.

are not associated with acute rheumatic fever; however, glomerulonephritis and reactive arthritis may rarely occur. Treatment is with oral antibiotics.

Lemierre syndrome is a rare complication of acute pharyngitis that involves septic thrombosis of the internal jugular vein. The initial infection spreads from the oropharynx into the parapharyngeal space and blood vessels leading to the internal jugular vein. This diagnosis should be considered in patients with antecedent pharyngitis and persistent fever despite antibiotic treatment. Soft-tissue CT of the neck with contrast typically shows a jugular vein thrombus with surrounding tissue enhancement. Treatment of Lemierre syndrome includes intravenous antibiotics. Surgical drainage may become necessary if an abscess forms. The need for anticoagulation should be determined on a case-by-case basis; its use in Lemierre syndrome has not been studied in clinical trials.

KEY POINTS

- In patients with symptoms of acute sinusitis, antibiotics are recommended only for those with 3 to 4 days of severe symptoms (fever, purulent drainage, and facial pain), worsening of symptoms that were initially improving, or failure to improve after 10 days.

- Allergic rhinitis is a clinical diagnosis, and effective initial treatments are intranasal glucocorticoids, antihistamines, or cromolyn.

- Diagnosis and treatment of patients with group A streptococcal pharyngitis is aided by the four-point Centor criteria: (1) fever, (2) absence of cough, (3) tonsillar exudates, and (4) tender anterior cervical lymphadenopathy.

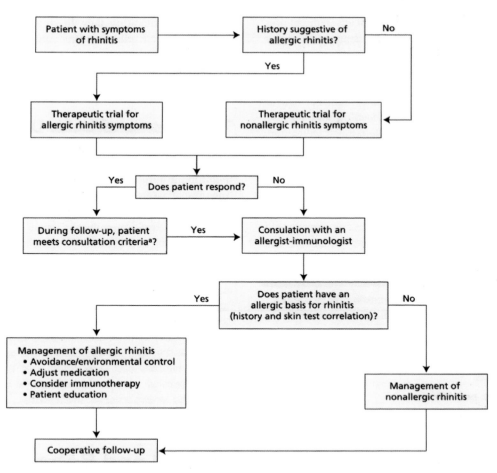

FIGURE 34. Algorithm for the management of rhinitis.

^aCharacteristics that should lead to consideration of consultation with an allergist-immunologist include the following:

- The patient has had prolonged manifestations of rhinitis; complications of rhinitis, such as otitis media, sinusitis, and/or nasal polyposis; and/or a comorbid condition, such as asthma and chronic sinusitis.
- The patient has required a systemic glucocorticoid for the treatment of rhinitis.
- The patient's symptoms or medication side effects interfere with ability to function or significantly decrease quality of life, such as a decrease in comfort and well-being, sleep disturbance, anosmia, or ageusia.
- Treatment with medications for rhinitis is ineffective or produces adverse events.
- The patient has been diagnosed with rhinitis medicamentosa.
- Allergic/environmental triggers causing the patient's rhinitis symptoms need further identification and clarification.
- There is a need for more complete education.
- The patient has required multiple and/or costly medications over a prolonged period.
- Specific allergy immunotherapy is a treatment consideration.

Epistaxis

Approximately 90% of nosebleeds originate along the anterior nasal septum, which is where four arterial supplies converge and anastomose as the Kiesselbach plexus. The remaining 10% of epistaxis episodes occur posteriorly (behind the posterior middle turbinate, requiring a nasopharyngoscope for visualization). The presentation of anterior epistaxis is usually obvious, whereas posterior epistaxis can be asymptomatic. Causes of epistaxis may include nose picking, intranasal medication use, dry nasal mucosa, rhinosinusitis, and neoplasms. Hematologic malignancies, hemophilia, acquired bleeding disorders, and anticoagulant or antiplatelet medication use are also associated with epistaxis due to their bleeding diatheses. Routine laboratory testing is not required. If there are symptoms of anemia or significant blood loss, a hemoglobin level should be obtained. A complete blood count, prothrombin time, and activated partial thromboplastin time might be considered in patients with symptoms or signs of a bleeding disorder and those with severe or recurrent epistaxis. CT imaging may be considered if a foreign body, tumor, or sinusitis is a suspected cause.

Initial treatment for anterior epistaxis is patient-exerted compression of the nasal ala against the septum for at least 15 minutes, which will stop most anterior bleeds. If direct pressure fails, visualization of the anterior septum should be attempted to find the source of bleeding. Removal of clots or foreign bodies can be done with suction, irrigation, or forceps. If a bleeding site is found, silver nitrate or a topical vasoconstrictor (oxymetolazone or phenylephrine) can be applied to control the bleeding. If the bleeding does not stop, anterior nasal packing should be applied. Electrical cautery by an otorhinolaryngologist may be necessary if these therapies fail. An otorhinolaryngologist should be consulted for patients with posterior bleeds that require packing. Most patients who require posterior packing should be hospitalized for observation and assessed for the need for further intervention. The packing typically remains in place for 4 to 5 days. An antibiotic is typically given to prevent sinusitis and otitis media. 🄷

KEY POINT

- Initial treatment for anterior epistaxis is patient-exerted compression of the nasal ala against the septum for at least 15 minutes.

Oral Health

Oral Infections and Ulcers

Oral mucosal findings are discussed in MKSAP 17 Dermatology.

Dental Infection

Dental infections may involve the tooth, bony structures, or gingiva. Infections of the tooth structure are typically asymptomatic until they involve the pulp cavity, at which point an abscess can develop. Dental pulp infection, as a result of caries, is the leading cause of odontogenic infection. Prompt referral to a dental specialist is warranted. Endodontic removal of diseased pulp (root canal) or extraction of the infected tooth is the definitive treatment. If dental care is not immediately available, therapy should focus on pain relief until the appropriate intervention (filling, root canal, local irrigation, incisional drainage) can be performed.

Periodontal disease involves inflammation of the gingiva, with or without accompanying destruction of supportive connective tissue and alveolar bone. Periodontal disease may be linked with an increase in atherosclerotic cardiovascular disease. Therapy should focus on performing proper oral hygiene.

Halitosis

Eighty percent to 90% of cases of halitosis originate in the mouth, principally as a result of microbial breakdown of food, saliva, and other substances. Halitosis can also be associated with sinusitis, nasal polyps, tonsillar stones, esophageal diverticula, and chronic pulmonary infections, as well as other systemic diseases leading to alterations in the odor of the breath, such as ketoacidosis or advanced liver disease or kidney failure. Treatment includes good oral hygiene, including daily flossing and scraping the posterior tongue. A chlorhexidine mouthwash used nightly may also be effective in reducing odor. Patients with dental caries, abscesses, or periodontal disease should receive dental care.

Temporomandibular Disorders

Temporomandibular disorders include articular disorders (derangements of the intra-articular disk of the temporomandibular joint [TMJ]) and masticatory muscle disorders (myofascial pain syndrome). TMJ disorder can present with jaw pain, headache, and clicking. Most TMJ symptoms are self-limited. Evaluation should involve exclusion of other disorders such as trigeminal neuralgia, mastoiditis, dental pain, temporal arteritis, or herpes zoster. Palpation of the TMJ may reveal tenderness, clicking, or crepitus. Generally, imaging is not indicated; however, CT is useful in diagnosing osteoarthritis of the TMJ, and MRI can provide information about soft tissues and vasculature. Treatment involves jaw relaxation with physical therapy exercises, cognitive-behavioral therapy, jaw appliances, and analgesic medications. In patients with osteoarthritis of the TMJ, glucocorticoid injection may be beneficial. In refractory cases, referral for arthrocentesis, arthroscopy, or joint replacement may be warranted.

Mental and Behavioral Health

Mood Disorders

Mood disorders are characterized by disturbed mood accompanied by cognitive, psychomotor, and vegetative symptoms and interpersonal difficulties. Mood disorders include depressive disorders and bipolar disorder.

Depressive Disorders

About 20% of women and 12% of men experience depression during their lifetimes; peak onset is approximately age 40 years for women and age 55 years for men. Depression is a leading cause of disability and a risk factor for suicide. Depression is common in persons with medical diseases; its presence adversely affects outcomes of the diseases.

Depression is a common reason for primary care visits but is often underrecognized. The U.S. Preventive Services Task Force recommends screening adults for depression when appropriate support for definitive diagnosis, effective treatment, and follow-up is available. Validated depression screening tools are available, the simplest being a two-question instrument ("Over the past 2 weeks, have you felt down, depressed, or hopeless?" and "Over the past 2 weeks, have you felt little interest or pleasure in doing things?"). A positive response to either question warrants further evaluation.

Some nonpsychiatric conditions manifest symptoms that mimic depression, including chronic infectious diseases (such as HIV), endocrine diseases and conditions (such as thyroid and adrenal gland diseases, androgen deficiency, or menopause), cancer, heart failure, neurologic diseases (such as Parkinson disease or multiple sclerosis), and sleep apnea. Medications can also cause symptoms of depression (such as glucocorticoids, hormone therapies, interferons, or anticancer drugs).

Diagnosis

Major Depressive Disorder

Major depressive disorder is diagnosed according to the DSM-5 by the presence of at least five of the following symptoms during the same 2-week period, at least one of which is depressed mood or loss of interest or pleasure:

1. Depressed mood most of the day, nearly every day by self-report (for example, feels sad, blue, or hopeless) or observed by others (for example, frequently tearful)

2. Markedly diminished interest or pleasure in all, or almost all, activities most of the day, nearly every day

3. Significant weight loss when not dieting or weight gain or decrease or increase in appetite nearly every day

4. Insomnia or hypersomnia nearly every day

5. Psychomotor agitation or retardation nearly every day

6. Fatigue or loss of energy nearly every day

7. Feelings of worthlessness or excessive inappropriate guilt nearly every day

8. Diminished ability to think or concentrate nearly every day

9. Recurrent thoughts of death (not just fear of dying); recurrent suicidal ideation with or without a specific plan; suicide attempt

Depressive symptoms cause work-related and social impairment and cannot be attributed to a medical condition, drug, or substance abuse. A tool for identifying and assessing the severity of depression is the PHQ-9 (www.integration.samhsa.gov/images/res/PHQ%20-%20 Questions.pdf); the items correlate with the DSM-5 criteria. Each item is scored from 0 (not bothered by the symptom) to 3 (bothered by the symptom every day); the maximum score is 27. A score of 5 to 9 indicates mild, 10 to 14 moderate, 15 to 19 moderately severe, and ≥20 severe depression. Physicians should determine whether the depressed patient has a history of abnormal elevation of mood (termed mania or hypomania based on the degree); this may indicate bipolar disorder, which is treated differently than depressive disorders. Notably, treating a patient with bipolar depression with an antidepressant drug alone (that is, without a mood stabilizer) may "switch" the patient's depression to mania.

Persistent Depressive Disorder

Symptoms of persistent depressive disorder (formerly known as dysthymia) are milder than those of major depressive disorder. DSM-5 diagnostic criteria are 1) depressed mood most of the day, more days than not, for at least 2 years and 2) the presence, while depressed, of two or more of the following symptoms: poor appetite or overeating, insomnia or hypersomnia, low energy or fatigue, low self-esteem, poor concentration or difficulty making decisions, and feelings of hopelessness. Symptoms do not abate for more than 2 months.

Seasonal Affective Disorder

Seasonal affective disorder is a subtype of major depressive disorder characterized by the onset of symptoms during autumn or winter, which resolve during the subsequent spring. It is more common in women than in men. Affected patients experience psychomotor retardation, overeating, and hypersomnia. Diagnosis requires 3 consecutive years of symptoms.

Premenstrual Dysphoric Disorder

Premenstrual dysphoric disorder affects 3% to 5% of menstruating women. It is characterized by the presence of specific symptoms occurring during the final week before the onset of menses, which improve within a few days after the onset of menses and become minimal or absent the week after menses. Primary symptoms required for diagnosis include one of the following: affective lability, irritability or anger with interpersonal conflict, depressed mood, or anxiety. Additional symptoms include decreased interest in usual activities, difficulty concentrating, lack of energy, appetite changes, sleep disturbance, a sense of loss of control, and other physical symptoms (such as breast tenderness, bloating, weight gain).

Peripartum Depression

The DSM-5 has changed the term *postpartum depression* to *peripartum depression* because nearly 50% of women develop these symptoms during pregnancy. Peripartum depression affects 10% to 15% of women within 6 months of giving birth. Single and poor mothers are at greatest risk. Although not considered an independent disorder, it is specified by DSM-5 as major depressive disorder that occurs during pregnancy or within 4 weeks following delivery, although clinical symptoms may not be recognized until after this period.

Persistent Complex Bereavement Disorder

Grief and bereavement are normal responses after the death of a loved one. Emotional lability, sadness, loneliness, sense of numbness, dreams of the deceased, and fleeting visual or auditory hallucinations of the deceased are all common during the normal grieving process. Normal grieving often occurs in fits and starts but gradually becomes less intense over time. Grieving that lasts for more than 12 months (6 months in children); is associated with persistent yearning, sorrow, or preoccupation with the deceased; disrupts normal function or social relationships; and is out of proportion to cultural norms is considered pathologic and is termed persistent complex bereavement disorder, formerly complicated grief disorder. Nearly 20% of all bereaved persons experience persistent complex bereavement disorder. Risk factors for the development of persistent complex bereavement disorder include pre-existing psychiatric illness, excess caregiver burden, and ongoing significant life stressors. The death of a loved one can also precipitate a true major depressive episode in a vulnerable individual, and the presence of grief does not necessarily exclude the existence of concomitant major depression.

Management

Most patients with mild or moderate depression (for example, PHQ-9 score <15) are treated by primary care physicians. In the United States, generalists prescribe 75% of all antidepressant medications; psychiatric referral is reserved for those with complex psychiatric comorbid conditions or when initial antidepressant treatments fail to achieve desired results. Before initiating treatment, medical illnesses, medications, and drug use that cause symptoms of depression and bipolar

disorder should be ruled out. Psychotherapy (cognitive-behavioral therapy [CBT], psychodynamic therapy, and interpersonal therapy) and psychopharmacology, alone or in combination, are mainstays of treatment and can prove synergistic. In addition to those refractory to initial treatment, referral to a psychiatrist is indicated for patients with homicidal or suicidal ideation, psychotic symptoms, or evidence of bipolar disorder. Diet, exercise, spiritual support, and other measures are adjuncts.

Several classes of antidepressant drugs are available (**Table 71**). Choice of drug is based on the patient's symptoms, the drug's side effects, and the patient's personal and family history of responses to antidepressant drugs. The initial dose should be low and subsequently increased based on clinical response. Patients should be informed of potential side effects and that side effects will likely occur before benefits. Patients who do not respond to full-dose antidepressant monotherapy for 6 weeks may respond to a different antidepressant drug, either from the same or a different class, or the addition of a second antidepressant drug. Another strategy is to add an antipsychotic drug. The FDA has approved

TABLE 71.	Characteristics of Selected Antidepressants	
Drug	**Advantages**	**Disadvantages**
SSRIs		
Citalopram	Few drug interactions	GI and sexual side effects
Escitalopram	Few drug interactions	GI and sexual side effects
Fluoxetine	Long half-life reduces risk for withdrawal syndrome; effective for anxiety disorders, OCD, PMDD	Long half-life increases risk for drug accumulation; drug interactions common; CYP2D6 substrate
Fluvoxamine	OCD, SAD, panic disorder	GI and sexual side effects; sleep disturbance
Paroxetine	Effective for anxiety disorders, panic disorder, PTSD, OCD	FDA pregnancy category D; weight gain; constipation; sedation; drug interaction; high risk for withdrawal syndrome
Sertraline	Few drug interactions; effective for panic disorder, PTSD, OCD, PMDD	GI and sexual side effects; sleep disturbance
SNRIs		
Venlafaxine	Effective for anxiety disorders	Nausea; elevated heart rate and blood pressure
Desvenlafaxine	Effective for anxiety disorders	Nausea; elevated blood pressure
Duloxetine	Effective for pain syndromes and GAD	Nausea; urinary retention
Tricyclic Antidepressants		
Nortriptyline	Analgesic effect; sedating	Cardiac toxicity with overdose; anticholinergic effects
Amitriptyline	Analgesic effect; sedating	Cardiac toxicity with overdose; anticholinergic effects; weight gain
Other Agents		
Bupropion	Fewer sexual side effects than SSRIs; energizing; improved concentration; less weight gain	Seizure risk; elevated blood pressure
Mirtazapine	Sedating; increased appetite	Sedation; weight gain
Trazodone	Sedating; increased sexual function	Sedation; orthostatic hypotension; priapism

GAD = generalized anxiety disorder; GI = gastrointestinal; OCD = obsessive-compulsive disorder; PMDD = premenstrual dysphoric disorder; PTSD = posttraumatic stress disorder; SAD = seasonal affective disorder; SNRI = serotonin-norepinephrine reuptake inhibitor; SSRI = selective serotonin reuptake inhibitor.

the following combinations of antidepressant and antipsychotic drugs for the treatment of depression: aripiprazole or quetiapine extended-release with any antidepressant, and olanzapine with fluoxetine.

About 50% of patients with unipolar depression successfully treated with acute pharmacotherapy followed by placebo and about 40% of patients successfully treated with acute CBT followed by no subsequent treatment experience relapse and recurrence of depression after 1 year. To prevent relapse, an American Psychiatric Association guideline recommends continuation therapy (4 to 9 months) for patients with unipolar depression who respond to acute therapy. In general, the dose of antidepressant drug used in the acute phase should be used in the continuation phase and depression-focused psychotherapy should be continued for those receiving it. Patients with severe depression or those who have experienced more than two depressive episodes are at increased risk for recurrent depression and should be considered for life-long treatment.

Antidepressant drugs should not be stopped abruptly; they should be tapered gradually to avoid discontinuation syndromes. Although some antidepressant drugs have been associated with precipitating suicidal ideation, the risk of suicide in untreated depression is likely greater.

The most widely prescribed antidepressant drugs are selective serotonin reuptake inhibitors (SSRIs). SSRIs have excellent safety profiles compared with tricyclic antidepressant drugs, but adverse sexual side effects (such as reduced libido, anorgasmia, or delayed orgasm) are common. Serotonin-norepinephrine reuptake inhibitors (SNRIs) are helpful in patients who also have pain syndromes. Bupropion is an alternative agent for patients with SSRI- or SNRI-associated sexual side effects; however, this agent is contraindicated in patients with seizure disorders. Monoamine oxidase inhibitors (MAOIs) are seldom used. SSRIs, SNRIs, and MAOIs, particularly if used in combination, can cause serotonin syndrome, which is characterized by altered mental status, autonomic instability, and neuromuscular hyperactivity and is potentially lethal. Patients who do not respond to a single SSRI may respond to another antidepressant drug from the same or different class, adding a second antidepressant, or adding psychotherapy. For some patients, electroconvulsive therapy may be indicated, which is safe (low mortality risk) and effective.

Treatment of seasonal affective disorder involves daily therapeutic exposure (30-60 minutes) to 10,000 lux of visible light; antidepressant drugs and CBT are also used.

Treatment of premenstrual and peripartum depression is similar to that of other forms of depression. Notably, there are no contraindications to breastfeeding while taking antidepressant drugs. However, SSRIs and SNRIs are FDA pregnancy category C (paroxetine is category D).

Persistent complex bereavement disorder does not usually require pharmacologic treatment; medications, when used, should target specific symptoms (such as hypnotics for sleep). Pastoral care, support groups, and counseling may be helpful.

KEY POINTS

- About 20% of women and 12% of men experience depression during their lifetimes; depression is a leading cause of disability and a risk factor for suicide.
- Depression is common in persons with medical diseases; its presence adversely affects outcomes of the diseases.
- The U.S. Preventive Services Task Force recommends screening adults for depression when appropriate support for definitive diagnosis, effective treatment, and follow-up is available.
- Psychotherapy (cognitive-behavioral therapy, psychodynamic therapy, and interpersonal therapy) and psychopharmacology, alone or in combination, are mainstays of treatment of depression.
- Referral to a psychiatrist is indicated in patients with depression refractory to initial treatment, homicidal or suicidal ideation, psychotic symptoms, or evidence of bipolar disorder.

Bipolar Disorder

Bipolar disorder is a mood disorder characterized by episodes of mania or hypomania. Prevalence is about 1%. Men and women are equally affected; onset is usually during early adulthood. It is rare for patients with bipolar disorder to have mania or hypomania only; most have recurrent depressive episodes. Lifetime risk for suicide is high (6%-15%).

Bipolar I disorder is defined as one or more manic episodes. A manic episode is characterized by at least 7 days of severe, abnormally expansive, euphoric, or irritable mood associated with at least three of the following symptoms (four if irritable mood only): grandiosity or inflated self-esteem, pressured speech, flight of ideas, distractibility, increased goal-directed activity or psychomotor agitation, excessive involvement in pleasurable activities with high potential for adverse consequences (for example, spending sprees, sexual encounters), and lessened need for sleep. Dysfunction is substantial. The episode is not attributable to the physiologic effects of a substance (for example, a drug of abuse, a medication, other treatment) or to another medical condition. Most patients with bipolar I disorder experience depressive episodes. Bipolar II disorder is defined as major depression and hypomania. Compared with mania, hypomania is less severe, results in less dysfunction, and is present for at least 4 days.

Psychiatrists should be involved in the management of patients suspected of having bipolar disorder. Pharmacotherapy involves mood stabilizers (such as lithium, valproic acid, and carbamazepine) or lamotrigine; these drugs are essential because risk for recurrent manic or depressive episodes in affected patients is high. Lithium has a narrow therapeutic window and may adversely affect kidney and thyroid function. Acute manic episodes are usually treated with lithium or valproic acid and an atypical antipsychotic drug (such as olanzapine, quetiapine, or aripiprazole). FDA-approved pharmacologic treatments for bipolar depression are quetiapine and combination olanzapine-fluoxetine. Psychotherapy is adjunctive.

KEY POINT

- Mood stabilizers are essential in the treatment of bipolar disorder because risk for recurrent manic or depressive episodes in affected patients is high.

Anxiety Disorders

Generalized Anxiety Disorder

Generalized anxiety disorder (GAD) is relatively common; the lifetime prevalence in U.S. adults is between 4% and 7%. GAD affects women more than men. Patients with GAD often experience sweats, dyspnea, palpitations, difficulty swallowing, nausea, chest and abdominal pain, loose stools, muscle tension, insomnia, fatigue, tachycardia, and tremor. Diagnosis should be considered in patients with multiple unexplained physical symptoms.

The DSM-5 diagnostic criteria for GAD are as follows: 1) excessive anxiety or worry about a number of events or activities (for example, school or work) occurring more days than not for 6 months or longer; 2) the patient recognizes it is difficult to control the worry; 3) the anxiety or worry is associated with three or more of the following symptoms: restlessness, easy fatigability, difficulty concentrating, irritability, muscle tension, and sleep disturbance; 4) the anxiety, worry, or symptoms cause impairment at school, work, or other settings and cannot be attributable to medical or other psychiatric conditions, medications, or substance use.

A tool for identifying and assessing the severity of GAD is the GAD-7 (www.adaa.org/sites/default/files/GAD-7_Anxiety-updated.pdf). Treatment options include psychotherapy and medications. CBT is the most effective psychotherapy for GAD and in trials has been shown to be as effective as medications. SSRIs, SNRIs, and tricyclic antidepressant agents are effective if needed. Benzodiazepines are often used for GAD but carry a risk for dependence. Nonetheless, benzodiazepines can be useful in the early stages (for example, the first 6 weeks) of SSRI treatment–the time often necessary for SSRIs to take effect. The GAD-7 can be used to monitor symptom severity over time, allowing clinicians to monitor treatment effectiveness.

Panic Disorder

The lifetime prevalence of panic attack is 10% to 30%. However, the prevalence of panic disorder is much lower (about 2% in women and 1% in men); onset usually occurs during early adulthood. Not all patients with panic attacks have panic disorder. Panic attacks occur in patients with panic disorder but can also occur in other depressive or anxiety disorders as well.

Panic disorder is characterized by recurrent, unexpected, and abrupt surges of extreme anxiety that peak within minutes and is accompanied by four or more of the following symptoms: palpitations, sweating, trembling, dyspnea, choking sensation, chest pain, nausea or abdominal pain, lightheadedness, chills or heat sensations, numbness or tingling, feeling detached from oneself, and fear of losing control or dying. Diagnosis requires that an attack be followed by at least 1 month of worry by the patient that he or she will experience a recurrent attack. Because of physical symptoms, patients with panic disorder often present to primary care physicians or emergency departments after a panic attack; however, panic disorder is often unrecognized. The diagnosis should be considered if medical mimics (for example, hyperthyroidism, pheochromocytoma, substance use) are unlikely or have been excluded.

The recommended treatment of panic disorder is an antidepressant (SSRI or SNRI) in combination with CBT. If needed, a short course of a long-acting benzodiazepine (clonazepam) can be used in the first few weeks as the antidepressant is escalated. Shorter-acting benzodiazepines should be used with caution and for short periods because there is increased addiction potential. Treatment duration for panic disorder is about 1 year after symptom control is achieved, then reassessed.

Social Anxiety Disorder

Social anxiety disorder (formerly known as social phobia) has a lifetime prevalence of about 2.5%. Social anxiety disorder is characterized by severe, persistent anxiety or fear of social or performance situations (public speaking, meeting unfamiliar people) lasting 6 months or longer. In these situations, affected patients experience anxiety and physical symptoms such as palpitations, dyspnea, and flushing. Patients recognize their anxiety is excessive but nonetheless avoid trigger situations (or endure them with extreme anxiety), resulting in impairments at home, work, and other settings.

Treatment of social anxiety disorder includes CBT and medications. SSRIs and the SNRI venlafaxine are first-line therapy for social anxiety disorder.

Posttraumatic Stress Disorder

The DSM-5 diagnostic criteria for posttraumatic stress disorder (PTSD) are complex. In general, PTSD occurs in response to directly experiencing or witnessing traumatic events (actual or threatened death, injury, or sexual violence), learning that such an event has occurred to a loved one, or experiencing repeated or extreme exposures to "aversive details" of traumatic events. PTSD is characterized as at least 1 month of symptoms, including intrusive memories of the traumatic event, recurrent nightmares or flashbacks, persistent avoidance of reminders, persistent negative changes in thoughts and mood associated with the event, and alterations in arousal and reactivity (exaggerated startle, hypervigilance, sleep disturbance, reckless behavior). PTSD usually presents within 1 month of the traumatic event, but symptoms can be delayed.

Risk factors for PTSD include greater severity of the stressor, poor social support in general and especially after the stressor, subsequent life stressors (for example, loss of employment), parental neglect, and family and personal history of psychiatric disorder. Among veterans, those with traumatic brain injury (TBI) have a higher prevalence of PTSD than veterans without TBI; information about evaluating for PTSD in veterans is available from the Veterans Administration (www.mentalhealth.va.gov/communityproviders/miniclinics.asp). Comorbid psychiatric conditions may include depression, anxiety, and substance abuse. Patients with PTSD are at increased risk for occupational and marital discord and suicide.

Treatment of PTSD includes psychotherapy and medications. A psychotherapist with experience in treating survivors of trauma can be very helpful. Antidepressant drugs, especially SSRIs, are useful. Trazodone is useful for insomnia and nightmares (usually used in combination with another drug such as an SSRI). Benzodiazepines are not effective for PTSD.

Obsessive-Compulsive Disorder

Obsessive-compulsive disorder (OCD) is characterized by obsessions (persistent and intrusive thoughts, images, or impulses that are associated with distress) and compulsions (repetitive behaviors such as hand washing, counting, and inspecting that are done in order to decrease distress caused by the obsession), resulting in wasted time, marked distress, or impaired social function. Obsessive traits often precede the disorder. Prevalence is 2% to 3%; men and women are affected equally.

CBT is the primary treatment for OCD. Medications for OCD include SSRIs (sertraline, paroxetine, fluoxetine, and fluvoxamine) and clomipramine. Benzodiazepines are sometimes used for acute exacerbations but not as monotherapy. Treatment should continue for 1 to 2 years, then be reassessed.

KEY POINTS

- Cognitive-behavioral therapy has been shown to be as effective as medications in the treatment of generalized anxiety disorder.
- Panic disorder should be considered as a diagnosis in patients who present to the emergency department with physical symptoms of a panic attack if medical mimics (for example, hyperthyroidism, pheochromocytoma, substance use) are unlikely or have been excluded.
- Cognitive-behavioral therapy is the primary treatment for obsessive-compulsive disorder.

Substance Abuse Disorders

Tobacco

At least 70% of smokers will visit a physician each year, thus providing a key opportunity for tobacco cessation interventions.

Patients should be asked about tobacco use at each visit, as it has been shown to increase the frequency of tobacco cessation discussions in the clinical setting and to increase tobacco cessation rates. The Agency for Healthcare Research and Quality (AHRQ) and others have endorsed using the "5 A's" approach to office tobacco counseling (see Screening Recommendations for Adults in Routine Care of the Healthy Patient). For smokers not ready to quit, motivational interviewing, with emphasis on nonconfrontational strategies and discussion of patient choices, has shown higher cessation rates than use of brief advice or usual care. High-intensity counseling (greater time and number of sessions) is more effective than low-intensity strategies; for clinicians with limited time, recommendations are to use adjunctive telephone counseling, as every state in the United States has telephone counseling quit line services (1-800-Quit-Now).

Pharmacotherapy has proven to be effective and should be offered to those without contraindications (**Table 72**). Bupropion is contraindicated in patients with seizures and other conditions that can lower seizure threshold. Varenicline should be dose adjusted in patients with severe kidney impairment. Both bupropion and varenicline can cause vivid dreams and can increase suicidality. Bupropion can be used with long-acting (nicotine patches) or short-acting (nicotine gum, lozenges, inhalers, nasal spray) nicotine replacement. Varenicline can be used with a short-acting nicotine replacement, although a few studies have demonstrated safety and efficacy in combining varenicline and long-acting nicotine replacement. Bupropion and varenicline can also be combined. Referral to a specialist is appropriate, especially in cases of relapse.

Alcohol

The DSM-5 combined alcohol abuse and alcohol dependence as a single entity, termed alcohol use disorder, which is characterized as problematic alcohol use causing significant distress or impairment within a 12-month period. Common features include continued alcohol use despite recurrent adverse consequences, craving and impaired control of alcohol use, tolerance, and withdrawal. Alcohol use disorder should be treated as a chronic disease. Excessive alcohol use is the third-leading preventable cause of death, behind smoking and obesity. Much of the mortality risk is related to an increased risk of accidental death, including motor-vehicle accidents and drowning. Suicide rates are also higher among frequent alcohol users. Given the health risks associated with alcohol use, screening all adults is recommended (see Screening Recommendations for Adults in Routine Care of the Healthy Patient). The primary treatment of alcohol use disorder is psychosocial interventions (counseling, motivational interviewing, CBT, residential care, peer support groups such as Alcoholics Anonymous). Pharmacotherapy (naltrexone and acamprosate) can be used in combination with psychosocial treatment. Naltrexone is contraindicated in patients receiving or withdrawing from any opioid and in those with liver failure or hepatitis. Acamprosate enhances abstinence but is contraindicated in kidney disease.

TABLE 72. Commonly Used Pharmacologic Therapies for Smoking Cessation

Agent	Mechanism	Effectiveness	Initial Prescription	Advantages	Disadvantages
Nicotine gum[a]	Prevents nicotine withdrawal[b]	Increases cessation rates about 1.5-2 times at 6 mo.	1 piece (2 mg) whenever urge to smoke, up to 30 pieces/d. Continuous use for >3 mo not recommended. Max dose: 24 pieces/d	Less expensive than other forms of nicotine replacement. Chewing replaces smoking habit. No prescription required. Associated with delay in weight gain.	Some patients find taste unpleasant.
Nicotine patch (24 h)[a,c]	Prevents nicotine withdrawal[b]	Increases cessation rates about 1.5-2 times at 6 mo.	Most patients: 21-mg patch for 4-8 wk (remove and replace every 24 h), then 14-mg patch for 2-4 wk, followed by 7-mg patch for 2-4 wk. Max dose: 22 mg/d. Adults weighing <100 lb (45.5 kg), smoking fewer than 10 cigarettes/d, and/or with cardiovascular disease: 14-mg patch for 4-8 wk, then 7-mg patch for 2-4 wk.	Less expensive than other forms of nicotine replacement. No prescription required.	Can cause skin irritation.
Nicotine nasal spray[a]	Prevents nicotine withdrawal[b]	Increases cessation rates about 1.5-2 times at 6 mo.	1 spray (0.5 mg) in each nostril 1-2 times/h whenever urge to smoke, up to 10 sprays/h or 80 sprays/d. Initially, encourage use of at least 16 sprays/d, the minimum effective dose. Recommended duration of therapy is 3 mo. Max dose: 80 sprays/d; do not exceed 10 sprays/h.	Some patients prefer this delivery method.	More expensive than other forms of nicotine replacement. Requires a prescription. Safety not established for use >6 mo.
Nicotine inhaler[a]	Prevents nicotine withdrawal[b]	Increases cessation rates about 1.5-2 times at 6 mo.	6-16 cartridges (containing 4 mg)/d for up to 12 wk, followed by gradual reduction in dosage over a period up to 12 wk.	Some patients prefer this delivery method.	More expensive than other forms of nicotine replacement. Requires a prescription. Use >6 mo not recommended.
Nicotine lozenge[a]	Prevents nicotine withdrawal[b]	Increases cessation rates about 1.5-2 times at 6 mo.	1 lozenge (2 mg or 4 mg) every 1-2 h during weeks 1-6, then 1 lozenge every 2-4 h during weeks 7-9, then 1 lozenge every 4-8 h during weeks 10-12. Patients who smoke within 30 min of waking require 4-mg lozenge; those who have first cigarette later in the day require 2-mg lozenge. Recommended duration of therapy is 12 wk.	Some patients prefer this delivery method.	Some patients find the taste unpleasant. Side effects include nausea, dyspepsia, and mouth tingling. Avoid acidic beverages (juice, soda) 15 min before use.

(Continued on the next page)

Alcohol withdrawal occurs with chronic heavy alcohol use within hours to days after alcohol cessation. Early withdrawal symptoms occur within a few hours of abstinence and include agitation, anxiety, tremulousness, headache, and symptoms of autonomic hyperactivity (fever, diaphoresis, tachycardia, hypertension). Generalized tonic-clonic seizures may occur usually within 6 to 24 hours and should be treated with benzodiazepines because if left untreated, up to one third of patients may progress to delirium tremens. In general, antiepileptic drugs are not required. Delirium tremens is characterized by fluctuating levels of consciousness, confusion, and agitation with marked autonomic overdrive and is associated with a 5% mortality rate.

TABLE 72.	Commonly Used Pharmacologic Therapies for Smoking Cessation *(Continued)*				
Agent	Mechanism	Effectiveness	Initial Prescription	Advantages	Disadvantages
Bupropion	Unclear	Increases cessation rates about 2 times at 1 y.	Begin 1-2 wk before quit date; start with 150 mg once daily for 3 days, then 150 mg twice daily through end of therapy (7-12 wk max). Max dose: 150 mg twice daily.	Some antidepressant activity; may be a good option for patients with a history of depression. Associated with a delay in weight gain.	Requires a prescription. Can interact with other drugs. Safety in pregnancy is unclear. Associated with hypertension. Avoid in patients with eating disorders, patients with seizure disorder or at risk for seizure, and in patients taking MAOIs. May cause vivid dreams and increase suicidality.
Varenicline	Reduces cravings via nicotine receptor agonist.	Increases cessation rates >3.5 times and almost 2 times over bupropion at 12 wk.	Begin 0.5 mg once daily on days 1-3, then 0.5 mg twice daily on days 4-7, then 1 mg twice daily through end of therapy (12 wk). Consider additional 12 wk of therapy to prevent relapse. Max dose: 1 mg twice daily.	No hepatic clearance. No clinically significant drug interactions reported.	Requires a prescription. Associated with hypertension. Safety in pregnancy is unclear. Caution in severe kidney disease. May cause nausea, insomnia, vivid dreams, and increased suicidality.

[a]Avoid nicotine replacement in patients with recent myocardial infarction, arrhythmia, or unstable angina. Safety of nicotine replacement in pregnancy is unclear.

[b]A standard cigarette contains approximately 1 mg of nicotine.

[c]Several formulations of patches are available. Dosing guidelines are for patches designed to stay in place for 24 h and that come in doses of 21 mg, 14 mg, and 7 mg. Clinicians should check prescribing information on nicotine patches that come in other doses or that are designed for use <24 h/d.

Adapted with permission from Wilson JF. In the clinic. Smoking cessation. Ann Intern Med. 2007 Feb 6;146(3):ITC2-1-ICT2-16. [PMID: 17283345]

Treatment of alcohol withdrawal includes thiamine and glucose to prevent Wernicke encephalopathy, intravenous fluids, multivitamins with folate, correction of electrolyte abnormalities, and long-acting benzodiazepines (short-acting benzodiazepines if there is severe liver disease). Benzodiazepines should be given as needed, rather than by scheduled dosing or continuous infusion.

The Clinical Institute Withdrawal Assessment (CIWA) scale may be useful to help monitor symptoms and deliver treatment. Patients with low CIWA scores can be monitored as an outpatient and may not require medication, whereas those with moderate scores should receive medication. Those with high CIWA scores, history of an alcohol withdrawal seizure or delirium tremens, or suicidal ideation should be hospitalized and in some cases require intensive care.

Drugs

Illicit drug use is common and affects 9% of the U.S. population yet often goes undetected. Any illicit drug use should be considered harmful given potential health and legal consequences of even infrequent use. Asking about illicit drug use and prescription drug misuse is recommended during initial medical visits and when clinically relevant (see Routine Care of the Healthy Patient). The approach to treatment is similar to that for tobacco and alcohol misuse, consisting primarily of behavioral interventions. Prevalence of co-occurring serious mental illnesses with substance abuse, high-risk sexual behavior, and polysubstance abuse is increased among illicit drug users. Veterans who have experienced combat, multiple deployments, and those with PTSD are at higher risk for substance abuse. The Veterans' Administration has created a series of veteran-focused mini clinics to help clinicians optimize mental health and wellness among veterans. Module topics include tobacco use, substance abuse, PTSD, mental illness, and suicide prevention and are available at www.mental-health.va.gov/communityproviders/miniclinics.asp.

KEY POINTS

- For smokers not ready to quit, motivational interviewing, with emphasis on nonconfrontational strategies and discussion of patient choices, has shown higher cessation rates than use of brief advice or usual care.

- Pharmacotherapy with nicotine replacement, bupropion, and/or varenicline has proven to be effective for smoking cessation and should be offered to those without contraindications.

- The primary treatment of alcohol use disorder is psychosocial interventions.

Personality Disorders

A personality disorder is characterized by persistent patterns of inner experiences and behaviors that digress substantially from the expectations of the affected person's culture. These disorders are entrenched, rigid, and stable over time, and lead to substantial impairment and distress. Onset is usually during adolescence or early adulthood. There are 10 specific personality disorders, which are grouped into 3 clusters based on symptoms (**Table 73**). Persons with personality disorders usually do not recognize their interactions with others as abnormal.

Patients with personality disorders often interface with the health care system. Physicians should balance the patient's need to be seen (for example, frequent, yet brief, visits) with clear boundaries. Patients with personality disorders often

TABLE 73. Personality Disorders
Cluster A: Odd or Eccentric Thinking and Behaviors
Paranoid: pervasive distrust of others; unjustified suspicion of others; unjustified suspicions regarding their partners or spouses; overly hostile reactions to perceived insults
Schizoid: prefer to be alone and lack interest in relationships; seem indifferent, cold, and unresponsive to social cues; take pleasure in few activities
Schizotypal: manifest odd thinking, beliefs (e.g., their thoughts are magical and can influence others, events have hidden meaning), dress, and other behaviors
Cluster B: Dramatic or Unpredictable Thinking and Behaviors, Emotional
Antisocial: engage in behaviors such as lying, stealing, and other aggressive and violent behaviors; disregard others' feelings, rights, and safety; lack remorse for these behaviors; often experience recurrent legal problems
Borderline: have chaotic relationships (idealized and devalued) and a fragile self-image; fear abandonment; experience labile and intense emotions (e.g., anger), sense of emptiness; engage in impulsive and risky behaviors (e.g., gambling, sex); may manifest self-injury and suicidality
Histrionic: excessive emotionality and attention-seeking behavior; dramatic; often seductive or sexually provocative; melodramatic
Narcissistic: grandiose and inflated self-perceptions; desire attention
Cluster C: Anxious and Fearful Thinking and Behaviors
Avoidant: feel inadequate and are sensitive to criticism; extremely shy and socially inhibited and avoid activities that involve interactions with others, especially strangers
Dependent: excessively dependent on others ("clingy") and fear being alone; lack self-confidence and tolerate poor treatment by others
Obsessive-compulsive: perfectionistic and preoccupied with orderliness and rules; controlling of situations and others; rigid regarding values; not the same as obsessive-compulsive disorder, which is an anxiety disorder

Reprinted with permission from Schneider RK, Levenson JL. Psychiatry Essentials for Primary Care. Philadelphia: American College of Physicians, 2008.

require more time than the primary care physician can realistically provide and may benefit from referral to a mental health professional. Affected persons may benefit from psychotherapy. There are no FDA-approved medications for personality disorders; medications are used to relieve symptoms (for example, mood stabilizers for mood swings and impulsivity).

Somatic Symptom and Related Disorders

The DSM-5 has reclassified the somatoform disorders under the term somatic symptom and related disorders (SSRDs). More commonly encountered in nonpsychiatric settings, these disorders may be seen in up to 20% of patients in primary care settings. Such patients have very high utilization of health care despite overall dissatisfaction with their medical care. Although patients with these disorders typically present with medically unexplained symptoms, this should not be used as the key diagnostic feature. Instead, the patient's interpretation of the symptoms causes functional impairment.

Diagnostic criteria for somatic symptom disorder are as follows: at least one somatic symptom causing distress or interference with daily life; excessive thoughts, behaviors, and feelings related to the somatic symptom(s) (disproportionate or persistent concern about seriousness of symptoms, persistent high level of anxiety about health, or excessive focus of time and energy on health concerns); and persistent somatic symptoms for at least 6 months (does not have to be the same symptom for 6 months).

When this disorder has pain as the main symptom, the specifier "with predominant pain" should be used because this diagnosis has replaced pain disorder. Illness anxiety disorder (previously known as hypochondriasis) is characterized by excessive worry about general health and preoccupation with health-related activities (such as measuring pulse). Unlike somatic symptom disorder, patients with illness anxiety disorder have no or only mild somatic symptoms. Conversion disorder (functional neurologic symptom disorder) involves one or more symptoms of abnormal sensation or motor function (such as limb weakness) that are not explained by a medical condition and are inconsistent with physical examination findings. Factitious disorder is a deliberate falsification of symptoms or infliction of injury on oneself or another, even in the absence of clear external benefit. Prior to diagnosing any of the somatic symptom and related disorders, excluding or optimizing treatment of organic disease or other psychiatric disorders (such as depression and generalized anxiety) is indicated.

These patients are challenging and difficult to treat. The symptoms are often chronic in nature and patients frequently undergo repetitive and unnecessary diagnostic testing, which often leads to unnecessary invasive medical and surgical interventions. Management begins with an open discussion of the diagnosis, scheduling of regular follow-up visits, and coordination of care with a psychiatrist. Diagnostic testing should be avoided as a means of reassurance. Antidepressants may be beneficial, but CBT has greater potential for managing the underlying behavioral disorder.

Eating Disorders

Types

The DSM-5 has reshaped the classification for eating disorders. Binge eating disorder (BED), now formally recognized as a separate entity, is defined as recurring episodes (on average ≥1 per week for 3 months) of eating significantly more food in a short period than most people would under similar circumstances while feeling a lack of control. Common features include eating more rapidly than normal, feeling uncomfortably full, eating large amounts when not hungry, eating alone due to embarrassment, and feeling disgust or guilt afterward. These features can help differentiate BED from the common occurrence of overeating.

Compared with BED, bulimia nervosa is characterized by frequent episodes (≥1 per week) of binge eating followed by inappropriate compensatory behaviors (self-induced vomiting or misuse of laxatives, diuretics, and enemas) due to fear of weight gain. Physical examination may reveal erosion of dental enamel, parotid gland swelling, xerosis, and Russell sign (scarring or calluses on the dorsum of the hand if used to induce vomiting).

Anorexia nervosa is an important entity to recognize because it is associated with high mortality. It is characterized by persistent caloric intake restriction leading to significantly low body weight, a distorted body image, and an intense fear of gaining weight or becoming fat. Subtypes include restricting type (no binge eating or purging behaviors) and binge eating/purging type (purging with or without binging). It primarily affects adolescent girls and young women but can also affect men and older women. In the DSM-5, amenorrhea is no longer included in the diagnostic criteria, although this still commonly occurs. Physical examination may reveal emaciation, brittle hair and nails, lanugo, xerosis, yellow skin especially of the palms (from hypercarotenemia), and edema.

Medical Complications

Anorexia nervosa is associated with multiple medical complications, nearly all of which are reversible with restoration of ideal body weight. Loss of bone density, seen in ≥30% of patients, often is not completely reversible, in part because anorexia nervosa often affects adolescents before peak bone mass is reached. Bone density measurement is often suggested after 6 to 12 months of continued symptoms. Vital sign abnormalities may also occur and are reflective of a hypometabolic

state, including sinus bradycardia, hypotension, and hypothermia. Electrolyte abnormalities (hypokalemia, hypomagnesemia, hypophosphatemia) are often seen and can contribute to life-threatening arrhythmias and prolonged corrected QT intervals. Other laboratory abnormalities include anemia, leukopenia, and elevation of liver chemistry tests. Refeeding syndrome is another serious complication and can be avoided by gradually increasing caloric intake according to basal metabolic rate during the first few weeks of the refeeding.

Bulimia nervosa can also cause electrolyte derangements leading to arrhythmias but also involves gastrointestinal-related complications, including esophagitis, Mallory-Weiss tears, and esophageal rupture. Purging and misuse of laxatives, diuretics, and enemas can cause electrolyte abnormalities.

Both anorexia nervosa and bulimia nervosa also impart an increased risk of depression, anxiety, substance abuse, and suicide risk.

Treatment

The primary treatment of eating disorders is restoration of normal weight and eating behaviors. This can be done in a combination of outpatient, residential, or inpatient settings involving a multidisciplinary team, including a primary care physician, dieticians, and mental health specialists.

Treatment of anorexia nervosa involves psychotherapy (including family therapy, especially in adolescents) and nutritional restoration (supervised meals, medical monitoring, and hospitalization in severe cases). Intense psychological support is often needed during the process of regaining weight. In bulimia nervosa and BED, CBT has been consistently shown to be beneficial. Antidepressants can be useful in bulimia nervosa (fluoxetine is FDA approved for bulimia nervosa) but have not demonstrated benefit in the treatment of anorexia nervosa. Olanzapine has shown recent promise in reducing obsessive-compulsive tendencies and improving weight gain in anorexia nervosa. Antidepressants and topiramate have shown benefit in BED.

Schizophrenia

Schizophrenia often begins in late adolescence and is characterized by at least two of the following symptoms: delusions, hallucinations, disorganized speech, disorganized or catatonic behavior, and negative symptoms (affective flattening, alogia, or avolition). These symptoms must affect one or more major areas of functioning (work, interpersonal relations, or self-care) and have been present for 6 months (including at least 1 month of active symptoms).

Schizophrenia is associated with a 2- to 3-fold increase in mortality, which is due to a 13-fold increased risk of suicide and greater than 2-fold increase in cardiovascular disease mortality. Rates of hypertension, dyslipidemia, diabetes mellitus, obesity, smoking, and metabolic syndrome are significantly increased. Atypical antipsychotics may contribute to metabolic complications. Furthermore, schizophrenia is often associated with undertreatment of chronic medical disorders and low rates of obtaining screening and preventive care.

Antipsychotic medications are first-line therapy for schizophrenia. Typical antipsychotics have a higher risk of sedation, anticholinergic effects, extrapyramidal symptoms, and hyperprolactinemia. Second-generation antipsychotics have fewer extrapyramidal symptoms and are more effective than typical antipsychotics. Clozapine has proved more effective than other antipsychotics but requires routine blood monitoring because it can cause agranulocytosis. Both clozapine and olanzapine are associated with high risk of weight gain and metabolic complications.

KEY POINT

- Antipsychotic medications are first-line therapy for schizophrenia; clozapine has proven more effective than other antipsychotics but requires routine blood monitoring because of the potential for agranulocytosis.

Attention-Deficit/Hyperactivity Disorder

The diagnosis of attention-deficit/hyperactivity disorder (ADHD) requires persistent inattention and/or hyperactivity-impulsivity that interfere with functioning or development in at least two areas of life (home, work, school, peer relationships). Although symptoms need to be present by the age of 12 years, a diagnosis is often not made until later. Up to 60% of children with ADHD continue to have symptoms as an adult, although adult ADHD remains underdiagnosed and undertreated. Symptoms of hyperactivity and impulsivity often lessen over time; adults with ADHD may be easily distracted, disorganized, and feel restless. Many adults have comorbid psychiatric problems such as sleep disorders, depression, anxiety, and substance abuse. Stimulants are first-line therapy in adults without a substance abuse history; given their cardiovascular side effects (hypertension, arrhythmias, cardiac arrest), routine blood pressure monitoring is necessary. In those with a history of substance abuse, the selective norepinephrine reuptake inhibitor atomoxetine may be useful. CBT is a useful adjunctive treatment.

Autism Spectrum Disorder

The DSM-5 has eliminated the subclassifications of autism (including Asperger syndrome) and merged these entities into autism spectrum disorder (ASD). ASD describes heterogeneous conditions characterized by repetitive behaviors and persistent deficits in communication and social interaction associated with impairment in function. Symptoms must be present in early childhood but may not manifest or may be masked by compensatory skills until later in life. ASD may be associated with intellectual or language impairment (some may have specific exceptional abilities). It is also associated with seizures, sleep disorders, and gastrointestinal and feeding problems. Acute changes in behavior may signal an underlying medical issue rather than a behavioral issue. If possible, internists should involve the patient's caregiver to optimize communication during the visit. Use of clear, brief language, visual aids, or alternative modes of communication may be helpful. Treatment involves specialists and community resources consisting of sustained behavioral and educational interventions, which may include speech, language, and occupational therapy, and should also involve caregivers. Pharmacotherapy (antipsychotics) and complementary therapies (diet modification, music therapy) can also be used. Early intervention improves outcomes. Adults with autism have normal life expectancies, but most continue to require at least some assistance, with some requiring life-long residential care. Follow-up care should be life-long.

Geriatric Medicine
Comprehensive Geriatric Assessment

The evaluation of geriatric patients must emphasize functional ability, independence, and quality of life. The comprehensive geriatric assessment prioritizes these outcomes through multidisciplinary review of physical health, functional status, sensory capacity, cognition, mental health, and environmental factors that affect patients and their caregivers. Performance of comprehensive geriatric assessment in the home and in dedicated geriatric inpatient hospital units has demonstrated improved morbidity and mortality and decreased rates of institutionalization. The impact of outpatient or inpatient consultative comprehensive geriatric assessment on outcomes is less clear.

Functional Assessment

Functional status can be evaluated by assessing basic activities of daily living (ADLs) and instrumental activities of daily living (IADLs). Basic ADLs refer to self-care tasks necessary to provide one's own personal care. IADLs are tasks necessary to maintain an independent household, such as using the telephone, preparing meals, and managing one's own medications. Identifying deficiencies in ADLs and IADLs allows for the provision of appropriate support services. There are several screening tools available that may be used to measure functional status in the older adult (**Table 74**).

TABLE 74.	Indices to Assess Basic and Instrumental Activities of Daily Living		
Index	**Assessed Functional Activity**	**Scoring**	**Comments**
Katz Index of Independence in Activities of Daily Living	Bathing Dressing Toileting Transferring Continence Feeding	The Katz Index is scored by assigning a score of 1 point to each activity if it can be performed independently, which is defined as requiring no supervision, direction, or personal assistance; scores are then added for a range of 0 to 6. (6 = fully functional; 4 = moderately impaired; 2 = severely impaired)	Simple to use/score; brief, takes only a few minutes to complete. Less discriminative at low levels of disability.
Modified Barthel Index	Feeding Bathing Grooming Dressing Bowels Bladder Toilet use Transfers Mobility Stairs	Each item in the Modified Barthel Index is scored on a range from 0 to 15, depending on how much the patient is able to do. Total scores range from 0 to 100, with 100 being fully independent. In stroke patients, a score of less than 60 is considered a poor outcome.	A form must be filled out; takes approximately 10 minutes to complete. Highly validated in multiple settings. Better discriminative function and very sensitive to change.
Lawton and Brody Instrumental Activities of Daily Living (IADL) Scale	Ability to use telephone Shopping Food preparation Housekeeping Laundry Transportation Medication management Ability to handle finances	The Lawton and Brody IADL Scale is scored by assigning a score of 1 point to each activity if it can be performed at all; scores are then added for a range of 0 to 8, with a score of 8 representing independence and 0 representing total dependence for IADLs.	Simple to use; brief, takes only a few minutes to complete.

Vision

Visual impairment, often resulting from cataracts, macular degeneration, presbyopia, glaucoma, or diabetic retinopathy, is common in the elderly, but frequently underrecognized by patient and physician alike. There is little evidence that standard vision screening tests actually improve outcomes in older adults. Vision screening tests, such as the Snellen eye chart, primarily measure visual acuity, which may help identify presbyopia but may miss visual deficits due to the other previously mentioned ocular disorders. Glaucoma and macular degeneration are difficult to detect in the primary care setting. A functional assessment of vision, such as having the patient read a paragraph of newsprint, seems reasonable, but there is no evidence to support its use as a screening measure. Therefore, although visual acuity screening is inexpensive and simple to perform, it may be insufficient alone to adequately assess elderly patients. Although the U.S. Preventive Services Task Force (USPSTF) has found inconclusive evidence to justify routine vision screening in older adults, the American Academy of Ophthalmology recommends a comprehensive medical eye examination by an eye professional in asymptomatic adults aged 65 years and older every 1 to 2 years; more frequent screening is recommended for patients with risk factors for diabetes mellitus or glaucoma.

Hearing

Hearing loss is common in the elderly, with a prevalence as high as 80% in those over 80 years of age. In this population, hearing loss results in significant impairment in quality of life and potentially leads to depression and social isolation, which may be further exacerbated by feelings of frustration that hearing loss can engender in caregivers. Because the patient may experience difficulties in understanding and communication, hearing loss in the elderly is frequently misdiagnosed as cognitive dysfunction. Presbycusis, age-related hearing loss, is the most common etiology, and its onset is subtle. Presbycusis begins as high-frequency hearing loss but progresses over time to encroach on frequencies important to hearing people speak. Often, patients report inability to understand speech rather than an inability to hear.

The USPSTF does not make a recommendation regarding screening for hearing loss in asymptomatic older patients.

However, patients who have cognitive or affective concerns that may be related to hearing should be evaluated for hearing loss. No one screening test has been shown to be superior to another. Whispered voice test, finger rub test, hearing loss questionnaire, and hand-held audiometry are all reasonable screening tests (see Ear, Nose, Mouth, and Throat Disorders). Patients who test positive in this clinical scenario or who report hearing loss should be referred for formal audiologic testing and consideration of hearing aids.

Hearing aids may improve communication abilities in older adults; however, they require considerable patient motivation to be used effectively, and cost may be a significant issue for many patients. In studies, the patients who have benefited from hearing aids have predominantly self-identified as having hearing loss. There is limited evidence suggesting that hearing aids may improve quality of life and mood and decrease social isolation.

Depression

Depression is common in older adults, although it is both underrecognized and undertreated. In the United States, depression is present in 5% of men aged 60 years and older and 7% of women aged 60 years and older. Additionally, older persons have higher rates of completed suicide than younger adults, although older adults attempt suicide less often. Depression should be suspected in the older adult if there are mood symptoms more intense than expected, poor response to medical therapy, low motivation, and lack of engagement with providers. In the elderly, depression can frequently masquerade as cognitive impairment or multiple somatic complaints, resulting in delayed diagnosis.

A simple two-question screen is highly sensitive (97%) but less specific (67%) for depression in the elderly. Using this tool, the clinician asks, "During the past month, have you been bothered by feeling down, depressed, or hopeless?" and "During the past month, have you been bothered by little interest or pleasure in doing things?" A positive response to either question constitutes a positive screening result. Because the specificity of the two-question screen is low, a positive result should be further evaluated with a more extensive diagnostic instrument, such as the Geriatric Depression Scale (GDS) or PHQ-9. Both the GDS and PHQ-9 have been validated in the elderly population and have similar positive predictive values for the diagnosis of depression. The GDS relies less on somatic symptoms and has a simplified yes-or-no format, which may be more conducive to screening those with cognitive impairment.

Selective serotonin reuptake inhibitors are considered first-line pharmacotherapy for the elderly. Further discussion on diagnosing and treating depression can be found in Mental and Behavioral Health.

Cognitive Function

Dementia affects more than 35% of persons age 90 years and older. It is characterized by a progressive decline in at least two cognitive domains (memory, attention, language, visuo-spatial, executive) that is severe enough to impair functioning. Mild cognitive impairment (MCI) represents cognitive deficits that do not affect daily functioning. In older patients who are asymptomatic, there is currently insufficient evidence to support routine screening for cognitive impairment. However, since patients with cognitive dysfunction are at increased risk for accidents, medical nonadherence, and behavioral disturbances, physicians should maintain a very low threshold for screening patients if there is any suspicion of cognitive impairment.

There are many simple, effective screening tests available. The Mini–Mental State Examination (MMSE) has the strongest evidence base, but recent proprietary restrictions have complicated its use clinically. The Mini-Cog screening tool is a simple, validated test that assesses both memory and executive function with a high degree of sensitivity and specificity across multiple settings. The Mini-Cog is also copyright protected, although it is available to clinicians for free use as a clinical and educational tool. The Mini-Cog involves a three-item recall and clock drawing test. Recall of all three items is normal, whereas recall of none of the items indicates dementia. If only one to two items are recalled, the results of the clock drawing test are used to classify the patient, with a normal clock drawing result indicating no dementia and an abnormal result indicating dementia. For further discussion of MCI and discussion of pharmacologic therapies for cognitive symptoms, see MKSAP 17 Neurology.

Fall Prevention

Thirty percent to 40% of community-dwelling adults older than 65 years experience a fall in a given year. The prevalence of falls increases to 50% for persons in long-term care facilities and to 60% for persons with cognitive dysfunction. In older adults, falls are a source of morbidity, mortality, decreased functionality, and premature institutionalization. Risk factors for falling are myriad; the strongest associations include lower extremity weakness, history of falls, gait or balance deficits, polypharmacy, low vitamin D level, and visual impairments. Many risk factors are amenable to remediation. **Figure 35** presents the American Geriatric Society's recommended algorithm for preventing falls in older persons.

Older patients should be routinely asked about falls. Patients who present with a fall, have a history of recurrent falls, or acknowledge gait or balance concerns should undergo a full fall evaluation. Patients with a history of one fall in the last year should be screened for balance or gait disturbance with a Timed Up and Go test, in which the patient is timed in the activity of rising from a chair, walking 10 feet (3 m), turning around, and returning to the chair. A time of longer than 20 seconds is abnormal, and the patient should be referred for full fall evaluation.

The full fall evaluation is a multidisciplinary assessment of risk, followed by a multicomponent intervention based on risk factor identification. Studies suggest that with intensive

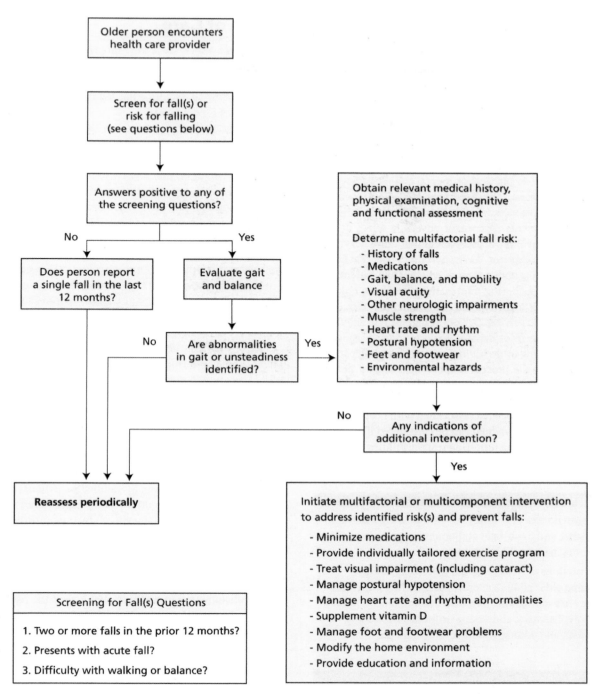

FIGURE 35. Prevention of falls in older persons living in a community.

Reprinted with permission from Panel on Prevention of Falls in Older Persons, American Geriatrics Society and British Geriatrics Society. Summary of the Updated American Geriatrics Society/British Geriatrics Society clinical practice guideline for prevention of falls in older persons. J Am Geriatr Soc. 2011 Jan;59(1):148-57. [PMID: 21226685] Copyright 2011, John Wiley & Sons, Inc.

intervention, those community-dwelling adults at the highest risk of falling can decrease their fall rates by 20%. Interventions for community-dwelling older adults include individualized exercise programs that emphasize balance, gait, and strength training, such as physical therapy or tai chi. Exercise programs do not seem to benefit institutionalized residents, however. Limiting polypharmacy (particularly psychoactive medications), addressing orthostasis, and assessing footwear and providing appropriate adaptive equipment should also be stressed. Ample evidence exists to support supplementation with 800 U/d of vitamin D to decrease fall risk in older adults, with a number needed to treat of only 15 irrespective of vitamin deficiency. Given that vitamin D is safe, inexpensive, and highly effective, some experts believe that vitamin D supplementation should be routine for all older adults. There is currently insufficient evidence to support any recommendations to reduce fall risk in the cognitively impaired. Modification of the home environment in isolation is ineffective, but when performed in addition to the previously mentioned interventions as part of a multimodal fall prevention program, it has been shown to be beneficial.

Assessment of the Older Driver

Older drivers are involved in more fatal car crashes per mile driven than any other age group excepting those under age 25 years. In older drivers, the accident rate can be at least partially attributed to physical or mental changes associated with aging or disease. The American Medical Association recommends that physicians assess older patients for physical or mental impairments that might adversely affect driving abilities. This is a qualitative assessment that relies heavily on physician clinical judgment. It is important to note that family assessment of driving ability is more reliable than patient self-assessment when gathering information. The more risk factors (**Table 75**) that a patient has, the higher the risk of an adverse event while driving. Drivers at highest risk should be counseled to retire from driving. Experts suggest using the terminology "retiring from driving" when counseling patients as this normalizes the process. Experts also suggest helping patients brainstorm alternative transportation options when counseling them against driving. A formal assessment by a driver rehabilitation specialist (associated with hospital occupational therapy departments) can be considered if the situation is unclear. Physician reporting responsibilities vary from state to state, and physicians should be aware of the laws in their own state.

KEY POINTS

HVC
- Whispered voice test, finger rub test, hearing loss questionnaire, and hand-held audiometry are all reasonable screening tests for hearing loss.

HVC
- Interventions that decrease fall risk in community-dwelling older adults include implementing individualized exercise programs (physical therapy, tai chi), limiting polypharmacy, addressing orthostasis, assessing footwear, and adding vitamin D supplements.

TABLE 75. Risk Factors for Impaired Driving

Cognitive dysfunction
Caregiver report of marginal or unsafe skills
History of citations or accidents
Driving <60 miles/week
Emotional aggression or impulsivity
Use of alcohol and/or medications that affect the central nervous system
Impaired mobility or coordination of neck or extremities
Medical disorders that predispose to loss of consciousness
Visual impairment

Levels of Care

In the United States, there are more than 43 million persons older than 65 years and more than 1.4 million nursing home residents. The economics of providing comprehensive, high-quality care for aging adults has led to an expansion of care options for this population.

Acutely ill elderly patients are cared for primarily in a hospital setting. Home hospital care is a service in which health care professionals provide active treatment in the home setting of a condition that otherwise would have required an inpatient hospital stay, and although the feasibility and safety of home hospital care have been established, the intensive resources required are not widely available. For patients with ongoing, high-intensity care needs who require regular physician input, such as chronic mechanical ventilation, multiple intravenous therapies, or complex wound care needs, a long-term acute care hospital (LTACH) is often the most appropriate site for care. When the patient no longer requires high-acuity care, there are a multitude of care options with varying levels of intensity depending on patient need.

Elderly patients often require posthospital rehabilitation, which can be performed in many different settings. The purpose of rehabilitation is to maximize functional recovery and independence. Conceptually, disability involves two domains—the patient's disease and the patient's environment. Both need to be addressed in order to maximize independent functioning. Free-standing rehabilitation hospitals provide intensive rehabilitation services under the direction of specialized physiatrists. To qualify, patients must require active, intensive rehabilitation services, usually defined as 3 hours per day, 5 days per week, from multiple therapy disciplines (physical therapy, occupational therapy, speech therapy, prosthetics services). Medicare covers the expense of this rehabilitation for patients who qualify. For patients unable to tolerate that level of therapy intensity, rehabilitation may be performed at a skilled nursing facility (SNF). Medicare covers all or part of the cost of rehabilitation in a SNF for 100 days if the patient has had a 3-day inpatient hospital stay before admission and makes continued progress towards rehabilitation goals during the stay. For patients who are more functional, rehabilitation services can be provided on an outpatient basis, either in the patient's own home if the patient is homebound or at an outpatient rehabilitation clinic. If the patient needs rehabilitation services for a specific disease, such as cardiac rehabilitation after acute myocardial infarction or pulmonary rehabilitation for chronic lung disease, this type of rehabilitation is generally done on an outpatient basis.

For patients who require increased assistance with ADLs, custodial services are available in many settings. Custodial care services are nonskilled personal care services such as bathing, dressing, toileting, and mobility services; they are not covered by Medicare but may be covered by Medicaid in some cases. Nursing homes, which may provide either skilled rehabilitation services or nonskilled custodial services, are the most familiar custodial care in the United States. Most patients in a nursing home require substantial assistance with several ADLs. Assisted living is a home-like living environment that provides some custodial services to residents. Types and intensity of services vary widely and may include meals, transportation, ADL assistance, and social interaction. Typically, residents in assisted living facilities are more functional than those in a nursing home but are not able to live independently. Adult foster care and group homes provide custodial care in a home-like setting for a smaller number of residents.

For some patients, care in the home is most ideal. Persons with financial means may hire full-time or part-time custodial care providers (skilled or unskilled, depending on need) to provide respite for family caregivers. For patients who are homebound and have a skilled care need such as medication management, wound care, intravenous infusions, or physical therapy, home care services are a covered medical benefit. Multidisciplinary services, with physician oversight, are provided in the home on an intermittent basis for patients who meet these criteria.

Adult day care is a community-based option that provides care for patients who require supervision while their primary caregiver is at work. Adult day care may also be used to provide caregiver respite. The adult day care model is often an alternative to in-home or nursing home care, and it is much less costly.

Complex patients with many comorbid conditions often require care in more than one setting, or may move between different settings depending on the status of their medical issues. This movement between settings of care increases the number of transfers of care between institutions and providers, and increases the risk of medication errors, duplication of services, or failure to understand the patient's medical conditions and treatments. Therefore, careful attention to these care transitions is extremely important. Information that should be conveyed during transitions includes a summary of the hospital course, list of problems and diagnoses, baseline and discharge functional and cognitive status, reconciled medication list, outstanding test results, follow-up appointments, and information about goals of care and advance directives. Direct communication between discharge and receiving physician should occur when there are critical test results pending or complexities in family dynamics or goals of care. Checklists are helpful to assure completion. **H**

KEY POINT

- The economics of providing comprehensive, high-quality care for aging adults has led to an expansion of care options for this population; complex patients with many comorbid conditions often require care in more than one setting or may move between different settings, and careful attention to these care transitions is essential.

Polypharmacy

Approximately 50% of patients over age 65 years take five or more medications each week. In a recent nationwide study, older adults frequently had multiple drugs started, stopped, or otherwise changed, with a median of four medication changes per patient in a 1-year period. The use of multiple medications increases the risk for inappropriate use, drug-drug interactions, duplication of therapy, adverse reactions, and medication errors. Polypharmacy is clearly associated with increased outpatient visits, increased risk for hospitalization, increased health care costs, and decreased functional status. Additionally, the risk for nonadherence increases, which can lead to treatment failure and disease progression.

In the elderly, drug dosing must be adjusted for age as well as kidney function, as drug metabolism may be altered due to decreased glomerular filtration, underlying illness, or altered pharmacokinetics related to aging. Certain medications have been found to particularly incur high risk for geriatric patients. In an effort to improve the care of older adults by reducing the use of potentially inappropriate medications, the American Geriatrics Society has compiled a list of high-risk drugs that must be carefully considered in terms of risk-to-benefit ratio in the elderly (available at http://geriatricscareonline.org/ProductAbstract/american-geriatrics-society-updated-beers-criteria-for-potentially-inappropriate-medication-use-in-older-adults/CL001).

Although treatment of multiple comorbid conditions often requires multiple medications, evidence shows that half of older adults take one or more medications that are not medically necessary (that is, not indicated, not effective, or therapeutically duplicative). Frequent, routine review to verify need for medication and appropriate dosing is an essential aspect of optimal geriatric care.

KEY POINT

- Polypharmacy increases the risk for inappropriate drug use, drug-drug interactions, duplication of therapy, nonadherence, adverse reactions, and medication errors.

Urinary Incontinence
Epidemiology

Urinary incontinence affects 25% to 45% of women, with 9% to 39% of women over age 60 years reporting daily urinary incontinence. The prevalence of urinary incontinence in men is roughly half of that in women; 11% to 34% of older men experience urinary incontinence, with 2% to 9% of older men experiencing daily incontinence. The true prevalence, however, may be higher, as many patients do not report incontinence due to embarrassment.

Urinary incontinence has a strong impact on quality of life, affecting the patient's psychological state, social and work functioning, and sexual activity. It increases the risk of falls and may lead to nursing home admission. Risk factors for urinary incontinence include age, female sex, obesity, parity, gynecologic surgery, benign prostatic hyperplasia, prostate surgery, pelvic floor muscle weakness, diabetes mellitus, high caffeine intake, tobacco use, and impairment in cognition or mobility. Most evidence on the management of urinary incontinence has been produced from studies on women, although principles can generally be applied to men.

Evaluation

There are four main classifications of urinary incontinence: (1) urge incontinence, characterized by loss of urine accompanied by sense of urgency; (2) stress incontinence, in which coughing, sneezing, or exertion causes urine loss; (3) mixed urge and stress incontinence; and (4) overflow incontinence, typified by continuous leakage or dribbling. Overflow incontinence is rare in women; it more frequently occurs in men due to prostate enlargement. Functional incontinence, which occurs in patients who cannot reach and use the toilet in a timely manner, may occur in patients with significant mobility or cognitive impairments. Classifying the type(s) of incontinence helps guide management.

Asking the older adult about urinary incontinence is recommended, as patients may be hesitant to openly discuss symptoms of urinary incontinence with their physician. A brief standardized questionnaire can be used to distinguish urge from stress incontinence (**Figure 36**). Voiding symptom diaries are helpful in determining symptom patterns and severity.

Before embarking on a more complicated path to diagnosis, reversible or transient causes of incontinence should be identified. A review of medications is essential, with attention to diuretic use, along with a review of possible situational, metabolic, cognitive, or infectious causes. Evaluation should incorporate a targeted history, including surgeries, instrumentations, and radiation. In women, an obstetric history should be obtained, and a pelvic examination should be performed to rule out atrophy or prolapse. Men should be asked about prostate symptoms and should undergo a digital rectal examination. Additionally, urinalysis should be performed. Post-void residual urine volume need not be determined unless there is high clinical suspicion for neurologic disease or bladder outlet obstruction. When possible, ultrasound bladder volume measurement is preferred to urethral catheterization.

Treatment

The treatment of urinary incontinence generally progresses in a stepwise manner. Lifestyle changes and behavioral therapy should be initiated first, followed by pharmacologic therapy and devices, and finally surgery if all other therapies have

1. During the last 3 months, have you leaked urine (even a small amount)?

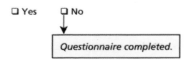

2. During the last 3 months, did you leak urine:
(*Check all that apply.*)

    ❑ a. When you were performing some physical activity, such as coughing, sneezing, lifting, or exercise?
    ❑ b. When you had the urge or the feeling that you needed to empty your bladder, but you could not get to the toilet fast enough?
    ❑ c. Without physical activity and without a sense of urgency?

3. During the last 3 months, did you leak urine *most often*:
(*Check only one.*)

    ❑ a. When you were performing some physical activity, such as coughing, sneezing, lifting, or exercise?
    ❑ b. When you had the urge or the feeling that you needed to empty your bladder, but you could not get to the toilet fast enough?
    ❑ c. Without physical activity and without a sense of urgency?
    ❑ d. About equally as often with physical activity as with a sense of urgency?

Definitions of type of urinary incontinence are based on responses to question 3:

Response to Question 3	Type of Incontinence
a. Most often with physical activity	Stress only or stress predominant
b. Most often with the urge to empty the bladder	Urge only or urge predominant
c. Without physical activity or sense of urgency	Other cause only or other cause predominant
d. About equally with physical activity and sense of urgency	Mixed

FIGURE 36. The 3 Incontinence Questions (3IQ) for evaluation of urinary incontinence.

failed. First-line lifestyle modifications, which may be used for all types of incontinence, include fluid and food management (avoidance of caffeine and alcohol) and weight loss. Excess fluid intake should be avoided, especially at nighttime. Any underlying causes should also be addressed. Subsequent treatment is guided by the type of urinary incontinence.

Behavioral Therapy

The two most effective behavioral therapies are pelvic floor muscle training (PFMT, or Kegel exercises) and bladder training/urge suppression techniques. The American College of Physicians (ACP) recommends PFMT as first-line therapy for women with stress incontinence and may also be of benefit in patients with mixed urge and stress incontinence. In men, PFMT may also be beneficial in those with postmicturition dribble. If performed correctly and diligently, PFMT exercises may strengthen the pelvic floor muscles and enhance urinary retention. The patient is advised to tighten the pelvic muscles as if trying to interrupt urination, although it should be emphasized to the patient that he or she should not habitually interrupt urine flow. Best results require three or four sets of ten contractions daily, with contractions lasting 10 seconds. The regimen should be continued for a minimum of 15 to 20 weeks. The ACP recommends bladder training and suppressive therapy for urge and mixed incontinence. With bladder training, patients are instructed to void regularly throughout the day, regardless of urge, and progressively increase the interval between voids. Suppression techniques are used to manage urge to void outside of the schedule. The patient is instructed to contract pelvic floor muscles quickly three or four times, use a distraction technique (counting backwards from 100), and, when the urge passes, walk to the bathroom to urinate. The ACP recommends weight loss and exercise for all obese women with urinary incontinence.

Prompted voiding is a useful technique for patients with cognitive impairment and is usually implemented in nursing homes. Prompted voiding involves regularly asking the patient to report on incontinence, asking the patient if he or she needs to void and providing assistance, and praising the patient for continence.

Pharmacologic Therapy

No drugs are recommended for the treatment of stress urinary incontinence. The ACP recommends antimuscarinic medications (oxybutynin, tolterodine, fesoterodine, darifenacin, solifenacin, and trospium) for urge incontinence if bladder training was unsuccessful. All of these drugs appear therapeutically equivalent and provide similar small benefits in continence rates, and choice should be guided by cost and side effect profile. There is a high incidence of anticholinergic adverse effects, including constipation and dry mouth, necessitating careful consideration of risk-to-benefit ratio. Anticholinergic agents are contraindicated in patients with angle-closure glaucoma.

Pharmacologic therapy for prostate-related lower urinary tract symptoms is addressed in further detail in Men's Health.

Devices, Injectable Agents, and Surgery

Patients who fail to respond to conservative behavioral and/or pharmacologic interventions should be referred to a urologist or urogynecologist for consideration of other treatment options. For patients with stress incontinence, medical devices, including pessaries and urethral plugs, can be considered as adjunctive treatments. Pessaries may be effective for stress incontinence and are safe and low cost, although they are underused and require fitting by experienced practitioners. Periurethral injection of bulking agents, such as collagen, silicone microparticles, or carbon beads, is a minimally invasive treatment for stress incontinence, with cure rates between 18% and 40% and improvement rates between 33% and 39%. Repeated injections are needed to maintain effectiveness. Urinary urgency, urinary tract infection, difficulty voiding, and urinary retention are possible adverse effects.

In women, the most beneficial surgeries for stress incontinence are sling procedures for intrinsic sphincter deficiency. The mid-urethral sling procedure is associated with objective and patient-perceived improvement of stress incontinence and fewer complications than other surgical approaches. The advent of laparoscopic procedures allows for speedier recovery, but relative safety and long-term effectiveness are not yet known. In men with stress incontinence, placement of an artificial urinary sphincter may be effective when other measures fail.

For the treatment of urge incontinence, injection of botulinum toxin into the detrusor muscle can be considered in patients who are unresponsive to conservative or pharmacologic measures. In a recent Cochrane review, botulinum toxin injection demonstrated superiority over placebo in reducing incontinence. Symptoms are typically reduced for a period of 3 to 6 months. Another option is continuous neuromodulation with transcutaneous tibial or surgically implanted sacral nerve stimulators, which inhibit detrusor muscle activity and have demonstrated efficacy. High cost is a deterrent, however, and long-term efficacy data are limited.

Chronic indwelling catheters are generally not advised, except as a palliative or temporizing measure, as they are associated with urethral injury, urinary tract infection, and kidney stones. Condom catheters have fewer associated complications than indwelling catheters; however, an incorrectly fitting condom catheter can result in skin irritation, leakage, and infection. **H**

KEY POINTS

- Pelvic floor muscle training is recommended as first-line therapy for stress urinary incontinence. **HVC**

- Bladder training is recommended as first-line therapy for urge urinary incontinence. **HVC**

- Antimuscarinic medications are recommended for urge urinary incontinence when bladder training is unsuccessful.

- Weight loss and exercise are recommended for obese women with urinary incontinence. **HVC**

Pressure Ulcers

Clinical Presentation

Pressure ulcers are a common occurrence in hospitals and long-term care settings, affecting up to 3 million patients and costing nearly $11 billion per year in the United States. In addition to the accompanying high costs, pressure ulcers can result in decreased quality of life, with associated depression, impaired mobility, and social isolation. The Centers for Medicare and Medicaid Services have selected the development of pressure ulcers as a sentinel health event (unexpected and preventable occurrences that result in serious patient injury) for health care facilities. In addition, Medicare no longer offers reimbursement for the treatment of stage III and IV pressure ulcers that develop in the inpatient setting.

Pressure ulcers are characterized by localized injury to the skin or soft tissue as a result of pressure and shear forces. Risk factors for the development of pressure ulcers include advanced age, cognitive impairment, reduced mobility, sensory impairment, and comorbid conditions that affect skin integrity (such as low body weight, incontinence, edema, poor microcirculation, and hypoalbuminemia). Pressure ulcers may be classified by use of a staging system (**Table 76**), with each stage distinguished by the amount of tissue loss.

Prevention and Management

In 2015, the American College of Physicians published a clinical practice guideline for risk assessment and prevention of pressure ulcers. This guideline recommends risk assessment to identify patients at risk for developing pressure ulcers; the National Pressure Ulcer Advisory Panel Guideline additionally recommends use of a validated risk assessment tool for this purpose. For those found to be at risk, skin inspection should occur regularly. Prevention of pressure ulcers should begin with a support surface that ensures pressure redistribution, shear reduction, and microclimate control. There is moderate evidence that the use of advanced static mattresses and overlays (such as foam, gel, or air mattresses/overlays) is associated with a lower risk for pressure ulcers compared with conventional bedding. No one advanced static mattress or overlay has been shown to be superior to another. There is no evidence to support the use of more sophisticated bed systems, such as alternating-pressure air mattresses or low–air-loss systems, in prevention of pressure ulcers, although they can be beneficial in the treatment of existing pressure ulcers. Although there is insufficient evidence to support repositioning, nutritional supplementation, creams, or dressings in prevention of pressure ulcers, these interventions are standard in most guidelines.

The ACP has also issued a clinical practice guideline for treatment of pressure ulcers. Treatment of pressure ulcers is aimed at addressing the factors that predisposed the patient to the development of the ulcer. Air-fluidized beds have been shown to enhance healing of pressure ulcers compared with standard hospital mattresses. Dressings, such as hydrocolloid dressings, are used to maintain a moist wound environment while also controlling exudate. Debridement of nonviable tissue via surgical or nonsurgical techniques (for example, wet-to-dry dressings) is also indicated. Nutritional supplementation to enhance wound healing remains controversial; however, there is weak evidence that protein or amino acid supplementation improves wound healing. There is insufficient evidence to support vitamin supplementation or zinc supplementation, although these interventions are considered very low risk. Conversely, at least in patients with advanced dementia, enteral feeding worsened pressure ulcers. There is low-level evidence supporting electrical stimulation and vacuum wound devices in reducing wound size, although the potential harms of vacuum wound devices are unclear. Evidence is insufficient to support electromagnetic, ultrasound, or hyperbaric treatment of pressure ulcers, even though these treatments remain widely utilized. Overall, the evidence for treating pressure ulcers is limited. **H**

TABLE 76.	Classification of Pressure Ulcers
Stage	**Description**
I	Intact skin with nonblanchable redness
II	Partial-thickness loss of dermis. Shallow open ulcer with red-pink wound bed without slough. May also present as intact or ruptured serum-filled blister.
III	Full-thickness tissue loss. Visible subcutaneous fat but not bone, tendon, or muscle. May include undermining or tunneling.
IV	Full-thickness tissue loss with exposed bone, tendon, or muscle.
Unstageable	Full-thickness tissue loss in which the base of the ulcer is covered by slough or eschar.
Suspected deep-tissue injury	Purple or maroon localized area of discolored but intact skin or a blood-filled blister due to damage of underlying soft tissue from pressure or shear.

Adapted from National Pressure Ulcer Advisory Panel. National Pressure Ulcer Advisory Panel, European Pressure Ulcer Advisory Panel, and Pan Pacific Pressure Injury Alliance. Prevention and Treatment of Pressure Ulcers: Quick Reference Guide. Cambridge Media: Perth, Australia; 2014.

KEY POINTS

- Prevention of pressure ulcers should begin with a support surface that ensures pressure redistribution, shear reduction, and microclimate control; special attention to patient positioning is also paramount.
- Air-fluidized beds and surgical or nonsurgical debridement may enhance healing rates of pressure ulcers.

Perioperative Medicine

General Recommendations

Rather than providing "clearance" for surgery, a comprehensive preoperative evaluation achieves three important objectives. First, it provides an opportunity to reassess and optimize the patient's baseline general health and chronic disease management. Second, risk assessment and subsequent discussion with the patient ensure that an informed choice is made about surgery. Third, a preoperative evaluation can identify potential postoperative risks and forms the basis of a care "handover" to those treating the patient after surgery.

Preoperative Testing

Routine diagnostic testing is not indicated preoperatively. Multiple studies have demonstrated low yield and poor risk correlation of routine preoperative diagnostic tests. The American Board of Internal Medicine Foundation's Choosing Wisely initiative (www.choosingwisely.org) and the American College of Physicians' (ACP) High Value Care initiative (http://hvc.acponline.org) include several recommendations against practices such as obtaining routine preoperative laboratory studies in healthy patients undergoing elective or low-risk surgery (such as eye surgery) or obtaining preoperative chest radiography in the absence of cardiopulmonary symptoms.

In most circumstances, patient-specific factors determine diagnostic testing needs. For example, serum electrolytes in patients who will undergo diuresis, and kidney function studies in those with chronic kidney disease (CKD), are reasonable testing indications. The American Society of Anesthesiology (ASA) does not recommend repeating laboratory studies obtained within 6 months of surgery in the absence of a clinical change.

A few studies may be indicated for surgery-related reasons. Pregnancy testing should be offered to women of childbearing age, and preoperative urinalysis should be performed in patients undergoing urologic procedures.

Perioperative Medication Management

Detailed medication reconciliation, the process of creating the most accurate list of medications a patient is actually taking (including over-the-counter medications) and comparing it with the list of medications currently ordered, can prevent complications as well as allow for reassessment of long-term benefits and risks.

Perioperative medication management begins with determination of medication indications. For agents with no clear benefit, the medication should be stopped before surgery (as long as there is no concern for withdrawal symptoms) and long-term use reconsidered. Unless specific surgery-related risks are identified, medications with a clear indication should be continued uninterrupted, with the patient taking the medications with sips of water while fasting for surgery. If risk outweighs benefit, the medication should be stopped long enough before surgery to ensure adequate clearance (usually 3-5 half-lives) and should not be restarted until the risk subsides.

Management of immunomodulators and disease-modifying antirheumatic drugs (DMARDs) is particularly challenging.

Risks of infection and poor wound healing need to be carefully balanced. Solid organ transplant recipients should generally have no medication changes, but an important exception to this is sirolimus, which has been associated with wound dehiscence and should be discontinued before surgery. For nontransplant patients, DMARDs and biologic agents should be stopped for at least 4 half-lives prior to surgery and not restarted until after wound healing is complete (usually 2-4 weeks after surgery); however, methotrexate and hydroxychloroquine are typically safe to continue perioperatively.

It is also important to consider specific drugs and their potential effect in certain clinical circumstances. For example, intraoperative floppy iris syndrome is a complication affecting 2% to 3% of patients undergoing cataract surgery who are taking α_1-antagonists (in particular, tamsulosin). This complication increases the risk of retinal detachment and endophthalmitis; therefore, the management of this agent in patients being evaluated for a cataract procedure should be discussed with the eye surgeon preoperatively.

Table 77 lists other medications with potential surgery-related risk and recommended time frames for withholding them. **H**

KEY POINTS

- Several organizations recommend against obtaining routine preoperative laboratory studies in healthy patients undergoing elective or low-risk surgery and against obtaining preoperative chest radiography in the absence of cardiopulmonary symptoms. **HVC**

- Unless specific surgery-related risks are identified, medications with a clear indication should be continued uninterrupted; if risk outweighs benefit, medications should be stopped long enough before surgery to assure adequate clearance.

Cardiovascular Perioperative Management

Cardiovascular Risk Assessment

The 2014 American College of Cardiology (ACC) and American Heart Association (AHA) perioperative cardiovascular guidelines provide comprehensive recommendations for managing noncardiac surgery in patients with all types of cardiac disease and those with unclear cardiovascular risk (**Figure 37**). Patients requiring emergency surgery cannot afford any delay for cardiac testing, whereas those experiencing an acute coronary syndrome (ACS) should not undergo surgery until they have received appropriate cardiac assessment and treatment. If a patient has no history, symptoms, or risk factors for coronary artery disease (CAD), no preoperative coronary evaluation is necessary.

For patients with risk factors for cardiovascular disease, the guidelines recommend determination of risk for a major adverse cardiac event (MACE). The Revised Cardiac Risk Index (RCRI)

TABLE 77. Suggested Perioperative Medication Management

Medication Class	Recommendation	Comments
Anticoagulant	Continue for minor surgery. Discontinue before major surgery: IV heparin: 4-6 h LMWH: 24 h (12 h for prophylactic dose) Warfarin: 5 days TSOAC: 1-2 d (normal kidney function), 3-6 d (eGFR <50 mL/min/1.73 m^2) (discontinue earlier for high bleeding risk procedures).	Bridging with heparin indicated for high-risk patients and possibly moderate-risk patients.
Antiplatelet	Clopidogrel: discontinue 5-7 d before surgery; patients with cardiac stent may require continuation. Aspirin: continue if minor surgery. Continue if indication is recent myocardial infarction (up to 6 months), cardiac stent, or high risk for coronary event; otherwise, discontinue 7-10 d before major surgery (other than CABG).	Aspirin and clopidogrel use in patients with cardiac stent and/or at high risk is controversial. Aspirin should be started before CABG.
Cardiovascular	Continue β-blockers, calcium channel blockers, nitrates, antiarrhythmia agents. ACE inhibitors and ARBs should be used with caution. Diuretics usually withheld on day of surgery.	ACE inhibitors and ARBs can promote intraoperative hypotension, especially in patients with hypovolemia; perioperative use, especially in persons with left ventricular dysfunction, is controversial.
Lipid lowering	Continue statins; withhold all other lipid-lowering agents on day of surgery.	
Pulmonary	Continue controller and rescue inhalers as well as systemic glucocorticoids (if used). Probably continue leukotriene antagonists and lipoxygenase inhibitors.	
Gastrointestinal	Continue H$_2$ receptor blockers and proton pump inhibitors.	
Hypoglycemic agents	Oral hypoglycemic agents: discontinue 12-72 h before surgery depending upon half-life of the drug and risk of hypoglycemia. Short-acting insulin: withhold morning of surgery; may need dose reduction preoperatively if modified diet (e.g., gastrointestinal surgery). Intermediate-acting insulin: reduce dose, typically to one half of usual dose. Long-acting insulin: continue at previous dose or reduce dose to two thirds.	Hypoglycemia is more dangerous than hyperglycemia; caution to always have some basal insulin present in patients with type 1 diabetes.
Thyroid	Continue thyroid replacement, propylthiouracil, methimazole.	
Glucocorticoids	Continue; increase to stress doses if indicated.	Stress-dose glucocorticoids for patients taking >10 mg/d prednisone for >3 weeks.
Estrogen	Discontinue several weeks before surgery if feasible; if continued, increase level of deep venous thrombosis prophylaxis.	
Psychiatric	Discontinue MAOIs 10-14 d before surgery; SSRIs and TCAs can either be continued or tapered 2-3 weeks before surgery. Continue antipsychotic medications. Can continue lithium, although some experts taper and discontinue several days before surgery.	Paucity of evidence, although most psychiatric agents confer at least some theoretical risk. Risk of serotonin syndrome with some anesthetic agents. Must weigh risks of continuing versus stopping. May wish to consult with psychiatrist.
Neurologic	Continue antiepileptic drugs. May continue antiparkinsonian agents, although some experts may discontinue the night before surgery. Discontinue dementia drugs.	
Herbal	Discontinue up to 1 week before surgery.	
Analgesic	NSAIDs and COX-2 inhibitors are usually discontinued 7 d before surgery. Long-acting narcotics continued or dose reduced.	

(Continued on the next page)

TABLE 77. Suggested Perioperative Medication Management *(Continued)*

Medication Class	Recommendation	Comments
Immunomodulators	For transplant recipients, continue all except sirolimus without interruption. For non-transplant patients, discontinue for at least 4 half-lives before and 2 weeks after surgery.	Paucity of data; risk of disease flare balanced against risk of adverse reaction from medication. Risk of perioperative wound complications may be lower for methotrexate, hydroxychloroquine, and sulfasalazine.

ARB = angiotensin receptor blocker; CABG = coronary artery bypass grafting; COX-2 = cyclooxygenase-2; eGFR = estimated glomerular filtration rate; IV = intravenous; LMWH = low-molecular-weight heparin; MAOI = monoamine oxidase inhibitor; SSRI = selective serotonin reuptake inhibitor; TCA = tricyclic antidepressant; TSOAC = target-specific oral anticoagulant.

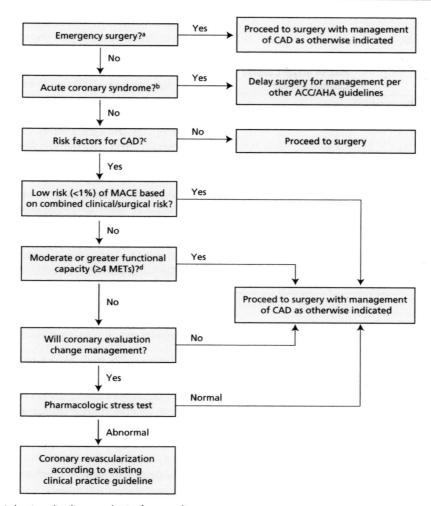

FIGURE 37. Perioperative ischemic cardiac disease evaluation for noncardiac surgery.

ACC = American College of Cardiology; AHA = American Heart Association; CAD = coronary artery disease; MACE = major adverse cardiac events; MET = metabolic equivalents.

[a]Emergency surgery required within 6 hours to avoid loss of life or limb.

[b]Acute coronary syndromes: myocardial infarction <30 days ago, unstable or severe angina.

[c]Risk factors for CAD: not specifically defined in ACC/AHA guidelines; examples include known CAD, cerebrovascular disease (that is, stroke or transient ischemic attack), chronic kidney disease, diabetes mellitus, and heart failure.

[d]Examples of activities requiring ≥4 METs include climbing a flight of stairs, walking up a hill, walking on level ground at 4 miles per hour, running for a short distance, and playing tennis.

Recommendations from Fleisher LA, Fleischmann KE, Auerbach A, et al. 2014 ACC/AHA guideline on perioperative cardiovascular evaluation and management of patients undergoing noncardiac surgery. J Am Coll Cardiol. 2014 Dec 9;64(22):e77-137. [PMID: 25091544]

has been the most utilized risk prediction model due to its simplicity and fairly effective risk stratification for major cardiac complications (**Table 78**). However, it was not developed or validated for use in low-risk or ambulatory surgery and significantly overestimates risk for these procedures.

Additionally, the RCRI has been shown to underestimate the risk in vascular surgery procedures. The RCRI may be used to estimate MACE risk, but it is important to recognize low-risk surgeries for which further cardiac testing is unnecessary even if the RCRI score is elevated (2 or higher). Low-risk procedures

TABLE 78. Revised Cardiac Risk Index and Predicted Rate of Major Cardiac Complications Perioperatively

Risk Factor (1 point for each)
High-risk surgery (intrathoracic, intraperitoneal, suprainguinal vascular)
Ischemic heart disease
Heart failure (compensated)
Diabetes mellitus (requiring insulin)
Cerebrovascular disease
Chronic kidney disease (serum creatinine >2.0 mg/dL [176.8 µmol/L])[a]

Number of Points	Risk of Major Cardiac Complications[b]
0	0.5%
1	2.6%
2	7.2%
≥3	14.4%

[a]Estimated glomerular filtration rate (eGFR) <30 mL/min/1.73 m² also shown to predict cardiovascular risk.

[b]Defined as myocardial infarction, pulmonary edema, or primary cardiac arrest.

Data from Lee TH, Marcantonio ER, Mangione CM, et al. Derivation and prospective validation of a simple index for prediction of cardiac risk of major noncardiac surgery. Circulation. 1999;100(10):1043-9. [PMID: 10477528] and Davis C, Tait G, Carroll J, et al. The Revised Cardiac Risk Index in the new millennium: a single-centre prospective cohort re-evaluation of the original variables in 9,519 consecutive elective surgical patients. Can J Anesth. 2013 Sept;60(9):855-63. [PMID: 23813289]

include cataract extraction, carpal tunnel release, breast biopsy, and inguinal hernia repair. Although not externally validated like the RCRI, the American College of Surgeons (ACS) National Surgical Quality Improvement Program (NSQIP) Surgical Risk Calculator (http://riskcalculator.facs.org/) has the potential to provide a procedure-specific estimate of MACE risk.

For patients with an elevated MACE risk (≥1%), an estimated functional capacity of <4 metabolic equivalents (METs) suggests that pharmacologic stress testing be considered if the results will change management. Examples of activities requiring the equivalent of ≥4 METs include climbing a flight of stairs or walking up a hill without stopping, running a short distance, lifting or moving heavy furniture, and participating in moderate-exertion sporting activities such as bowling or golf.

Prior to proceeding with pharmacologic stress testing in an asymptomatic patient undergoing noncardiac surgery, the purpose of testing and how it might change management must be carefully considered. In most instances, preoperative coronary evaluation will not influence medical management. However, for patients faced with different surgical options (higher versus lower risk) or in whom the risk-benefit ratio for elective surgery is uncertain, coronary evaluation may provide useful data for decision-making. Studies have failed to demonstrate survival benefit with percutaneous coronary intervention (PCI) in stable patients or improved postoperative outcomes in most patients who undergo preoperative coronary revascularization. Instead, for stable (including asymptomatic) patients with ischemia on stress testing, the ACC/AHA recommend that revascularization prior to noncardiac surgery be reserved for the same indications as in the general setting according to existing guidelines.

Echocardiography may also be beneficial in specific circumstances for assessment of left ventricular function or valvular heart disease. For patients with symptoms suggestive of undiagnosed heart failure or with a history of heart failure and a change in symptoms, the ACC/AHA recommend obtaining an echocardiogram. Reassessment of left ventricular function in patients with clinically stable heart failure who have not had an echocardiogram within the past year is also reasonable. The ACC/AHA also recommend echocardiography for patients with suspected or known moderate to severe valvular disease if the patient has had a change in clinical status (or physical examination findings) or if there is no echocardiogram within the past year.

The ACC/AHA state that it is reasonable to obtain an electrocardiogram (ECG) within 1 to 3 months of surgery in any patient with CAD, significant arrhythmias, cerebrovascular disease (stroke or transient ischemic attack), peripheral arterial disease, or other structural heart disease unless they are undergoing low-risk surgery. A preoperative ECG may also be considered in asymptomatic patients without known CAD, except in those undergoing low-risk surgery. Routine ECG is not useful in asymptomatic patients undergoing low-risk surgical procedures.

At this time, it is still unclear what role cardiac biomarkers (troponin and B-type natriuretic peptides) and CT coronary angiography should play in perioperative cardiovascular care.

Cardiovascular Risk Management

Patients with known CAD should not undergo elective noncardiac surgery within 30 days of bare metal stent implantation or 12 months of drug-eluting stent (DES) placement, and dual antiplatelet therapy should not be interrupted during this time frame. Optimally, surgery should be delayed for 12 months after DES placement. However, if the risk of further surgical delay is thought to be greater than the expected risk of ischemia and stent thrombosis, noncardiac surgery after DES implantation may be considered after 180 days; in this case, aspirin should be continued and if the second antiplatelet agent is withheld, the window of time off the agent should be as short as possible. Antiplatelet therapy must also be managed carefully to balance the bleeding risks of perioperative continuation and the thrombotic risks of cessation (see Perioperative Management of Antiplatelet Medications).

Perioperative β-blocker therapy remains controversial. At present, the strongest ACC/AHA recommendation for perioperative β-blockade indicates that it should be continued uninterrupted in patients who are already on a β-blocker. For patients who have moderate- to high-risk ischemia on preoperative testing or three or more RCRI factors, starting a β-blocker at least 1 day (preferably ≥1 week) prior to surgery is reasonable after consideration of potential adverse effects (for example, increased stroke risk and heart failure decompensation).

Statins may also provide perioperative cardiac risk reduction, and limited data suggest this benefit can be seen even when initiated shortly before surgery. Individuals who qualify for statin therapy according to the 2013 ACC/AHA cholesterol treatment guidelines (see Dyslipidemia) should begin this therapy preoperatively. Statins should also be continued perioperatively in patients already taking them.

ACC/AHA guidelines do not recommend routine postoperative surveillance with ECG or measurement of cardiac biomarkers unless symptoms of an acute coronary syndrome are present. This recommendation is based upon the lack of data supporting specific risk reduction measures for patients with perioperative asymptomatic myocardial infarction or isolated cardiac biomarker elevation.

ACC/AHA guidelines also provide suggestions and evidence-based recommendations for other forms of cardiac disease, including cardiomyopathies, pulmonary hypertension, valvular heart disease, and arrhythmias. In general, these conditions should be medically optimized as much as possible prior to surgery and need careful attention to postoperative hemodynamic management. Perioperative care planning for patients with congenital heart disease, cardiomyopathy, or significant arrhythmias should include collaboration with the appropriate subspecialists (cardiology and electrophysiology), and a specific perioperative management plan should be obtained from the clinician who manages the patient's implanted cardiac devices. Severe valvular disease should be repaired if intervention criteria are met; if repair is not indicated, elective noncardiac surgery is reasonable to perform with close perioperative hemodynamic monitoring. **H**

KEY POINTS

- Patients without coronary artery disease (CAD) or CAD risk factors with an estimated major adverse cardiac event risk of <1% or with a functional capacity ≥4 metabolic equivalents do not require preoperative coronary evaluation.

- Preoperative coronary revascularization in asymptomatic patients has not been shown to reduce postoperative cardiac complications and should be reserved for the same indications as in the general setting.

- Current recommendations indicate that perioperative β-blockade should be continued uninterrupted in patients who are already on a β-blocker.

Pulmonary Perioperative Management

Pulmonary complications account for more than 50% of adverse perioperative events and have higher mortality and cost than postoperative cardiac problems. The pulmonary complications of greatest clinical concern are respiratory failure and pneumonia; risk factors can be divided into procedure-specific and patient-specific factors (**Table 79**).

TABLE 79. Major Risk Factors for Postoperative Pulmonary Complications

Procedure-Specific
Emergency surgery
Prolonged surgery (>3 h)
Thoracic surgery
Abdominal surgery
Head and neck surgery
Aortic surgery (open)
General anesthesia

Patient-Specific
Advanced age[a]
ADL functional limitations
ASA class 2 or higher[b]
COPD
Smoking within past year
Preoperative sepsis; obstructive sleep apnea; pulmonary hypertension

ADL = activities of daily living; ASA = American Society of Anesthesiologists.

[a]Incremental risk increase with every decade above age 50 years.

[b]ASA classes are as follows: class 1, normal healthy patient; class 2, patient with mild systemic disease; class 3, patient with severe systemic disease; class 4, patient with systemic disease that is a constant threat to life; and class 5, moribund patient who is not expected to survive for 24 hours with or without operation.

Several models and risk calculators have been developed for predicting pulmonary risk. Although these calculators may provide a fairly reliable estimate of general pulmonary complications, they have limitations because they were derived from surgical data that did not capture information on obstructive sleep apnea (OSA) or pulmonary hypertension, both of which have been shown to significantly increase the risk of postoperative pulmonary complications. Most interventions for pulmonary risk reduction have minimal potential adverse effects and are not specific for any particular level of risk or risk factor. Therefore, clinical assessment of risk factors without a validated risk calculator is likely sufficient in most clinical situations. The exception is assessment of OSA risk, for which there are specific perioperative considerations. All surgical patients should be screened for OSA with a validated tool such as the STOP-BANG survey (**Table 80**).

Spirometry is no more predictive of complications than clinical assessment alone and should be performed only for dyspnea or hypoxia of uncertain cause. Arterial blood gas analysis and chest radiograph results rarely alter perioperative management when obtained in clinically stable patients.

Surgery should be delayed whenever possible to treat acute respiratory disease, and medical management of chronic pulmonary problems should be fully optimized. Smoking cessation should be strongly encouraged; the greatest benefit comes from quitting more than 8 weeks before surgery. The ASA suggests pursuing polysomnography and initiation of

TABLE 80. STOP-BANG Obstructive Sleep Apnea Screening Tool

Survey Items (1 point for each)	
Snoring	
Tiredness or sleepiness during the day	
Observed apnea during sleep	
Pressure, high blood	
BMI >35	
Age >50 years	
Neck circumference >40 cm	
Gender = male	

STOP-BANG Score	Risk Correlation
0-2	Low risk of OSA
≥3	Increased risk of OSA
≥5	Increased risk of moderate-severe OSA

OSA = obstructive sleep apnea.

Adapted with permission from Chung F, Yegneswaran B, Liao P, et al. STOP questionnaire: a tool to screen patients for obstructive sleep apnea. Anesthesiology. 2008 May;108(5):812-21. [PMID: 18431116] and Chung F, Subramanyam R, Liao P, Sasaki E, Shapiro C, Sun Y. High STOP-Bang score indicates a high probability of obstructive sleep apnoea. Br J Anaesth. 2012 May;108(5):768-75. [PMID: 22401881]

continuous positive airway pressure (CPAP) therapy for patients with presumed severe OSA. For a patient with suspected OSA who is scheduled for outpatient surgery, discussion with the anesthesiologist and surgeon is important to determine whether the surgical procedure is most appropriately performed on an inpatient or outpatient basis.

The mainstay of risk management is lung expansion maneuvers, including deep breathing exercises, incentive spirometry, intermittent positive pressure breathing, and CPAP therapy. Each of these is equally effective, and a combination of modalities provides no additive benefit. Selective use of nasogastric intubation is also effective at preventing pulmonary complications. Regional and neuraxial anesthesia and analgesia, intraoperative protective lung ventilation, and laparoscopic surgical approaches are other available risk reduction methods. Patients with suspected or diagnosed OSA should receive nonsupine positioning (unless contraindicated) and continuous pulse oximetry. **H**

KEY POINTS

- All surgical patients must be screened for obstructive sleep apnea with a validated tool such as the STOP-BANG survey.
- **HVC** Preoperative spirometry should be performed only for dyspnea or hypoxia of uncertain cause.
- **HVC** The mainstay of perioperative pulmonary risk management is lung expansion maneuvers, including deep breathing exercises and incentive spirometry.

Hematologic Perioperative Management

Venous Thromboembolism Prophylaxis

Venous thromboembolism (VTE) is estimated to cause more than 50,000 postoperative deaths per year in the United States. The American College of Chest Physicians (ACCP) antithrombotic guidelines provide recommendations for VTE prophylaxis after many types of surgery and incorporate use of the Caprini model for perioperative VTE risk stratification (**Table 81** and **Table 82**). The Caprini model has been validated in multiple types of surgery (excluding orthopedic and gynecologic oncology surgery) and provides a relatively simple objective assessment of postoperative VTE risk. Prophylactic antithrombotic agents should be withheld until the risk of surgical bleeding has sufficiently subsided (at least 12 hours after surgery) and should be continued until hospital discharge. Major orthopedic and abdominal-pelvic surgery for cancer carries especially high VTE risk and requires extended-duration prophylaxis (up to 35 days after surgery).

Evidence does not support the use of inferior vena cava (IVC) filters for primary prophylaxis. Instead, IVC filters should be reserved for patients with an acute VTE event and an absolute contraindication for anticoagulation. This includes patients with VTE within 3 months before necessary surgery for which anticoagulation must be withheld. Removable IVC filters are preferred, and the perioperative management plan should include a timeline for when anticoagulation can be resumed and the filter extracted.

Perioperative Management of Anticoagulant Therapy

Surgical patients on chronic anticoagulant therapy confront the challenge of balancing their baseline thrombotic risk with the added thromboembolic and bleeding risks associated with invasive procedures. Anticoagulation management must address the following: (1) need for temporary anticoagulant cessation, (2) potential benefit of bridging anticoagulation if cessation is necessary, and (3) appropriate timing for anticoagulant resumption after surgery.

Anticoagulation must be stopped for most surgical procedures except those with minimal expected blood loss (for example, cataract surgery, dermatologic procedures, dental procedures, and endoscopic procedures without biopsy). If temporary cessation is warranted, therapy should be withheld for a sufficient period of time to leave minimal residual anticoagulant activity. Stopping warfarin 5 days prior to surgery usually achieves the standard target of an INR of less than 1.5. Much less data are available for the perioperative management of target-specific oral anticoagulants. Most experts recommend a conservative approach to ensure elimination by the time of surgery (**Table 83**). Although normal activated partial thromboplastin time (aPTT) in patients taking dabigatran and normal INR in patients taking apixaban or rivaroxaban correlate with minimal residual activity, such

TABLE 81. Postoperative Venous Thromboembolism Prophylaxis Recommendations for Common Noncardiothoracic Surgeries

Surgery and Risks		Recommended Prophylaxis[a]
General, abdominal-pelvic, urologic, plastic, vascular	Caprini[b] score 0	Early ambulation
	Caprini score 1-2	IPC
	Caprini score 3-4 — Average bleeding risk	LMWH, LDUH, IPC
	High bleeding risk[c]	IPC
	Caprini score ≥5 — Average bleeding risk	LMWH or LDUH (+ IPC)
	High bleeding risk[c]	IPC
	Cancer surgery	LMWH for 4 weeks
Orthopedic	Hip or knee arthroplasty[d]	IPC + LMWH, LDUH, aspirin, TSOAC, fondaparinux, warfarin, or IPC alone if high bleeding risk; continue for 10-35 d
	Hip fracture repair[c]	IPC + LMWH, LDUH, warfarin, fondaparinux, or IPC alone if high bleeding risk; continue for 10-35 d
	Isolated lower leg fracture repairs	None
	Knee arthroscopy with no previous VTE	Early ambulation
Spine (elective)	Average VTE risk	IPC
	High VTE risk (e.g., malignancy, anterior-posterior approach)	IPC + LMWH (when bleeding risk sufficiently low)
Major trauma	Average VTE risk	LMWH, LDUH, IPC
	High VTE risk (e.g., spinal cord or brain injury)	LMWH or LDUH (+ IPC)
	High bleeding risk[c]	IPC
Intracranial	Average VTE risk	IPC
	High VTE risk (e.g., malignancy)	LMWH or LDUH (+ IPC)

IPC = intermittent pneumatic compression; LDUH = low-dose unfractionated heparin; LMWH = low-molecular-weight heparin; TSOAC = target-specific oral anticoagulant (dabigatran, rivaroxaban, apixaban); VTE = venous thromboembolism.

[a]Duration is for postoperative hospitalization unless noted otherwise.

[b]See Table 82 for the Caprini Risk Assessment Scoring method.

[c]Risk factors suggesting high bleeding risk: concurrent antithrombotic therapy (e.g., aspirin for cardiac disease), known or suspected bleeding disorder, active bleeding, liver or kidney disease, and sepsis.

[d]LMWH is preferred.

Recommendations from Gould MK, Garcia DA, Wren SM, et al. Prevention of VTE in nonorthopedic surgical patients: Antithrombotic Therapy and Prevention of Thrombosis, 9th ed: American College of Chest Physicians Evidence-Based Clinical Practice Guidelines. Chest. 2012 Feb;141(2 Suppl):e227S-e277S. [PMID: 22315263] and Falck-Ytter Y, Francis CW, Johanson NA, et al; American College of Chest Physicians. Prevention of VTE in orthopedic surgery patients: Antithrombotic Therapy and Prevention of Thrombosis, 9th ed: American College of Chest Physicians Evidence-Based Clinical Practice Guidelines. Chest. 2012 Feb;141(2 Suppl):e278S-325S. [PMID: 22315265]

testing is not routinely recommended. There are no approved reversal strategies for these agents. Rapid reversal of warfarin for urgent surgery can be accomplished with vitamin K, fresh frozen plasma, or prothrombin complex concentrates, but the potential thrombotic complications of this approach must be considered.

Bridging anticoagulation is not currently recommended for patients stopping dabigatran, rivaroxaban, or apixaban. For patients chronically taking warfarin, the decision to provide alternative anticoagulation while off this drug is based upon the indication for chronic anticoagulation and level of thromboembolic risk (**Table 84**). For patients with low thromboembolic risk, warfarin therapy is stopped with no bridging anti-

coagulation, whereas high-risk patients should receive bridging anticoagulation with intravenous unfractionated heparin (UFH) or therapeutic-dose low-molecular-weight heparin (LMWH). For all other patients, the decision for bridging is individualized based on patient and surgical considerations. Although the CHA_2DS_2-VASc risk score is the preferred method for long-term thromboembolic risk stratification in atrial fibrillation patients, its utility for perioperative risk stratification is unknown, and current ACCP guidelines for perioperative anticoagulation management utilize the $CHADS_2$ system for perioperative risk stratification (see MKSAP 17 Cardiovascular Medicine). LMWH should be avoided in patients with an estimated glomerular filtration

TABLE 82. Caprini Venous Thromboembolism Risk Assessment Scoring Method

Number of Points for Each Risk Factor	Risk Factors
1	Age 41-60 y; minor surgery; BMI >25; leg edema; varicose veins; recent or current pregnancy; estrogen use; recurrent spontaneous abortion; recent sepsis (<1 mo)/pneumonia (<1 mo); severe lung disease; abnormal pulmonary function; inflammatory bowel disease; acute MI; recent HF (<1 mo); medical patient at bed rest
2	Age 61-74 y; arthroscopic surgery; major surgery lasting >45 min; malignancy; bed rest for >72 h; immobilizing cast; central venous access
3	Age ≥75 y; personal history of VTE; family history of VTE; congenital or acquired thrombophilia; HIT
5	Stroke or spinal cord injury within 1 mo; elective arthroplasty; hip, pelvis, or leg fracture

HF = heart failure; HIT = heparin-induced thrombocytopenia; MI = myocardial infarction; VTE = venous thromboembolism.

Adapted from Bahl V, Hu HM, Henke PK, Wakefield TW, Campbell DA Jr, Caprini JA. A validation study of a retrospective venous thromboembolism risk scoring method. Ann Surg. 2010 Feb;251(2):344-50. [PMID: 19779324]

TABLE 83. Cessation of Target-Specific Oral Anticoagulants Before Surgery

Agent	Duration of Preoperative Cessation by Kidney Function[a]		
	eGFR >50 mL/min/ 1.73 m²	eGFR 31-50 mL/ min/1.73 m²	eGFR ≤30 mL/min/ 1.73 m²
Apixaban	1-2 d	2-3 d	>3 d
Rivaroxaban	1-2 d	1-2 d	2-3 d
Dabigatran	1-2 d	2-4 d	>4 d

eGFR = estimated glomerular filtration rate.

[a]For surgeries with high bleeding risk, use longer duration. All target-specific oral anticoagulants should not be restarted postoperatively until 24 hours after low bleeding risk surgery and 48 to 72 hours after high bleeding risk procedures.

rate <30 mL/min/1.73 m². If bridging is utilized, UFH or LMWH should be started approximately 36 hours after the last dose of warfarin. In patients receiving bridging with UFH, the last presurgical dose should be 4 to 6 hours before surgery. In those being bridged with LMWH, the last dose should be given no sooner than 12 hours before surgery if being dosed at prophylactic levels, or no sooner than 24 hours if being given at therapeutic dosing levels.

Warfarin can be safely restarted 12 to 24 hours after surgery if there are no major bleeding concerns. Therapeutic-dose LMWH and UFH may be started 24 hours after surgery with low operative blood loss (<500 mL) but should be withheld for at least 48 to 72 hours after surgery with greater blood loss. In the latter situation, it may be advisable to provide prophylactic-dose LMWH (which can be resumed within 12 hours after surgery) until therapeutic doses are possible. Dabigatran, rivaroxaban, and apixaban all have rapid onset of action and should be restarted using the same guidelines as LMWH.

TABLE 84. Perioperative Warfarin Bridging Strategies

TE Risk (rate per year)	Patient Characteristics	Bridging Strategy
Low (<5%)	Bileaflet mechanical aortic valve without atrial fibrillation, CVA, or other risk factors	No bridging
	Atrial fibrillation with CHADS₂ score ≤2 and no prior CVA	No bridging
	VTE >12 mo previously with no other risk factors	No bridging
Intermediate (5%-10%)	Bileaflet mechanical aortic valve with atrial fibrillation or CHADS₂ score >0	Bridging on case-by-case basis; use therapeutic- or prophylactic-dose[a] LMWH or UFH
	Atrial fibrillation with CHADS₂ score 3-4	Bridging on case-by-case basis; use therapeutic- or prophylactic-dose[a] LMWH or UFH
	Recurrent VTE or VTE within past 3-12 mo or associated with nonsevere thrombophilia or active cancer	Bridging on case-by-case basis; use therapeutic- or prophylactic-dose[a] LMWH or UFH
High (>10%)	Mitral or caged ball or tilting disc mechanical aortic valve, or bileaflet mechanical aortic valve with recent CVA	Bridge with therapeutic LMWH or UFH
	Atrial fibrillation with CHADS₂ score >4, rheumatic valvular heart disease, or recent CVA or TIA	Bridge with therapeutic LMWH or UFH
	VTE within past 3 mo or with severe thrombophilia	Bridge with therapeutic LMWH or UFH

CVA = cerebrovascular accident; LMWH = low-molecular-weight heparin; TE = thromboembolism; TIA = transient ischemic attack; UFH = unfractionated heparin; VTE = venous thromboembolism.

[a]Prophylactic-dose LMWH is only an option in patients with VTE as their indication for chronic anticoagulation.

Adapted from Douketis JD, Spyropoulos AC, Spencer FA, et al. Perioperative management of antithrombotic therapy: Antithrombotic Therapy and Prevention of Thrombosis, 9th ed: American College of Chest Physicians Evidence-Based Clinical Practice Guidelines. Chest. 2012;141(2 suppl):e326S-e350S. [PMID: 22315266]

Perioperative Management of Antiplatelet Medications

For patients who take aspirin for primary prevention or analgesia, the risks of surgical bleeding most likely outweigh any benefits, and aspirin should be stopped 7 to 10 days before surgery. In patients with CAD on dual antiplatelet therapy with aspirin and another agent (clopidogrel, ticagrelor, ticlopidine, or prasugrel), neither should be stopped within 12 months of drug-eluting stent placement or 4 to 6 weeks of bare metal stent placement. If a patient requires surgery during these intervals, dual antiplatelet therapy, or at least aspirin alone, should be continued perioperatively. Following these time periods, the non-aspirin antiplatelet can be temporarily discontinued 5 to 7 days before surgery, but aspirin should be continued uninterrupted unless the risk of surgical bleeding is excessive (such as intracranial surgery). The timing and safety of antiplatelet cessation for surgery within 1 year after acute myocardial infarction or surgical coronary revascularization should be discussed with a cardiologist. Management of patients taking antiplatelet agents for other secondary prevention (such as history of stroke) is less clear, but the ACC/AHA and ACCP suggest considering the perioperative continuation of aspirin based on assessment if the ischemic risk is considered greater than the bleeding risk.

If antiplatelet therapy is withheld for surgery, it can be safely restarted 24 hours after surgery unless there is persistent risk for surgical bleeding. However, careful consideration should be given to the benefits and risks of restarting dual antiplatelet therapy for patients who will receive concomitant postoperative anticoagulation.

Perioperative Management of Anemia, Coagulopathies, and Thrombocytopenia

All patients should undergo a thorough personal and family history and physical examination to identify underlying anemia or bleeding diatheses. Laboratory testing for coagulation and platelet disorders should not be done routinely due to very low yield and poor correlation with surgical bleeding risk. Hemoglobin and hematocrit should be measured in the setting of signs or symptoms of anemia or surgery with a large expected blood loss. For the patient with a history suggestive of a bleeding disorder, preoperative prothrombin time, activated partial thromboplastin time, and platelet count measurements are indicated.

Preoperative anemia is associated with increased surgical morbidity and mortality and reversible causes, such as iron or vitamin B_{12} deficiency, and should be treated whenever possible. Preoperative autologous blood donation is rarely used because it increases the risk of preoperative anemia and results in the waste of up to 50% of donated units.

Erythrocyte transfusion thresholds have been the focus of much recent research. For multiple types of surgeries and patient characteristics (including those with cardiovascular disease), studies have shown that a conservative transfusion protocol (transfusing for signs or symptoms attributable to anemia or a hemoglobin level <7-8 g/dL [70-80 g/L]) is as good, if not better, than transfusing at a higher hemoglobin level. Studies of patients with cardiovascular disease have also suggested no benefit from more liberal transfusion strategies. One specific exception to a conservative blood management approach is patients with sickle cell disease who benefit from perioperative maintenance of a hemoglobin level of 10 g/dL (100 g/L), either through exchange or traditional erythrocyte transfusions.

A platelet count of greater than $50,000/\mu L$ ($50 \times 10^9/L$) is sufficient to achieve hemostasis in most surgeries. In patients with immune-mediated thrombocytopenia, glucocorticoids and intravenous immune globulin can temporarily boost platelet counts. Patients with platelet function defects may be given prophylactic desmopressin, factor VIII/von Willebrand factor concentrates, or platelet transfusions, depending on their specific disorder. Known coagulation factor deficiencies are treated with specific factor replacement (hemophilia A and B) or fresh frozen plasma (factor XI deficiency). The complexity of platelet function disorders and coagulopathies makes consultation with a hematologist advised in most cases. **H**

KEY POINTS

- Anticoagulation must be stopped prior to most surgical procedures except those with minimal expected blood loss.
- Preoperatively, for patients with low thromboembolic risk, warfarin therapy is stopped with no bridging anticoagulation, whereas high-risk patients should receive bridging anticoagulation. **HVC**
- In patients with coronary artery disease on dual antiplatelet therapy, neither agent should be stopped within 12 months of drug-eluting stent placement or 4 to 6 weeks of bare metal stent placement, acute myocardial infarction, or surgical coronary revascularization.

Perioperative Management of Endocrine Diseases
Diabetes Mellitus

Diabetes mellitus is a risk factor for several perioperative complications, although the link between glucose levels and risk remains indistinct. In cardiac surgery, poor glycemic control, both preoperatively and postoperatively, has been associated with worse cardiovascular, infectious, and neurologic outcomes. For other types of surgery, hyperglycemia is an inconsistent risk factor for complications, and postoperative hyperglycemia (even in patients without a preoperative diagnosis of diabetes) appears to be most predictive of adverse events.

Preoperatively, the status of glycemic control and diabetic complications in patients with diabetes should be assessed, which includes obtaining a hemoglobin A_{1c} measurement and kidney function assay if not tested recently. Although no evidence-based hemoglobin A_{1c} cutoff for elective surgery exists, reasonably good glycemic control (hemoglobin A_{1c} <8%-9%) should be achieved before nonurgent surgery.

Patients on insulin will likely have different insulin needs postoperatively and need close perioperative monitoring. Long-acting insulins (glargine or detemir) should be continued unchanged or at two thirds of their usual dose, depending on risk factors for hypoglycemia and duration of fasting state and procedure. On the morning of surgery and while fasting, neutral protamine Hagedorn (NPH) insulin can be given at half of the usual dose. Short-acting insulins should usually be withheld on the morning of surgery. Patients with type 1 diabetes require at least some insulin at all times to prevent ketoacidosis.

Oral hypoglycemic agents (OHAs) should be withheld for 12 to 72 hours depending on the half-life of the medication. Due to potential side effects and unpredictable postoperative nutrition, these agents should be withheld until the patient has resumed a normal diet. Insulin is the preferred therapy and likely the safest choice for achieving inpatient glycemic control. The recommended insulin regimen should incorporate both basal and prandial coverage. In the setting of preprandial hyperglycemia, prandial coverage can be supplemented with additional insulin (correction factor insulin). Sliding-scale insulin is not recommended. Patients with good preoperative glycemic control (hemoglobin A_{1c} <7%) can resume OHAs on discharge, even if they required significant amounts of insulin while hospitalized. Patients with poor preoperative glycemic control on OHAs meet American Diabetes Association (ADA) criteria for insulin therapy, and the postoperative period can be used to transition to long-term insulin therapy.

Specific postoperative glycemic control targets remain unclear. Recent literature has demonstrated that intensive insulin therapy may not necessarily improve outcomes in hospitalized patients. The ADA and ACP guidelines for managing hyperglycemia in the hospital setting are described in MKSAP 17 Endocrinology and Metabolism.

Thyroid Disease

For patients with stable thyroid disease, thyroid function testing within 6 months before surgery is usually sufficient for preoperative evaluation. Clinicians should order thyroid function tests for any patient with symptoms suggestive of unstable or new thyroid disease. Patients with mild to moderate hypothyroidism generally tolerate surgery well, but those with severe hypothyroidism (overt symptoms related to thyroid hormone deficiency and/or free thyroxine [T_4] level <1.0 ng/dL [12.9 pmol/L]) are at risk for multiple complications. Elective surgery should be postponed for patients who have severe hypothyroidism or those with hypothyroidism who are undergoing high-risk elective surgery. Hyperthyroidism is problematic in the perioperative setting because it is more likely to cause arrhythmias and heart failure. Elective surgery should be delayed to achieve a euthyroid state in patients with clinical hyperthyroidism. If surgery is urgently required, patients should be managed with aggressive β-blocker therapy. Consultation with an endocrine specialist is also warranted to determine other appropriate therapy.

Adrenal Insufficiency

There is minimal evidence on best management of patients at risk for adrenal insufficiency. A practical approach utilizes risk stratification based upon assessment of the physiologic stress of surgery and patient characteristics (**Table 85**). Patients with no risk factors and those undergoing low-risk procedures (such as surgery lasting <45 minutes or without general or neuraxial anesthesia) require only their usual dose of glucocorticoid on the day of surgery. If such patients develop signs or symptoms of adrenal insufficiency, increased doses of glucocorticoids should be provided. Even for those patients at high risk for adrenal insufficiency or undergoing high-risk procedures (such as intrathoracic and intra-abdominal surgery), "stress-dose" glucocorticoids should be rapidly de-escalated within the first few days after surgery. Although adrenocorticotropin hormone stimulation testing can be used to objectively assess the responsiveness of the hypothalamic-pituitary-adrenal axis to surgical stress, such testing is generally not employed because it is expensive and logistically difficult. **H**

KEY POINTS

- In patients with diabetes mellitus, short-acting insulins should usually be withheld on the morning of surgery, and long-acting insulins should usually be continued at two thirds to 100% of the usual dose.

- Elective surgery should be postponed for patients with severe hypothyroidism or those with hypothyroidism undergoing high-risk elective surgery.

- Patient-related risk factors for perioperative adrenal insufficiency include primary adrenal insufficiency and a daily prednisone dose of ≥10 mg for ≥3 weeks in the previous year.

TABLE 85. Management of Perioperative Adrenal Insufficiency Risk

Patient Risk		Management Based on Surgical Risk	
		High	Low
High	Primary adrenal insufficiency; ≥10 mg of daily prednisone[a] for ≥3 weeks in past year	Hydrocortisone, 50-100 mg IV, before surgery, then 25-50 mg IV every 8 h for 24-48 h	Give usual dose of glucocorticoid on day of surgery
Low	Any other glucocorticoid exposure	Give usual dose of glucocorticoid on day of surgery	Give usual dose of glucocorticoid on day of surgery

[a]Or other glucocorticoid of equivalent dose.

Perioperative Management of Kidney Disease

Up to 7% of surgical patients with chronic kidney disease (CKD) experience acute kidney injury (AKI), and even small decrements in kidney function increase morbidity and mortality. Patients should be counseled on these risks.

All patients with CKD should have a recent basic metabolic panel and optimization of blood pressure control and volume status preoperatively. Patients on chronic dialysis should have the timing of dialysis and surgery carefully coordinated. Ideally, dialysis should be performed the day before surgery to allow for re-equilibration of electrolytes and stabilization of blood pressure; dialysis the day after surgery is often necessary if intravascular volume is an issue.

A recent Cochrane systematic review found no significant evidence that specific interventions preserve kidney function perioperatively. However, adequate preoperative hydration, avoidance of nephrotoxic agents (such as NSAIDs), and minimization of perioperative hypotension are useful for patients with kidney disease. It is also important to emphasize the need to maintain adequate hydration during perioperative fasting. ASA fasting guidelines permit clear liquid intake until up to 2 hours before the surgical procedure.

In the postoperative period, kidney function, blood pressure, electrolyte levels, and volume status should be monitored closely in patients with CKD. Urine output poorly correlates with kidney function and should not be used as the sole means of assessing intravascular volume status. Medications should be appropriately dosed for kidney function; morphine, LMWH, and other agents highly dependent on kidney clearance should be used with caution or avoided completely.

KEY POINT

- Patients on chronic dialysis should ideally have dialysis performed the day before surgery to allow for re-equilibration of electrolytes and stabilization of blood pressure.

Perioperative Management of Liver Disease

Abnormal liver function predisposes patients to bleeding, poor wound healing, and infections, and many common perioperative medications, including anesthetics and sedatives, are hepatically metabolized and prone to prolonged effects. Patients with newly diagnosed or worsened liver disease should have elective surgery postponed. If elective surgery is undertaken, patients with stable viral hepatitis and cirrhosis need to be fully apprised of the risks, including the potential for further liver decompensation. For patients with cirrhosis, postoperative mortality is up to 10% for patients with Child-Turcotte-Pugh class A disease and 80% for class C disease. Postoperative mortality for major surgery in patients with cirrhosis can be estimated using a calculator incorporating the Mayo End-stage Liver Disease (MELD) score, patient age, and

ASA classification (www.mayoclinic.org/meld/mayomodel9.html). In general, elective surgeries are safe in patients with a MELD score of less than 8 and are generally not recommended in patients with a MELD score ≥15.

For patients with cirrhosis who do proceed to surgery, liver disease management should be fully optimized (see MKSAP 17 Gastroenterology and Hepatology, Disorders of the Liver). It is advisable to enlist the help of a hepatologist or gastroenterologist in the perioperative management of these patients due to the high perioperative risk of sepsis, kidney failure, liver failure, bleeding, encephalopathy, hypotension, cholestasis, ascites, and pulmonary edema.

KEY POINTS

- Patients with newly diagnosed or worsened liver disease should have elective surgery postponed.
- In general, elective surgeries are safe in patients with a Mayo End-stage Liver Disease (MELD) score of less than 8 and are not recommended in patients with a MELD score ≥15.

Perioperative Management of Neurologic Disease

Patients with chronic neurologic disease are at risk for decompensation in the surgical setting. In general, all medications for chronic neurologic disease should be continued uninterrupted. This is especially important for antiepileptic drugs and Parkinson disease agents. Missing doses of the latter can precipitate a syndrome similar to the neuroleptic malignant syndrome, with severe muscle rigidity and respiratory compromise. For patients likely to be unable to take oral medications, preoperative planning for alternative routes of administration (nasogastric, parenteral, sublingual, transdermal, rectal) should be coordinated with a neurologist.

Even with proper medication management, patients with neuromuscular disease or Parkinson disease remain at risk for complications. Respiratory and oropharyngeal muscle weakness is common in these conditions and may be exacerbated by surgery. Close monitoring for respiratory failure, aspiration, and pneumonia are necessary. Delirium is particularly common in elderly surgical patients, but perioperative risk factors and treatment are similar to those for delirium in the general hospital setting (see MKSAP 17 Neurology).

Postoperative stroke occurs in 0.5% of major surgical procedures and is most common in patients with other cardiovascular risk factors. The contribution of asymptomatic carotid stenosis to the risk of perioperative stroke remains unclear, and prophylactic intervention is not advised prior to noncardiac surgery. Further information on perioperative stroke management is covered in MKSAP 17 Neurology.

KEY POINT

- In general, all medications for chronic neurologic disease should be continued uninterrupted perioperatively.

Bibliography

High Value Care in Internal Medicine

Institute of Medicine (US) Roundtable on Evidence-Based Medicine; Yong PL, Saunders RS, Olsen LA, editors. The Healthcare Imperative: Lowering Costs and Improving Outcomes: Workshop Series Summary. Washington (DC): National Academies Press (US); 2010. [PMID: 21595114]

Murray CJ, Atkinson C, Bhalla K, et al; U.S. Burden of Disease Collaborators. The state of US health, 1990-2010: burden of diseases, injuries, and risk factors. JAMA. 2013 Aug 14;310(6):591-608. [PMID: 23842577]

Sager A, Socolar D. Health Costs Absorb One-Quarter of Economic Growth, 2000-2005. Boston University School of Public Health Web site. February 2005. Available at www.bu.edu/news/2005/02/09/health-costs-absorb-one-quarter-of-economic-growth-2000-05/. Accessed June 8, 2015.

Interpretation of the Medical Literature

Hulley SB, Cummings SR, Browner WS, et al. Designing Clinical Research. 4th ed. Philadelphia, PA: Lippincott, Williams & Wilkins; 2013.

MacMahon B, Yen S, Trichopoulos D, Warren K, Nardi G. Coffee and cancer of the pancreas. N Engl J Med. 1981 Mar 12;304(11):630-3. [PMID: 7453739]

West CP, Dupras DM. 5 ways statistics can fool you–tips for practicing clinicians. Vaccine. 2013 Mar 15;31(12):1550-2. [PMID: 23246309]

Routine Care of the Healthy Patient

Bellcross CA, Page PZ, Meaney-Delman D. Direct-to-consumer personal genome testing and cancer risk prediction. Cancer J. 2012 Jul-Aug;18(4):293-302. [PMID: 22846729]

Bloomfield HE, Olson A, Greer N, et al. Screening pelvic examinations in asymptomatic, average-risk adult women: an evidence report for a clinical practice guideline from the American College of Physicians. Ann Intern Med. 2014 Jul 1;161(1):46-53. [PMID: 24979449]

Centers for Disease Control and Prevention (CDC). Prevention and control of seasonal influenza with vaccines. Recommendations of the Advisory Committee on Immunization Practices–United States, 2013-2014. MMWR Recomm Rep. 2013 Sep 20;62(RR-07):1-43. Erratum in: MMWR Recomm Rep. 2013 Nov 15;62(45):906. [PMID: 24048214]

Cohn AC, MacNeil JR, Clark TA, et al; Centers for Disease Control and Prevention (CDC). Prevention and control of meningococcal disease: recommendations of the Advisory Committee on Immunization Practices (ACIP). MMWR Recomm Rep. 2013 Mar 22;62(RR-2):1-28. [PMID: 23515099]

Cornetta K, Brown CG. Balancing personalized medicine and personalized care. Acad Med. 2013 Mar;88(3):309-13. [PMID: 23348082]

Fenton JJ, Cai Y, Weiss NS, et al. Delivery of cancer screening: how important is the preventive health examination? Arch Intern Med. 2007 Mar 26;167(6):580-5. [PMID: 17389289]

Fitzmaurice DA, Hobbs FD, Jowett S, et al. Screening versus routine practice in detection of atrial fibrillation in patients aged 65 or over: cluster randomised controlled trial. BMJ. 2007 Aug 25;335(7616):383. [PMID: 17673732]

Goldstein MG, Whitlock EP, DePue J; Planning Committee of the Addressing Multiple Behavioral Risk Factors in Primary Care Project. Multiple behavioral risk factor interventions in primary care. Summary of research evidence. Am J Prev Med. 2004 Aug;27(2 Suppl):61-79. [PMID: 15275675]

Gøtzsche PC, Jørgensen KJ. Screening for breast cancer with mammography. Cochrane Database Syst Rev. 2013 Jun 4;6:CD001877. [PMID: 23737396]

Hayes JH, Barry MJ. Screening for prostate cancer with the prostate-specific antigen test: a review of current evidence. JAMA. 2014 Mar 19;311(11):1143-9. [PMID: 24643604]

Humphrey LL, Deffebach M, Pappas M, et al. Screening for lung cancer with low-dose computed tomography: a systematic review to update the US Preventive Services Task Force recommendation. Ann Intern Med. 2013 Sep 17;159(6):411-20. [PMID: 23897166]

Hye RJ, Smith AE, Wong GH, et al. Leveraging the electronic medical record to implement an abdominal aortic aneurysm screening program. J Vasc Surg. 2014 Jun;59(6):1535-42. [PMID: 24507825]

Independent UK Panel on Breast Cancer Screening. The benefits and harms of breast cancer screening: an independent review. Lancet. 2012 Nov 17;380(9855):1778-86. [PMID: 23117178]

Kim DK, Bridges CB, Harriman KH, on behalf of the Advisory Committee on Immunization Practices. Advisory Committee on Immunization Practices Recommended Immunization Schedule for Adults Aged 19 Years or Older: United States, 2015*. Ann Intern Med. 2015;162:214-223.

Krogsbøll LT, Jørgensen KJ, Grønhøj Larsen C, et al. General health checks in adults for reducing morbidity and mortality from disease: Cochrane systematic review and meta-analysis. BMJ. 2012 Nov 20;345:e7191. [PMID: 23169868]

LeFevre ML; U.S. Preventive Services Task Force. Screening for abdominal aortic aneurysm: U.S. Preventive Services Task Force recommendation statement. Ann Intern Med. 2014 Aug 19;161(4):281-90. [PMID: 24957320]

Lieberman DA. Clinical practice. Screening for colorectal cancer. N Engl J Med. 2009 Sep 17;361(12):1179-87. [PMID: 19759380]

Moyer VA; U.S. Preventive Services Task Force. Behavioral counseling interventions to promote a healthful diet and physical activity for cardiovascular disease prevention in adults: U.S. Preventive Services Task Force recommendation statement. Ann Intern Med. 2012 Sep 4;157(5):367-71. [PMID: 22733153]

Moyer VA; U.S. Preventive Services Task Force. Risk assessment, genetic counseling, and genetic testing for BRCA-related cancer in women: U.S. Preventive Services Task Force recommendation statement. Ann Intern Med. 2014 Feb 18;160(4):271-81. [PMID: 24366376]

Moyer VA; U.S. Preventive Services Task Force. Vitamin, mineral, and multivitamin supplements for the primary prevention of cardiovascular disease and cancer: U.S. Preventive services Task Force recommendation statement. Ann Intern Med. 2014 Apr 15;160(8):558-64. [PMID: 24566474]

National Center for Immunization and Respiratory Diseases. General recommendations on immunization–recommendations of the Advisory Committee on Immunization Practices (ACIP). MMWR Recomm Rep. 2011 Jan 28;60(2):1-64. Erratum in: MMWR Recomm Rep. 2011 Jul 29;60:993. [PMID: 21293327]

Nelson HD, Tyne K, Naik A, et al; U.S. Preventive Services Task Force. Screening for breast cancer: an update for the U.S. Preventive Services Task Force. Ann Intern Med. 2009 Nov 17;151(10):727-37, W237-42. [PMID: 19920273]

Oboler SK, LaForce FM. The periodic physical examination in asymptomatic adults. Ann Intern Med. 1989 Feb 1;110(3):214-26. [PMID: 2643379]

Patient Safety and Quality Improvement

Christensen M, Lundh A. Medication review in hospitalised patients to reduce morbidity and mortality. Cochrane Database Syst Rev. 2013 Feb 28;2:CD008986. [PMID: 23450593]

Croskerry P. The importance of cognitive errors in diagnosis and strategies to minimize them. Acad Med. 2003 Aug;78(8):775-80. [PMID: 12915363]

Gallagher TH, Garbutt JM, Waterman AD, et al. Choosing your words carefully: how physicians would disclose harmful medical errors to patients. Arch Intern Med. 2006 Aug 14-28;166(15):1585-93. [PMID: 16908791]

Institute of Medicine (US) Committee on Quality of Health Care in America; Kohn LT, Corrigan JM, Donaldson MS, editors. To Err is Human: Building a Safer Health System. Washington (DC): National Academies Press (US); 2000. [PMID: 25077248]

Kachalia A, Kaufman SR, Boothman R, et al. Liability claims and costs before and after implementation of a medical error disclosure program. Ann Intern Med. 2010 Aug 17;153(4):213-21. [PMID: 20713789]

Makaryus AN, Friedman EA. Patients' understanding of their treatment plans and diagnosis at discharge. Mayo Clin Proc. 2005 Aug;80(8):991-4. [PMID: 16092576]

Roy CL, Poon EG, Karson AS, et al. Patient safety concerns arising from test results that return after hospital discharge. Ann Intern Med. 2005 Jul 19;143(2):121-8. [PMID: 16027454]

Saber Tehrani AS, Lee H, Mathews SC, et al. 25-Year summary of US malpractice claims for diagnostic errors 1986-2010: an analysis from the National Practitioner Data Bank. BMJ Qual Saf. 2013 Aug;22(8):672-80. [PMID: 23610443]

Seminerio MJ, Ratain MJ. Preventing adverse drug-drug interactions: a need for improved data and logistics. Mayo Clin Proc. 2013 Feb;88(2):126-8. [PMID: 23374616]

Varkey P, Reller MK, Resar RK. Basics of quality improvement in health care. Mayo Clin Proc. 2007 Jun;82(6):735-9. [PMID: 17550754]

Professionalism and Ethics

ABIM Foundation. American Board of Internal Medicine; ACP-ASIM Foundation. American College of Physicians-American Society of Internal Medicine; European Federation of Internal Medicine. Medical professionalism in the new millennium: a physician charter. Ann Intern Med. 2002 Feb 5;136(3):243-6. [PMID: 11827500]

Brennan TA, Rothman DJ, Blank L, et al. Health industry practices that create conflicts of interest: a policy proposal for academic medical centers. JAMA. 2006 Jan 25;295(4):429-33. [PMID: 16434633]

Farnan JM, Snyder Sulmasy L, Worster BK, Chaudhry HJ, Rhyne JA, Arora VM; American College of Physicians Ethics, Professionalism and Human Rights Committee; American College of Physicians Council of Associates; Federation of State Medical Boards Special Committee on Ethics and

Professionalism*. Online medical professionalism: patient and public relationships: policy statement from the American College of Physicians and the Federation of State Medical Boards. Ann Intern Med. 2013 Apr 16;158(8):620-7. [PMID: 23579867]

Jonsen AR, Siegler M, Winslade WJ. Clinical Ethics: A Practical Approach to Ethical Decisions in Clinical Medicine. 5th ed. New York: McGraw-Hill; 2002.

Murphy JG, McEvoy MT. Revealing medical errors to your patients. Chest. 2008 May;133(5):1064-5. [PMID: 18460511]

Snyder L; American College of Physicians Ethics, Professionalism, and Human Rights Committee. American College of Physicians Ethics Manual: sixth edition. Ann Intern Med. 2012 Jan 3;156(1 Pt 2):73-104. [PMID: 22213573]

Topazian RJ, Hook CC, Mueller PS. Duty to speak up in the health care setting a professionalism and ethics analysis. Minn Med. 2013 Nov;96(11):40-3. [PMID: 24428018]

Palliative Care

Block SD. Assessing and managing depression in the terminally ill patient. ACP-ASIM End-of-Life Care Consensus Panel. American College of Physicians - American Society of Internal Medicine. Ann Intern Med. 2000 Feb 1;132(3):209-18. [PMID: 10651602]

Evans WG, Tulsky JA, Back AL, Arnold RM. Communication at times of transitions: how to help patients cope with loss and re-define hope. Cancer J. 2006 Sep-Oct;12(5):417-24. [PMID: 17034677]

Strand JJ, Kamdar MM, Carey EC. Top 10 things palliative care clinicians wished everyone knew about palliative care. Mayo Clin Proc. 2013 Aug;88(8):859-65. [PMID: 23910412]

Swetz KM, Kamal AH. In the clinic. Palliative care. Ann Intern Med. 2012 Feb 7; 156(3):ITC2-1. [PMID: 22312158]

Wood GJ, Shega JW, Lynch B, Von Roenn JH. Management of intractable nausea and vomiting in patients at the end of life: "I was feeling nauseous all of the time . . . nothing was working". JAMA. 2007 Sep 12;298(10):1196-207. [PMID: 17848654]

Common Symptoms

Barnett ML, Linder JA. Antibiotic prescribing for adults with acute bronchitis in the United States, 1996-2010. JAMA. 2014 May 21;311(19):2020-2. [PMID: 24846041]

Belgrade MJ, Schamber CD, Lindgren BR. The DIRE score: predicting outcomes of opioid prescribing for chronic pain. J Pain. 2006 Sep;7(9):671-81. [PMID: 16942953]

Brignole M, Hamdan MH. New concepts in the assessment of syncope. J Am Coll Cardiol. 2012 May 1;59(18):1583-91. [PMID: 22538328]

Committee on the Diagnostic Criteria for Myalgic Encephalomyelitis/Chronic Fatigue Syndrome, Board on the Health of Select Populations, Institute of Medicine. Beyond Myalgic Encephalomyelitis/Chronic Fatigue Syndrome: Redefining an Illness. Washington (DC): National Academies Press (US); 2015. [PMID: 25695122]

Ebell MH. Risk stratification of patients presenting with syncope. Am Fam Physician. 2012 Jun 1;85(11):1047-52. [PMID: 22962874]

Edwards TM, Stern A, Clarke DD, Ivbijaro G, Kasney LM. The treatment of patients with medically unexplained symptoms in primary care: a review of the literature. Ment Health Fam Med. 2010 Dec;7(4):209-21. [PMID: 22477945]

Hatcher S, Arroll B. Assessment and management of medically unexplained symptoms. BMJ. 2008 May 17;336(7653):1124-8. [PMID: 18483055]

Hillier SL, McDonnell M. Vestibular rehabilitation for unilateral peripheral vestibular dysfunction. Cochrane Database Syst Rev. 2011 Feb 16;(2):CD005397. [PMID: 21328277]

Hooten WM, Timming R, Belgrade M, et al. Institute for Clinical Systems Improvement. Assessment and management of chronic pain. Available at https://www.icsi.org/_asset/bw798b/ChronicPain.pdf. Updated November 2013. Accessed April 24, 2015.

Howard L, Wessely S, Leese M, et al. Are investigations anxiolytic or anxiogenic? A randomised controlled trial of neuroimaging to provide reassurance in chronic daily headache. J Neurol Neurosurg Psychiatry. 2005 Nov;76(11):1558-64. [PMID: 16227551]

Irwin RS, Baumann MH, Bolser DC, et al; American College of Chest Physicians (ACCP). Diagnosis and management of cough executive summary: ACCP evidence-based clinical practice guidelines. Chest. 2006 Jan;129(1 Suppl):1S-23S. [PMID: 16428686]

Kahn SR, Shapiro S, Wells PS, et al; Compression stockings to prevent post-thrombotic syndrome: a randomised placebo-controlled trial. Lancet. 2014 March;282(9920):880-8. [PMID: 24315521]

Kim JS, Zee DS. Clinical practice. Benign paroxysmal positional vertigo. N Engl J Med. 2014 Mar 20;370(12):1138-47. [PMID: 24645946]

Kripke DF, Langer RD, Kline LE. Hypnotics' association with mortality or cancer: a matched cohort study. BMJ Open. 2012 Feb 27;2(1):e000850. [PMID: 22371848]

Makani H, Bangalore S, Romero J, et al. Peripheral edema associated with calcium channel blockers: incidence and withdrawal rate–a meta-analysis of randomized trials. J Hypertens. 2011 Jul;29(7):1270-80. [PMID: 21558959]

Manchikanti L, Abdi S, Atluri S, et al; American Society of Interventional Pain Physicians. American Society of Interventional Pain Physicians (ASIPP) guidelines for responsible opioid prescribing in chronic non-cancer pain: Part I–evidence assessment. Pain Physician. 2012 Jul;15(3 Suppl):S1-65. [PMID: 22786448]

Manchikanti L, Abdi S, Atluri S, et al; American Society of Interventional Pain Physicians. American Society of Interventional Pain Physicians (ASIPP) guidelines for responsible opioid prescribing in chronic non-cancer pain: Part 2–guidance. Pain Physician. 2012 Jul;15(3 Suppl):S67-116. [PMID: 22786449]

Masters PA. In the clinic. Insomnia. Ann Intern Med. 2014 Oct 7;161(7):ITC1-15. [PMID: 25285559]

Morgenthaler T, Kramer M, Alessi C, et al; American Academy of Sleep Medicine. Practice parameters for the psychological and behavioral treatment of insomnia: an update. An american academy of sleep medicine report. Sleep. 2006 Nov;29(11):1415-9. [PMID: 17162987]

Nuckols TK, Anderson L, Popescu I, et al. Opioid prescribing: a systematic review and critical appraisal of guidelines for chronic pain. Ann Intern Med. 2014 Jan 7;160(1):38-47. [PMID: 24217469]

Qaseem A, Alguire P, Dallas P, et al. Appropriate use of screening and diagnostic tests to foster high-value, cost-conscious care. Ann Intern Med. 2012 Jan 17;156(2):147-9. [PMID: 22250146]

Rosanio S, Schwarz ER, Ware DL, Vitarelli A. Syncope in adults: systematic review and proposal of a diagnostic and therapeutic algorithm. Int J Cardiol. 2013 Jan 20;162(3):149-57. [PMID: 22188993]

Ryan NM, Birring SS, Gibson PG. Gabapentin for refractory chronic cough: a randomised, double-blind, placebo-controlled trial. Lancet. 2012 Nov 3;380(9853):1583-9. [PMID: 22951084]

Smith ME, Haney E, McDonagh M, et al. Treatment of myalgic encephalomyelitis/chronic fatigue syndrome: a systematic review for a National Institutes of Health Pathways to Prevention Workshop. Ann Intern Med. 2015 Jun 16;162(12):841-50. [PMID: 26075755]

Smith RC, Lyles JS, Gardiner JC, et al. Primary care clinicians treat patients with medically unexplained symptoms: a randomized controlled trial. J Gen Intern Med. 2006 Jul;21(7):671-7. [PMID: 16808764]

Tarnutzer AA, Berkowitz AL, Robinson KA, Hsieh YH, Newman-Toker DE. Does my dizzy patient have a stroke? A systematic review of bedside diagnosis in acute vestibular syndrome. CMAJ. 2011 Jun 14;183(9):E571-92. [PMID: 21576300]

Task Force for the Diagnosis and Management of Syncope; European Society of Cardiology (ESC); European Heart Rhythm Association (EHRA); Heart Failure Association (HFA); Heart Rhythm Society (HRS), Moya A, Sutton R, Ammirati F, et al. Guidelines for the diagnosis and management of syncope (version 2009). Eur Heart J. 2009 Nov;30(21):2631-71. [PMID: 19713422]

Wilt TJ, Harris RP, Qaseem A; High Value Care Task Force of the American College of Physicians. Screening for cancer: advice for high-value care from the American College of Physicians. Ann Intern Med. 2015 May 19;162(10):718-25. [PMID: 25984847]

Yancy WS Jr, McCrory DC, Coeytaux RR, et al. Efficacy and tolerability of treatments for chronic cough: a systematic review and meta-analysis. Chest. 2013 Dec;144(6):1827-38. [PMID: 23928798]

Musculoskeletal Pain

Atroshi I, Flondell M, Hofer M, Ranstam J. Methylprednisolone injections for the carpal tunnel syndrome: a randomized, placebo-controlled trial. Ann Intern Med. 2013 Sep 3;159(5):309-17. [PMID: 24026316]

Chou R, Qaseem A, Snow V, et al; Clinical Efficacy Assessment Subcommittee of the American College of Physicians; American College of Physicians; American Pain Society Low Back Pain Guidelines Panel. Diagnosis and treatment of low back pain: a joint clinical practice guideline from the American College of Physicians and the American Pain Society. Ann Intern Med. 2007 Oct 2;147(7):478-91. Erratum in: Ann Intern Med. 2008 Feb 5;148(3):247-8. [PMID: 17909209]

Delitto A, George SZ, Van Dillen LR, et al; Orthopaedic Section of the American Physical Therapy Association. Low back pain. J Orthop Sports Phys Ther. 2012 Apr;42(4):A1-57. [PMID: 22466247]

Hegedus EJ, Goode AP, Cooke CE. Which physical examination tests provide clinicians with the most value when examining the shoulder? Update of a systematic review with meta-analysis of individual tests. Br J Sports Med. 2012 Nov;46(14):964-78. [PMID: 22773322]

Henschke N, Ostelo RW, van Tulder MW, et al. Behavioural treatment for chronic low-back pain. Cochrane Database Syst Rev. 2010 Jul 7;(7): CD002014. [PMID: 20614428]

Hermans J, Luime JJ, Meuffels DE, Reijman M, Simel DL, Bierma-Zeinstra SMA. Does this patient with shoulder pain have rotator cuff disease? The rational clinical examination review. JAMA. 2013 Aug 28;310(8):837-47. [PMID: 23982370]

Kay TM, Gross A, Goldsmith CH, et al. Exercises for mechanical neck disorders. Cochrane Database Syst Rev. 2012 Aug 15;8:CD004250. [PMID: 22895940]

Lankhorst NE, Bierma-Zeinstra SM, van Middelkoop M. Factors associated with patellofemoral pain syndrome: a systematic review. Br J Sports Med. 2013 Mar;47(4):193-206. [PMID: 22815424]

Pattanittum P, Turner T, Green S, Buchbinder R. Non-steroidal anti-inflammatory drugs (NSAIDs) for treating lateral elbow pain in adults. Cochrane Database Syst Rev. 2013 May 31;5:CD003686. [PMID: 23728646]

Soroceanu A, Sidhwa F, Aarabi S, Kaufman A, Glazebrook M. Surgical versus nonsurgical treatment of acute Achilles tendon rupture: a meta-analysis of randomized trials. J Bone Joint Surg Am. 2012 Dec 5;94:2136-43. [PMID: 23224384]

Williams CM, Maher CG, Latimer J, et al. Efficacy of paracetamol for acute low-back pain: a double-blind, randomized controlled trial. Lancet. 2014 Nov 1;384(9954):1586-96. [PMID: 25064594]

Young C. In the clinic: plantar fasciitis. Ann Int Med. 2012;156(1 Pt 1):ITC1-1-ITC1-15. [PMID: 22213510]

Dyslipidemia

Alberti KG, Eckel RH, Grundy SM, et al. Harmonizing the metabolic syndrome: a joint interim statement of the International Diabetes Federation Task Force on Epidemiology and Prevention; National Heart, Lung, and Blood Institute; American Heart Association; World Heart Federation; International Atherosclerosis Society; and International Association for the Study of Obesity. Circulation. 2009 Oct 20; 120(16):1640-5. [PMID: 19805654]

Eckel RH, Jakicic JM, Ard JD, et al; American College of Cardiology/American Heart Association Task Force on Practice Guidelines. 2013 AHA/ACC guideline on lifestyle management to reduce cardiovascular risk: a report of the American College of Cardiology/American Heart Association Task Force on Practice Guidelines. J Am Coll Cardiol. 2014 Jul 1;63(25 Pt B):2960-84. Erratum in: J Am Coll Cardiol. 2014 Jul 1;63(25 Pt B):3027-3028. [PMID: 24239922]

Goff DC Jr, Lloyd-Jones DM, Bennett G, et al; American College of Cardiology/American Heart Association Task Force on Practice Guidelines. 2013 ACC/AHA guideline on the assessment of cardiovascular risk: a report of the American College of Cardiology/American Heart Association Task Force on Practice Guidelines. Circulation. 2014 Jun 24;129(25 Suppl 2):S49-73. Erratum in: Circulation. 2014 Jun 24;129(25 Suppl 2):S74-5. [PMID: 24222018]

Miller M, Stone NJ, Ballantyne C, et al. Triglycerides and cardiovascular disease: a scientific statement from the American Heart Association. Circulation. 2011 May 24;123(20):2292-333. [PMID: 21502576]

Stone NJ, Robinson JG, Lichtenstein AH, et al; American College of Cardiology/American Heart Association Task Force on Practice Guidelines. 2013 ACC/AHA guideline on the treatment of blood cholesterol to reduce atherosclerotic cardiovascular risk in adults: a report of the American College of Cardiology/American Heart Association Task Force on Practice Guidelines. J Am Coll Cardiol. 2014 Jul 1;63(25 Pt B):2889-934. Erratum in: J Am Coll Cardiol. 2014 Jul 1;63(25 Pt B):3024-3025. [PMID: 24239923]

Obesity

Adams TD, Gress RE, Smith SC, et al. Long-term mortality after gastric bypass surgery. N Engl J Med. 2007 Aug 23;357(8):753-61. [PMID: 17715409]

Gloy VL, Briel M, Bhatt DL, et al. Bariatric surgery versus non-surgical treatment for obesity: a systematic review and meta-analysis of randomised controlled trials. BMJ. 2013 Oct 22;347:f5934. [PMID: 24149519]

Greenway FL, Fujioka K, Plodkowski RA, et al; COR-I Study Group. Effect of naltrexone plus bupropion on weight loss in overweight and obese adults (COR-I): a multicentre, randomised, double-blind, placebo-controlled, phase 3 trial. Lancet. 2010 Aug 21;376(9741):595-605. Erratum in: Lancet. 2010 Oct 23;376(9750):1392. Lancet. 2010 Aug 21;376(9741):594. [PMID: 20673995]

Jensen MD, Ryan DH, Apovian CM, et al; American College of Cardiology/American Heart Association Task Force on Practice Guidelines; Obesity Society. 2013 AHA/ACC/TOS guideline for the management of overweight and obesity in adults: a report of the American College of Cardiology/American Heart Association Task Force on Practice Guidelines and The Obesity Society. Circulation. 2014 Jun 24;129(25 Suppl 2):S102-38. Erratum in: Circulation. 2014 Jun 24;129(25 Suppl 2):S139-40. [PMID: 24222017]

Johnston BC, Kanters S, Bandayrel K, et al. Comparison of weight loss among named diet programs in overweight and obese adults: a meta-analysis. JAMA. 2014 Sep 3;312(9):923-33. [PMID: 25182101]

Leblanc ES, O'Connor E, Whitlock EP, Patnode CD, Kapka T. Effectiveness of primary care-relevant treatments for obesity in adults: a systematic evidence review for the U.S. Preventive Services Task Force. Ann Intern Med. 2011 Oct 4;155(7):434-47. [PMID: 21969342]

Mechanick JI, Youdim A, Jones DB, et al; American Association of Clinical Endocrinologists; Obesity Society; American Society for Metabolic & Bariatric Surgery. Clinical practice guidelines for the perioperative nutritional, metabolic, and nonsurgical support of the bariatric surgery patient-2013 update: cosponsored by American Association of Clinical Endocrinologists, The Obesity Society, and American Society for Metabolic & Bariatric Surgery. Obesity (Silver Spring). 2013 Mar;21 Suppl 1:S1-27. [PMID: 23529939]

Moyer VA; U.S. Preventive Services Task Force. Screening for and management of obesity in adults: U.S. Preventive Services Task Force recommendation statement. Ann Intern Med. 2012 Sep 4;157(5):373-8. [PMID: 22733087]

Rucker D, Padwal R, Li SK, Curioni C, Lau DC. Long term pharmacotherapy for obesity and overweight: updated meta-analysis. BMJ. 2007 Dec 8;335(7631):1194-9. Erratum in: BMJ. 2007 Nov 24;335(7629). [PMID: 18006966]

Shyh G, Cheng-Lai A. New antiobesity agents: lorcaserin (Belviq) and phentermine/topiramate ER (Qsymia). Cardiol Rev. 2014 Jan-Feb;22(1):43-50. [PMID: 24304809]

Snow V, Barry P, Fitterman N, Qaseem A, Weiss K; Clinical Efficacy Assessment Subcommittee of the American College of Physicians. Pharmacologic and surgical management of obesity in primary care: a clinical practice guideline from the American College of Physicians. Ann Intern Med. 2005 Apr 5;142(7):525-31. [PMID: 15809464]

Thompson WG, Cook DA, Clark MM, Bardia A, Levine JA. Treatment of obesity. Mayo Clin Proc. 2007 Jan;82(1):93-101. [PMID: 17285790]

Men's Health

AUA Practice Guidelines Committee. AUA guideline on management of benign prostatic hyperplasia (2003). Chapter 1: diagnosis and treatment recommendations. J Urol. 2003 Aug;170(2 Pt 1):530-47. [PMID: 12853821]

Bacon CG, Mittleman MA, Kawachi I, Giovannucci E, Glasser DB, Rimm EB. Sexual function in men older than 50 years of age: results from the health professions follow-up study. Ann Intern Med. 2003 Aug 5;139(3):161-68. [PMID: 12899583]

Barry MJ, Fowler FJ Jr, O'Leary MP, et al. The American Urological Association symptom index for benign prostatic hyperplasia. The Measurement Committee of the American Urological Association. J Urol. 1992 Nov;148(5):1549-57. [PMID: 1279218]

Beckman TJ, Abu-Lebdeh HS, Mynderse LA. Evaluation and medical management of erectile dysfunction. Mayo Clin Proc. 2006 Mar;81(3):385-90. [PMID: 16529142]

Beckman TJ, Mynderse LA. Evaluation and medical management of benign prostatic hyperplasia. Mayo Clin Proc. 2005 Nov;80(10):1356-62. [PMID: 16212149]

Esposito K, Giugliano F, Di Palo C, et al. Effect of lifestyle changes on erectile function in obese men: a randomized controlled trial. JAMA. 2004 Jun 23;291(24):2978-84. [PMID: 15213209]

U.S. Food and Drug Administration. FDA warns consumers about dangerous ingredients in "dietary supplements" promoted for sexual enhancement. www.fda.gov/NewsEvents/Newsroom/PressAnnouncements/2006/ucm108690.htm#. Accessed September 27, 2014.

Women's Health

ACOG Practice Bulletin No. 141: management of menopausal symptoms. Obstet Gynecol. 2014 Jan;123(1):202-16. [PMID: 24463691]

Dawood MY. Primary dysmenorrhea: advances in pathogenesis and management. Obstet Gynecol. 2006 Aug;108(2):428-41. [PMID: 16880317]

Division of Reproductive Health, National Center for Chronic Disease Prevention and Health Promotion, Centers for Disease Control and Prevention (CDC). U.S. Selected Practice Recommendations for Contraceptive Use, 2013: adapted from the World Health Organization selected practice recommendations for contraceptive use, 2nd edition. MMWR Recomm Rep. 2013 Jun 21;62(RR-05):1-60. [PMID: 23784109]

John M. Eisenberg Center for Clinical Decisions and Communications Science. Effectiveness of Treatments for Noncyclic Chronic Pelvic Pain in Adult Women. 2012 Apr 16. Comparative Effectiveness Review Summary Guides for Clinicians. Rockville (MD): Agency for Healthcare Research and Quality (US); 2007-2012. Available at www.ncbi.nlm.nih.gov/books/NBK95339/. [PMID: 22624166]

Manson JE, Chlebowski RT, Stefanick ML, et al. Menopausal hormone therapy and health outcomes during the intervention and extended poststopping phases of the Women's Health Initiative randomized trials. JAMA. 2013 Oct 2;310(13):1353-68. [PMID: 24084921]

Marjoribanks J, Brown J, O'Brien PM, Wyatt K. Selective serotonin reuptake inhibitors for premenstrual syndrome. Cochrane Database Syst Rev. 2013 Jun 7;6:CD001396. [PMID: 23744611]

North American Menopause Society. The 2012 hormone therapy position statement of: The North American Menopause Society. Menopause. 2012 Mar;19(3):257-71. [PMID: 22367731]

Powell AM, Nyirjesy P. Recurrent vulvovaginitis. Best Pract Res Clin Obstet Gynaecol. 2014 Oct;28(7):967-76. [PMID: 25220102]

Shufelt CL, Merz CN, Prentice RL, et al. Hormone therapy dose, formulation, route of delivery, and risk of cardiovascular events in women: findings from the Women's Health Initiative Observational Study. Menopause. 2014 Mar;21(3):260-6. [PMID: 24045672]

Sweet MG, Schmidt-Dalton TA, Weiss PM, Madsen KP. Evaluation and management of abnormal uterine bleeding in premenopausal women. Am Fam Physician. 2012 Jan 1;85(1):35-43. [PMID: 22230306]

Sweetland S, Beral V, Balkwill A, et al; Million Women Study Collaborators. Venous thromboembolism risk in relation to use of different types of postmenopausal hormone therapy in a large prospective study. J Thromb Haemost. 2012 Nov;10(11):2277-86. [PMID: 22963114]

Workowski KA, Bolan GA. Sexually transmitted diseases treatment guidelines, 2015. MMWR Recomm Rep. 2015 Jun 5;64(RR-03):1-137. [PMID: 26042815]

Eye Disorders

Alward WL. Medical management of glaucoma. N Engl J Med. 1998 Oct 29;339(18):1298-307. [PMID: 9791148]

Bal SK, Hollingworth GR. Red eye. BMJ. 2005 Aug 20;331(7514):438. [PMID: 16110072]

Pokhrel PK, Loftus SA. Ocular emergencies. Am Fam Physician. 2007 Sep 15;76(6):829-36. Erratum in: Am Fam Physician. 2008 Apr 1;77(7):920. [PMID: 17910297]

Wirbelauer C. Management of the red eye for the primary care physician. Am J Med. 2006 Apr;119(4):302-6. [PMID: 16564769]

Ear, Nose, Mouth, and Throat Disorders

Chow AW, Benninger MS, Brook I, et al. IDSA clinical practice guideline for acute bacterial rhinosinusitis in children and adults. Clin Infect Dis. 2012 Apr;54(8):e72-e112. [PMID: 22438350]

Lieberthal AS, Carroll AE, Chonmaitree T, et al. The diagnosis and management of acute otitis media. Pediatrics. 2013 Mar;131(3):e964-99. Erratum in: Pediatrics. 2014 Feb;133(2):346. Dosage error in article text. [PMID: 23439909]

Osguthorpe JD, Nielsen DR. Otitis externa: Review and clinical update. Am Fam Physician. 2006 Nov 1;74(9):1510-6. [PMID: 17111889]

Roland PS, Smith TL, Schwartz SR, et al. Clinical practice guideline: cerumen impaction. Otolaryngol Head Neck Surg. 2008 Sep;139(3 Suppl 2):S1-S21. [PMID: 18707628]

Schlosser RJ. Clinical practice. Epistaxis. N Engl J Med. 2009 Feb 19;360(8):784-9. [PMID: 19228621]

Scrivani SJ, Keith DA, Kaban LB. Temporomandibular disorders. N Engl J Med. 2008 Dec 18;359(25):2693-705. [PMID: 19092154]

Walling AD, Dickson GM. Hearing loss in older adults. Am Fam Physician. 2012 Jun 15;85(12):1150-6. [PMID: 22962895]

Wei BP, Stathopoulos D, O'Leary S. Steroids for idiopathic sudden sensorineural hearing loss. Cochrane Database Syst Rev. 2013 Jul 2;7:CD003998. [PMID: 23818120]

Mental and Behavioral Health

American Psychiatric Association. Diagnostic and Statistical Manual of Mental Disorders, 5th ed: DSM-5. Arlington, VA: American Psychiatric Association; 2013.

American Psychiatric Association. Practice guideline for the treatment of patients with major depressive disorder. 3rd ed. Arlington, VA: American Psychiatric Association; 2010. Available at http://psychiatryonline.org/pb/assets/raw/sitewide/practice_guidelines/guidelines/mdd.pdf. Accessed November 10, 2014.

Belmaker RH. Treatment of bipolar depression. N Engl J Med. 2007 Apr 26;356(17):1771-73. [PMID: 17392296]

Bostwick JM. A generalist's guide to treating patients with depression with an emphasis on using side effects to tailor antidepressant therapy. Mayo Clin Proc. 2010 Jun;85(6):538-50. [PMID: 20431115]

Cahill K, Stevens S, Perera R, Lancaster T. Pharmacological interventions for smoking cessation: an overview and network meta-analysis. Cochrane Database Syst Rev. 2013 May 31;5:CD009329. [PMID: 23728690]

Fiore MC, Baker TB. Clinical practice. Treating smokers in the health care setting. N Engl J Med. 2011 Sept 29;365(13):1222-31. [PMID: 21991895]

Kosten TR, O'Connor PG. Management of drug and alcohol withdrawal. N Engl J Med. 2003 May 1;348(18):1786-95. [PMID: 12724485]

Kroenke K, Spitzer RL, Williams JB. The PHQ-9: validity of a brief depression severity measure. J Gen Intern Med. 2001 Sept;16(9):606-13. [PMID: 11556941]

Leucht S, Cipriani A, Spineli L, et al. Comparative efficacy and tolerability of 15 antipsychotic drugs in schizophrenia: a multiple-treatments meta-analysis. Erratum in: Lancet. 2013 Sep 14;382(9896):940. Lancet. 2013 Sep 14;382(9896):951-62. [PMID: 23810019]

Schneider RK, Levenson JL. Psychiatry Essentials for Primary Care. Philadelphia: American College of Physicians; 2008.

Spitzer RL, Kroenke K, Williams JBW, Löwe B. A brief measure for assessing generalized anxiety disorder: the GAD-7. Arch Intern Med 2006 May 22;166(10):1092-97. [PMID: 16717171]

U.S. Preventive Services Task Force. Screening for depression in adults. Available at www.uspreventiveservicestaskforce.org/uspstf/uspsaddepr.htm. Accessed April 2, 2014.

Viron M, Baggett T, Hill M, Freudenreich O. Schizophrenia for primary care providers: how to contribute to the care of a vulnerable patient population. Am J Med. 2012 Mar;125(3):223-30. [PMID: 22340915]

Geriatric Medicine

American Geriatrics Society 2012 Beers Criteria Update Expert Panel. American Geriatrics Society updated Beers Criteria for potentially inappropriate medication use in older adults. J Am Geriatr Soc. 2012 Apr;60(4):616-31. [PMID: 22376048]

Cameron AP, Heidelbaugh JJ, Jimbo M. Diagnosis and office-based treatment of urinary incontinence in adults. Part one: diagnosis and testing. Ther Adv Urol. 2013 Aug;5(4):181-7. [PMID: 23904857]

Cameron AP, Jimbo M, Heidelbaugh JJ. Diagnosis and office-based treatment of urinary incontinence in adults. Part two: treatment. Ther Adv Urol. 2013 Aug;5(4):189-200. [PMID: 23904858]

Coleman EA, Boult C; American Geriatrics Society Health Care Systems Committee. Improving the quality of transitional care for persons with complex care needs. J Am Geriatr Soc. 2003 Apr;51(4):556-7. [PMID: 12657079]

Dumoulin C, Hay-Smith EJ, Mac Habée-Séguin G. Pelvic floor muscle training versus no treatment, or inactive control treatments, for urinary incontinence in women. Cochrane Database Syst Rev. 2014 May 14;5:CD005654. [PMID: 24823491]

Ellis G, Whitehead MA, O'Neill D, Langhorne P, Robinson D. Comprehensive geriatric assessment for older adults admitted to hospital. Cochrane Database Syst Rev. 2011 Jul 6;(7):CD006211. [PMID: 21735403]

Iverson DJ, Gronseth GS, Reger MA, et al; Quality Standards Subcommittee of the American Academy of Neurology. Practice parameter update: evaluation and management of driving risk in dementia: report of the Quality Standards Subcommittee of the American Academy of Neurology. Neurology. 2010 Apr 20;74(16):1316-24. [PMID: 20385882]

Lin JS, O'Connor E, Rossom RC, Perdue LA, Eckstrom E. Screening for cognitive impairment in older adults: A systematic review for the U.S. Preventive Services Task Force. Ann Intern Med. 2013 Nov 5;159(9):601-12. Erratum in: Ann Intern Med. 2014 Jan 7;160(1):72. [PMID: 24145578]

Moyer VA; U.S. Preventive Services Task Force. Screening for hearing loss in older adults: U.S. Preventive Services Task Force recommendation statement. Ann Intern Med. 2012 Nov 6;157(9):655-61. [PMID: 22893115]

National Pressure Ulcer Advisory Panel, European Pressure Ulcer Advisory Panel and Pan Pacific Pressure Injury Alliance. Prevention and Treatment of Pressure Ulcers: Quick Reference Guide. Perth, Australia: Cambridge Media; 2014.

Panel on Prevention of Falls in Older Persons, American Geriatrics Society and British Geriatrics Society. Summary of the Updated American Geriatrics Society/British Geriatrics Society clinical practice guideline for prevention of falls in older persons. J Am Geriatr Soc. 2011 Jan;59(1):148-57. [PMID: 21226685]

Qaseem A, Dallas P, Forciea MA, Starkey M, Denberg TD, Shekelle P; Clinical Guidelines Committee of the American College of Physicians. Nonsurgical management of urinary incontinence in women: a clinical practice guideline from the American College of Physicians. Ann Intern Med. 2014 Sep 16;161(6):429-40. [PMID: 25222388]

Qaseem A, Humphrey LL, Forciea MA, Starkey M, Denberg TD; Clinical Guidelines Committee of the American College of Physicians. Treatment of pressure ulcers: a clinical practice guideline from the American College of Physicians. Ann Intern Med. 2015 Mar 3;162(5):370-9. [PMID: 25732279]

Qaseem A, Mir TP, Starkey M, Denberg TD; Clinical Guidelines Committee of the American College of Physicians. Risk assessment and prevention of pressure ulcers: a clinical practice guideline from the American College of Physicians. Ann Intern Med. 2015 Mar 3;162(5):359-69. [PMID: 25732278]

Teno JM, Gozalo P, Mitchell SL, et al. Feeding tubes and the prevention or healing of pressure ulcers. Arch Intern Med. 2012 May 14;172(9):697-701. [PMID: 22782196]

U.S. Preventive Services Task Force. Screening for impaired visual acuity in older adults: U.S. Preventive Services Task Force recommendation statement. Ann Intern Med. 2009 Jul 7;151(1):37-43, W10. [PMID: 19581645]

Perioperative Medicine

American Society of Anesthesiologists Task Force on Perioperative Management of patients with obstructive sleep apnea. Practice guidelines for the perioperative management of patients with obstructive sleep apnea: an updated report by the American Society of Anesthesiologists Task Force on Perioperative Management of patients with obstructive sleep apnea. Anesthesiology. 2014 Feb;120(2):268-86. [PMID: 24346178]

Carson JL, Grossman BJ, Kleinman S, et al; Clinical Transfusion Medicine Committee of the AABB. Red blood cell transfusion: a clinical practice guideline from the AABB. Ann Intern Med. 2012 Jul 3;157(1):49-58. [PMID: 22751760]

Committee on Standards and Practice Parameters, Apfelbaum JL, Connis RT, et al. Practice advisory for preanesthesia evaluation: an updated report by the American Society of Anesthesiologists Task Force on Preanesthesia Evaluation. Anesthesiology. 2012 Mar;116(3):522-38. [PMID: 22273990]

Douketis JD, Spyropoulos AC, Spencer FA, et al; American College of Chest Physicians. Perioperative management of antithrombotic therapy: Antithrombotic Therapy and Prevention of Thrombosis, 9th ed: American College of Chest Physicians Evidence-Based Clinical Practice Guidelines. Chest. 2012 Feb;141(2 Suppl):e326S-50S. [PMID: 22315266]

Falck-Ytter Y, Francis CW, Johanson NA, et al; American College of Chest Physicians. Prevention of VTE in orthopedic surgery patients: Antithrombotic Therapy and Prevention of Thrombosis, 9th ed: American College of Chest Physicians Evidence-Based Clinical Practice Guidelines. Chest. 2012 Feb;141(2 Suppl):e278S-325S. [PMID: 22315265]

Fleisher LA, Fleischmann KE, Auerbach AD, et al; American College of Cardiology; American Heart Association. 2014 ACC/AHA Guideline on perioperative cardiovascular evaluation and management of patients undergoing noncardiac surgery: a report of the American College of Cardiology/American Heart Association Task Force on practice guidelines. J Am Coll Cardiol. 2014 Dec 9;64(22):e77-137. [PMID: 25091544]

Gould MK, Garcia DA, Wren SM, et al; American College of Chest Physicians. Prevention of VTE in nonorthopedic surgical patients: Antithrombotic Therapy and Prevention of Thrombosis, 9th ed: American College of Chest Physicians Evidence-Based Clinical Practice Guidelines. Chest. 2012 Feb;141(2 Suppl):e227S-77S. [PMID: 22315263]

Kalamas AG, Niemann CU. Patients with chronic kidney disease. Med Clin North Am. 2013 Nov;97(6):1109-22. [PMID: 24182722]

Pieringer H, Stuby U, Biesenbach G. Patients with rheumatoid arthritis undergoing surgery: how should we deal with antirheumatic treatment? Semin Arthritis Rheum. 2007 Apr;36(5):278-86. [PMID: 17204310]

Smetana GW, Lawrence VA, Cornell JE. Preoperative pulmonary risk stratification for noncardiothoracic surgery: systematic review for the American College of Physicians. Ann Intern Med. 2006 Apr 18;144(8):581-95. [PMID: 16618956]

General Internal Medicine Self-Assessment Test

This self-assessment test contains one-best-answer multiple-choice questions. Please read these directions carefully before answering the questions. Answers, critiques, and bibliographies immediately follow these multiple-choice questions. The American College of Physicians is accredited by the Accreditation Council for Continuing Medical Education (ACCME) to provide continuing medical education for physicians.

The American College of Physicians designates MKSAP 17 **General Internal Medicine** for a maximum of **26** *AMA PRA Category 1 Credits*™. Physicians should claim only the credit commensurate with the extent of their participation in the activity.

Earn "Instantaneous" CME Credits Online

Print subscribers can enter their answers online to earn CME credits instantaneously. You can submit your answers using online answer sheets that are provided at mksap.acponline.org, where a record of your MKSAP 17 credits will be available. To earn CME credits, you need to answer all of the questions in a test and earn a score of at least 50% correct (number of correct answers divided by the total number of questions). Take any of the following approaches:

> ➤ Use the printed answer sheet at the back of this book to record your answers. Go to mksap.acponline.org, access the appropriate online answer sheet, transcribe your answers, and submit your test for instantaneous CME credits. There is no additional fee for this service.

> ➤ Go to mksap.acponline.org, access the appropriate online answer sheet, directly enter your answers, and submit your test for instantaneous CME credits. There is no additional fee for this service.

> ➤ Pay a $15 processing fee per answer sheet and submit the printed answer sheet at the back of this book by mail or fax, as instructed on the answer sheet. Make sure you calculate your score and fax the answer sheet to 215-351-2799 or mail the answer sheet to Member and Customer Service, American College of Physicians, 190 N. Independence Mall West, Philadelphia, PA 19106-1572, using the courtesy envelope provided in your MKSAP 17 slipcase. You will need your 10-digit order number and 8-digit ACP ID number, which are printed on your packing slip. Please allow 4 to 6 weeks for your score report to be emailed back to you. Be sure to include your email address for a response.

If you do not have a 10-digit order number and 8-digit ACP ID number or if you need help creating a username and password to access the MKSAP 17 online answer sheets, go to mksap.acponline.org or email custserv@acponline.org.

CME credit is available from the publication date of December 31, 2015, until December 31, 2018. You may submit your answer sheets at any time during this period.

*Each of the numbered items is followed by lettered answers. Select the **ONE** lettered answer that is **BEST** in each case.*

Item 1

A 58-year-old woman is evaluated during a routine examination. She is asymptomatic. Medical history is unremarkable. She smoked cigarettes socially in her 20s but is currently a nonsmoker. Family history is significant for her mother who had a hip fracture in her 70s and two cousins who have hypothyroidism. She takes no medications.

On physical examination, temperature is normal, blood pressure is 118/72 mm Hg, and pulse rate is 72/min. BMI is 24. The remainder of the physical examination is normal.

A lipid panel and fasting plasma glucose level obtained 1 year ago were normal. Pap smear and human papillomavirus testing performed 3 years ago were negative. Her Fracture Risk Assessment Tool (FRAX) score indicates a 13% risk for major osteoporotic fracture over the next 10 years.

Which of the following is the most appropriate screening test for this patient?

(A) Dual-energy x-ray absorptiometry scan
(B) Fasting lipid panel
(C) Fasting plasma glucose level
(D) Pap smear
(E) Thyroid-stimulating hormone level

Item 2

A 38-year-old woman is evaluated during a routine examination. She is a mother of two children and works full time at a high-stress job. She smokes 10 cigarettes daily, eats fast food three times per week, and drinks two alcoholic beverages most nights. She does not exercise. Family history is noncontributory. She takes no medications.

On physical examination, the patient is afebrile, blood pressure is 122/76 mm Hg, and pulse rate is 80/min. BMI is 26. The remainder of the physical examination is normal.

Which of the following interventions will have the largest impact on this patient's health?

(A) Decrease alcohol consumption
(B) Exercise 30 minutes daily, 5 days per week
(C) Healthful diet including fruits and vegetables
(D) Smoking cessation
(E) Stress management and relaxation techniques

Item 3

A 62-year-old woman is evaluated for a 4-hour episode of dizziness. Upon arising from bed in the morning, she noted the abrupt onset of a spinning sensation and imbalance. She has moderate nausea but no vomiting. Symptoms are markedly accentuated when she positions her head backward or forward, such as when bending down to tie her shoe. She reports no dysarthria, diplopia, dysphagia, weakness, numbness, tinnitus, headache, recent head trauma, otalgia, or recent upper respiratory tract infection.

She had a similar episode several years ago. Medical history is remarkable for osteoporosis. Her medications are alendronate, calcium, and vitamin D.

On physical examination, the patient is afebrile, blood pressure is 137/84 mm Hg and pulse rate is 78/min without orthostasis, and respiration rate is 13/min. BMI is 25. Tympanic membranes, external auditory canals, and gross auditory acuity are normal. Cardiopulmonary and neurologic examinations are normal. The Dix-Hallpike maneuver results in mild vertigo with nausea, and after 10 seconds, there are five beats of upbeat nystagmus with a rotatory component with the upper pole of the eyes beating toward the lower ear. The nystagmus lasts for 10 seconds and then abates.

Which of the following is the most appropriate next step in management?

(A) Diazepam
(B) Epley maneuver
(C) Meclizine
(D) Vestibular rehabilitation therapy

Item 4

A 52-year-old woman is seen for preoperative evaluation for open total abdominal hysterectomy. She is an active smoker with a 30-pack-year smoking history but no cough, dyspnea, or chest pain. She reports no daytime fatigue and has never been told she snores or stops breathing in her sleep. She exercises by running for 2 miles on a treadmill every other day. She takes no medications.

On physical examination, respiration rate is 14/min. Oxygen saturation on pulse oximetry is 98% with the patient breathing ambient air. BMI is 28. Cardiovascular examination is normal. Lungs are clear to auscultation and percussion. There is no clubbing or cyanosis of the digits.

In addition to smoking cessation counseling, which of the following is the most appropriate diagnostic test to perform next?

(A) Chest radiography
(B) Chest radiography and spirometry
(C) Chest radiography, spirometry, and arterial blood gas analysis
(D) No further diagnostic tests

Item 5

A 42-year-old woman is evaluated for a 6-day history of right elbow pain that started after lifting a heavy box. The pain is often worse at night and sometimes radiates to the wrist. Her medical and family histories are unremarkable. Her only medication is ibuprofen as needed for the elbow pain, and she has no allergies.

On physical examination, vital signs are normal. There is tenderness over the right lateral epicondyle, but there is normal elbow range of motion and no elbow swelling.

Pain is elicited with resisted wrist extension. The neck and shoulder examinations are normal.

Which of the following is the most appropriate management?

(A) Advise limiting pain-inducing activities
(B) Evaluation for surgical treatment
(C) Glucocorticoid injection
(D) MRI of the right elbow

Item 6

In recent patient satisfaction surveys, a clinical laboratory scored poorly with regard to waiting times for patients. A quality improvement team is created to study the problem and reduce patient waiting times.

Which of the following quality improvement methods would be most useful to help reduce waiting times?

(A) Define, Measure, Analyze, Improve, Control (DMAIC) process
(B) Lean
(C) Plan, Do, Study, Act (PDSA) cycle
(D) Six Sigma

Item 7

A 24-year-old woman is evaluated for severe cramps associated with her menstrual periods. The cramps have worsened over the past year, and the discomfort is severe enough that she has periodically missed work. She reports no abnormal vaginal discharge. Menses are unchanged from her baseline pattern. She has tried ibuprofen and naproxen for pain relief, but these medications cause stomach upset. The patient is sexually active with several male partners. She has no history of sexually transmitted infection and is up to date with her immunizations and gynecologic screening. Medical history is otherwise unremarkable, and she takes no medications.

On physical examination, vital signs are normal. On pelvic examination, there is no cervical motion tenderness, adnexal tenderness, masses, or abnormal discharge. The cervix appears normal. Bimanual examination is unremarkable, and the remainder of the physical examination is normal.

A urine pregnancy test is negative. Tests for *Chlamydia trachomatis* and *Neisseria gonorrhoeae* are negative.

Which of the following is the most appropriate treatment for this patient's dysmenorrhea?

(A) Combined estrogen-progestin contraceptive pill
(B) Depot medroxyprogesterone acetate
(C) Low-dose selective serotonin reuptake inhibitor
(D) Progestin-only contraceptive pill
(E) Tranexamic acid

 ## Item 8

A 91-year-old woman with advanced dementia is examined in her extended-care facility for a routine evaluation. She is nonverbal, incontinent of urine and stool, largely bedbound, and dependent on others for all activities of daily living. The patient's nurse notes that the patient has continued to lose weight despite being actively fed but raises no other concerns. Medical history is significant for hypertension, and her only medication is amlodipine.

On physical examination, blood pressure is 132/87 mm Hg; other vital signs are normal. The patient appears cachectic with temporal wasting. She is awake but is unresponsive to questions. Mucous membranes are moist. She does not appear to have any pain. There are mild early contractures of her ankles and hips. The remainder of the examination, including skin examination, is unremarkable.

Which of the following is the most appropriate intervention for preventing pressure ulcers in this patient?

(A) Alternating-air mattress
(B) Enteral nutrition
(C) Foam mattress overlay
(D) Frequent repositioning

Item 9

A 75-year-old woman is evaluated during a follow-up examination. Medical history is significant for hypertension, type 2 diabetes mellitus, and end-stage kidney disease. She has been treated with hemodialysis for the past year and is not considered a candidate for kidney transplantation. She is currently asymptomatic. Family history is significant for a maternal aunt who was diagnosed with breast cancer at age 70 years. Current medications are lisinopril, nifedipine, sevelamer, aspirin, and regular and neutral protamine Hagedorn (NPH) insulin.

On physical examination, the patient is afebrile, blood pressure is 142/76 mm Hg, and pulse rate is 82/min. An arteriovenous hemodialysis graft is present in the left upper extremity. The remainder of her examination is unremarkable.

The patient's last mammogram, performed 1 year ago, was normal.

Which of the following is the most appropriate management of this patient's breast cancer screening?

(A) Begin annual mammography with breast MRI
(B) Continue annual mammography
(C) Switch to biennial mammography
(D) Discontinue breast cancer screening

Item 10

A 17-year-old teenager is evaluated during an office visit. She is brought in by her mother who is concerned about her focus on diet and weight. The patient states that she believes that she is obese and feels as though she needs to diet to achieve a more appropriate body weight. She also reports exercising on a daily basis to help her lose weight. Dietary history suggests that most of the time she consumes very little food, but at least twice per week she will eat large amounts of high-calorie desserts over the course of 1 to 2 hours. She describes feeling guilty after doing so and will make herself vomit. Medical history is otherwise unremarkable, although she indicates that her menstrual periods are highly irregular.

On physical examination, vital signs are normal. BMI is 23. The parotid glands are enlarged, but the remainder of the examination is unremarkable.

Which of the following is the most likely diagnosis?

(A) Anorexia, purging subtype

(B) Anorexia, restricting subtype

(C) Binge eating disorder

(D) Bulimia nervosa

Item 11

A 28-year-old man is evaluated for a 3-week history of "stuffiness," decreased hearing, and discomfort in his left ear. He has no other symptoms and otherwise feels well except for mild nasal congestion that he attributes to seasonal allergies. Medical history is unremarkable, and he takes no medications.

On physical examination, temperature is normal, blood pressure is 122/62 mm Hg, pulse rate is 90/min, and respiration rate is 11/min. Examination of the left ear is shown. There is no lymphadenopathy. The remainder of the examination is unremarkable.

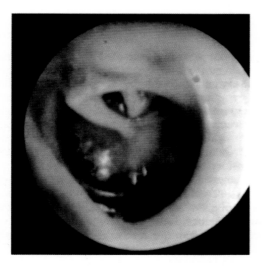

Which of the following is the most appropriate next step in management?

(A) Amoxicillin

(B) Neomycin, polymyxin B, and hydrocortisone ear drops

(C) Tympanostomy tube placement

(D) Clinical observation

Item 12

An 86-year-old woman is evaluated in her assisted-living facility for pain. Four weeks ago, she developed herpetic lesions on her right posterior thorax in a T7 distribution. She was treated with acyclovir, and the lesions healed; however, she has persistent severe burning pain. The pain is so severe that she is unable to leave her bed to attend meals. Medical history is remarkable for hypertension, mild cognitive impairment, and osteoporosis. She ambulates short distances but uses a walker for longer distances. Medications are amlodipine and as-needed acetaminophen. She cannot tolerate opioid medications because they have caused delirium in the past.

On physical examination, the patient is afebrile, blood pressure is 140/86 mm Hg, pulse rate is 62/min, and respiration rate is 14/min. BMI is 18. Examination of the back reveals allodynia and hyperalgesia in the right posterior T7 dermatome. All zoster skin lesions have resolved. On neurologic examination, she exhibits short-term memory impairment, which her family reports is her baseline. The remainder of the examination is unremarkable.

Which of the following medications is the most appropriate pharmacologic therapy for this patient's pain?

(A) Fentanyl patch

(B) Oral gabapentin

(C) Oral tramadol

(D) Topical lidocaine

Item 13

A 26-year-old woman is evaluated for a 3-day history of pain and redness of the left eye. She also notes increased pain when looking at bright objects with that eye. Her symptoms have been progressively worsening since onset. Medical history is unremarkable, although she reports generalized fatigue, chronic low back pain, and stiffness over the past several months. The back pain awakens her at night and improves throughout the day with activity. Her only medication is as-needed ibuprofen for her back pain, which provides some relief.

On physical examination, temperature is normal, blood pressure is 126/64 mm Hg, and pulse rate is 54/min. BMI is 27. On ophthalmologic examination, extraocular muscle movements and visual acuity are normal. There is pronounced redness of the sclera surrounding the border where it meets the cornea in the left eye. The left pupil is constricted, and there is photophobia with illumination of the left eye. The right eye is normal. The physical examination is normal except for tenderness to palpation over the buttocks in the region of the sacroiliac joints.

Which of the following is the most likely diagnosis?

(A) Corneal ulcer

(B) Episcleritis

(C) Scleritis

(D) Uveitis

Item 14

A 49-year-old woman is evaluated during a follow-up visit. She is overweight and has hypertension and type 2 diabetes mellitus, both of which are well controlled. For several years, she has attempted to lose weight through various commercial diets; dietician-monitored, calorie-restricted diets; and physical activity. She has worked with a behavioral therapist, and although she has not achieved weight loss, her weight has remained stable. She exercises 30 minutes daily. Medical history is also remarkable for glaucoma, generalized anxiety disorder, and chronic constipation. Medications are lisinopril, metformin, timolol eye drops, and sertraline.

On physical examination, temperature is normal, blood pressure is 128/74 mm Hg, pulse rate is 70/min, and respiration rate is 12/min. BMI is 29. Waist circumference is 92 cm (36 in). Head, neck, lung, and heart examinations are normal. The abdomen is obese without striae.

In addition to continuing calorie restriction and exercise, which of the following is the most appropriate management to help this patient achieve weight loss?

(A) Lorcaserin
(B) Orlistat
(C) Phentermine-topiramate
(D) Roux-en-Y gastric bypass

Item 15

A 94-year-old woman is brought to the office by her two daughters, who are concerned about her ability to drive. The patient lives independently and drives fewer than 30 miles per week, only during daylight hours. She has no history of traffic tickets or accidents. She feels that she is a very capable driver, although her daughters cite several "near misses," which she dismisses as irrelevant. Medical history is remarkable for mild cognitive impairment, osteoarthritis, and macular degeneration. She sees an ophthalmologist every 3 months, and her corrected vision was stable at her last visit, allowing her to pass the driver's vision test with a restriction to daytime driving at low speeds. She consumes alcohol only occasionally and does not smoke. Her only medication is as-needed acetaminophen.

On physical examination, vital signs and general examination are normal. On musculoskeletal examination, the lateral range of motion of her neck is mildly limited. Gait is antalgic, and she is slow to arise from a seated position. Mini-Mental State Examination score is 24/30.

Which of the following is the most appropriate management of this patient's driving?

(A) Accept the patient's assessment of her ability to drive safely
(B) Advise the patient that she should no longer drive
(C) Ask the patient's ophthalmologist for an assessment of her ability to drive safely
(D) Obtain formal neuropsychiatric testing

Item 16

A 35-year-old woman is evaluated for a several-year history of multiple symptoms, including chronic headaches, dizziness, lightheadedness, shortness of breath, back pain, insomnia, generalized abdominal pain, and numbness. She reports no depressed mood, anhedonia, or problems with concentration or memory. She has been seen by multiple physicians for her symptoms and has been treated in the past with paroxetine, sumatriptan, gabapentin, and

an as-needed albuterol inhaler without improvement of her symptoms.

Review of previous records shows laboratory studies significant for normal comprehensive metabolic profile, complete blood count, thyroid function tests, and antinuclear antibody test. Other studies include an unremarkable mammogram, chest radiograph, abdominal and pelvic CT scans, and MRI of the lumbar spine. Upper endoscopy is unremarkable, and pulmonary function tests are normal.

Medical history is significant for depression in college. She does not smoke, drink alcohol, or use illicit drugs. She is currently unemployed and on disability due to her symptoms. She reports allergies to multiple medications, including penicillin, sulfa-containing drugs, and macrolide and fluoroquinolone antibiotics. Medications are as-needed ibuprofen and multiple herbal preparations.

Physical examination is unremarkable.

Which of the following is the most appropriate management of this patient?

(A) Brain MRI
(B) Citalopram
(C) Cognitive-behavioral therapy
(D) Evaluation by a neurologist
(E) Follow-up in 6 months

Item 17

A 56-year-old woman is evaluated for a painless lump in her right breast that she first noticed 6 weeks ago. She has not had any nipple discharge. She has no history of breast lumps or abnormal mammograms; her last screening mammogram was 8 months ago and was negative. Medical history is unremarkable. She experienced menarche at age 12 years and menopause at age 53 years, and she is gravida 4, para 3. There is no breast, ovarian, or colon cancer in her family history. She takes no medications.

On physical examination, she is afebrile, blood pressure is 134/82 mm Hg, pulse rate is 72/min, and respiration rate is 12/min. BMI is 25. Examination of the breasts reveals a firm, nontender, 1-cm mass on the right upper outer quadrant 3 cm from the areolar edge. There is no nipple discharge or skin change, and no supraclavicular or axillary lymphadenopathy.

A mammogram is obtained and is read as benign (Breast Imaging Reporting and Data System [BI-RADS] category 1).

Which of the following is the most appropriate management?

(A) Breast MRI
(B) Clinical reassessment in 4 weeks
(C) Core needle biopsy
(D) Resume regular mammographic screening

Item 18

An 88-year-old woman living in a nursing home is evaluated for worsening dizziness, weakness, and gait unsteadiness of several weeks' duration. She also reports occasional vague lightheadedness and feeling like her legs are "wobbly." She reports no vertigo, chest pain, palpitations, loss of consciousness, leg or arm weakness, numbness, tingling, tinnitus, headaches, neck or other joint pain, or falls or head trauma. She was provided with a cane, but she feels too weak to use it. Medical history is also remarkable for cataract, hearing loss, osteoporosis, and hypertension. Medications are alendronate, lisinopril, and vitamin D.

On physical examination, the patient is alert and oriented. She is afebrile. Blood pressure is 142/70 mm Hg supine and 136/70 mm Hg standing, precipitating symptoms of lightheadedness; pulse rate is 86/min supine and 88/min standing; and respiration rate is 16/min. BMI is 20. On neurologic examination, she has 20/200 vision, diminished hearing, and 4/5 motor strength in both upper and lower extremities. The remainder of the examination is normal.

Laboratory studies reveal a hemoglobin level of 11.6 g/dL (116 g/L) and normal vitamin B_{12} and thyroid-stimulating hormone levels. Results of a comprehensive metabolic profile are normal.

Electrocardiogram shows normal sinus rhythm with first-degree atrioventricular block and left ventricular hypertrophy.

Referrals are made to address her auditory and visual impairments.

Which of the following is the most appropriate additional management?

(A) CT scan of the head
(B) 24-Hour ambulatory electrocardiography
(C) Physical therapy
(D) Provide a walker

Item 19

A 66-year-old man is evaluated following a multilevel lumbar spine laminectomy and fusion 2 days ago. He tolerated general anesthesia well and had approximately 1200 mL of intraoperative blood loss. Postoperative recovery has been uneventful. He has been fully participating in physical therapy without symptoms of lightheadedness, shortness of breath, or chest pain. His surgical site pain is well controlled and gradually receding. Medical history is notable for hypertension, hyperlipidemia, anemia of chronic disease, and coronary artery disease with placement of a bare metal stent 4 years ago. Medications are carvedilol, atorvastatin, aspirin, and as-needed oxycodone and acetaminophen.

On physical examination, the patient is afebrile. Blood pressure is 140/86 mm Hg, and pulse rate is 60/min. The surgical site is intact with no surrounding erythema, tenderness, or induration. The remainder of the examination is normal.

Laboratory studies are significant for a hemoglobin level of 9.1 g/dL (91 g/L). Prior to surgery, the hemoglobin level was 13.1 g/dL (131 g/L). Leukocyte count and platelet count are normal.

Which of the following is the most appropriate management of this patient's anemia?

(A) Administer intravenous iron
(B) Transfusion of one unit of packed red blood cells
(C) Transfusion of two units of packed red blood cells
(D) Clinical observation

Item 20

A 68-year-old man is evaluated for a 3-month history of pain on the superior aspect of the right shoulder. The pain developed insidiously and has progressively worsened. He reports no trauma or other symptoms. Medical history is unremarkable. The patient has tried both acetaminophen and ibuprofen, with only minimal pain relief.

On physical examination, the patient is afebrile, blood pressure is 134/84 mm Hg, pulse rate is 92/min, and respiration rate is 16/min. BMI is 28. The right shoulder is normal in appearance. Pain is reproduced with adduction of the right arm across the body. The painful arc test and drop-arm test are negative. There is full active and passive range of motion; strength is 5/5 throughout the right arm. The remainder of the examination is unremarkable.

Which of the following is the most likely diagnosis?

(A) Acromioclavicular joint degeneration
(B) Adhesive capsulitis
(C) Rotator cuff tear
(D) Supraspinatus tendinitis

Item 21

A 77-year-old man is evaluated in follow-up for prostate cancer. He is asymptomatic and feels well. He was diagnosed with high-grade prostate cancer 3 years ago and was treated with external-beam radiation therapy. Since that time, he has undergone regular surveillance.

His most recent serum prostate-specific antigen level rose from undetectable to 120 ng/mL (120 µg/L). A subsequent abdominopelvic CT scan showed an increase in regional lymphadenopathy and multiple sclerotic bony lesions in the visualized pelvis and spine.

The patient has been actively engaged in his medical care and has expressed a desire to be made aware of all information about his health status. The patient has scheduled this visit to discuss the results of his prostate cancer surveillance testing, and the physician indicates to the patient that, unfortunately, he has bad news to convey.

Which of the following is the most appropriate approach to conveying this news to the patient?

(A) Explain that the planned surveillance has done what was intended and that it has led to the finding of possible recurrent tumors
(B) Indicate that there are several abnormal lesions in his bones that will require further evaluation
(C) Note that the cancer has likely returned but that hormonal therapy and chemotherapy are usually effective treatments
(D) State that the cancer has returned

Item 22

A 59-year-old man is evaluated during a health maintenance visit. He is asymptomatic. He has a 35-pack-year smoking history, but he quit smoking 5 years ago. He takes no medications.

Vital signs and the results of the physical examination are normal.

Which of the following is the most appropriate screening test to obtain?

(A) Abdominal ultrasonography
(B) Chest radiography
(C) Low-dose chest CT
(D) Spirometry

Item 23

A 78-year-old man is evaluated for low back pain that has worsened over the past 24 hours. The patient has had chronic low back pain localized to the lumbar spine without radiation for many years. He reports no trauma but notes that his low back pain has rapidly increased in intensity and that he now has a "pins and needles" sensation over the inner thighs and intermittent radiation of pain down both legs. Treatment with over-the-counter analgesics and anti-inflammatory agents usually resolves his pain, but these medications have not helped his current symptoms. He has not had fever, chills, or other systemic symptoms. He has had urinary retention but no bowel incontinence. Medical history is significant for hypertension and hyperlipidemia. Current medications are hydrochlorothiazide, atorvastatin, and as-needed acetaminophen and naproxen.

On physical examination, temperature is 37.1 °C (98.7 °F), blood pressure is 148/70 mm Hg, and pulse rate is 95/min. BMI is 26. The general medical examination is unremarkable. On musculoskeletal examination, the major lower extremity muscle groups show normal bulk and tone with normal or slightly decreased strength. Neurologic examination shows a decrease in anal tone and saddle anesthesia. The patellar reflexes are normal, but ankle reflexes are absent bilaterally.

MRI of the lumbosacral spine shows vertebral endplate osteophytosis, facet joint hypertrophy, and thickening of the ligamentum flavum resulting in narrowing of the spinal canal at multiple levels but without evidence of mass or hemorrhage.

Which of the following is the most appropriate management?

(A) Epidural glucocorticoid injection
(B) High-dose intravenous glucocorticoid therapy
(C) Lumbar puncture
(D) Surgical evaluation

Item 24

A 55-year-old man is evaluated for the gradual onset of erectile dysfunction over the past year. He reports a satisfying marriage, but during most sexual encounters, he is unable to achieve an erection that is satisfactory for vaginal penetration. He has been spending longer hours at work, and he no longer exercises regularly. Nonetheless, he describes his mood as excellent and continues to enjoy time with his family. He sleeps well, and his energy level is good. He reports no chest pain or dyspnea. He does not have nocturnal erections. He does not smoke cigarettes.

On physical examination, the patient appears alert and comfortable. Blood pressure is 134/60 mm Hg. BMI is 32. Cardiopulmonary examination is normal. The penis, testicles, and prostate are normal.

Which of the following is the most appropriate next step in management?

(A) Intraurethral alprostadil
(B) Marriage counseling
(C) Venlafaxine
(D) Weight loss

Item 25

An 80-year-old man was hospitalized 1 week ago for a 5-day history of acute leg ischemia treated with angioplasty and stenting. He is now asymptomatic. The patient has a history of stage 3 chronic kidney disease and hypertension that is well controlled with diltiazem and lisinopril. Other medications are aspirin and clopidogrel.

On physical examination, the patient is afebrile, and blood pressure is 130/78 mm Hg. The remainder of the examination is unremarkable.

Laboratory studies:

Alanine aminotransferase	20 U/L
Total cholesterol	170 mg/dL (4.40 mmol/L)
LDL cholesterol	97 mg/dL (2.51 mmol/L)
HDL cholesterol	44 mg/dL (1.14 mmol/L)
Serum creatinine	1.8 mg/dL (159 µmol/L)
Triglycerides	147 mg/dL (1.67 mmol/L)
Estimated glomerular filtration rate	35 mL/min/1.73 m²

Which of the following is the most appropriate therapy for secondary prevention of cardiovascular disease in this patient?

(A) High-intensity rosuvastatin
(B) Moderate-intensity rosuvastatin
(C) Niacin
(D) No additional treatment

Item 26

A physician reviews a study in which investigators attempted to determine whether tadalafil improved erectile function following radiation treatment for prostate cancer. The researchers reviewed the records of 940 patients with prostate cancer who had undergone radiation therapy. Three hundred patients received daily tadalafil following radiation, and 640 patients did not receive tadalafil. There was no significant difference in the overall International Index of Erectile Function scores ($P < 0.15$) between the two groups.

Which of the following would be the most appropriate outcome measure for this study?

(A) Confidence interval
(B) Number needed to treat
(C) Odds ratio
(D) Relative risk

Item 27

An 88-year-old man is evaluated at an assisted-living facility. Staff members have noticed that the patient seems more withdrawn than usual, is less interactive with other residents, and no longer attends social functions. At times, he seems confused and answers questions nonsensically or has difficulty navigating simple conversations. At other times, he seems normal and cheerful. The staff has not observed any crying spells. He appropriately manages his own medications and finances. There have been no recent changes in his medications. He has had no recent falls, illness, or fever.

On physical examination, vital signs are normal. The patient is appropriately conversant. The general medical examination is unremarkable. On neurologic examination, Mini-Mental State Examination score is 25/30, which is unchanged over the past 18 months. A two-question depression screen is negative. The remainder of the neurologic examination is unremarkable.

Which of the following is the most appropriate management of this patient?

(A) Donepezil
(B) PHQ-9 depression assessment
(C) Whispered voice test
(D) Clinical observation

Item 28

A 79-year-old man is evaluated for a 3-month history of right hip pain. He points to the center of his right buttock when asked to identify the location of the pain. He has no radicular symptoms. He reports no focal trauma but believes his symptoms began after he stepped off a curb that was higher than anticipated. Medical history is otherwise unremarkable. His only medication is as-needed acetaminophen for pain.

On physical examination, vital signs are normal. The general medical examination is unremarkable. There is no tenderness to palpation over the lateral right hip, and he notes mild discomfort when the "dimple" areas of the posterior surface of the buttocks are palpated. There is no pain with passive range of motion of both hips. Straight-leg raise test is negative. When either hip is flexed, abducted, and externally rotated with downward pressure applied to the knee, his pain is reproduced.

Which of the following is the most likely diagnosis?

(A) Hip joint osteoarthritis
(B) Piriformis syndrome
(C) Sacroiliitis
(D) Trochanteric bursitis

Item 29

A 26-year-old woman is evaluated during a routine follow-up visit. She recently underwent direct-to-consumer genetic testing that offered risk screening for more than 200 different conditions. Her results indicate that her genetic breast cancer risk is 52.5% greater than that of the average woman, and she is interested in discussing what should be done next. She feels well and has no symptoms. Three-generation family history is negative for breast and ovarian cancer. She takes no medications.

The physical examination is normal.

Which of the following is the most appropriate next diagnostic test?

(A) Biennial breast MRI screening
(B) *BRCA* genetic testing
(C) Monthly breast self-examination
(D) No further testing

Item 30

An 88-year-old woman with severe emphysema is evaluated in the hospital for dyspnea. This is her seventh hospitalization in the last 6 months for similar symptoms. Her ability to perform basic daily activities between hospitalizations is markedly limited, and she reports uncomfortable shortness of breath both at rest and with minimal activity. Medical history is otherwise significant only for hypertension. Medications are tiotropium, mometasone/formoterol, as-needed albuterol, hydrochlorothiazide, and supplemental oxygen.

On physical examination, the patient is notably dyspneic with increased work of breathing at rest. She is afebrile, blood pressure is 148/84 mm Hg, pulse rate is 98/min, and respiration rate is 22/min. Oxygen saturation is 86% breathing 6 L of oxygen by nasal cannula. BMI is 17. There is no jugular venous distention. The lungs show markedly decreased air movement but no focal findings. There is trace bipedal edema. The remainder of the examination is unremarkable.

Following extensive discussion with the patient, she indicates a desire to pursue a palliative approach with a focus on symptom control given her advanced disease and lack of response to maximal medical therapy.

Which of the following is the most appropriate treatment of this patient's dyspnea?

(A) Nebulized lidocaine
(B) Nebulized morphine
(C) Oral lorazepam
(D) Oral morphine

Item 31

A 68-year-old man is evaluated in the hospital for a right intertrochanteric fracture sustained in a mechanical fall. He reports right hip pain but no other symptoms. He has hypertension and type 2 diabetes mellitus and was in his usual state of health prior to the fall. He checks his blood glucose level several times daily; his average blood glucose level is 150 mg/dL (8.3 mmol/L), with a low of 92 mg/dL (5.1 mmol/L) and a high of 208 mg/dL (11.5 mmol/L). Surgical repair is scheduled for tomorrow at 7:00 AM with an anticipated length of surgery of 1.5 hours; use of spinal anesthesia is planned. Medications are enalapril; extended-release metformin; insulin glargine, 20 units nightly; and insulin lispro, 8 units with each meal. It is 8:00 PM, and the patient took his usual morning medications and insulin lispro prior to dinner but has not yet taken insulin glargine.

On physical examination, vital signs are normal. An ecchymosis is noted over the right hip. The right leg is externally rotated. The remainder of the examination is unremarkable.

Laboratory studies are significant for a hemoglobin A_{1c} level of 8.2% and a plasma glucose level of 182 mg/dL (10.1 mmol/L).

In addition to discontinuing metformin, which of the following is the most appropriate preoperative diabetic management for this patient?

(A) Administer insulin glargine as usual; withhold scheduled insulin lispro

(B) Continue both insulin glargine and insulin lispro uninterrupted

(C) Stop insulin glargine and insulin lispro; start intravenous insulin infusion

(D) No further insulin until after surgery

Item 32

A 26-year-old man is evaluated for a 3-month history of depressed mood, poor concentration, decreased energy, increased sleep, and weight gain. He reports missing many days at work and that his work performance has lagged. He has no suicidal ideation. He states that his current symptoms differ markedly from his usual state of being "highly upbeat and energetic" and having high job performance. He has experienced several 30- to 40-day periods of high energy during which he sleeps little and makes "bad choices" (such as spending sprees and "one-night stands"). He has not experienced hallucinations. Medical history is notable for treatment of depression during college with a 6-month course of sertraline. He stopped the drug when he felt "energetic." He is currently taking no medications.

Physical examination is unremarkable.

Laboratory studies are normal.

Which of the following is the most appropriate treatment?

(A) Desipramine

(B) Paroxetine

(C) Quetiapine

(D) Venlafaxine

Item 33

A 66-year-old man who was admitted to the hospital after undergoing urgent sigmoid colectomy for a perforated diverticulum is evaluated for co-management of his medical problems. He tolerated general anesthesia well and had no immediate perioperative complications. He is fully awake, alert, and breathing comfortably with adequate control of postoperative pain. Additional history provided by his wife indicates that he snores loudly when sleeping and occasionally seems to gag and stop breathing. He reports no daytime somnolence. Medical history includes hypertension and hyperlipidemia. Medications are lisinopril, simvastatin, and as-needed oxycodone.

On physical examination, blood pressure is 156/94 mm Hg, and respiration rate is 18/min. Oxygen saturation on pulse oximetry is 97% with the patient breathing ambient air. BMI is 45. Cardiovascular examination is normal. The lungs are clear to auscultation. The left lower quadrant surgical incision is intact with minimal tenderness to palpation; bowel sounds are present, and the abdomen is not distended.

Laboratory studies on admission were significant for a hemoglobin level of 14.6 g/dL (146 g/L), a leukocyte count of 18,000/μL (18×10^9/L) with 95% neutrophils, and a normal basic metabolic panel.

In addition to continuous pulse oximetry, which of the following is the most appropriate respiratory management of this patient?

(A) Insert a nasogastric tube

(B) Keep the head of the bed elevated at 30 degrees

(C) Start nebulized albuterol

(D) Start nocturnal continuous positive airway pressure ventilation

Item 34

A 65-year-old man is scheduled to undergo staged bilateral cataract extractions under conscious sedation. Medical history is notable for hypertension and asthma. Medications are amlodipine, an albuterol inhaler as needed, and a fluticasone inhaler.

On physical examination, blood pressure is 122/74 mm Hg. The cardiac examination is normal. The lungs are clear.

Laboratory studies from 1 year ago show normal serum electrolyte and serum creatinine levels.

Which of the following is the most appropriate diagnostic test to perform next?

(A) Chest radiography

(B) Complete blood count, prothrombin time, and activated partial thromboplastin time

(C) Electrocardiography

(D) Serum electrolytes and creatinine

(E) No diagnostic studies

Item 35

A 29-year-old woman is evaluated for a 2-week history of a tender lump in the left breast. She has not noticed skin changes, swollen glands, or nipple discharge, and there is no history of trauma to the breast. She had a similar problem last year with a breast biopsy that was negative for cancer and was told she has fibrocystic breasts. She takes a monocyclic oral contraceptive and her menses are regular, with her last menstrual period starting 1 week ago. She underwent menarche at age 12 years, and she has never been pregnant. She has no family history of breast cancer.

On physical examination, all vital signs are normal. BMI is 25. Examination of the breasts reveals a 2-cm round, mobile, tender mass in the upper outer quadrant of the left breast. There are no skin changes and no supraclavicular or axillary lymphadenopathy. The remainder of the physical examination is unremarkable.

Which of the following is the most appropriate management?

(A) Diagnostic ultrasonography

(B) Digital diagnostic mammography

(C) Fine needle aspiration biopsy

(D) Stop hormonal contraception

Item 36

A 39-year-old woman presents for a second opinion following a recent diagnosis of systemic exertion intolerance disease (formerly known as chronic fatigue syndrome), which was made after a thorough evaluation. Her symptoms are interfering with her daily personal and professional activities. She reports generalized myalgia, arthralgia, difficulty concentrating, unrefreshing sleep, and chronic headaches but no anhedonia or thoughts of self-harm. Review of previous records shows a normal physical examination. Complete blood count, erythrocyte sedimentation rate, thyroid function tests, electrolytes, kidney function tests, glucose level, creatine kinase level, serum creatinine level, liver chemistry studies, antinuclear antibody test, and urine drug screen were all normal within the past several months. A sleep study and imaging studies of the chest, abdomen, and pelvis were normal. Medical history is significant for hypertension. Family history is remarkable for hypertension in both parents. Her only medication is ramipril.

Physical examination is unremarkable.

Which of the following is the most appropriate next step in management?

(A) Citalopram

(B) Cognitive-behavioral therapy

(C) Methylphenidate

(D) Valacyclovir

Item 37

A 28-year-old woman visits to discuss her contraceptive options. She is sexually active and is in a monogamous relationship with a new partner. She has been using depot medroxyprogesterone acetate for the past 2 years but has unpredictable breakthrough bleeding, which she finds unacceptable; in addition, she reports mood changes and weight gain. She does not plan to have children for several years and is interested in trying birth control pills. Medical history is significant for episodic migraine associated with photophobia and visual aura. She has never smoked. Her only medication is as-needed sumatriptan.

On physical examination, vital signs are normal. BMI is 21. The general medical examination is unremarkable.

In addition to recommending condom use to reduce risk of sexually transmitted infections, which of the following is the most appropriate contraceptive method to recommend?

(A) Estrogen-progestin oral contraceptive

(B) Estrogen-progestin vaginal ring

(C) Intrauterine device

(D) Progestin-only oral contraceptive

(E) Progestin subcutaneous implant

Item 38

A 65-year-old man is evaluated during a follow-up examination. The patient is asymptomatic. He expresses interest in being screened for prostate cancer with a new screening test. The patient brings in a printout of a study of the screening test, which used a randomly selected population of men and divided them into two groups: one that was screened for prostate cancer using the new test and another that did not undergo screening and in whom any cases of prostate cancer were diagnosed by detection of symptoms and signs of the disease. The researchers, including outcome assessors, were blinded.

The study found that prostate cancer survival was increased by 2 years in the screened group compared with the non-screened group. The study mostly included healthy white men with an average age of 66 years. There was little crossover between groups. In the group that was screened for prostate cancer, there were more cases of prostate cancer diagnosed overall, most of which were low-grade cancers. In the group that was not screened, there were significantly fewer cases of prostate cancer diagnosed overall; however, those that were diagnosed were more aggressive.

Which of the following is the most likely cause of the increased survival in the screen-detected cohort?

(A) Contamination bias

(B) Length-time bias

(C) Observer bias

(D) Selection bias

Item 39

A 48-year-old man is evaluated for a 2-day history of right anterior knee pain and swelling. The pain began suddenly and has increased in intensity. He currently rates his pain as an 8 on a 10-point scale. He has no knee instability and reports no fever or chills. He has no history of trauma and has never had this problem before. Other than his right knee pain and swelling, he feels well. He is employed as a carpet layer. His only medication is ibuprofen, which provides minimal relief.

On physical examination, vital signs are normal. BMI is 28. On examination of the right knee, there is a palpable fluid collection that is located anterior to the patella. The right knee has full range of motion. There is no medial or lateral joint line tenderness or laxity with varus or valgus forces. Anterior drawer, posterior drawer, and Lachman tests are all negative.

Which of the following is the most appropriate next step in management?

(A) Aspiration

(B) Compression

(C) Glucocorticoid injection

(D) Right knee radiographs

(E) Ultrasound

Item 40

A 35-year-old woman is scheduled for right carpal tunnel release to be performed with local anesthesia and mild sedation. Anticipated duration of surgery is less than 1 hour. She is physically active and otherwise feels well with no lightheadedness, weight changes, fatigue, or shortness of breath. She received a living-related kidney transplant 5 years ago for polycystic kidney disease; she also has hypertension. Medications are amlodipine, tacrolimus, mycophenolate, and prednisone, 5 mg/d. She has not had any recent changes in her medications.

On physical examination, she is afebrile. Blood pressure is 128/80 mm Hg, and pulse rate is 68/min. Except for paresthesias in the right hand following the distribution of the median nerve, the physical examination is unremarkable.

Laboratory studies show a normal basic chemistry panel and kidney function tests.

Which of the following is the most appropriate preoperative management of this patient's glucocorticoid therapy on the day of surgery?

(A) Continue current prednisone dose
(B) Double the current prednisone dose
(C) Substitute intravenous hydrocortisone, 50 mg, for daily prednisone
(D) Withhold prednisone

Item 41

An 81-year-old man is admitted to the hospital with an acute coronary syndrome. Immediate coronary angiography with possible angioplasty and stent placement is indicated. The patient has mild dementia treated with donepezil. He is married, and his wife is his designated surrogate decision maker. The patient is informed of the risks, benefits, and alternatives to the procedure. He expresses understanding of these elements in basic terms and is able to reflect back the risks, benefits, and alternatives to the procedure. He consents to coronary angiography, and when asked again, his decision is unchanged. His wife is currently unavailable.

Which of the following is the most appropriate next step?

(A) Obtain consent from the patient's spouse
(B) Perform a Mini-Mental State Examination
(C) Proceed with coronary angiography
(D) Request that a colleague assess and confirm the patient's decision-making capacity

Item 42

A 27-year-old man is evaluated in the emergency department for dull, throbbing, left testicular pain occurring over the past week. He also notes urinary frequency and dysuria, but no penile discharge. He reports no back pain, weight loss, or fever. Medical history is unremarkable. His only medication is ibuprofen, which he takes as needed for pain. He is sexually active with several different partners and uses barrier protection only intermittently. He reports no testicular trauma.

On physical examination, blood pressure is 126/64 mm Hg, and pulse rate is 90/min. BMI is 22. The penis appears normal without discharge at the meatus. The left testicle is boggy and exquisitely tender to palpation over the superior pole. The testicular pain lessens with elevation of the testis.

Laboratory studies reveal a normal complete blood count, and urinalysis with microscopy shows 2 leukocytes/hpf.

Which of the following is the most likely diagnosis?

(A) Epididymitis
(B) Testicular torsion
(C) Urinary tract infection
(D) Varicocele

Item 43

A 64-year-old woman is evaluated for difficulty controlling her urine. The patient works and maintains a very active lifestyle; the urinary leakage is restricting her activities. She needs to wear pads because of involuntary loss of urine with coughing, sneezing, and laughing, and occasionally with physical exertion. There is no dysuria or increased urinary frequency. She does not smoke and does not drink alcoholic beverages. Medical history is remarkable for hypertension, and her only medication is lisinopril.

On physical examination, temperature is normal, blood pressure is 130/78 mm Hg, pulse rate is 72/min, and respiration rate is 14/min; BMI is 29. General examination is unremarkable. Pelvic examination is normal except for mild anterior wall prolapse.

Urinalysis is normal.

In addition to suggesting weight loss, which of the following is the most appropriate management?

(A) Oxybutynin
(B) Pelvic floor muscle training
(C) Postvoid residual urine volume measurement
(D) Prompted voiding
(E) Urodynamic study

Item 44

A 26-year-old woman is evaluated during a routine examination. Her last Pap smear was performed 1 year ago and was normal. She has received a complete human papillomavirus (HPV) quadrivalent vaccine series. Medical history is unremarkable. Family history is noncontributory. She takes no medications.

On physical examination, temperature is normal, blood pressure is 110/72 mm Hg, and pulse rate is 78/min. The remainder of the physical examination is normal.

Which of the following is the most appropriate management of this patient's cervical cancer screening?

(A) Obtain HPV testing in 2 years
(B) Obtain Pap smear in 2 years
(C) Obtain Pap smear and HPV testing now
(D) Obtain Pap smear and HPV testing in 2 years

Item 45

A 67-year-old man is evaluated following a recent diagnosis of type 2 diabetes mellitus. He is sedentary but is without cardiopulmonary symptoms. Family history is significant for myocardial infarction in his father at age 50 years and stroke in his mother at age 54 years. He takes no medications.

On physical examination, the patient is afebrile, and blood pressure is 144/96 mm Hg. BMI is 40. Other than obesity, his physical examination is normal.

Laboratory studies:

Alanine aminotransferase	31 U/L
Total cholesterol	203 mg/dL (5.26 mmol/L)
LDL cholesterol	123 mg/dL (3.19 mmol/L)
HDL cholesterol	40 mg/dL (1.04 mmol/L)
Serum creatinine	0.75 mg/dL (66.3 µmol/L)
Glucose	194 mg/dL (10.8 mmol/L)
Triglycerides	201 mg/dL (2.27 mmol/L)
Hemoglobin A$_{1c}$	6.7%

Electrocardiogram is normal.

His 10-year atherosclerotic cardiovascular disease risk based on the Pooled Cohort Equations is 25%.

The patient is counseled on lifestyle changes to reduce cardiovascular risk, and management of his diabetes and hypertension is initiated with metformin and ramipril.

Which of the following is the most appropriate treatment of this patient's hyperlipidemia?

(A) Gemfibrozil
(B) High-intensity atorvastatin
(C) Moderate-intensity simvastatin
(D) No additional treatment

Item 46

A 49-year-old man is evaluated during a routine examination. He is asymptomatic but is concerned about his risk for cardiovascular disease. Medical history is notable for hypertension. He is a nonsmoker, and he works as an executive at a highly successful company. Family history is noncontributory. His only medication is hydrochlorothiazide.

On physical examination, the patient is afebrile, blood pressure is 118/78 mm Hg, and pulse rate is 78/min. BMI is 31. The remainder of the physical examination is normal.

Results of laboratory studies show a serum total cholesterol level of 190 mg/dL (4.92 mmol/L) and a serum HDL cholesterol level of 46 mg/dL (1.19 mmol/L). Fasting plasma glucose level is 95 mg/dL (5.27 mmol/L).

His estimated 10-year risk of atherosclerotic cardiovascular disease using the Pooled Cohort Equations is 3.2%.

In addition to diet and exercise, which of the following is the most appropriate next step in management?

(A) Coronary artery calcium scoring
(B) Exercise electrocardiography
(C) Resting electrocardiography
(D) No further testing

Item 47

A 91-year-old man is brought to the office by his daughter following two recent falls. He lives independently in his own home, and both falls occurred at home while the patient was using a walker. He had no serious injuries with either fall. He cannot recall what led to the falls, but he was able to get himself up after each one. He has a known multifactorial gait disturbance and has routinely used a walker for the last 2 years. He reports that his balance has worsened in the last few months and that his activity level has been "slowing down." He reports no lightheadedness or specific weakness. His cognition is normal. Medical history is remarkable for diffuse osteoarthritis with minimal discomfort and a small stroke 10 years ago without any residual deficits. He does not drink alcohol. Medications are daily aspirin, as-needed acetaminophen, and topical menthol ointment for occasional joint pain.

On physical examination, the patient is afebrile. Blood pressure is 138/82 mm Hg sitting and 140/84 mm Hg standing, and pulse rate is 84/min sitting and 80/min standing. His corrected vision is 20/25 in both eyes. He has a slow, wide-based gait with use of his walker. Neurologic examination is normal with no parkinsonian features. No detectable asymmetries in muscle strength are noted. He is wearing flip flops, which are his preferred footwear.

A multimodal intervention to prevent falls is initiated, and the patient is referred to physical therapy for an individualized exercise program. A home safety evaluation is ordered to optimize his home environment, and he is educated on proper footwear.

Which of the following additional treatments is most likely to decrease this patient's risk of falls?

(A) Compression stockings
(B) Hip protectors
(C) Mineralocorticoid supplementation
(D) Vitamin D supplementation

Item 48

A 39-year-old man in hospice is evaluated for depressed mood. He has progressive amyotrophic lateral sclerosis, with an estimated life expectancy of weeks to months. His wife is his primary caregiver, and he has two teenage sons still at home. The patient is tearful and reports feeling sad and overwhelmed at times. He is fatigued, his appetite is poor, and he has lost weight. He admits to sometimes wishing death would come quickly but has no plan to act on these feelings. He attributes his illness to past illicit drug use and feels guilty that his sons will come of age without their father.

Which of the following is the most likely diagnosis?

(A) Adjustment disorder with depressed mood
(B) Anticipatory grief
(C) Major depression
(D) Persistent complex bereavement disorder

Item 49

A 77-year-old man is evaluated for a 6-month history of fatigue, weakness, and erectile dysfunction. He previously had an enjoyable sex life with his wife but more recently has experienced low interest in sexual activity. He is unable to engage in his regular exercise routine due to reduced energy and muscle weakness. He reports no weight loss or depressed mood.

On physical examination, the patient is afebrile, blood pressure is 142/88 mm Hg, and pulse rate is 90/min. BMI is 32. Examination of the heart and lungs is normal. Musculoskeletal and nervous system examinations are normal. Normal-appearing testes and circumcised penis are noted.

Laboratory studies show an 8:00 AM serum total testosterone level of 195 ng/dL (6.8 nmol/L). Serum thyroid-stimulating hormone level is within normal limits.

Which of the following is the most appropriate next step in management?

(A) Begin testosterone replacement therapy
(B) Measure follicle-stimulating hormone and luteinizing hormone levels
(C) Measure prolactin level
(D) Obtain a pituitary MRI
(E) Repeat 8:00 AM testosterone level

Item 50

A 46-year-old man is evaluated for a 3-week history of right foot pain. The pain is located near the medial inferior heel without radiation. He describes the pain as sharp and occurring with the first few steps taken after awakening in the morning or after prolonged rest. The pain improves with continued walking. He reports no edema, erythema, or ecchymoses in this area, and he has no history of trauma. Medical history is significant for obesity. He has tried ibuprofen without pain relief.

On physical examination, vital signs are normal. BMI is 35. Strength and sensation in the foot are normal. There is pain on palpation of the medial tubercle of the calcaneus. Pain is also reproduced with passive dorsiflexion of the toes. Pain is not present on palpation of the posterior heel or with tapping inferior to the medial malleolus. There is no atrophy of the heel fat pad. Pes planus is present.

Which of the following is the most likely diagnosis?

(A) Achilles tendinopathy
(B) Heel pad syndrome
(C) Plantar fasciitis
(D) Stress fracture of the tarsal navicular bone

Item 51

A 48-year-old woman is evaluated for a 6-week history of persistent low back pain. The patient is a nurse and has had continuous pain ever since helping lift a patient. The pain is localized to the lumbar back, is bilateral, and does not radiate. She has not had fever or bowel or bladder dysfunction. The patient was involved in a motor vehicle accident 10 years ago and sustained a back injury that has subsequently healed. Medical history is otherwise unremarkable, and her only medication is as-needed naproxen for pain control.

On physical examination, vital signs are normal. BMI is 27. The general medical examination is normal. Musculoskeletal examination shows pain induced with palpation over the lumbar paraspinal muscles. Range of motion with back flexion and extension is limited. Results of the straight-leg raise test are negative bilaterally. Lower extremity muscle strength and reflexes are normal.

Which of the following is the most appropriate treatment?

(A) Bed rest
(B) Glucocorticoid taper
(C) Lumbar support
(D) Massage therapy

Item 52

A 50-year-old man is evaluated in the emergency department after sustaining a complex right tibia fracture in a motor vehicle accident at 9:00 PM. He underwent splinting of the fracture and was admitted to the hospital for wound debridement and internal fixation to occur the next morning. Medical history is notable for hypertension, hyperlipidemia, and type 2 diabetes mellitus. Medications are extended-release metoprolol every morning, pravastatin every evening, and metformin twice daily. He took all of his usual medications today (both morning and evening doses). He was in his usual state of health with no symptoms prior to the accident.

On physical examination, the patient has a splint on the right lower extremity. Blood pressure is 138/86 mm Hg, and pulse rate is 78/min. The remainder of the physical examination is normal.

Laboratory studies show normal serum bicarbonate, blood urea nitrogen, serum creatinine, and serum potassium levels; random plasma glucose level is 119 mg/dL (6.6 mmol/L).

Which of the patient's medications should be taken the morning of surgery?

(A) Metformin
(B) Metoprolol
(C) Metoprolol and metformin
(D) No medications

Item 53

A 28-year-old man is evaluated for right knee pain that began 2 days ago. He was playing football when he stopped suddenly and pivoted to make a catch. He heard a popping sound and immediately developed severe pain in his right knee. Within 30 minutes, the knee became swollen. Since the injury, he has been able to bear weight, but he has discomfort with ambulation and reports feeling that his right knee is going to buckle. He has also been unable to participate in any further sports activities. Medical history is unremarkable. He takes no medications.

On physical examination, vital signs are normal. BMI is 24. The right knee is swollen with a palpable effusion. There is no overlying erythema, medial or lateral joint line tenderness, or increased laxity with varus and valgus forces. Anterior drawer and Lachman tests are positive. Posterior drawer test is negative.

Which of the following is the most likely diagnosis?

(A) Anterior cruciate ligament tear
(B) Lateral collateral ligament tear
(C) Medial collateral ligament tear
(D) Meniscal tear

Item 54

At a morbidity and mortality conference, a case is presented in which an older man died because of a delay in the diagnosis of cholecystitis. He was admitted to the medical service for evaluation of abdominal discomfort. The care team diagnosed constipation based on the history of abdominal bloating and an abdominal radiograph showing a large amount of stool. Treatment with stool softeners and laxatives was initiated. The patient later developed vomiting, fever, escalating abdominal pain, and leukocytosis; however, no additional studies were performed, and his treatment was not significantly altered. He subsequently died.

Which of the following cognitive errors contributed most to the outcome?

(A) Anchoring
(B) Confirmation bias
(C) Framing bias
(D) Triage cueing

Item 55

A 68-year-old woman is evaluated for sinus symptoms of 2 to 3 days' duration. She reports nasal congestion and a whitish nasal discharge, a full sensation over both maxillary sinuses, and pain in her upper teeth. She does not have fever or ear or throat pain and has had no sick contacts. Medical history is significant for hypertension and type 2 diabetes mellitus. She has no known drug allergies. Her medications are fosinopril and metformin.

On physical examination, temperature is 37.2 °C (98.9 °F), blood pressure is 122/72 mm Hg, and pulse rate is 68/min. BMI is 26. There is tenderness to palpation over both maxillary sinuses. Dentition and tympanic membranes are normal. The oropharynx is mildly erythematous without exudates. There is no cervical lymphadenopathy. The lungs are clear. The remainder of the examination is normal.

Which of the following is the most appropriate management?

(A) Amoxicillin-clavulanate
(B) Doxycycline
(C) Sinus CT scan
(D) Supportive care

Item 56

A 57-year-old woman is evaluated for a 2-month history of bothersome hot flushes multiple times daily, with night sweats disrupting sleep about two to three times nightly. She also reports irritability and mood lability and reports worsening vaginal dryness with dyspareunia. Her last menstrual period was 13 months ago. Medical history is

significant only for hypothyroidism. Personal and family histories are negative for breast and ovarian cancer. Her only medication is levothyroxine. Mammography and cervical cancer screening are up to date.

On physical examination, vital signs are normal. The general medical examination is unremarkable. Breast examination is negative. On pelvic examination, the vaginal mucosa is pale with decreased rugae with petechial hemorrhages present. Decreased vaginal lubrication is noted.

Which of the following is the most appropriate next step in management?

(A) Measure serum follicle-stimulating hormone level
(B) Measure serum estradiol level
(C) Prescribe estradiol-progestin combination
(D) Prescribe low-dose paroxetine
(E) Prescribe vaginal estradiol cream

Item 57

A nursing care facility is noted to have a higher than expected rate of infections related to use of urinary catheters. To address this finding, a quality improvement team performs a root cause analysis that discovers multiple issues that are possibly contributing to the high rate of infection.

Which of the following quality improvement tools should be used to organize the results of the root cause analysis?

(A) Cause-and-effect (fishbone) diagram
(B) Control chart
(C) Pareto chart
(D) Spaghetti diagram

Item 58

A 68-year-old man is seen for a preoperative evaluation for a total left knee arthroplasty. He engages in no exercise and does minimal walking due to his knee pain. He reports no other symptoms. Medical history is notable for hypertension, for which he takes losartan.

On physical examination, blood pressure is 130/74 mm Hg. Cardiovascular examination is normal. The left knee shows changes compatible with severe osteoarthritis.

Laboratory studies show a normal serum creatinine level.

Which of the following should be performed preoperatively?

(A) Noninvasive pharmacologic cardiac stress testing
(B) Resting echocardiography
(C) Serum troponin measurement
(D) No further diagnostic testing

Item 59

A 42-year-old woman is evaluated in the emergency department for an episode of transient loss of consciousness. Two hours ago, she was standing in line at the grocery store and began to feel warm, flushed, and nauseated. After

H
CONT.

about a minute, she remembers becoming lightheaded with "graying" of her vision, after which she fell to the ground. She immediately regained consciousness and had no residual symptoms. She reports no chest pain, palpitations, nausea, numbness, tingling, weakness, vertigo, or headache. There was no apparent seizure activity or bowel or bladder incontinence.

On physical examination, temperature is 36.8 °C (98.2 °F). Blood pressure is 110/80 mm Hg supine and 102/68 mm Hg standing, pulse rate is 78/min supine and 88/min standing, and respiration rate is 14/min. BMI is 28. The lungs are clear, and examination of the heart is normal and without murmurs. The remainder of the general medical examination is unremarkable. Neurologic examination is normal.

Laboratory test results reveal a hemoglobin level of 13.2 g/dL (132 g/L). Pregnancy test is negative.

Which of the following is the most appropriate diagnostic test to perform next?

(A) Echocardiography
(B) Electrocardiography
(C) Head CT
(D) No additional testing

Item 60

A 61-year-old man is seen for preoperative evaluation before left total hip arthroplasty scheduled in 2 weeks. He was hospitalized 4 months ago for an ST-elevation myocardial infarction related to a completely occluded proximal left circumflex artery. He underwent percutaneous coronary intervention and stenting with an everolimus-eluting coronary stent. He has since done well with no symptoms with daily activities, and an echocardiogram 1 month ago showed preserved left ventricular function and no structural heart disease. Medical history is also notable for hypertension and hyperlipidemia. Medications are aspirin, clopidogrel, carvedilol, atorvastatin, and lisinopril.

On physical examination, blood pressure is 126/76 mm Hg, and pulse rate is 64/min. Central venous pressure is normal. Cardiac and pulmonary examinations are normal. There is no peripheral edema.

Laboratory studies show a normal basic metabolic panel and complete blood count.

Electrocardiogram shows normal sinus rhythm.

Which of the following is the optimal preoperative management?

(A) Continue clopidogrel and aspirin throughout surgery
(B) Delay surgery for at least 8 months
(C) Stop aspirin and clopidogrel 5 to 7 days before surgery
(D) Stop clopidogrel 5 to 7 days before surgery; continue aspirin

Item 61

A 26-year-old man is evaluated for almost daily unexpected episodes of sweating, palpitations, tremulousness, shortness of breath, and numbness in his fingers and toes. During these episodes, he feels as if he is going to die. Episodes have occurred during lectures at medical school and

while watching films in movie theaters; symptoms can be so severe that he must leave "to get air." All of the episodes resolve after 15 to 20 minutes. Because of fear of future episodes, he has withdrawn from social activities. His sleep has been poor, and he is fatigued. Medical history is otherwise unremarkable. He does not smoke, drink alcohol, or use illicit drugs.

On physical examination, the patient appears anxious. Blood pressure is 124/76 mm Hg, pulse rate is 94/min, and respiration rate is 16/min. BMI is 23. The remainder of the physical examination, including heart, lung, and nervous system examinations, is unremarkable.

Laboratory studies, including thyroid function tests, are normal.

In addition to cognitive-behavioral therapy, which of the following is the most appropriate long-term pharmacologic treatment for this patient?

(A) Alprazolam
(B) Buspirone
(C) Propranolol
(D) Sertraline

Item 62

A 40-year-old woman is evaluated during a routine visit and asks to start on contraception. She had been sexually inactive since her divorce several years ago but is in a new sexual relationship and is interested in starting an oral contraceptive. Medical history is unremarkable, with no history of thromboembolism, heart disease, or headache. She is a never-smoker and takes no medications. Her last Pap smear was 1 year ago and was normal. Menses are regular; her most recent period began approximately 3 weeks ago.

On physical examination, vital signs are normal. BMI is 27. The general medical examination, including breast examination, is unremarkable.

Which of the following is the most appropriate management prior to starting hormonal contraception in this patient?

(A) Lipid profile
(B) Mammogram
(C) Pelvic examination and Pap smear
(D) Pregnancy test
(E) No additional testing

Item 63

A 28-year-old man is evaluated for a 3-day history of cough, rhinorrhea, sore throat, generalized malaise, and low-grade fever. His nasal discharge is slightly yellow, and his cough is productive of small amounts of yellow sputum. He reports no wheezing or shortness of breath. He does not smoke cigarettes and has no new environmental exposures. He is an elementary school teacher, and many of his students have had similar symptoms over the previous week. Medications are acetaminophen and ibuprofen as needed. He has no allergies. The patient requests a prescription for a medication that will help manage his symptoms.

On physical examination, temperature is 37.8 °C (100.0 °F), blood pressure is 132/70 mm Hg, pulse rate is 90/min, and respiration rate is 18/min. BMI is 24. There is mild bilateral conjunctival injection. Ear examination is normal. The posterior pharynx is erythematous without tonsillar enlargement or exudate. Nasal turbinates are mildly swollen, and there is a copious amount of clear nasal drainage. Lung examination reveals no wheezing or rhonchi, and there is no dullness to percussion. The remainder of the examination is normal.

Which of the following is the most appropriate treatment?

(A) Azithromycin
(B) Chlorpheniramine-pseudoephedrine
(C) Codeine
(D) Inhaled albuterol

Item 64

A 38-year-old woman is evaluated in the emergency department for a 1-day history of right shoulder pain, which began after she fell on her right shoulder while running. She reports no shoulder problems before the fall. She is a highly active athlete who enjoys running, biking, and playing racquetball. Medical history is unremarkable. Her only medication is acetaminophen as needed for pain.

On physical examination, vital signs are normal. BMI is 21. Findings on general medical examination are unremarkable. On musculoskeletal examination, the neck is normal. The right shoulder is normal in appearance, and there is no tenderness to palpation of bony structures. The patient is unable to actively abduct her right shoulder beyond 90 degrees. When asked to lower her arm progressively once it has been passively abducted to 90 degrees, her arm falls to her waist. When her arm is passively abducted to 20 degrees and externally rotated, she is unable to maintain external rotation. There is no pain with internal or external rotation. Grip strength and sensation in the hand are normal.

Plain radiographs of the right shoulder show no dislocation or fracture.

Which of the following is the most appropriate next step in management?

(A) Glucocorticoid injection
(B) MRI of the right shoulder
(C) Physical therapy
(D) Right upper extremity nerve conduction study

Item 65

A 38-year-old man is evaluated during a follow-up visit. Eight weeks ago, he was diagnosed with a first episode of depression based on symptoms of depressed mood, fatigue, increased sleep, anhedonia, and weight gain. His score on the PHQ-9 was 15 (moderately severe depression). Citalopram, 20 mg/d, was initiated at that time. Six weeks ago, he was tolerating the medication with no significant side effects but without improvement of symptoms; citalopram was therefore increased to the maximum dose of 40 mg/d. Currently,

he reports no improvement of his depressive symptoms, and his PHQ-9 score remains 15. He has no suicidal ideation.

On physical examination, the patient has a mildly depressed affect but responds appropriately. Vital signs are normal, and the remainder of the examination is unremarkable.

Which of the following is the most appropriate next step in management?

(A) Add liothyronine
(B) Discontinue citalopram and begin bupropion
(C) Discontinue citalopram and begin olanzapine
(D) Refer for electroconvulsive therapy

Item 66

A physician group practice recently hired a new graduate of an internal medicine residency training program. The new physician had excellent references, and her performance in the practice has been exemplary. She is well liked by patients, her clinical care is considered excellent, and staff members indicate that she is an outstanding team player.

A physician colleague in the practice discovers that the new physician's social media page contains disparaging comments about obese patients, patients with somatoform disorders, and nonadherent patients, although there is no mention of specific patients in the practice. Her social media page also contains photographs of her drinking alcohol at various parties.

Which of the following is the most appropriate course of action for this physician to take regarding the colleague's social media use?

(A) Meet with the colleague and advise that she remove the inappropriate content
(B) Notify the head physician in the practice of the inappropriate posts
(C) Post a comment on the colleague's social media page indicating that the content is unprofessional
(D) No action is required

Item 67

A 45-year-old man is evaluated for a 1-year history of cough. The cough is described as episodic throughout the day and nonproductive. He believes his cough may worsen after a heavy meal. He reports no postnasal drip, shortness of breath, wheezing, chest pain, paroxysmal nocturnal dyspnea, or lower extremity edema, although he experiences occasional heartburn. He smokes one pack of cigarettes per day with a 15-pack-year history, and he drinks one alcoholic beverage and three cups of coffee daily. He has no history of environmental exposures. Medical history is otherwise unremarkable, and he takes no medications.

On physical examination, temperature is 37.2 °C (98.9 °F), blood pressure is 140/70 mm Hg, pulse rate is 70/min, and respiration rate is 16/min. BMI is 35. Lung examination reveals normal breath sounds. Cardiovascular examination is normal; there is no S_3. Abdomen is obese, and no pedal edema is noted.

A posteroanterior/lateral chest radiograph is normal.

In addition to smoking cessation and weight reduction counseling, which of the following is the most appropriate management of this patient?

(A) Antihistamine-decongestant
(B) Bronchoscopy
(C) Echocardiography
(D) Proton pump inhibitor

Item 68

A 65-year-old man is evaluated during a routine examination. He is asymptomatic. The patient has a 15-pack-year smoking history, and family history is noncontributory. He takes no medications.

Which of the following is the most effective screening maneuver?

(A) Abdominal aorta palpation
(B) Carotid artery auscultation
(C) Pulse palpation
(D) Testicular examination

Item 69

A 63-year-old woman is evaluated for a 3-week history of vaginal discharge. The discharge is described as yellowish and malodorous and is accompanied by burning and dyspareunia. She is postmenopausal and is sexually active with a new male partner. Her last Pap smear was 2 years ago and was normal. Medical history is significant for hypertension, and her only medication is hydrochlorothiazide.

On physical examination, the patient is afebrile, blood pressure is 128/78 mm Hg, pulse rate is 72/min, and respiration rate is 12/min. BMI is 26. On pelvic examination, a frothy, yellowish discharge is present in the vaginal vault. The cervix is without lesions, although there is contact bleeding with speculum placement. There is no cervical motion tenderness or adnexal tenderness. The remainder of the examination is unremarkable.

Laboratory studies show a vaginal pH is 6.0; whiff test is negative. Saline microscopy is shown. Potassium hydroxide microscopy is negative. Testing for *Chlamydia trachomatis* and *Neisseria gonorrhoeae* is negative.

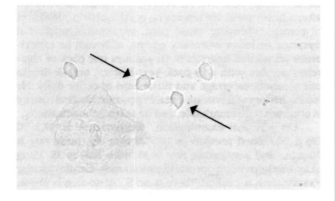

Treatment with single-dose metronidazole is planned.

Which of the following is the most appropriate additional intervention?

(A) Confirm infection with a nucleic acid amplification test
(B) Perform repeat Pap smear following treatment
(C) Test for cure following treatment
(D) Treat the patient's sexual partner

Item 70

A 55-year-old man is evaluated during a new patient visit. He feels well and has no specific symptoms, but he asks for advice on reducing his risk for cardiovascular disease because his younger brother recently had a myocardial infarction. He leads a sedentary lifestyle but has no cardiopulmonary symptoms. Medical history is significant for obesity and hypertension. Medications are hydrochlorothiazide and lisinopril.

On physical examination, he is afebrile, and blood pressure is 136/82 mm Hg. BMI is 34. Waist circumference is 99 cm (39 in). The remainder of the physical examination is normal.

Laboratory studies:

Alanine aminotransferase	Normal
Total cholesterol	207 mg/dL (5.36 mmol/L)
LDL cholesterol	137 mg/dL (3.55 mmol/L)
HDL cholesterol	34 mg/dL (0.88 mmol/L)
Creatine kinase	Normal
Serum creatinine	Normal
Triglycerides	180 mg/dL (2.03 mmol/L)
Hemoglobin A_{1c}	Normal

His 10-year risk for a major cardiovascular event based on the Framingham risk calculator is 12%.

The patient is instructed on lifestyle modifications and is started on moderate-intensity simvastatin.

Which of the following is the most appropriate additional treatment for reduction of this patient's cardiovascular risk?

(A) Aspirin
(B) Diltiazem
(C) Fenofibrate
(D) Metformin

Item 71

A 54-year-old woman is evaluated for severe hot flushes that started about 12 months ago. They occur several times each night, waking her from sleep. They also occur throughout the day, disturbing her concentration at work. She reports being tired with emotional lability. She does not feel depressed but is very frustrated by her symptoms and moodiness. She also reports vaginal dryness with intermittent dyspareunia and is using lubricants with minimal relief. She does not have dysuria and has not noted any abnormal vaginal discharge. She has tried black cohosh, yoga, and increased exercise, but her discomfort persists. Medical history is otherwise significant for hypertension and negative for thromboembolism or cardiac disease. She underwent hysterectomy 5 years ago for fibroids. She is up to date with scheduled health screening interventions, including mammography. Her only medication is hydrochlorothiazide.

On physical examination, blood pressure is 136/80 mm Hg, and her other vital signs are normal. Speculum examination shows pale vaginal mucosa with decreased rugae. The remainder of the physical examination, including the breast examination, is normal.

Which of the following is the most appropriate treatment?

(A) Oral estradiol-progestin
(B) Oral progestin
(C) Transdermal estradiol
(D) Vaginal estradiol

Item 72

A 32-year-old woman is evaluated during a follow-up visit. She indicates that she and her husband are contemplating pregnancy, and she discontinued her oral contraceptive 2 months ago. Medical history is significant for hypertension, type 2 diabetes mellitus, and severe depression, which is currently in remission. Medications are lisinopril, metformin, atorvastatin, and sertraline. She does not smoke or use alcohol or illicit drugs. A normal Pap smear was obtained 1 year ago, no high-risk behaviors are identified, and her vaccinations are up to date.

On physical examination, blood pressure is 114/70 mm Hg. BMI is 24. The remainder of the examination is unremarkable.

A urine pregnancy test is negative.

Her lisinopril is discontinued, and she is started on a prenatal vitamin with folate.

Which of the following medications also needs to be discontinued?

(A) Atorvastatin
(B) Metformin
(C) Sertraline
(D) No additional changes needed

Item 73

A 27-year-old woman is evaluated for overweight. Her weight has steadily increased over the past 10 years, and she has attempted weight loss through commercial diets and increased physical activity. Additionally, she has met with a dietician for nutritional guidance. She frequently eats fast food, and she snacks at work, before meals, and especially when she is under stress. She currently exercises 30 minutes daily. She does not smoke and rarely consumes alcohol. Medical history is otherwise unremarkable, and she takes no medications.

On physical examination, the patient is afebrile, blood pressure is 138/74 mm Hg, and pulse rate is 76/min. BMI is 29. Waist circumference is 92 cm (36 in). Head, neck, lung,

and heart examinations are normal. The abdomen is obese without striae.

Laboratory studies, including fasting plasma glucose, total cholesterol, and thyroid-stimulating hormone levels, are normal.

In addition to calorie restriction and continued regular exercise, which of the following is the most appropriate next step to help this patient achieve sustained weight loss?

(A) Behavioral therapy
(B) Laparoscopic adjustable gastric banding
(C) Orlistat
(D) Phentermine

Item 74

A 47-year-old woman is evaluated for a 2-year history of cramping lower abdominal pain that is not associated with nausea or changes in bowel movements. She also notes a 1-year history of right-sided chest pain that is intermittent, lasting for 2 to 3 hours and resolving spontaneously. Her chest pain is not associated with exertion but is sometimes triggered by stress. She has seen six different physicians for these symptoms and has undergone multiple examinations and diagnostic studies, which have been unrevealing. She has taken several sick days from work and almost daily researches her symptoms online. She voices frustration over her previous medical care and is afraid that she has cancer or some other serious illness that no one can diagnose. She has no family history of cancer. Medications are acetaminophen and probiotic tablets.

A complete physical examination, including vital signs and pelvic examination, is normal.

Which of the following is the most likely diagnosis?

(A) Conversion disorder
(B) Factitious disorder
(C) Illness anxiety disorder
(D) Somatic symptom disorder

Item 75

A 40-year-old woman presents for a second opinion for her chronic pain. She has had widespread pain consistent with fibromyalgia for several years. She describes her pain as achy in nature, constant, and worsening with strenuous activity. It is associated with poor sleep quality and "foggy" thinking but no clear deficits on cognitive testing. She has not responded to adequate trials of gabapentin, pregabalin, topiramate, amitriptyline, nortriptyline, duloxetine, and venlafaxine. Additionally, she has tried many complementary and integrative therapies to help manage her pain, and she has not responded to numerous herbal supplements and bioidentical hormones. She finds acupuncture helpful for short periods of time, but she cannot afford it in the long term. She is frustrated by the inability of her previous physicians to find a medication that relieves her pain. Her only medication is trazodone for sleep.

Physical examination is unremarkable except for widespread muscle tenderness.

Which of the following is the most appropriate treatment for this patient?

(A) Cognitive-behavioral therapy
(B) Lidocaine patch
(C) NSAID therapy
(D) Opioid therapy

Item 76

A 32-year-old woman visits to discuss genetic testing. She inquires whether she should be tested for the *BRCA* gene mutation after having read a magazine article that recommended testing. She feels well with no symptoms. She reports no palpable breast masses, nipple discharge, or breast skin changes. She takes no medications.

On physical examination, the patient is afebrile, blood pressure is 112/72 mm Hg, pulse rate is 66/min, and respiration rate is 16/min. BMI is 23. The remainder of the physical examination, including breast examination, is normal.

Which of the following is the most appropriate management?

(A) Obtain a three-generation family history
(B) Order screening mammography
(C) Perform *BRCA* genetic testing
(D) Refer for genetic counseling

Item 77

A 98-year-old woman is evaluated in the emergency department after falling on her left hip at home. The patient lives with her daughter, and she uses a walker and requires assistance for most of her activities of daily living. Her daughter cares for the patient full time and is very conscientious and attentive. Medical history is significant for moderate dementia, osteoarthritis, and osteoporosis. She has mild vision loss that is maximally corrected with glasses. Medications are supplemental calcium, vitamin D, and as-needed acetaminophen.

On physical examination, she is pleasant but frail appearing. Vital signs are normal without orthostatic changes. BMI is 17. She is oriented only to person but can name her daughter. Her general physical examination, including skin examination, is unremarkable. Her vision is maximally corrected. On musculoskeletal examination, there is bruising about her left hip, but otherwise she has full painless range of motion of the hip. Her gait is antalgic and unsteady, and she requires one-person assist for transfers.

Pelvic and left hip and leg radiographs show joint osteoarthritis but are negative for fracture.

Which of the following is the most appropriate management of this patient to decrease future falls?

(A) Initiate an individualized exercise program
(B) Initiate risperidone
(C) Recommend nursing home placement
(D) Continue current care

Item 78

A 62-year-old man is evaluated during a new patient visit. He reports never having received influenza vaccination because of an egg allergy. The allergy was diagnosed many years ago after he developed hives upon eating eggs. His medical history is otherwise unremarkable. He currently feels well and takes no medications.

Physical examination, including vital signs, is normal.

Which of the following is the most appropriate management of this patient's influenza vaccination?

(A) Administer inactivated influenza vaccine
(B) Administer live attenuated influenza vaccine
(C) Perform influenza vaccine skin testing
(D) Do not vaccinate the patient against influenza

Item 79

A 45-year-old man is evaluated during a routine examination. He is interested in quitting smoking. He has a history of seizures but has not had a seizure in 15 years and discontinued his seizure medication 4 years ago. He also has hypertension. His only medication is amlodipine.

Physical examination is unremarkable.

Which of the following will most likely give this patient the greatest chance of success in quitting smoking?

(A) Bupropion
(B) Electronic cigarettes
(C) Nicotine replacement patches
(D) Varenicline

Item 80

A 78-year-old man is evaluated for vertigo that began abruptly 2 days ago. The vertigo waxes and wanes in severity, with each episode lasting several hours, and is accompanied by visual blurring, nausea, low-grade headache, and unsteadiness on his feet. He reports no chest pain, shortness of breath, or recent head trauma. He does not smoke cigarettes and drinks one 4-ounce glass of wine daily. Medical history is remarkable for myocardial infarction 5 years ago, type 1 diabetes mellitus, hypertension, and hyperlipidemia. Medications are insulin glargine, lisinopril, atorvastatin, and aspirin.

On physical examination, temperature is 37.5 °C (99.5 °F), blood pressure is 162/80 mm Hg, pulse rate is 78/min, and respiration rate is 15/min. BMI is 24. The neurologic examination is notable for impaired near vision, a Dix-Hallpike maneuver that reveals 8 beats of lateral nystagmus without delay, and an unsteady gait with leaning to his right side. The remainder of the physical examination is normal.

Laboratory studies show a plasma glucose level of 244 mg/dL (13.5 mmol/L).

Electrocardiogram reveals a normal sinus rhythm, evidence of an old inferior myocardial infarction, and no acute ST- or T-wave changes.

Which of the following is the most appropriate diagnostic test to perform next?

(A) Carotid Doppler ultrasonography
(B) CT scan of the head

(C) Lumbar puncture

(D) MRI of the brain

Item 81

A 26-year-old man is evaluated during a routine follow-up visit. He inquires about undergoing genetic testing because his father and paternal grandfather both died of Huntington disease. His older brother recently underwent genetic testing, which confirmed the *HD* gene mutation; however, his older brother is not yet manifesting any symptoms. His younger brother was also tested, but the results were negative for the mutant gene. The patient is asymptomatic and takes no medications.

The physical examination is normal.

Which of the following is the most appropriate management of this patient?

(A) Obtain electromyogram

(B) Obtain genetic testing

(C) Refer the patient for genetic counseling

(D) Tell the patient that testing is unnecessary

Item 82

An 83-year-old man is admitted to the hospital with fever, severe dyspnea, and hypoxemia due to pneumonia. He is lethargic, disoriented, and lacks capacity to make decisions. Medical history is significant for chronic bronchitis. Respiratory failure and need for mechanical ventilation are imminent. There is no advance directive. Two surviving adult children are struggling with making decisions about his care, especially regarding mechanical ventilation.

Which of the following is the most appropriate course of action to facilitate a decision on this patient's care?

(A) Ask the patient's children to make a decision based on the patient's best interests

(B) Ask the patient's children to make a decision based on what they feel is correct

(C) Ask the patient's children what the patient would do if he were able to make a decision

(D) Encourage the patient's children to speak to a social worker

(E) Wait for the court to appoint a guardian who will make a decision

Item 83

A 52-year-old woman is evaluated during a routine examination. She is healthy with no symptoms. The patient underwent menarche at age 14 years. She is gravida 1, para 1, with pregnancy at age 30 years. She has no family history of breast or ovarian cancer. Medical history is otherwise negative, and she takes no medications.

Vital signs are normal, and the remainder of the physical examination is unremarkable.

A film screening mammogram shows heterogeneously dense breast tissue using the Breast Imaging Reporting and Data System (BI-RADS) breast density categories; the mammogram is otherwise normal.

Which of the following imaging modalities is the most appropriate for subsequent breast cancer screening in this patient?

(A) Breast MRI

(B) Digital mammography

(C) Film mammography

(D) Whole breast ultrasonography

Item 84

A 58-year-old man is evaluated for a 1-year history of slowly progressive bilateral leg swelling. He notes that the swelling is minimal in the morning and is most pronounced at the end of the day. He reports no calf pain but does note a sensation of heaviness in both legs that is worse at night. He has no dyspnea, orthopnea, paroxysmal nocturnal dyspnea, or abdominal distention. He uses alcohol socially and is a never-smoker. He works as a police officer. Medical history is otherwise unremarkable, and he takes no medications.

On physical examination, the patient is afebrile, blood pressure is 112/76 mm Hg, pulse rate is 76/min, and respiration rate is 16/min. BMI is 31. There is no elevation in central venous pressure. The lungs are clear. No murmurs or extra heart sounds are noted on cardiac examination. The abdominal examination is normal. There is no inguinal lymphadenopathy. Pitting edema of the lower extremities extends to approximately 3 inches above the ankles.

Laboratory studies are significant for normal kidney function and liver chemistry tests; the serum albumin level is 4.0 g/dL (40 g/L). Urinalysis is normal.

Which of the following is the most appropriate next diagnostic study?

(A) Abdominal/pelvic CT

(B) Lower extremity venous duplex ultrasonography

(C) Transthoracic echocardiogram

(D) No additional testing

Item 85

An 86-year-old woman is evaluated for increasing urinary incontinence. The patient has dementia and lives with her daughter, who is her primary caregiver. She previously had occasional urinary incontinence but now needs to wear a diaper. Her daughter is concerned about mild skin irritation she has noticed on the patient's buttocks. In addition to dementia, the patient has osteoarthritis and hypothyroidism. Medications are levothyroxine and as-needed acetaminophen.

On physical examination, vital signs are normal. BMI is 21. The patient is confused but cooperative. She appears frail and uses a walker for balance when standing and ambulating. Cardiopulmonary examination is normal. The abdomen shows no tenderness or suprapubic fullness. Erythema is present around the groin and buttocks, but no pressure ulcers are seen.

Urinalysis is normal.

Which of the following is the most appropriate management?

(A) Antimuscarinic agent
(B) Pelvic floor muscle training
(C) Prompted voiding
(D) Transdermal estradiol

Item 86

A 79-year-old man is evaluated for pain in the buttocks region. He was diagnosed with non-Hodgkin large B-cell lymphoma 6 months ago. Although his lymphoma has responded well to therapy and he is without evidence of active disease, he required hospitalization three times for chemotherapy-associated complications during his treatment course. He has been bedbound at home during his lymphoma treatment. He describes the pain as severe when sitting and has difficulty finding a comfortable position lying down as well. He has the least pain when standing, but he is unable to stand for very long. He has had no fever. Medical history is otherwise remarkable for hypertension, hyperlipidemia, type 2 diabetes mellitus, and advanced chronic kidney disease being treated with in-center hemodialysis. Medications are felodipine, insulin, calcium carbonate, calcitriol, and erythropoietin.

On physical examination, the patient is afebrile, blood pressure is 104/58 mm Hg, and pulse rate is 64/min supine. BMI is 18. Weight is 58 kg (128 lb), decreased from 77 kg (170 lb) 5 months ago. He appears cachectic with temporal wasting. Examination of his back shows no vertebral tenderness to palpation. There is wasting of the gluteal muscles. Examination of the sacrum reveals a shallow ulcer that is 5 cm in diameter with a hard black eschar covering the base. There is no wound drainage and no surrounding erythema.

Which of the following is the most appropriate management of this patient's lesion?

(A) Biopsy of the lesion
(B) Intravenous antibiotics
(C) Leave the wound open to air
(D) Surgical debridement

Item 87

A 25-year-old man is evaluated during a follow-up visit for a diagnosis of schizophrenia. He was diagnosed after his affect became increasingly flat, he would express little emotion, and he developed a feeling that his thoughts were actively being broadcast over the radio. He was started on chlorpromazine 3 months ago with improvement in his psychiatric symptoms. However, his family notes that he has started exhibiting involuntary, repetitive body movements. His medical history is otherwise normal, and his family history is notable for his father who also has schizophrenia.

On physical examination, the patient is afebrile, blood pressure is 125/76 mm Hg, and pulse rate is 82/min. BMI is 24. He looks unkempt and has little facial expression, poor eye contact, monotone speech, and occasional grimacing and lip smacking. The remainder of his examination is unremarkable.

Which of the following is the most appropriate management of this patient's medication?

(A) Continue chlorpromazine
(B) Switch chlorpromazine to clozapine
(C) Switch chlorpromazine to haloperidol
(D) Switch chlorpromazine to thioridazine

Item 88

A 53-year-old woman is evaluated for increasing vaginal dryness, itching, and dyspareunia. She notes a slight vaginal discharge, sometimes yellowish, but reports no odor, dysuria, urinary frequency, or abnormal bleeding. She has tried vaginal lubricants, but they offer minimal relief. Intercourse is so uncomfortable that she is avoiding sex, and this is putting a strain on her marriage.

Medical history is unremarkable, and she takes no medications. She is gravida 3, para 2, and has been menopausal since age 51 years. She reports occasional hot flushes, but they do not wake her at night. Her last cervical cancer screening was 2 years ago and was negative.

On physical examination, vital signs are normal. The general medical examination is unremarkable. Pelvic examination demonstrates pale vaginal mucosa with decreased rugae. There is scant yellow-orange discharge. The cervix appears normal. Bimanual examination is normal with no tenderness or masses.

Vaginal pH is 5.5. Microscopy shows 3 to 5 leukocytes and 2 to 3 erythrocytes/hpf and is negative for clue cells, and a potassium hydroxide preparation is negative for yeast. Whiff test is negative.

Which of the following is the most appropriate treatment?

(A) Estradiol vaginal tablets
(B) Metronidazole vaginal gel
(C) Miconazole vaginal cream
(D) Transdermal estradiol with oral progestin

Item 89

A 97-year-old woman is evaluated in the emergency department for acute abdominal pain radiating to her back. She is found to have a ruptured aortic aneurysm. Following discussion with the patient and her family, she declines any attempt at endovascular or surgical intervention and requests that care be focused on keeping her comfortable. Her estimated life expectancy is hours to days. Medical history is significant for hypertension, and her only medication prior to admission was felodipine.

On physical examination, temperature is normal, blood pressure is 90/48 mm Hg, pulse rate is 115/min, and respiration rate is 24/min. BMI is 22. She is awake, alert, and able to answer questions. She appears frail and is in obvious pain. Her abdomen is tender to palpation with guarding. No bowel sounds are detected.

Laboratory studies are significant for a hemoglobin level of 8.0 g/dL (80 g/L) and serum creatinine level of 5.9 mg/dL (521 µmol/L).

Her antihypertensive medication is held.

CONT.

Which of the following is the most appropriate treatment of this patient's pain?

(A) Fentanyl, transdermally

(B) Hydromorphone, intravenously

(C) Morphine, intravenously

(D) Tramadol, orally

Item 90

A physician has observed that a colleague with whom he has worked for many years has arrived late for and been absent from work with increasing frequency in recent months. While at work, the colleague appears disengaged, distracted, moody, and forgetful. The physician has also noticed lapses in his colleague's judgment and errors which, if unnoticed, might have resulted in patient harm. The physician met with the colleague in private and told him of his observations. He asked his colleague if something is wrong and was rebuffed, being told that he is fine.

Which of the following is the most appropriate course of action for the physician to take regarding his colleague?

(A) Ask other physicians if they have made similar observations of the colleague

(B) Inform the colleague's supervisor of the observations and outcome of the private meeting

(C) Review the colleague's patient care notes for evidence of negligent care

(D) Continue close observation of the colleague

Item 91

A 40-year-old woman is evaluated following several recurrent witnessed episodes of syncope. The patient is an orthopedic surgeon and has experienced loss of consciousness on three separate occasions over the past 6 months after prolonged standing in the operating room. Each episode was brief, was preceded by darkening of peripheral vision, and occurred approximately 2 hours into each surgical procedure. She reports no chest pain, palpitations, weakness, headache, sensory symptoms, flushing, or nausea before the episodes, and no bladder or bowel incontinence or postevent confusion were seen following syncope. She had a normal evaluation in the emergency department after each episode with a normal physical examination, laboratory studies, and electrocardiogram. A 24-hour electrocardiographic monitor placed after her second episode was normal. Medical history is otherwise unremarkable, and she takes no medications.

On physical examination, the patient is afebrile. Blood pressure is 132/74 mm Hg supine and 128/68 mm Hg standing, pulse rate is 66/min supine and 76/min standing, and respiration rate is 14/min. BMI is 22. Cardiac, pulmonary, abdominal, and neurologic examinations are normal.

Laboratory studies are significant for a normal complete blood count and comprehensive metabolic profile, including a fasting plasma glucose level and kidney function studies. A urine pregnancy test is negative.

Which of the following is the most appropriate diagnostic test to perform next?

(A) Brain MRI

(B) Echocardiography

(C) 48-Hour ambulatory electrocardiography

(D) Tilt-table testing

(E) No further testing

Item 92

A 31-year-old man is evaluated for a 9-month history of worry, irritability, restlessness, poor sleep, and fatigue. He feels "keyed up," has difficulty concentrating on tasks, and worries constantly about his health, job performance, and financial matters. In a recent job performance evaluation, his work was rated "poor." He has withdrawn from social circles and is sedentary. He experiences frequent headaches, loose stools, and rapid heartbeat. Because of his symptoms, he worries that he has an undiagnosed medical condition. His PHQ-9 score is 9, and his Generalized Anxiety Disorder 7-item scale score is 13. When asked about the impact of his symptoms on his ability to work, take care of things at home, or get along with other people, he indicates that they have made these activities very difficult. He does not smoke cigarettes or use illicit drugs; he drinks one alcoholic beverage per day.

On physical examination, blood pressure is 138/84 mm Hg, and pulse rate is 100/min. BMI is 28. The remainder of the physical examination is unremarkable.

Laboratory studies, including thyroid function tests, are normal.

Which of the following is the most likely diagnosis?

(A) Attention-deficit/hyperactivity disorder

(B) Generalized anxiety disorder

(C) Major depression

(D) Obsessive-compulsive disorder

Item 93

A 27-year-old woman is evaluated during a follow-up visit. She is planning a trip to China, and her immunization status is being reviewed. She received the first dose of the hepatitis B virus (HBV) vaccine series 18 months ago and the second dose 1 month thereafter. However, she has not received the third dose, which was scheduled for administration 3 months ago. Medical history is unremarkable, and she takes no medications.

Results of the physical examination are unremarkable.

Which of the following is the most appropriate management?

(A) Administer the third dose of the HBV vaccine series now

(B) Order hepatitis B surface antibody titers to assess for immunity

(C) Restart the HBV vaccine series

(D) No additional HBV vaccination is required

Item 94

A 43-year-old man is evaluated for pain and swelling of the left elbow of several weeks' duration. He is a taxi driver and has been working more than usual. When driving, he tends to move his elbow back and forth across the armrest, and the swelling has developed progressively. He notes no acute trauma, skin breaks, rash, or fever. He also reports no history of gout or alcohol use. Medical history is unremarkable, and he takes no medications.

On physical examination, vital signs are normal. BMI is 26. The left olecranon bursa is fluctuant but nontender, and there is no redness or warmth. The left elbow has full range of motion. The remainder of the examination is normal.

In addition to protection of the elbow area, which of the following is the most appropriate therapy?

(A) Glucocorticoid injection
(B) NSAID therapy
(C) Topical lidocaine
(D) Tramadol

Item 95

A 36-year-old woman is evaluated for a 5-year history of multiple symptoms, including back pain, food intolerances, headaches, pelvic pain, nausea, myalgia, joint stiffness, lightheadedness, and fatigue. She reports that her most bothersome symptom is mid/low back pain. She reports no trauma, fever, weight loss, rash, or bladder or bowel incontinence. She notes that if she removes highly processed foods from her diet, her symptoms seem to improve, especially the fatigue.

During the past 3 years, the patient has been evaluated by an orthopedic surgeon, allergist, neurologist, gastroenterologist, gynecologist, and rheumatologist, along with three different internists. She is married with no history of intimate partner violence. She does not smoke, drink alcohol, or use illicit drugs. Medications are citalopram, gabapentin, tramadol, and several herbal preparations.

On physical examination, vital signs are normal. BMI is 21. Back examination shows mild tenderness to palpation along the paraspinal muscles. Straight-leg raise test is negative for radicular symptoms but does reproduce her low back discomfort. The remainder of the examination is unremarkable.

Previous records show a normal comprehensive metabolic profile, creatine kinase level, complete blood count, and thyroid-stimulating hormone level within the past year. An erythrocyte sedimentation rate measured 1 month ago was 25 mm/h, and Lyme serology performed at the same time was negative. A lumbosacral spine radiograph 6 months ago was normal.

Which of the following is the most appropriate diagnostic test to perform next?

(A) Food allergy testing
(B) MRI of the lumbosacral spine
(C) Repeat Lyme serology
(D) No additional testing

Item 96

A 59-year-old man is evaluated in the emergency department for an episode of syncope. He experienced lightheadedness upon arising from a chair, which was followed by a witnessed transient loss of consciousness. He was immediately arousable and alert within 10 seconds. There was no loss of bladder or bowel function. He was otherwise asymptomatic prior to the event. Medical history is significant for hypertension and poorly controlled type 2 diabetes mellitus. Medications are benazepril, insulin glargine, and rosuvastatin.

On physical examination, the patient is afebrile. Blood pressure is 147/72 mm Hg supine and 120/76 mm Hg standing, pulse rate is 72/min supine and 94/min standing, and respiration rate is 14/min. BMI is 27. There is no jugular venous distention. Cardiopulmonary and abdominal examinations are normal. On neurologic examination, he is alert and oriented. Neurologic examination is unremarkable except for decreased sensation to touch in the feet bilaterally.

Laboratory studies are significant for a plasma glucose level of 338 mg/dL (18.8 mmol/L).

A 12-lead electrocardiogram shows normal sinus rhythm with normal axis and intervals and no acute ST- or T-wave changes.

Which of the following is the most likely cause of this patient's syncope?

(A) Orthostatic hypotension
(B) Seizure
(C) Silent cardiac ischemia
(D) Ventricular arrhythmia

Item 97

A 62-year-old woman is evaluated during a routine examination. She is asymptomatic. Her most recent Pap smear and human papillomavirus test were performed 3 years ago and were negative. A lipid panel and fasting plasma glucose level obtained last year were normal. She has never smoked cigarettes. Family history is noncontributory. She takes no medications.

On physical examination, the patient is afebrile, blood pressure is 116/78 mm Hg, and pulse rate is 78/min. BMI is 24. The remainder of the physical examination is normal.

Which of the following is the most appropriate screening test for this patient?

(A) Fasting lipid panel
(B) Fasting plasma glucose
(C) HIV testing
(D) Pap smear

Item 98

An 85-year-old woman is evaluated during a follow-up examination. She lives independently and is the primary caretaker of her elderly husband, who has dementia. Over the last 6 months, she has noticed increased difficulty reading the print on her husband's prescription pill bottles. She has worn glasses for many years and has had stable corrected vision, with her last prescription for glasses around 9 months ago. She reports no headache, jaw claudication, or muscle aches. Medical history is significant for hypertension and osteoporosis. She has never smoked and does not use alcohol. Medications are amlodipine, calcium, vitamin D, and alendronate.

On physical examination, she is afebrile, blood pressure is 137/82 mm Hg, pulse rate is 77/min, and respiration rate is 13/min. BMI is 23. The general physical examination is unremarkable, and there are no focal neurologic findings. There are no findings on undilated ophthalmoscopic examination.

Which of the following is the most appropriate next step in managing this patient's vision?

(A) Erythrocyte sedimentation rate
(B) Pinhole testing
(C) Referral to an eye professional
(D) Snellen eye chart testing

Item 99

A 37-year-old woman is evaluated for a 4-month history of anterior left knee pain that developed after she started training for a marathon. The pain was gradual in onset and has slowly worsened. She rates the pain as a 5 on a 10-point scale when at its worst. The pain increases when she climbs stairs or when she sits for an extended period of time. She reports no knee instability or recent trauma. Due to her pain, she has cut back on her running. Medical history is unremarkable. Her only medication is ibuprofen as needed for pain.

On physical examination, vital signs are normal. BMI is 25. Pain is reproduced by applying direct pressure to the left patella, and there is increased patellar laxity with lateral and medial displacement. There is no varus or valgus laxity, medial or lateral joint line tenderness, palpable joint effusion or swelling, or other tenderness to palpation. Anterior drawer, posterior drawer, and Lachman tests are negative. The remainder of the examination is unremarkable.

Which of the following is the most likely diagnosis?

(A) Iliotibial band syndrome
(B) Patellofemoral pain syndrome
(C) Pes anserine bursitis
(D) Prepatellar bursitis

Item 100

A 68-year-old woman in hospice care is evaluated for cachexia. She has widely metastatic breast cancer, which has progressed through multiple cycles of chemotherapy. Her estimated life expectancy is months. She reports anorexia and has lost 8% of her body weight despite attempts to increase her caloric intake with dietary measures and high-calorie supplements. Her pain is well controlled, and she reports no symptoms of sedation, depression, nausea, or constipation. The patient, her husband, and her daughter all express concern about her loss of appetite and weight loss, and they request information on pharmacologic options for weight gain. Current medications are extended-release morphine and bisacodyl.

On physical examination, the patient appears comfortable but very thin with notable temporal wasting. Temperature is normal, blood pressure is 112/72 mm Hg, and pulse rate is 66/min. BMI is 17. The mucous membranes are moist. Abdominal examination shows an enlarged liver that is nontender to palpation. Bowel sounds are normal. The remainder of the examination is unremarkable.

Which of the following is the most appropriate management of this patient's cachexia?

(A) Dronabinol
(B) Enteral nutrition
(C) Megestrol
(D) Continue current care

Item 101

A 29-year-old woman is evaluated for a 5-month history of widespread muscle aching. The pain was insidious in onset and has gradually worsened over time. The patient describes the pain as aching in nature and worsening after prolonged activity. She reports no sensations of burning, tingling, or numbness. Her symptoms have interfered with her ability to do household chores as well as her job as a bank teller because she is unable to stand for long periods of time due to the pain. She notes that her sleep is poor and that she awakens feeling unrefreshed. She reports no depressed mood, and her PHQ-9 score is not indicative of depression. She has not had any recent stressors in her life, and she enjoys her job. Medical history is otherwise unremarkable. There is no family history of rheumatologic diseases. She takes no medications.

On physical examination, vital signs are normal. On musculoskeletal examination, there is widespread muscle tenderness involving her deltoid, rhomboid, trapezius, paraspinal, and gluteal muscles, and thighs and calves bilaterally. There is no pain with joint range of motion and no joint synovitis. Strength is normal in all muscle groups. Reflexes are normal throughout. No rash is present.

Laboratory testing reveals a normal erythrocyte sedimentation rate and normal C-reactive protein level.

Which of the following types of pain is responsible for the patient's condition?

(A) Central pain
(B) Neuropathic pain
(C) Nociceptive pain
(D) Psychological pain

Item 102

A 35-year-old man is evaluated in the emergency department following a motor vehicle accident. The patient experienced significant abdominal trauma and multiple lacerations and contusions. Abdominal imaging shows a splenic laceration with intra-abdominal bleeding. Urgent laparotomy for splenectomy is planned. Medical history is unremarkable, and he has no known allergies. He takes no medications.

On physical examination, the patient is alert and oriented and reports moderate pain. He is afebrile, blood pressure is 124/76 mm Hg, pulse rate is 105/min, and respiration rate is 16/min. BMI is 23. Cardiopulmonary examination is normal. There is significant abdominal tenderness in the left upper quadrant. Scattered lacerations are noted across the chest and abdomen. The remainder of the physical examination is unremarkable.

Which of the following is the most appropriate pneumococcal vaccination strategy in this patient?

(A) Administer pneumococcal conjugate vaccine (PCV13) and pneumococcal polysaccharide vaccine (PPSV23) now

(B) Administer PCV13 now, followed by PPSV23 in 8 weeks

(C) Administer PPSV23 now

(D) Administer PPSV23 now, followed by PCV13 in 8 weeks

Item 103

A 29-year-old woman is evaluated for increasing nervousness associated with public speaking. She recently was promoted to a leadership position at work; her previous position required little interaction with others and no public speaking. When required to speak to a group of people, she becomes extremely anxious and is increasingly seeking ways to avoid this responsibility. When she must do so, she becomes sweaty and tachycardic, and she worries that she will be seen as appearing nervous and incompetent. She states that she "would rather die" than speak publicly and "does not want to be the center of attention." She relates that she has always been uncomfortable around others, avoiding social gatherings and rarely dating. She recognizes her fear of public speaking is excessive. Her PHQ-9 score is 2, and her Generalized Anxiety Disorder 7-item scale score is 4. She otherwise has no worries or health concerns.

On physical examination, blood pressure is 118/72 mm Hg, and pulse rate is 84/min. BMI is 23. The remainder of the physical examination is unremarkable.

Which of the following is the most appropriate pharmacologic treatment for this patient?

(A) Clonazepam

(B) Diazepam

(C) Propranolol

(D) Sertraline

Item 104

A 74-year-old woman is seen for preoperative evaluation for arthroscopic repair of a right rotator cuff tear. The pain and weakness significantly limit her activities of daily living and have been unresponsive to acetaminophen, NSAIDs, and physical therapy. Medical history is notable for severe aortic stenosis diagnosed 6 months ago. She

reports no cardiac symptoms, and her functional status has not changed in the last 6 months. She does not currently meet criteria for aortic valve replacement. Current medications are acetaminophen and ibuprofen.

On physical examination, blood pressure is 142/78 mm Hg, and pulse rate is 76/min. There is a grade 3/6 crescendo-decrescendo murmur at the cardiac base with radiation to the carotid arteries and a diminished S_2. Right shoulder findings include supraspinatus muscle weakness, weakness with external rotation, and a positive drop-arm test in the right arm.

An echocardiogram from 6 months ago reveals an ejection fraction of 65% and severe aortic stenosis (aortic valve area: 1 cm²; aortic valve mean gradient: 42 mm Hg; aortic valve peak velocity: 4.1 m/s).

An electrocardiogram from 5 months ago is normal. Treadmill exercise stress testing as part of aortic stenosis evaluation and risk stratification 5 months ago showed the patient achieving 4 metabolic equivalents (METs) and 90% of maximum predicted heart rate; she stopped the test due to knee pain but had normal blood pressure response to exercise and no symptoms or electrocardiographic changes with exercise.

Which of the following is the most appropriate management?

(A) Cancel surgery

(B) Perform dobutamine stress echocardiography

(C) Proceed to surgery

(D) Repeat echocardiography

Item 105

A 48-year-old man is evaluated for a 3-month history of bilateral lower extremity edema, mostly of the ankles. The edema does not seem to vary during the day and has been getting progressively worse. He reports no leg pain. He notes no dyspnea, orthopnea, abdominal distention, or constitutional symptoms. He has not had any recent surgical procedures or travel. Medical history is significant for hypertension. His current medications are amlodipine and hydrochlorothiazide.

On physical examination, the patient is afebrile, blood pressure is 132/76 mm Hg, pulse rate is 76/min, and respiration rate is 16/min. BMI is 28. There is no elevation in central venous pressure. The lungs are clear. No extra heart sounds or murmurs are noted. The abdomen shows no hepatomegaly, shifting dullness, fluid wave, or bulging flanks. No inguinal lymphadenopathy is present. There is pitting edema to the level of the ankles bilaterally.

Laboratory studies are significant for normal liver chemistry and kidney function tests; the serum albumin level is 4.1 g/dL (41 g/L). Urinalysis is normal.

Which of the following is the most appropriate next step in management?

(A) Compression stockings

(B) Lower extremity venous duplex ultrasonography

(C) Switch amlodipine to lisinopril

(D) Switch hydrochlorothiazide to furosemide

Item 106

A 30-year-old woman is evaluated for severe breast discomfort that is worse in the week before her menstrual periods. Both breasts ache and hurt with movement, and to the touch, the left breast is more painful than the right. She has not noted any lumps, skin changes, or nipple discharge. She otherwise feels well with no fever, cough, or joint pain. Her menses are regular. She has never been pregnant, and she does not smoke or use illicit drugs. She drinks one to two cups of coffee each morning. Her maternal aunt had breast cancer at age 52 years. She takes vitamin D daily but no other medications.

On physical examination, vital signs are normal. BMI is 27. Except for diffuse tenderness, the results of the breast examination are normal bilaterally, with no skin changes or dimpling, no focal abnormalities or masses, no nipple discharge, and no supraclavicular, cervical, or axillary lymphadenopathy. There is diffuse symmetric nodularity, which is most prominent in the upper outer quadrant of both breasts. There is no chest wall tenderness, and the heart and lungs are normal to examination.

Which of the following is the most appropriate management?

- (A) Breast ultrasonography
- (B) Caffeine-free diet
- (C) Combined hormonal oral contraceptive
- (D) Danazol
- (E) Support bra

Item 107

A 72-year-old man is evaluated in the emergency department for a witnessed syncopal episode. The patient was sitting in church when he noted acute onset lightheadedness accompanied by a rapid heartbeat. He abruptly lost consciousness and was unresponsive for 1 minute. There was no apparent seizure activity, bladder or bowel incontinence, or tongue biting. Upon regaining consciousness, he was groggy but alert with no retrograde amnesia, chest pain, shortness of breath, or weakness. He is a current smoker with a 50-pack-year history. Medical history is remarkable for type 2 diabetes mellitus, hypertension, and hyperlipidemia. Medications are metformin, lisinopril, and simvastatin.

On physical examination, temperature is 36.7 °C (98.0 °F), blood pressure is 138/86 mm Hg without orthostatic change, pulse rate is 56/min and regular, and respiration rate is 15/min. BMI is 33. Oxygen saturation is 93% with the patient breathing ambient air. Carotid upstrokes are normal and without bruits. The lungs are clear. Cardiac examination shows occasional premature beats but is otherwise normal.

Electrocardiogram reveals normal sinus rhythm with a left axis shift, QRS interval of 140 ms, and complete left bundle branch block pattern (unchanged from 1 year ago). Chest radiograph is normal.

Which of the following is the most appropriate next step in management?

- (A) 24-Hour ambulatory event monitor
- (B) Implantable loop recorder
- (C) Inpatient cardiac monitoring
- (D) Pacemaker insertion

Item 108

A 46-year-old man is evaluated for left shoulder pain that began suddenly 2 weeks ago. The pain worsens with overhead activities and at night. He notes limited range of motion and pain with lifting his arm. He reports no trauma to his shoulder and has never had this pain before. He is employed as a painter, and the pain is interfering with his ability to work. Medical history is unremarkable. His only medication is ibuprofen, which provides modest relief.

On physical examination, vital signs are normal. The left shoulder is normal in appearance, and there is no tenderness to palpation of bony structures. Examination reveals a positive painful arc test. Pain is elicited over the anterolateral aspect of his left shoulder with active but not passive shoulder abduction. External rotation resistance, external rotation lag, and internal rotation lag tests are negative. He has no pain with his left arm in full flexion, and he is able to slowly and smoothly lower his left arm to his waist. When the patient is asked to hold the arm flexed at 90 degrees with the forearm bent to 90 degrees (at 12 o'clock), he does not have pain with the arm internally rotated to cross in front of the body (negative Hawkins test). When his left shoulder is abducted to 90 degrees and then adducted 30 degrees in the scapular plane with the thumb pointed downward and downward pressure is applied at the elbow against resistance, he does not have any pain or weakness (negative empty can test). Strength is 5/5 throughout.

Which of the following is the most appropriate next step in management?

- (A) Conservative therapy
- (B) MRI of the left shoulder
- (C) Orthopedic surgery evaluation
- (D) Radiographs of the left shoulder

Item 109

A 32-year-old man is evaluated for a 2-week history of non-radiating low back pain. He notes that the pain developed insidiously and worsens with increased physical activity, such as playing basketball. He has no morning stiffness. He has not had any trauma and reports no weakness or abnormal sensation in the lower extremities. He otherwise feels well and has no other symptoms. Medical history is unremarkable. He does not use alcohol excessively, and he does not smoke or use illicit drugs. He takes no medications except for as-needed ibuprofen, which provides only modest pain relief.

On physical examination, vital signs are normal. BMI is 23. The general medical evaluation, including eye and skin examinations, is unremarkable. Musculoskeletal examination shows no scoliosis or kyphosis and no tenderness to palpation across the lower back and spine. There is normal muscle bulk and tone and normal sensation in the lower extremities. Flexion and extension of the back are limited by pain. Straight-leg raise test is negative. Examination of the joints is unremarkable, and deep tendon reflexes are normal.

Which of the following is the most appropriate diagnostic test to perform next?

(A) Erythrocyte sedimentation rate
(B) HLA-B27 testing
(C) Radiography of the lumbar spine
(D) No additional testing

Item 110

A 64-year-old man is evaluated for the gradual onset of lower urinary tract symptoms over the past year. He notes a weak urinary stream and nocturia once nightly. He drinks two cups of coffee each morning and does not drink fluids within 3 hours of retiring to sleep. He reports no dysuria, hematuria, or fever. Medical history is notable for hyperlipidemia and osteoarthritis. He drinks two alcoholic beverages each week, and his social history is otherwise noncontributory. Medications are simvastatin and aspirin.

On physical examination, the patient is afebrile, blood pressure is 100/54 mm Hg, and pulse rate is 60/min. BMI is 27. The prostate is diffusely enlarged to approximately 30 mL in volume (normal, 20 mL); no nodules are detected. Cardiac and pulmonary examinations are normal. The penis is normal. The patient's American Urological Association Symptom Index score is 4.

Urinalysis with microscopy shows 2 leukocytes/hpf and is otherwise unremarkable.

Which of the following is the most appropriate management?

(A) Ciprofloxacin
(B) Finasteride
(C) Tamsulosin
(D) Observation

Item 111

A 52-year-old man is evaluated for the sudden onset of erectile dysfunction that has persisted for 6 months. He reports having erections that are inadequate for vaginal penetration. He feels guilty about not being able to satisfy his wife's requests for sexual intercourse, although he still has sexual desires. He has been sleeping poorly and feeling fatigued throughout the day. He reports no snoring or daytime somnolence, and his review of systems is otherwise negative. His wife does not report that the patient has episodes of nocturnal gasping or apnea. He has firm erections upon waking in the morning. For years, he has run 2 miles daily without chest pain or exercise-limiting dyspnea, although he has not been interested in exercise

over recent weeks. Medical history is notable for hypertension. Family history is notable for his father who died of a myocardial infarction at age 70 years and his mother who died of complications from a stroke at the age of 94 years. He has never smoked cigarettes. His 10-year risk of atherosclerotic cardiovascular disease is calculated to be 5% using the Pooled Cohort Equations. Medications are hydrochlorothiazide and lisinopril. He has taken these medications for 6 years without interruption.

On physical examination, the patient is afebrile, and blood pressure is 132/64 mm Hg. BMI is 26. Heart, lung, and abdominal examinations are normal. The penis is uncircumcised without abnormalities, and the testes are normal size.

Laboratory studies show a fasting plasma glucose level of 98 mg/dL (5.4 mmol/L).

Which of the following is the most likely cause of this patient's erectile dysfunction?

(A) Hypogonadism
(B) Mood disorder
(C) Obstructive sleep apnea
(D) Prolactinoma

Item 112

A study in which researchers randomized 150 patients with asthma to a program of mindfulness meditation and 150 patients with asthma to a mock intervention of reading in a quiet room is reviewed. All subjects were patients at the same academic medical center. The intervention group was enrolled in a meditation program that was administered in July, whereas the control group participated in the mock intervention during the months of January through March. Outcomes, which were measured 1 hour after meditation and mock intervention, included peak-flow rates and validated health care quality-of-life scores. The researchers found that patients with asthma randomized to meditation had significantly better peak-flow rates and quality-of-life scores than control subjects.

Which of the following would improve the validity of this study's results?

(A) Include patients with COPD
(B) Increase the sample size
(C) Measure the outcomes of both study groups concurrently
(D) Use a more precise measure of airway function

Item 113

A 43-year-old woman is evaluated for acute-onset vertigo of 3 days' duration. She reports that severe vertigo accompanied by nausea and vomiting began abruptly and has been persistent. There are no maneuvers that accentuate or totally relieve her symptoms, and the severity of the vertigo prevents her from conducting her usual activities at work and home. She prefers to lie in bed with her eyes closed. She has had neither head trauma nor headaches and reports no motor weakness, numbness, tingling, otalgia, dysarthria, diplopia, hearing loss, tinnitus, fevers, or chills. Ten days ago, she had an upper respiratory tract infection. Medical history is otherwise unremarkable, and she takes no medications.

On physical examination, the patient is afebrile, blood pressure is 135/80 mm Hg, pulse rate is 98/min, and respiration rate is 14/min. BMI is 22. She appears uncomfortable and is lying down on the examination table with her eyes closed. She is unable to walk because of the vertigo. Hearing is normal. Pupils are equal, round, and reactive to light. Funduscopic examination reveals normal discs and vasculature. The remainder of the general medical examination is normal. On neurologic examination, finger-to-nose, rapid alternating movements, and heel-to-knee-to-shin tests are normal. The Dix-Hallpike maneuver evokes mixed upbeat-torsional nystagmus after 6 seconds that lasts for about 30 seconds; she then becomes very symptomatic and vomits. The remainder of the neurologic examination is normal.

Which of the following is the most likely diagnosis?

(A) Benign paroxysmal positional vertigo
(B) Brainstem infarction
(C) Labyrinthitis
(D) Vestibular neuronitis

Item 114

A 46-year-old man visits to discuss preventive measures. He feels well and has no current symptoms, although he asks whether he should be taking vitamin supplements to decrease his risk for cardiovascular disease and cancer. He reports exercising regularly and eating a healthy diet that includes fruits and vegetables. Family history is significant for his father who had a myocardial infarction at age 72 years and a paternal uncle who developed colon cancer in his 70s. He takes no medications.

On physical examination, the patient is afebrile, blood pressure is 118/78 mm Hg, pulse rate is 76/min, and respiration rate is 16/min. BMI is 25. The remainder of the examination is unremarkable.

Which of the following is the most appropriate recommendation for this patient to reduce his risk for cardiovascular disease and cancer?

(A) β-Carotene
(B) Multivitamin with minerals
(C) Vitamin C
(D) No vitamin supplementation

Item 115

A 28-year-old woman is evaluated for bilateral eye pain and redness of 3 months' duration, which has recently worsened. She describes the pain as deep and constant and notes that it worsens at night. She also reports photophobia. She does not wear contact lenses. She has tried several types of over-the-counter eye drops without improvement in her symptoms. She is otherwise healthy and takes no medications.

On physical examination, the patient is afebrile, blood pressure is 100/62 mm Hg, and pulse rate is 94/min. BMI is 24. Ophthalmologic examination shows diffuse redness bilaterally, sparing the lids and iris. Visual acuity is normal. A nondilated funduscopic examination is unremarkable. The remainder of the examination is normal.

Which of the following is the most likely diagnosis?

(A) Episcleritis
(B) Keratoconjunctivitis sicca
(C) Scleritis
(D) Subconjunctival hemorrhage

Item 116

A 30-year-old woman is evaluated for a 2-week history of irritability, inability to sleep, feelings of emptiness, and suicidal thoughts. Just prior to the onset of her symptoms, her boyfriend, whom she describes as a "loser," broke up with her. The patient was seen 1 month ago for a preventive services evaluation, including a pelvic examination and Pap smear. At that time, she described her then-new boyfriend, whom she met online, as "perfect" even though he was unemployed and had previously been incarcerated. Immediately after meeting, they spent nearly all of their time together, and she described herself as the happiest she has ever been. However, they quickly engaged in arguments, and he broke up with her. Over the years, she has had similar relationships associated with emotional ups and downs. Medical history is notable for previous hospitalizations for suicide attempts.

Which of the following is the most likely primary diagnosis?

(A) Bipolar disorder
(B) Borderline personality disorder
(C) Depression
(D) Generalized anxiety disorder

Item 117

A 61-year-old man is evaluated for a gradual onset of difficulty achieving erections over the past year. He reports a good relationship with his wife and a strong interest in having sexual intercourse and does not have a depressed mood. He no longer has nocturnal erections. Over the past several months, he becomes fatigued and dyspneic with any regular exertion; these symptoms resolve after 10 minutes of rest. He normally has a sedentary lifestyle. He is a lifetime nonsmoker. Medical history is notable for hyperlipidemia treated with diet only and benign prostatic hyperplasia treated with tamsulosin.

On physical examination, the patient's affect is normal. Blood pressure is 104/64 mm Hg. BMI is 25. Examination of the heart, lungs, prostate, penis, and testicles is normal.

Electrocardiogram shows normal sinus rhythm and is otherwise normal. Chest radiograph is normal.

Which of the following is the most appropriate next step in management?

(A) Initiate tadalafil

(B) Obtain cardiac stress test

(C) Psychiatric evaluation

(D) Recommend weight loss through diet and exercise

Item 118

A 16-year-old teenager is evaluated during an office visit. He was brought to the office by his mother who has concerns about his behavior. She has noticed that since he was a toddler, he has been unable to make friends and prefers to be alone. He has difficulty engaging in social conversation and reading nonverbal cues and thus avoids social interactions. He has had significant difficulty with school because of his hesitation to communicate with others. She also describes that he is adamant about sticking to routines and gets frustrated with change. As an example, she states that he has to turn the light on and off three times before closing the door to his room. He also has a collection of shoelaces that he lines up nightly before bed and carries his teddy bear with him everywhere.

On physical examination, the patient is awake and alert but minimally communicative. Vital signs are normal, and the remainder of the physical examination is unremarkable.

Which of the following is the most likely diagnosis?

(A) Antisocial personality disorder

(B) Autism spectrum disorder

(C) Obsessive-compulsive disorder

(D) Social anxiety disorder

Item 119

A 35-year-old woman is evaluated in follow-up after treatment of her fourth episode of vulvovaginal candidiasis within the past year. Her usual symptoms include a thick, white vaginal discharge associated with severe itching, burning, and dyspareunia. Her last episode was 2 weeks ago and was treated with a single dose of oral fluconazole with complete resolution of symptoms. However, she wishes to discuss her options for avoiding future infections. Medical and gynecologic histories are otherwise unremarkable, and she takes no medications. She has one male sexual partner and uses an oral contraceptive.

On physical examination, vital signs are normal. BMI is 24. The general medical and gynecologic examinations are unremarkable.

Which of the following is the most appropriate recommendation to decrease recurrent infections?

(A) Antifungal treatment of her sexual partner

(B) Extended-course antifungal therapy

(C) *Lactobacillus* recolonization

(D) Switch to an alternative contraceptive method

Item 120

A 55-year-old man is evaluated for a 2-week history of visual symptoms in the left eye. He reports seeing black spots that move across his eye and flashes of light, followed by a progressive loss of vision over the lateral field, as if half of his vision is covered by a shadow. He reports no headaches or trauma. He does not wear contact lenses; however, he does wear glasses for the correction of myopia. He is a nonsmoker. Medical history is otherwise unremarkable, and he takes no medications.

On physical examination, vital signs are normal. BMI is 28. Visual acuity is intact. The pupils appear normal and are equally reactive to light. On dilated ophthalmoscopy, the left fundus is undulating and out of focus. There is no retinal pallor, and there are no cotton wool spots or hemorrhages. The remainder of the physical examination is normal.

Which of the following is the most likely diagnosis?

(A) Age-related macular degeneration

(B) Branch retinal vein occlusion

(C) Central retinal artery occlusion

(D) Retinal detachment

Item 121

A 78-year-old man is evaluated for low back and leg pain. He first noticed symptoms about 2 years ago, and they have steadily worsened. He describes a dull ache in the low back and pain that radiates down both legs. The leg pain is worse when ambulating and absent when seated, and his symptoms are particularly noticeable when walking up steps. He notes no previous trauma, weakness, or systemic symptoms. Medical history is significant for hypertension, hyperlipidemia, and obesity. He is a retired carpenter. Medications are ramipril, rosuvastatin, and as-needed acetaminophen and naproxen.

On physical examination, vital signs are normal. BMI is 31. The general medical examination is unremarkable. There is normal muscle bulk and tone in the lower extremities, and the distal extremities are warm with palpable dorsalis pedis and posterior tibialis pulses. No point tenderness is detected with palpation of the spine. Hyperextension of the back exacerbates the pain. There is no lower extremity weakness, and reflexes and sensory examination findings are normal.

Which of the following is the most likely cause of this patient's symptoms?

(A) Compression fracture

(B) Hip osteoarthritis

(C) Peripheral arterial disease

(D) Spinal stenosis

Item 122

A 40-year-old woman is evaluated during a follow-up visit for a 4-year history of medically unexplained symptoms. She reports shortness of breath, generalized pain, fatigue, arthralgia, nausea, headaches, and migratory dysesthesia. She has been evaluated by multiple primary care and specialty physicians and has had more than 20 emergency department visits during this time; all studies have been normal. Trials of two different antidepressant medications were unsuccessful. Her quality of life has significantly declined over the past several years. Medical history is otherwise unremarkable. Family history is significant for fibromyalgia in her mother. Medications are tramadol, albuterol, and ibuprofen, all taken as needed.

On physical examination, temperature is 36.0 °C (96.8 °F), blood pressure is 125/80 mm Hg, pulse rate is 88/min, and respiration rate is 16/min. BMI is 28. The remainder of the physical examination is normal.

Which of the following is the most appropriate management of this patient?

(A) Long-acting benzodiazepine
(B) Neuropsychological testing
(C) Physical therapy
(D) Regular primary care visits

Item 123

A 45-year-old man is hospitalized for fever and cough and started on appropriate antibiotic treatment for community-acquired pneumonia. While in the hospital, he develops a headache and begins to feel restless and agitated. He drinks four beers nightly on weekdays and eight beers daily on weekends. He has chronic liver disease and has had alcohol withdrawal seizures in the past. His last drink was 12 hours ago. Outpatient medications are lactulose and propranolol, but he has not been adherent with this regimen. He is given thiamine, glucose, intravenous fluids, and multivitamins.

On physical examination, the patient is diaphoretic. He is alert and oriented but tremulous. Temperature is 38.4 °C (101.1 °F), blood pressure is 182/94 mm Hg, pulse rate is 118/min, and respiration rate is 20/min. Jaundice is present. Numerous spider angiomas and palmar erythema are present. Other than tachycardia, the cardiac examination is normal. Crackles are heard in the left lower lung field. There is a small amount of ascites. The liver is not palpable, but the spleen tip is easily palpable. The deep tendon reflexes are brisk. There is no clonus.

Which of the following is the most appropriate treatment of this patient's current symptoms?

(A) Chlordiazepoxide
(B) Clonidine
(C) Lorazepam
(D) Propranolol

Item 124

A 35-year-old man is evaluated during a routine examination. He is asymptomatic but is interested in starting a diet and exercise program. In high school, he was athletic, thin, and fit, but since then, he has gradually gained weight. He works very long hours in a sedentary job, does not exercise,

and occasionally smokes a cigar. He drinks two to three alcoholic beverages per day on weekends, and he often eats fast food. He reports occasional snoring, but he feels refreshed when awaking in the morning. He reports no daytime somnolence or sleep intrusions. He does not have exertion-associated symptoms suggestive of cardiac ischemia. Medical history is unremarkable. He takes no medications.

On physical examination, the patient is afebrile, blood pressure is 126/76 mm Hg, and pulse rate is 78/min. BMI is 31. The abdomen is protuberant without pathologic striae. The remainder of the examination is normal.

Which of the following is the most appropriate cardiovascular risk stratification strategy?

(A) Exercise stress testing
(B) Overnight oximetry
(C) Resting electrocardiography
(D) Waist circumference measurement

Item 125

A 48-year-old man is evaluated during a follow-up appointment. Three months ago, he sustained an ST-elevation myocardial infarction and underwent percutaneous coronary intervention and bare metal stenting of his left circumflex artery. He was started on high-intensity rosuvastatin at the time of his myocardial infarction; his alanine aminotransferase and serum creatinine levels were normal. His recovery has been uneventful. He follows a heart-healthy diet and exercises regularly with no chest pain, dyspnea, palpitations, or lightheadedness. He reports no fatigue, muscle pains, abdominal pain, or changes in skin color. Medical history is significant for hypertension. Medications are aspirin, metoprolol, lisinopril, and rosuvastatin.

On physical examination, vital signs are normal. There is no muscle or abdominal tenderness. The remainder of the physical examination is unremarkable.

Which of the following is the most appropriate laboratory study to obtain at this visit?

(A) Alanine aminotransferase level
(B) Creatine kinase level
(C) Fasting lipid panel
(D) High-sensitivity C-reactive protein level

Item 126

A 65-year-old woman is evaluated during a routine examination. She is asymptomatic. Her most recent cervical cancer screening was 2 years ago at age 63 years and included a normal Pap smear. She has received regular Pap smears for the past 30 years, and all previous Pap smears have been negative. She is a widow and has had one new sexual partner in the last 2 years. Medical history is unremarkable. Family history is noncontributory. She takes no medications.

On physical examination, the patient is afebrile, blood pressure is 122/74 mm Hg, and pulse rate is 82/min. BMI is 28. The remainder of the physical examination is normal.

Which of the following is the most appropriate recommendation for cervical cancer screening?

(A) Obtain Pap smear in 1 year
(B) Obtain Pap smear in 3 years
(C) Obtain Pap smear now
(D) Discontinue screening

Item 127

A 58-year-old woman is evaluated for an 8-week history of persistent posterior neck pain. The patient describes the pain as a burning and tingling sensation that will occasionally radiate down both arms. She reports no headache, changes in vision, or upper extremity muscle weakness. There is no history of trauma. Medical history is otherwise unremarkable. Her only medications are acetaminophen and naproxen, which do not effectively relieve the pain.

On physical examination, vital signs are normal. The general medical examination is unremarkable. On musculoskeletal examination, range of motion of the neck is limited. There is no pain to palpation over the neck and upper back. Upper extremity muscle strength is normal, and there is no upper extremity spasticity or hyperreflexia. Extension and rotation of the patient's neck toward either side with pressure applied to the top of her head reproduces the discomfort. The remainder of the examination is unremarkable.

A plain radiograph of the neck shows osteoarthritis. Cervical spine MRI shows evidence of extensive degenerative changes, facet hypertrophy, and disk space narrowing.

Which of the following is the most appropriate next step in management?

(A) Diazepam
(B) Epidural glucocorticoid injections
(C) Erythrocyte sedimentation rate
(D) Gabapentin

Item 128

An 87-year-old woman is admitted to the hospital with altered mental status. Prior to her illness, she lived in an assisted-living facility. She has a history of mild cognitive impairment, and she now lacks the capacity to make decisions. The patient has an advance directive that names her daughter as the surrogate decision maker. The patient's daughter requests a do-not-resuscitate (DNR) order in accordance with the patient's previously expressed preferences.

Urinalysis reveals greater than 100 leukocytes/hpf and bacteria. The findings suggest that the patient's altered mental status may be due to a urinary tract infection and therefore may be reversible. Blood and urine cultures and intravenous fluids and antibiotics are recommended; however, the patient's daughter refuses, stating that her mother has a DNR order.

Which of the following is the most appropriate next step in management?

(A) Assess the daughter's understanding of her mother's condition and wishes
(B) Obtain an emergency court-appointed guardian

(C) Request an ethics consultation
(D) Withhold further testing and treatment

Item 129

A 59-year-old man is evaluated for hyperlipidemia. The physician suggests initiating a statin medication, and the patient asks how effective the medication will be at preventing myocardial infarction (MI). The physician reviews a randomized controlled trial that was conducted to determine whether statin medications reduce the risk of death from MI. A total of 2146 patients were randomized to receive a statin medication or placebo. After 5 years, the researchers determined the number of deaths from MI in each study group. The findings revealed that 93 of 1093 patients in the placebo group died of MI, whereas only 53 of 1053 patients in the statin group died of MI.

Based on the study results, what is the absolute risk reduction in mortality from a myocardial infarction after taking a statin medication for 5 years?

(A) 4%
(B) 14%
(C) 24%
(D) 94%

Item 130

A 48-year-old woman is evaluated during a routine gynecologic examination. Menstruation is generally regular; her last period was 3 weeks ago. She has had no abnormal bleeding or discharge and no dysuria. She is gravida 2, para 2. She has no history of sexual trauma or pelvic surgery.

When asked an open-ended screening question about sexual concerns, she hesitantly admits that she has been having a hard time in her marriage because she has lost interest in sex over the past 2 years. She engages in sexual activity to keep her partner happy but she does not enjoy intercourse. She has been increasingly avoiding sexual intimacy, and this has become a source of friction in her marriage. She uses a lubricant for intercourse, which has been adequate for reducing discomfort.

Results of the physical examination, including the pelvic examination, are unremarkable.

Which of the following is the most likely diagnosis?

(A) Genitopelvic pain/penetration disorder
(B) Orgasmic disorder
(C) Sexual interest/arousal disorder
(D) Vulvodynia

Item 131

An 18-year-old man is seen for a preparticipation sports evaluation. The patient has no specific symptoms. He has played varsity basketball for the past 3 years without any limitation and remains active in the off-season by participating in cross-country running and soccer.

Hypertension was recently diagnosed in his father; his two younger siblings are both healthy. He has no family history of cardiomyopathy or unexplained sudden death.

On physical examination, blood pressure is 112/62 mm Hg, and pulse rate is 52/min. The lungs are clear to auscultation. The jugular venous pulse shows a normal contour, and the carotid upstroke is normal. Precordial examination shows a prominent apical impulse that is not sustained or enlarged. The intensity of S_1 is slightly increased, and S_2 is normally split. No murmurs, rubs, or gallops are present. The remainder of the physical examination is unremarkable.

Which of the following is the most appropriate next step in management?

(A) Echocardiography

(B) Electrocardiographic stress testing

(C) Electrocardiography

(D) No further testing

Item 132

A 52-year-old man is evaluated during a follow-up visit for chronic back pain due to spinal injuries sustained in a motor vehicle accident 1 year ago. He underwent spinal stabilization surgery at the time of the accident and has experienced significant pain since recovery. His pain has not responded to appropriate trials of nonopioid pain medications, glucocorticoid injections, and physical therapy. Repeat orthopedic and neurosurgical evaluations indicate that no additional surgical interventions are indicated. He attended an intensive, multimodal pain rehabilitation program and continues to practice mindfulness-based stress reduction techniques. He exercises daily in the form of swimming. Although these interventions have helped to some degree, he remains functionally impaired due to his pain. He fears he will lose his job as a computer programmer due to his inability to sit in a chair all day. The patient has been reliable and engaged.

On physical examination, vital signs are normal. The general physical examination is unremarkable except for postsurgical changes in the back. The neurologic examination is normal.

The patient scores in the low-risk category for opioid therapy on DIRE (Diagnosis, Intractability, Risk, and Efficacy) risk assessment. Baseline screening urine drug testing is negative. The patient and physician both sign an opioid treatment agreement, and the patient is started on long-term opioid therapy.

Which of the following is the most appropriate method for monitoring the patient's opioid therapy?

(A) Documentation of functional assessment twice annually

(B) Office visits monthly for 3 months, followed by as-needed visits

(C) Regular 3-month office visits with urine drug testing at every office visit

(D) Use of a prescription drug monitoring program at every visit

Item 133

A 41-year-old man is evaluated during an examination to establish care. The patient reports being generally healthy and has no symptoms, although he leads a sedentary lifestyle and is obese. Medical and family histories are noncontributory. He does not smoke, drink alcohol excessively, or use illicit drugs. He takes no medications.

On physical examination, the patient is afebrile, blood pressure is 132/82 mm Hg, pulse rate is 80/min, and respiration rate is 11/min. BMI is 32. The remainder of the physical examination is unremarkable.

Laboratory studies:

Total cholesterol	251 mg/dL (6.50 mmol/L)
LDL cholesterol	172 mg/dL (4.45 mmol/L)
HDL cholesterol	35 mg/dL (0.91 mmol/L)
Triglycerides	220 mg/dL (2.49 mmol/L)
Hemoglobin A_{1c}	5%

The patient's estimated 10-year risk for atherosclerotic cardiovascular disease using the Pooled Cohort Equations is 3.4%.

Which of the following is the most appropriate management of this patient's hyperlipidemia?

(A) Ezetimibe

(B) High-intensity rosuvastatin

(C) Moderate-intensity rosuvastatin

(D) Niacin

(E) Therapeutic lifestyle modification

Item 134

A 28-year-old woman is admitted to the hospital with toxic epidermal necrolysis. Two weeks prior to admission, the patient was seen in the outpatient setting by the attending physician's colleague, and she was prescribed trimethoprim-sulfamethoxazole for a urinary tract infection. The patient's medical record indicates that she has a sulfa allergy. In the hospital, the patient is informed of the new findings and treatment plan, and the patient expresses concern that she was initially prescribed a sulfa drug. She asks if the attending physician's colleague made a mistake.

In addition to acknowledging that an error occurred, which of the following is the most appropriate course of action?

(A) Advise the patient to share her concerns with the physician who committed the error

(B) Inform the patient that the pharmacy was at fault for not preventing the error

(C) Offer to transfer the patient's care to a physician at another hospital

(D) Tell the patient that the colleague will be informed of the error and steps will be taken to prevent future errors

Item 135

A 58-year-old man is seen for preoperative evaluation prior to umbilical hernia repair scheduled in 1 week. He has been in good health except for increasing pain at the site of his umbilical hernia. He has experienced no incarceration of his hernia. He exercises regularly without symptoms. He has no history of stroke or transient ischemic attack. Medical history is notable for aortic valve replacement with bileaflet mechanical prosthesis performed 3 years ago for a bicuspid aortic valve and decreasing exercise capacity. Medications are warfarin and low-dose aspirin.

On physical examination, blood pressure is 124/72 mm Hg, and pulse rate is 70/min. Cardiovascular examination reveals a regular rhythm, a mechanical S_2, and a grade 1/6 early systolic crescendo-decrescendo murmur at the cardiac base without radiation.

Laboratory studies show a normal serum creatinine level.

An electrocardiogram performed 2 months ago showed normal sinus rhythm with normal intervals. An echocardiogram from 2 months ago showed normal left ventricular function and normal function of the mechanical aortic valve prosthesis.

In addition to continuing aspirin and stopping warfarin 5 days before surgery, which of the following is the most appropriate management for preoperative anticoagulation bridging?

(A) Intravenous unfractionated heparin

(B) Prophylactic-dose subcutaneous enoxaparin

(C) Therapeutic-dose subcutaneous enoxaparin

(D) No bridging anticoagulation

Item 136

A 42-year-old man is evaluated for a 3-month history of cough. He describes the cough as nonproductive and associated with sinus congestion. He also notes increased mucus production with frequent throat clearing. He has no shortness of breath, wheezing, hemoptysis, or chest pain. He does not notice any change in cough with exercise. He reports that he has had similar extended periods of cough in the past, usually in either the fall or spring. He has tried over-the-counter dextromethorphan and decongestants, alone and in combination, without noticeable improvement. Medical history is otherwise unremarkable. He is a never-smoker and takes no medications.

On physical examination, the patient is afebrile, blood pressure is 124/84 mm Hg, pulse rate is 68/min, and respiration rate is 15/min. Nasal turbinates are boggy. The lungs are clear to auscultation. The remainder of the examination is normal.

Which of the following is the most appropriate treatment?

(A) Antibiotic therapy

(B) Antihistamine-decongestant

(C) Inhaled bronchodilator

(D) Intranasal glucocorticoid

Item 137

A 38-year-old man is evaluated during a routine examination. Since high school, the patient has gradually gained 25 kg (55 lb). He has a sedentary job, does not exercise, and eats fast food for lunch and dinner and snacks throughout the day. The patient has never been treated with pharmacologic agents for weight loss, and he wonders if he is a candidate for gastric banding bariatric surgery. He reports no exertion-associated symptoms suggestive of cardiac ischemia and is otherwise healthy. Medical history and review of systems are unremarkable. He takes no medications.

On physical examination, temperature is normal, blood pressure is 122/70 mm Hg, pulse rate is 78/min, and respiration rate is 12/min. BMI is 36. Waist circumference is 106 cm (42 in). Head, neck, lung, and heart examinations are normal. The abdomen is protuberant without pathologic striae.

In addition to increasing physical activity, which of the following is the most appropriate next step in management?

(A) Laparoscopic adjustable gastric banding

(B) Lorcaserin

(C) Orlistat

(D) Reduce caloric intake to maintain a deficit of 500 kcal/d

Item 138

A 60-year-old man is evaluated for urinary frequency of several years' duration. His symptoms have worsened over the past 6 to 12 months, and he notes several episodes of nocturia over the past 3 months. He reports no fever or dysuria. Medical history is notable for hypertension, and his only medication is amlodipine; he takes no over-the-counter medications.

On physical examination, blood pressure is 140/60 mm Hg, and pulse rate is 64/min. BMI is 30. There is no evidence of suprapubic bladder distention. The prostate is diffusely enlarged, firm, and nontender without nodules. The penis appears normal. The remainder of the examination is normal.

Which of the following is the most appropriate next step in management?

(A) Postvoid residual urine volume

(B) Prostate ultrasonography

(C) Urinalysis

(D) Urine flow studies

Item 139

A 42-year-old man is evaluated for a lifelong history of insomnia. He reports always having had trouble sleeping, but sleep initiation and maintenance have become more difficult over the past few years. He experiences daytime sleepiness but does not have the opportunity to nap. He reports no depressed mood or anhedonia. His wife has not noticed excessive snoring or abnormal or absent breathing during sleep. He drinks one cup of coffee in the morning and drinks one alcoholic beverage 3 to 4 nights per week. Medical history is otherwise unremarkable. He takes no medications.

On physical examination, the patient is afebrile, blood pressure is 142/82 mm Hg, pulse rate is 78/min, and respiration rate is 14/min. BMI is 27. The remainder of the physical examination is normal.

Which of the following is the most appropriate next step in management?

(A) Alcohol cessation counseling

(B) Sleep hygiene counseling

(C) Trazodone

(D) Zolpidem

Item 140

A 27-year-old man is evaluated during a pre-employment examination. He is asymptomatic. Review of systems is negative, including no hearing loss, tinnitus, or ear pain. Medical history is otherwise unremarkable. He takes no medications.

On physical examination, vital signs are normal. BMI is 21. General examination is normal except for cerumen impaction of both auditory canals. The tympanic membranes cannot be visualized. Gross auditory acuity is normal. The remainder of the examination is unremarkable.

Which of the following is the most appropriate management?

(A) Ceruminolytic agent

(B) Ear irrigation

(C) Manual cerumen removal

(D) Clinical observation

Item 141

A 52-year-old man is evaluated in follow-up for a large, inoperable pelvic osteosarcoma that is currently being treated palliatively. He reports increasingly worsening pelvic and abdominal pain. His pain had previously been controlled with as-needed nonopioid analgesics, although he is experiencing increased pain with tumor growth. Except for pain, he has no other symptoms. Medical history is otherwise unremarkable, and his current medications are as-needed naproxen and acetaminophen.

On physical examination, the patient appears to be in mild painful distress. Vital signs are normal. BMI is 22. There is a mass in the right pelvis that is moderately tender to palpation. The remainder of the examination is unremarkable.

Scheduled oral hydromorphone is prescribed for pain control.

Which of the following daily adjunctive treatments should be given to this patient?

(A) Docusate

(B) Fiber supplementation

(C) Methylnaltrexone

(D) Senna

Item 142

A 66-year-old man was diagnosed with stage III colon cancer and underwent laparotomy with resection of the tumor and colostomy placement yesterday. He tolerated general

anesthesia without complications and had approximately 100 mL of blood loss during the procedure. He is ambulating, eating, and voiding without problems. He has been wearing intermittent pneumatic compression devices on his legs when in bed since admission. He is also prescribed acetaminophen and oxycodone as needed for postoperative pain.

On physical examination, vital signs are normal. The abdominal incision is intact with no surrounding erythema, induration, tenderness, or exudate. The abdomen is soft and nontender with normal bowel sounds. There is no peripheral edema.

Laboratory studies are significant for a hemoglobin level of 13.8 g/dL (138 g/L) (14.2 g/dL [142 g/L] before surgery), a platelet count of 308,000/μL (308 × 10^9/L), and a normal serum creatinine level.

Which of the following is the most appropriate management for venous thromboembolism prophylaxis?

(A) Continue intermittent pneumatic compression only until hospital discharge

(B) Initiate aspirin for up to 35 days after surgery

(C) Initiate prophylactic-dose enoxaparin for up to 28 days after surgery

(D) Initiate prophylactic-dose enoxaparin only until hospital discharge

(E) Initiate therapeutic warfarin for up to 35 days after surgery

Item 143

A 50-year-old man with a new diagnosis of non–small cell lung cancer is seen in follow-up. At the time of diagnosis, his disease was found to be metastatic to the liver, bone, and brain. He has completed whole-brain radiation for his brain metastases, and he is scheduled to begin chemotherapy. He states that he currently feels well, and his bone pain is well controlled with as-needed acetaminophen and NSAIDs.

In discussing his management, he indicates that he understands that his disease is incurable, and his overall goal is to live as long as possible comfortably so that he can spend as much quality time with his children as he can.

Which of the following is the most appropriate approach to management of this patient's care?

(A) Admit the patient to hospice

(B) Begin palliative care following completion of active treatment

(C) Begin palliative care if pain control becomes ineffective

(D) Begin palliative care now

(E) Continue current management

Item 144

An 88-year-old woman was admitted to the hospital 17 days ago with a small-bowel obstruction due to adhesions. She did not respond to conservative management and required surgical intervention. Her hospital course was complicated by atrial fibrillation, non–ST-elevation myocardial infarction, and acute kidney injury that is improving without the need for renal replacement therapy. Her bowel function has been slowly recovering, and she is increasingly taking food and fluids by mouth. Before admission, she had been living at home independently. The patient's children checked on her daily and brought her most meals. She used a walker but spent most of her day in a chair watching television or reading. She had a home health nurse who assisted with her medications.

In the hospital, she is fatigued and weak; she is participating in therapy but tires after 30 minutes. She requires one-person assist for transfers and to reach the bedside commode. The patient's family is not able to accommodate her in their home during her recovery but would be able to continue their previous level of support following discharge.

Which of the following discharge options is most appropriate for this patient?

(A) Home with family care and in-home rehabilitation services

(B) Rehabilitation at a long-term acute care hospital

(C) Short-term rehabilitation in a skilled nursing facility

(D) Short-term rehabilitation in a specialized rehabilitation hospital

Item 145

An 82-year-old man is evaluated during a follow-up visit. He was initially evaluated for a report of difficulty with his vision when he drives, which he describes as blurriness in both eyes, but reports no other vision problems. Medical history is significant for a 45-pack-year smoking history, and he is a current smoker. His only medication is a daily low-dose aspirin.

On physical examination, the patient is afebrile, blood pressure is 134/82 mm Hg, pulse rate is 82/min, and respiration rate is 16/min. BMI is 32. Large drusen are present bilaterally on funduscopic examination. There are no other ophthalmologic findings. The remainder of the physical examination is normal.

An ophthalmologic evaluation confirms bilateral moderate dry age-related macular degeneration.

In addition to encouraging the patient to stop smoking, which of the following is the most appropriate therapy?

(A) High-dose antioxidant vitamins

(B) Laser therapy

(C) Vascular endothelial growth factor inhibitor therapy

(D) Clinical observation

Item 146

A 79-year-old woman is admitted to the hospital with shortness of breath due to volume overload, hyperkalemia, and acidemia. She has stage 4 chronic kidney disease. Based on her history and physical examination, urgent hemodialysis is clinically indicated, and this is discussed with the patient. She articulates an understanding of the indications for hemodialysis and the consequences of refusing treatment, including possible death. She decides to decline hemodialysis, stating that she is at peace with her life and her God. The patient has an advance directive, which names her son as her surrogate decision maker.

Which of the following is the most appropriate management of this patient?

(A) Obtain a psychiatric assessment to determine competency

(B) Order hemodialysis

(C) Seek permission from the patient's son to perform hemodialysis

(D) Withhold hemodialysis

Item 147

A 24-year-old man is evaluated for a 1-week history of left posterior heel pain and stiffness. The pain developed gradually, and the patient rates the pain as an 8 on a 10-point scale when at its worst. He describes the pain as burning in character and notes that it worsens with activity and improves with rest. He reports no recent trauma but does note that he has been running more in preparation for a marathon. Medical history is unremarkable. His only medication is ibuprofen, which provides some improvement in his pain.

On physical examination, vital signs are normal. BMI is 23. There is tenderness to palpation approximately 2 to 3 cm proximal to the left calcaneus. No Achilles tendon defect is appreciated. Dorsiflexion and plantar flexion of the foot are intact. When the patient's calf is squeezed while the patient kneels with the feet hanging over the edge of the examining table, there is plantar flexion (negative Thompson test). There is no tenderness to palpation of the medial plantar surface. There is no pain with medial-lateral compression of the left leg at the mid-calf (negative squeeze test) or when the patient crosses his legs and places the mid-calf of the left leg on the right knee (negative crossed-leg test).

Which of the following is the most likely diagnosis?

(A) Achilles tendinopathy

(B) Achilles tendon rupture

(C) High ankle sprain

(D) Tarsal tunnel syndrome

Item 148

A 53-year-old woman is evaluated for a 1-year history of dyspareunia. She has tried using lubricants, but she still has discomfort and has lost interest in sexual intercourse. She reports vaginal itching but no vaginal discharge, bleeding, or odor. She reached menopause 2 years ago and notes occasional hot flushes, but they are not troublesome. There is no history of sexual trauma, sexually transmitted infection, or pelvic surgery. She reports no marital problems. Medical history is otherwise remarkable for hypertension. Her only medication is benazepril.

On physical examination, the patient is afebrile, blood pressure is 130/78 mm Hg, pulse rate is 72/min, and respiration rate is 14/min. BMI is 27. The general medical examination is unremarkable. On pelvic examination, she can only tolerate insertion of a narrow speculum, and the vaginal mucosa is pale and dry with smooth vaginal walls and decreased rugae. There is scant vaginal discharge. Bimanual examination is normal.

Microscopic evaluation of a vaginal preparation reveals no hyphae, yeast, or clue cells.

Which of the following is the most appropriate management?

(A) Discontinue benazepril

(B) Systemic estrogen and progestin therapy

(C) Topical testosterone

(D) Topical vaginal estradiol

Item 149

A 78-year-old man is evaluated for a 6-month history of bilateral tinnitus. The tinnitus is high-pitched, continuous, and nonpulsatile and does not disturb his sleep. There is no associated fever, dizziness, vertigo, or headache. The patient is now retired but has a history of occupational noise exposure after working in a factory for 30 years. He has some difficulty hearing conversations if there is background noise. Medical history is significant for hypertension and hyperlipidemia, and his only medications are benazepril and pravastatin.

On physical examination, vital signs are normal. BMI is 28. Examination of the ears shows normal tympanic membranes and no cerumen impaction. When a vibrating tuning fork is placed at the midline of the patient's forehead (Weber test), the vibration is heard equally in both ears. When placed against the mastoid process until it can no longer be heard and then moved to directly outside the ear (Rinne test), the tuning fork is best heard after removal from the mastoid.

The remainder of the physical and neurologic examinations is unremarkable.

Which of the following is the most likely cause of this patient's tinnitus?

(A) Acoustic neuroma

(B) Meniere disease

(C) Otosclerosis

(D) Sensorineural hearing loss

Item 150

A 50-year-old man is evaluated for a 1-year history of reduced vision in both eyes. Over the course of this time, he has noticed a decrease in peripheral vision, most apparent when driving his car. He has no eye pain, redness, or other symptoms. He wears only reading glasses and does not wear contact lenses. Medical history is remarkable for hypertension and hyperlipidemia. He has a 35-pack-year smoking history and is a current smoker. Medications are losartan and simvastatin.

On physical examination, temperature is normal, blood pressure is 138/88 mm Hg, and pulse rate is 84/min. BMI is 32. The eyes appear normal upon inspection. There is mild loss of peripheral vision on clinical visual field testing. Funduscopic examination findings are shown. Intraocular pressure is 35 mm Hg bilaterally. The remainder of the examination is unremarkable.

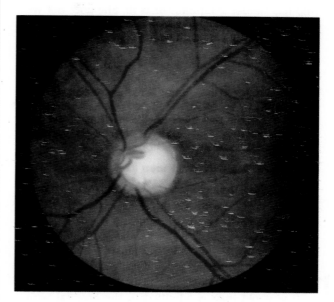

Which of the following is the most likely diagnosis?

(A) Ophthalmic artery occlusion

(B) Optic neuritis

(C) Papilledema

(D) Primary open angle glaucoma

Item 151

A 56-year-old woman is evaluated for an 8-month history of insomnia. She has difficulty falling asleep and maintaining sleep for longer than 3 hours; once she awakens, she often lies in bed for as long as 1 hour trying to fall back asleep. Her symptoms seem worse during the work week and are impairing her wakefulness during the day. She reports no new stressful events in her life or symptoms suggestive of sleep-disordered breathing or restless legs syndrome. She does not drink caffeinated beverages or alcohol. She exercises for 30 minutes five times weekly on her way home from work. She does not take daytime naps, has tried a relaxing bedtime regimen, does not watch television or use electronic devices in bed, and keeps the room quiet and dark at bedtime without improvement of her insomnia. Medical history is otherwise unremarkable, and she takes no medications.

Physical examination is normal.

Which of the following is the most appropriate next step in the management of this patient's insomnia?

(A) Diphenhydramine

(B) Shift exercise regimen to before bedtime

(C) Sleep restriction counseling

(D) Zolpidem

Item 152

A 32-year-old woman is evaluated for a 4-week history of eye symptoms. She notes redness of both eyes with itchiness and irritation. There is a watery discharge and mild crusting, mostly in the morning. Vision is normal, and she notes no other symptoms except for intermittent sneezing. She has not had contact with anyone who has similar symptoms or is ill. She does not wear contact lenses. Medical history is remarkable for hypothyroidism. Her medications are levothyroxine and an oral contraceptive.

On physical examination, she is afebrile, blood pressure is 124/60 mm Hg, and pulse rate is 62/min. Skin examination is normal. There is redness with edematous swelling of the conjunctivae in both eyes. A watery discharge is present, and there is mild swelling of the upper eyelids bilaterally. Visual acuity is normal. The remainder of the physical examination is normal.

Which of the following is the most likely diagnosis?

(A) Allergic conjunctivitis
(B) Bacterial conjunctivitis
(C) Blepharitis
(D) Viral conjunctivitis

Item 153

A 70-year-old man is admitted to the hospital with a 1-hour episode of left arm and left leg weakness. He is diagnosed with a transient ischemic attack. The patient has a history of hypertension and type 2 diabetes mellitus and a 30-pack-year history of smoking. Family history is noncontributory. His medications are metformin and lisinopril.

On physical examination, the patient is afebrile, and blood pressure is 148/88 mm Hg. The remainder of the examination is unremarkable.

Laboratory studies:

Alanine aminotransferase	28 U/L
Total cholesterol	239 mg/dL (6.19 mmol/L)
LDL cholesterol	140 mg/dL (3.63 mmol/L)
HDL cholesterol	38 mg/dL (0.98 mmol/L)
Serum creatinine	0.8 mg/dL (70.7 µmol/L)
Triglycerides	302 mg/dL (3.41 mmol/L)

In addition to aspirin, which of the following is the most appropriate treatment?

(A) Atorvastatin, high-intensity dosage
(B) Atorvastatin, moderate-intensity dosage
(C) Fenofibrate
(D) Fenofibrate and atorvastatin, high-intensity dosage

Item 154

A 27-year-old man is evaluated for a 4-day history of sore throat, malaise, rhinitis, and fever. He reports no cough, diarrhea, or vomiting. His 4-year-old daughter, who attends preschool, has similar symptoms. Medical history is noncontributory, and he has no allergies. His only medication is ibuprofen.

On physical examination, the patient is in no distress and has no shortness of breath. Temperature is 38.1 °C (100.6 °F), blood pressure is 112/52 mm Hg, pulse rate is 99/min, and respiration rate is 12/min. BMI is 23. The tympanic membranes are normal. The oropharynx shows tonsillar exudates. Tender anterior cervical lymphadenopathy is present. The lungs are clear with no evidence of consolidation. Abdominal examination is normal. The remainder of the examination is unremarkable.

Which of the following is the most appropriate management?

(A) Penicillin
(B) Rapid streptococcal antigen test
(C) Throat culture
(D) Clinical observation

Item 155

An 81-year-old woman is admitted to the hospital with intractable pain in the setting of metastatic breast cancer. Medical history is significant for ischemic cardiomyopathy. She has an implantable cardioverter-defibrillator (ICD) for the prevention of sudden cardiac death, and the ICD has fired in the past. The patient is started on intravenous morphine, and her pain diminishes. The patient knows that she is dying, and she requests comfort care only. She also requests that her ICD be deactivated so that it cannot deliver shocks. She understands the consequences of ICD deactivation and is steadfast in her decision. The patient has an advance directive, which names her daughter as her surrogate decision maker.

Which of the following is the most appropriate management of this patient's request?

(A) Continue the ICD
(B) Deactivate the ICD
(C) Obtain psychiatric assessment of competence prior to ICD deactivation
(D) Seek permission from the patient's daughter to continue the ICD

Item 156

A 27-year-old woman at 30 weeks' gestation is evaluated during a routine examination. She is gravida 2, para 1, and delivered her first child vaginally without complications 20 months ago. During her first pregnancy, she received the tetanus, diphtheria, and acellular pertussis (Tdap) vaccine. Her only medication is a daily prenatal vitamin.

Findings on physical examination are unremarkable.

Which of the following is the most appropriate management of this patient's vaccination status?

(A) Administer the Tdap vaccine after 36 weeks' gestation
(B) Administer the Tdap vaccine now
(C) Administer the tetanus and diphtheria (Td) vaccine now
(D) Administer the Td vaccine after 36 weeks' gestation
(E) Do not administer the Td or Tdap vaccines during this pregnancy

Item 157

A 36-year-old man is evaluated for a 1-year history of fatigue, intermittent headaches, sore throat, and joint and muscle pain. He reports no difficulties falling asleep and gets 10 hours of uninterrupted but nonrestorative sleep each night. He has seen several physicians over the past year. Evaluation has included a complete blood count with differential, thyroid-stimulating hormone level, and plasma glucose level that were normal at the time of initial presentation and again 2 months ago. HIV testing performed 4 months ago was negative. He is in a monogamous heterosexual relationship, and there is no history of blood transfusions or injection drug use. Medical history is otherwise unremarkable. Family history is significant for depression and type 2 diabetes mellitus. He takes no medications.

On physical examination, the patient appears anxious. Vital signs and the remainder of the physical examination are normal. The patient's evaluation for sleep disorders is normal. A screening test for depression is negative.

Which of the following is the most appropriate diagnostic test to perform next?

(A) Epstein-Barr virus titer
(B) Lyme disease titer
(C) Repeat HIV testing
(D) No further testing

Item 158

A 78-year-old man is evaluated for gradual hearing loss in the left ear over the past several years. Although hearing in his right ear seems normal, he has noticed that it is more difficult to hear men's voices or lower voices with his left ear. He reports no dizziness, tinnitus, or previous infection or exposure to loud noise in that ear. Medical history is significant for hypertension, hyperlipidemia, and coronary artery disease. Medications are losartan, rosuvastatin, and low-dose aspirin.

On physical examination, the patient is afebrile, blood pressure is 134/82 mm Hg, pulse rate is 85/min, and respiration rate is 13/min. BMI is 29. The tympanic membranes are normal. The remainder of the general medical examination is unremarkable. On neurologic examination, a vibrating tuning fork placed in contact with the patient's forehead at the midline results in vibrations being heard more loudly in the left ear.

Which of the following is the most likely diagnosis?

(A) Drug-induced hearing loss
(B) Meniere disease
(C) Otosclerosis
(D) Presbycusis

Item 159

A 47-year-old man is evaluated during a follow-up examination. He is obese and has hypertension, type 2 diabetes mellitus, and obstructive sleep apnea. He reports that he has always has been overweight, and over the years, his weight has gradually increased to 123 kg (271 lb). During the past 2 years, he has tried several commercial diets; a dietician-monitored, calorie-restricted diet; increased physical activity; orlistat; and a combination of these interventions, all without achieving sustained weight loss. Medical history is also significant for bilateral knee pain and depression. He uses continuous positive airway pressure for his obstructive sleep apnea, and his medications are lisinopril, amlodipine, metformin, paroxetine, and as-needed ibuprofen.

On physical examination, the patient is afebrile, blood pressure is 144/78 mm Hg, pulse rate is 86/min, and respiration rate is 18/min. BMI is 36. Cardiovascular and pulmonary examinations are normal. The abdomen is protuberant without pathologic striae. The knees show bony hypertrophy with crepitus, and there is trace bilateral lower extremity edema.

Laboratory studies are significant for a hemoglobin A_{1c} level of 9.1%.

Which of the following is the most appropriate management to help this patient achieve sustained weight loss?

(A) Bariatric surgery
(B) Hypnosis
(C) Lorcaserin
(D) Very-low-calorie, physician-monitored diet

Item 160

A 90-year-old woman is brought to the emergency department by her son for a 1-week history of worsening cognition, weakness, dizziness, and anorexia. She lives in an assisted-care facility and is generally alert. She is ambulatory when using a cane. Medical history includes hypertension, chronic heart failure, chronic kidney disease, osteoarthritis, allergic rhinitis, hyperlipidemia, and urinary stress incontinence. Current medications are lisinopril, bisoprolol, oxybutynin, loratadine, acetaminophen, pravastatin, and omeprazole.

On physical examination, she appears frail but is in no acute distress. Temperature is normal, blood pressure is 100/60 mm Hg, pulse rate is 88/min, and respiration rate is 14/min. BMI is 20. Oxygen saturation is 97% with the patient breathing ambient air. There is no orthostasis. Cardiac examination discloses an irregularly irregular rate. Pulmonary examination reveals slightly diminished breath sounds bilaterally but no crackles. The abdomen is mildly distended but nontender. Rectal examination reveals hard stool that is negative for occult blood. There is no edema. Neurologic examination is nonfocal, and the patient scores 24/30 on the Mini–Mental State Examination.

Laboratory studies:

Hematocrit	34%
Leukocyte count	7100/µl (7.1 × 10⁹/L); normal differential
Creatinine	1.6 mg/dL (141 µmol/L) (2 months ago: 1.3 mg/dL [114 µmol/L])
Electrolytes	Normal
Glucose	78 mg/dL (4.3 mmol/L)
Urinalysis	Trace protein, trace ketones, no cells

Chest radiograph shows no evidence of heart failure or pulmonary infiltrates.

Which of the following is the most likely cause of this patient's recent symptoms?

(A) Acute kidney injury
(B) Adverse medication effects
(C) Occult pneumonia
(D) Urinary tract infection

Item 161

A 32-year-old woman is evaluated during a follow-up visit for treatment of depression. She presented 3 months ago with depressed mood, decreased energy, increased sleep, and anhedonia but without suicidal ideation. Her PHQ-9 score was 13, indicating moderate depression. Citalopram, 20 mg/d, was initiated and titrated upward to 40 mg/d 6 weeks ago. She notes improved mood, energy, and sleep with a 6-point improvement in her PHQ-9 score. However, she reports persistent nausea and heartburn coupled with complete anorgasmia while taking this medication. Her medical history is notable for being overweight but is otherwise unremarkable. She takes no other medications.

On physical examination, blood pressure is 126/78 mm Hg. BMI is 29. Examination of the heart reveals physiologic splitting of the S_2. The abdomen is soft and nontender with normal bowel sounds. The remainder of the examination is normal.

Which of the following is the most appropriate alternative antidepressant to recommend for this patient?

(A) Amitriptyline
(B) Bupropion
(C) Buspirone
(D) Mirtazapine

Item 162

A 62-year-old man is evaluated during a routine follow-up visit. He expresses concern about developing prostate cancer because his father was diagnosed with the disease at age 55 years. He has read that the 5α-reductase inhibitor finasteride may prevent prostate cancer and asks whether he would be an appropriate candidate for treatment with this drug.

The physician reviews a study to determine whether finasteride prevents prostate cancer. In the study, investigators randomized 2000 patients equally to treatment with finasteride or placebo. Seven years later, all patients underwent a prostate biopsy. Results showed that prostate cancer occurred in 200 of 1000 (20%) patients taking finasteride compared with 300 of 1000 (30%) patients taking placebo.

Based on this study, how many patients need to be treated (number needed to treat) with finasteride for 7 years to prevent one case of prostate cancer?

(A) 2
(B) 3
(C) 5
(D) 10

Item 163

A 54-year-old man is seen for preoperative evaluation. Cervical spine laminectomy is planned. Despite his neck pain, he continues to do all activities of daily living, which includes doing laundry in his basement and carrying loads up and down the stairs. He has no chest pain, dyspnea, palpitations, or lightheadedness with this activity or at rest. He has no orthopnea or nocturnal dyspnea. Medical history is notable for a previous non–ST-elevation myocardial infarction with drug-eluting stent placement in his left circumflex artery 3 years ago; an echocardiogram following his myocardial infarction showed normal left ventricular function. He also has type 2 diabetes mellitus, hypertension, and hyperlipidemia. Medications are aspirin, lisinopril, atorvastatin, and metformin.

On physical examination, blood pressure is 138/82 mm Hg, and pulse rate is 62/min. Central venous pressure is 6 cm H_2O. Cardiac and pulmonary examinations are normal. There is trace bilateral pedal edema.

Laboratory studies show a hemoglobin A_{1c} level of 6.3% and a normal serum creatinine level.

Which of the following is the most appropriate diagnostic test to perform next?

(A) Electrocardiography
(B) Noninvasive pharmacologic cardiac stress testing
(C) Resting echocardiography
(D) Treadmill stress echocardiography

Item 164

A 52-year-old man is evaluated for a 3-year history of multiple symptoms, including fatigue, dizziness, headache, upper back pain, shortness of breath, and abdominal pain. He has undergone extensive evaluation of his symptoms with laboratory testing revealing type 2 diabetes mellitus and hyperlipidemia. Radiographic evaluation and consultation with a neurologist, cardiologist, and gastroenterologist have failed to identify a cause of his symptoms. He continues to follow up with his internist monthly; there have been no changes in his symptoms or physical examination findings.

He feels frustrated and dejected because of the lack of a diagnosis and the negative impact of his symptoms on his life. Over the past year, he has withdrawn from family activities, slept excessively during the day, and become relatively hopeless that he will ever regain his health. Recently, he took a leave of absence from work at the request of his boss due to failing productivity. He is anxious that he will be unable to afford college tuition for his son and is having trouble sleeping at night. Medications are ferrous sulfate, vitamin B_{12}, rosuvastatin, and metformin.

On physical examination, vital signs are normal. BMI is 24. The remainder of the physical examination is unremarkable.

Which of the following is the most appropriate treatment?

(A) Alprazolam
(B) Citalopram
(C) Lithium
(D) Methylphenidate

Item 165

A 20-year-old woman is evaluated for a 3-day history of pain, swelling, and redness of the right eye. She cannot open her eye because of the swelling. One week ago, she developed a fever with sinus congestion and postnasal drainage. Except for a continued subjective fever, these symptoms have resolved. She has no history of eye trauma or surgery. She takes no medications.

On physical examination, temperature is 38.0 °C (100.4 °F), blood pressure is 100/62 mm Hg, and pulse rate is 88/min. BMI is 23. Examination of the right eye shows red and edematous upper and lower lids with conjunctival erythema. Pupillary reflex to light is intact. Inspection reveals no foreign bodies. She is unable to move her eye. A limited funduscopic examination is normal. The left eye is normal, and the remainder of the physical examination is unremarkable.

Which of the following is the most likely diagnosis?

(A) Blepharitis
(B) Endophthalmitis
(C) Orbital cellulitis
(D) Preseptal cellulitis

Item 166

A 40-year-old woman is evaluated for intermittent heavy vaginal bleeding for the past year. Her menses had been regular until the past 2 years, when they became irregular and would sometimes skip for several months. Her last period was 3 months ago and lasted for almost 3 weeks. Menarche occurred when she was age 12 years. She has never been pregnant and is not currently sexually active. Her most recent cervical cancer screening was 2 years ago. Medical history is otherwise unremarkable, and she takes no medications.

On physical examination, vital signs are normal. BMI is 29. The general medical examination is unremarkable, as is the pelvic examination. A urine pregnancy test is negative.

Which of the following is the most appropriate diagnostic test to perform next?

(A) Endometrial biopsy
(B) Follicle-stimulating hormone level
(C) Serum β-human chorionic gonadotropin level
(D) Transvaginal ultrasonography

Item 167

A 68-year-old woman is evaluated for neck pain of 4 days' duration. The pain developed abruptly and awakened her from sleep. It is located in the posterior neck without radiation down the arms and worsens with neck movement but improves with recumbency. She reports no trauma, fever, muscle weakness, or weight loss. Medical history is significant for ductal carcinoma in situ treated 10 years ago without evidence of recurrence. Her only medication is naproxen for control of pain.

On physical examination, vital signs are normal. Both passive and active range of motion of the neck are severely reduced. Rotation of her head is limited by pain. The cervical paraspinal muscles are tight and tender to palpation. Upper extremity muscle strength and reflexes are normal.

Which of the following is the most appropriate management of this patient?

(A) CT myelography
(B) MRI of the cervical spine
(C) Plain radiography of the cervical spine
(D) Symptomatic care

Item 168

A 52-year-old man is evaluated for colon cancer screening. He feels well with no symptoms. His uncle experienced respiratory arrest with sedation during a screening colonoscopy, and the patient is adamant that he will not undergo colonoscopy. There is no family history of colon cancer or colon polyps.

On physical examination, vital signs are normal. The remainder of the physical examination is normal.

Which of the following is the most appropriate strategy for colon cancer screening in this patient?

(A) CT colonography every 10 years
(B) Fecal immunochemical testing every year
(C) Flexible sigmoidoscopy every 5 years with fecal occult blood testing every year
(D) Stool DNA testing every year

Answers and Critiques

Item 1   Answer: A

Educational Objective: Screen for osteoporosis in a patient with risk factors.

This patient should be screened for osteoporosis with dual-energy x-ray absorptiometry (DEXA). The U.S. Preventive Services Task Force (USPSTF) recommends screening for osteoporosis by measurement of bone mineral density in women aged 65 years and older and in younger women who have a fracture risk equal to or higher than a 65-year-old white woman (9.3%). The Fracture Risk Assessment Tool (FRAX) (available at www.shef.ac.uk/FRAX/) can be used to determine if the 10-year fracture risk for younger women is greater than or equal to 9.3%. Risk factors that can increase the FRAX score include a first-degree relative with a history of hip fracture, alcohol abuse, smoking, low body mass, and glucocorticoid use. Although this patient is younger than 65 years, her parental history of hip fracture increases her risk of fracture to 13%; therefore, she should be screened for osteoporosis using DEXA.

The USPSTF suggests screening for lipid disorders every 5 years in all men 35 years of age and older and all women 45 years of age and older who are at increased risk of coronary heart disease. This interval should be tailored to individual risk. Since this patient's lipid panel was normal when tested last year, screening in this patient would not be appropriate.

Although the optimal screening interval for diabetes mellitus is unknown, the American Diabetes Association recommends screening for diabetes every 3 years in adults 45 years and older and adults younger than 45 years with a BMI of 25 or higher and one risk factor for diabetes. In 2008, the USPSTF recommended screening for type 2 diabetes only in asymptomatic adults with sustained blood pressure higher than 135/80 mm Hg. An updated draft guideline, issued in October 2014, recommends screening for abnormal blood glucose and type 2 diabetes in adults with risk factors, including age 45 years or older, obesity or overweight, first-degree relative with diabetes, history of gestational diabetes or polycystic ovary syndrome, and certain high-risk ethnic backgrounds (African Americans, American Indians/Alaska Natives, Asian Americans, Hispanics/Latinos, and Native Hawaiians/Pacific Islanders). This patient was screened for diabetes last year, and therefore, she does not need to be screened again now.

A combination of cytology (Pap smear) and human papillomavirus (HPV) testing can be performed every 5 years in women aged 30 to 65 years to screen for cervical cancer. Screening with a Pap smear alone every 3 years is also acceptable. This patient had a normal Pap smear and HPV test 3 years ago.

The USPSTF concludes that there is insufficient evidence to recommend for or against screening for thyroid disease. The American College of Physicians recommends screening women over age 50 years who have at least one symptom that can be attributed to thyroid disease. The American Thyroid Association and the American Association of Clinical Endocrinologists recommend measuring thyroid-stimulating hormone (TSH) level in individuals with risk factors for hypothyroidism (for example, personal history of autoimmune disease, neck radiation, or thyroid surgery) and consideration of TSH testing in adults age 60 years and older. This patient does not have any symptoms of thyroid disease and therefore should not be screened.

KEY POINT

- Women aged 65 years and older and younger women who have a fracture risk of 9.3% or higher should be screened for osteoporosis.

Bibliography

U.S. Preventive Services Task Force. Screening for osteoporosis: U.S. Preventive Services Task Force recommendation statement. Ann Intern Med. 2011 Mar 1;154(5):356-64. [PMID: 21242341]

Item 2   Answer: D

Educational Objective: Identify the relatively large impact of smoking cessation on improving health.

This patient would most benefit from smoking cessation counseling. Cigarette smoking increases the risk of cancer, heart disease, stroke, and lung disease and is the leading preventable cause of death in the United States. Quitting smoking is the single most important thing that smokers can do to improve their quality and quantity of life. Smoking cessation before age 40 years reduces the risk of death associated with continued tobacco use by approximately 90%. The U.S. Preventive Services Task Force (USPSTF) recommends that clinicians ask all adults about tobacco use and provide tobacco cessation interventions for tobacco users. Behavioral counseling for smoking cessation in primary care settings has been found to improve quit rates and sustained abstinence at 1 year. Even minimal in-office interventions, defined as less than 3 minutes in duration, are effective in improving smoking cessation rates.

A meta-analysis suggested that women who consume an average of two or more alcoholic drinks per day had an increased mortality rate compared with nondrinkers; therefore, this patient may benefit from counseling regarding reducing her alcohol consumption. Nonetheless, the benefit of brief intervention for smoking cessation is still likely to be more impactful in this patient.

Exercising and eating a healthful diet both have a significantly positive impact on health and have been strongly linked with decreased incidence of cardiovascular disease.

However, the effect of behavioral counseling in promoting healthful diet and physical activity in adults without known cardiovascular disease, hypertension, hyperlipidemia, or diabetes is small. Given small potential effect, time limitations, and opportunity costs, the USPSTF recommends offering dietary and exercise behavioral counseling based only on individual patient circumstances. In this patient, smoking cessation counseling will have a greater benefit than counseling that promotes a healthful diet and physical activity.

Stress reduction and relaxation techniques have the potential to improve this patient's health; however, the health benefits of smoking cessation are likely to be greater.

KEY POINT

- The U.S. Preventive Services Task Force recommends that clinicians ask all adults about tobacco use and provide tobacco cessation interventions for tobacco users.

Bibliography

Jha P, Ramasundarahettige C, Landsman V, et al. 21st-century hazards of smoking and benefits of cessation in the United States. N Engl J Med. 2013 Jan 24;368(4):341-50. [PMID: 23343063]

Item 3   Answer: B

Educational Objective: Treat a patient with benign paroxysmal positional vertigo.

The Epley maneuver should be performed in this patient presenting with symptoms of benign paroxysmal positional vertigo (BPPV). In patients with vertigo, the Dix-Hallpike maneuver can assist in distinguishing peripheral from central causes. In peripheral vertigo, the maneuver will result in nystagmus that begins after a brief period of latency (2-40 seconds) and lasts less than 1 minute. With repeated trials, the nystagmus may not be further provoked. In vertigo of central origin, the nystagmus is not associated with latency, typically lasts longer than 1 minute, and does not fatigue with repeated trials. BPPV is the most common cause of vertigo and is attributed to debris (canalithiasis), usually in the posterior semicircular canal, perturbing labyrinthine sensory receptors and resulting in the erroneous perception of angular head acceleration. BPPV is characterized by abrupt episodes of vertigo that last less than 1 minute and is provoked by a sudden change in head position. The Epley maneuver, which is performed to reposition otoliths from the semicircular canal into the vestibule, can be curative in patients with BPPV. The maneuver involves sequentially positioning the patient to encourage movement of the otoliths, and modified versions of the procedure allow patients to perform the maneuver themselves for recurrent episodes. A meta-analysis demonstrated that patients with BPPV who were treated with the Epley maneuver had significantly higher rates of improvement in symptoms compared with those who received sham treatment (odds ratio [OR] 4.4; 95% CI, 2.6-7.2).

Pharmacologic therapy for BPPV, including centrally acting antihistamines (such as meclizine), vestibular sup-

pressants (such as diazepam), and antiemetics, may help symptoms transiently but, in general, is ineffective for long-term management or cure.

Vestibular rehabilitation therapy, when delivered by trained physical or occupational therapists, is beneficial in patients with peripheral vertigo, particularly those with recurrent or refractory symptoms; however, the initial management of this patient presenting with BPPV is to perform the Epley maneuver.

KEY POINT

- Benign paroxysmal positional vertigo can be effectively treated with the Epley maneuver, which is performed to reposition otoliths from the semicircular canal into the vestibule of the ear.

Bibliography

Kim JS, Zee DS. Clinical practice. Benign paroxysmal positional vertigo. N Engl J Med. 2014 Mar 20;370(12):1138-47. [PMID: 24645946]

Item 4   Answer: D

Educational Objective: Evaluate pulmonary risk in a preoperative patient.

No further diagnostic studies are needed for this asymptomatic patient scheduled for surgery. For patients with no history of cardiopulmonary disease and no cardiac or respiratory symptoms, preoperative pulmonary diagnostic testing is not beneficial. Moreover, these studies add considerable cost and potential risk (for example, radiation exposure with chest radiography). Although smoking is a risk factor for postoperative pulmonary complications, a history of smoking without other evidence of disease is not an indication for chest radiography, spirometry, or arterial blood gas analysis in the general or preoperative setting. Several studies have demonstrated that these studies do not offer improved prognostic value beyond clinical assessment alone and rarely alter management.

Chest radiography may be considered in patients with known cardiopulmonary disease or symptoms. Spirometry assessment is frequently done prior to cardiothoracic surgery, but its value is limited for other types of surgery. For nonthoracic surgery, spirometry should be performed for the same reasons as in a nonoperative situation (for example, evaluation of dyspnea or hypoxia). Similarly, preoperative arterial blood gas analysis may identify hypercapnia in patients at risk for carbon dioxide retention, but studies have not shown an incremental diagnostic benefit with this testing.

KEY POINT

- For patients with no history of cardiopulmonary disease and no cardiac or respiratory symptoms, preoperative pulmonary diagnostic testing is not beneficial.

Bibliography

Joo HS, Wong J, Naik VN, Savoldelli GL. The value of screening preoperative chest x-rays. Can J Anaesth. 2005 Jun-Jul;52(6):568-74. [PMID: 15983140]

Item 5   Answer: A

Educational Objective: Treat lateral epicondylosis (lateral epicondylitis).

This patient with signs and symptoms consistent with lateral epicondylosis (lateral epicondylitis) should be advised to limit pain-inducing activities. Lateral epicondylosis, also known as tennis elbow, is induced by activities that require repetitive wrist extension, such as prolonged computer use or racquet sports. Pain is located over the lateral elbow but may also radiate to the dorsal forearm. Tenderness over the lateral elbow and pain with resisted wrist extension are characteristic examination findings. Increasing evidence suggests that epicondylosis is a chronic tendinosis with disorganization and neovascularization of the tissues, instead of an acute or chronic inflammatory process as traditionally believed. Because the primary mechanism of injury appears to be mechanical strain, and repetitive use of injured tissues diminishes healing, the primary treatment is avoidance of those activities that cause pain and continued injury to the affected area. Braces may be useful when exacerbating activities cannot be avoided, and counterforce bracing, which alters the mechanical strain on the elbow tendons, may be helpful. With rest, pain usually subsides, although performance of resistance exercises may also be beneficial. The analgesic effect of topical or oral NSAIDs may provide short-term symptomatic relief.

Surgical treatment is indicated only for refractory cases of epicondylosis. Patients should first be treated with appropriate conservative measures, including rest and NSAIDs. The risks of surgical intervention would be warranted in this patient only if she had not responded to all nonsurgical therapy.

Glucocorticoid injections may improve symptoms in the short term, but data are conflicting on long-term benefits. Additionally, there is some evidence that glucocorticoid injections may lead to an increased risk of recurrence. There are associated risks (hyperglycemia in patients with diabetes mellitus, infection) that must also be considered. Glucocorticoid injections cannot be justified in this patient who has not received an adequate trial of conservative therapy.

Imaging, including MRI, is not necessary for diagnosis of lateral epicondylosis if the patient has clinical findings consistent with this disorder. MRI would be indicated if this patient had atypical findings or did not respond to initial treatment.

KEY POINT

- The primary treatment of lateral epicondylosis is avoidance of activities that cause pain.

Bibliography

Ahmad Z, Siddiqui N, Malik SS, et al. Lateral epicondylitis: a review of pathology and management. Bone Joint J. 2013;95-B(9):1158-64. [PMID: 23997125]

Item 6   Answer: B

Educational Objective: Select an appropriate quality improvement method to reduce waiting times.

The Lean model would be the most useful method for reducing waiting times. A number of quality improvement models that apply rigorous processes to identify, measure, and correct areas in need of improvement are in use by health care systems. Understanding the appropriate application of these models is important in achieving optimal quality improvement outcomes. The Lean model is a quality improvement method that focuses on eliminating non–value-added activities, or waste, within a system. Lean uses value stream mapping, a tool that graphically displays the steps of a process and the time required for each step from beginning to end. This allows identification of steps in the process that may be problematic. The Lean model is particularly well suited for analyzing apparent inefficient or redundant processes, such as prolonged waiting times, by identifying where in the system the delays are occurring.

The Define, Measure, Analyze, Improve, Control (DMAIC) process is a five-step approach used within the Six Sigma model, a quality improvement model initially developed to improve industrial manufacturing quality that has since been adapted to optimize health care system function. It tends to focus more on quality control in each step of a process rather than on optimizing the overall efficiency of a system.

Plan, Do, Study, Act (PDSA) cycles are rapid tests of change in which baseline data are collected, an intervention is planned and then implemented on a small scale, the results are analyzed, and an action plan is made. PDSA cycles tend to focus on specific points in a system and are not typically used for studying overall system function and efficiency.

Six Sigma is a quality improvement model that is designed to reduce variation and drive a process toward near perfection. The name Six Sigma is derived from a statistical measure indicating the number of standard deviations from the mean in which no production defects occur. Thus, a Six Sigma measure indicates almost perfect production quality. Several practical methodologies that are oriented toward the quality of each step in a process are used within Six Sigma. As an example, an ICU may have an unacceptably high rate of infections; the Six Sigma model could be used to decrease the defect (infection) rate. Because Six Sigma is highly focused on the quality of each step in a process, it would not be optimal for evaluating factors leading to system inefficiencies, such as patient waiting times.

KEY POINT

- The Lean model is a quality improvement method that focuses on eliminating non–value-added activities, or waste, within a system.

Bibliography

Varkey P, Reller MK, Resar RK. Basics of quality improvement in health care. Mayo Clin Proc. 2007 Jun;82(6):735-9. [PMID: 17550754]

Item 7   Answer: A

Educational Objective: Treat primary dysmenorrhea.

The most appropriate treatment for this patient is a combined estrogen-progestin contraceptive pill. Her history of cyclic pain and normal findings on pelvic examination are consistent with primary dysmenorrhea, which occurs in up to 50% of menstruating women and causes significant discomfort and disruption of activities. Etiology is thought to be associated with prostaglandin release that induces uterine contractions as a part of menses, resulting in increased uterine basal tone. This increase in tone may decrease uterine microvascular blood flow with relative ischemia and resulting pain. Evidence supports the efficacy of prostaglandin inhibitors (NSAIDs and cyclooxygenase-2 inhibitors) in treating dysmenorrhea; however, because this patient did not tolerate the gastrointestinal adverse effects associated with NSAID use, the next step is a trial of combined estrogen-progestin contraceptive pills, which frequently provide clinical relief.

Depot medroxyprogesterone acetate and progestin-only contraceptive pills are effective forms of contraception that can cause menstrual suppression, although bleeding patterns are very variable. Data for treatment of primary dysmenorrhea with depot medroxyprogesterone acetate or progestin-only contraceptive pills are lacking.

Selective serotonin reuptake inhibitors (SSRIs) may be considered for the treatment of premenstrual syndrome (PMS), in which disruptive physical or behavioral symptoms occur repetitively during the second half of the menstrual cycle, or premenstrual dysphoric disorder (PMDD), which is characterized by severe symptoms of irritability, mood swings, depression, anxiety, sleep disturbance, headache, fatigue, and musculoskeletal pain. Whereas PMS occurs in 30% to 80% of menstruating younger women, PMDD is less prevalent, occurring in 3% to 8% of women of reproductive age. This patient's symptoms are related to her menstrual period and do not support a diagnosis of PMS or PMDD; therefore, initiation of an SSRI is not appropriate.

Tranexamic acid is an antifibrinolytic drug that is used to treat severe menstrual bleeding. It is not an appropriate treatment for dysmenorrhea.

KEY POINT

- NSAIDs and cyclooxygenase-2 inhibitors are an effective treatment for primary dysmenorrhea; however, in patients who cannot tolerate NSAIDs or have incomplete relief of symptoms, use of combined estrogen-progestin hormonal contraceptive therapy is effective.

Bibliography

Osayande AS, Mehulic S. Diagnosis and initial management of dysmenorrhea. Am Fam Physician. 2014 Mar 1;89(5):341-6. [PMID: 24695505]

Item 8   Answer: C

Educational Objective: Prevent pressure ulcers in an older patient.

A foam mattress overlay is the most appropriate intervention in this patient at risk for a pressure ulcer. Pressure ulcers are a common occurrence in hospitals and long-term care settings, affecting up to 3 million patients and costing nearly $11 billion per year in the United States. It is far less costly to prevent pressure ulcers than to treat them; therefore, physicians need to be proactive in assessing risk for pressure ulcers and instituting evidence-based preventive measures. Risk factors include advanced age, cognitive impairment, reduced mobility, sensory impairment, and comorbid conditions that affect skin integrity (such as low body weight, incontinence, edema, poor microcirculation, and hypoalbuminemia). Intervention is warranted in this patient with multiple risk factors, including older age, advanced dementia, bedbound status, and urinary and fecal incontinence. A clinical practice guideline issued by the American College of Physicians (ACP) recommends the use of advanced static mattresses (a mattress made of foam or gel that does not move when a person lies on it) or an advanced static overlay (a material such as sheepskin or a pad filled with air, water, gel, or foam that is secured to the top of a bed mattress) to prevent pressure ulcers in at-risk individuals. These interventions have been found to lower the risk of pressure ulcers relative to standard hospital mattresses. Advanced static mattresses and overlays work by redistributing pressure and reducing shear that may lead to development of ulcers.

Dynamic support surfaces, such as low-air-loss beds or alternating-air mattresses or overlays, have no demonstrated benefit in preventing pressure ulcers, and the ACP guideline recommends against their use in pressure ulcer prevention. Additionally, these dynamic systems are very costly and their use for this purpose represents a low value care intervention. The role of dynamic support surfaces is also unclear in treating patients with established pressure ulcers, as they have not definitively been shown to improve outcomes relative to advanced static support surfaces and frequent repositioning.

Although malnutrition is clearly a risk factor for pressures ulcers, there are minimal data supporting the effectiveness of enteral feeding as an intervention to prevent pressure ulcers. In some studies, the risk of ulcer development appeared higher in patients placed on enteral feedings than in those not receiving enteral nutrition. Additionally, enteral feeding is not without complications and may negatively influence quality of life. Although there is evidence that protein and amino acid supplementation are of benefit in patients with established pressure ulcers, the role of nutritional supplementation, and specifically enteral nutrition, for prevention of pressure ulcers has not been determined.

Frequent repositioning is often performed as a component of multimodal interventions to prevent pressure ulcers.

H CONT.

Such multimodal interventions have been shown to be beneficial; however, there is a paucity of studies of repositioning alone and no good evidence to support repositioning alone as a pressure ulcer prevention tool. Nonetheless, repositioning should always be a part of a multimodal approach to pressure ulcer prevention.

KEY POINT

- Advanced static mattresses or overlays reduce the risk of pressure ulcers in at-risk patients.

Bibliography

Qaseem A, Mir TP, Starkey M, Denberg TD; Clinical Guidelines Committee of the American College of Physicians. Risk assessment and prevention of pressure ulcers: a clinical practice guideline from the American College of Physicians. Ann Intern Med. 2015 Mar 3;162(5):359-69. [PMID: 25732278]

Item 9   Answer: D

Educational Objective: Recognize when to discontinue breast cancer screening.

Recommending discontinuation of breast cancer screening is appropriate in this patient. Clinical trials of screening mammography in women 75 years of age and older are not available; therefore, the survival benefit of screening mammography for breast cancer in these women is not known. Additionally, observational studies suggest a potential benefit of breast cancer screening in women 75 years of age and older only if life expectancy exceeds 10 years. In this older patient with end-stage kidney disease, life expectancy is estimated to be approximately 3 years. There are also considerable potential harms to screening, including false-positive results that lead to overtreatment and psychological distress. Because of these factors, the American Society of Nephrology, through the Choosing Wisely campaign, recommends against performing routine cancer screening in patients on dialysis with limited life expectancies and no signs or symptoms of cancer. Therefore, continuing breast cancer screening with mammography in this patient, either annually or biennially, is likely to cause harm without significant benefit, and recommending discontinuation of screening is appropriate.

Breast MRI in addition to mammography is indicated for screening only in women with a lifetime risk of breast cancer of 20% to 25% or higher as calculated by models largely dependent on family history or other clinical circumstances. The use of breast MRI would not be appropriate in this patient who is not at high risk and without a clear indication for continued screening.

KEY POINT

- Women should have a life expectancy of at least 10 years to benefit from screening mammography.

Bibliography

Walter LC, Schonberg MA. Screening mammography in older women: a review. JAMA. 2014 Apr 2;311(13):1336-47. [PMID: 24691609]

Item 10   Answer: D

Educational Objective: Diagnose bulimia nervosa.

The most likely diagnosis is bulimia nervosa. It is important to differentiate between types of eating disorders as the treatment varies depending on the diagnosis. Bulimia nervosa is characterized by frequent episodes (≥1 per week) of binge eating followed by inappropriate compensatory behaviors (self-induced vomiting or misuse of laxatives, diuretics, and enemas) due to fear of weight gain. Physical examination may reveal erosion of dental enamel, parotid gland swelling, xerosis, and Russell sign (scarring or calluses on the dorsum of the hand if used to induce vomiting). This patient meets diagnostic criteria for bulimia nervosa because she has recurrent episodes of binge eating with recurrent purging to try to compensate for the intake of calories.

Anorexia nervosa is characterized by persistent caloric intake restriction leading to significantly low body weight, a distorted body image, and an intense fear of gaining weight or becoming fat. Subtypes include restricting type (no binge eating or purging behaviors) and binge eating/purging type (purging with or without binging). The differentiating factor between bulimia nervosa and the purging subtype of anorexia nervosa is BMI. Because both purging and laxative abuse are ineffective in removing calories (although they may cause loss of water weight), patients with bulimia nervosa tend to be normal weight to slightly overweight, as seen in this patient. Conversely, the diagnostic criteria for anorexia require that the patient be underweight, generally with a BMI less than 18.5. Menstrual irregularities occur in both anorexia nervosa and bulimia nervosa and are present in approximately one half to one third of patients with bulimia. Although amenorrhea previously was a requirement for the diagnosis of anorexia nervosa, it has been removed from the diagnostic criteria in the DSM-5. Many experts consider anorexia nervosa and bulimia nervosa as a continuum, as one condition often develops from the other.

Binge eating disorder is defined as episodes of eating significantly more food in a short period than most people at least once per week over 3 months, while feeling a lack of control, and is often accompanied by feelings of disgust or guilt afterward but without attempted compensatory behaviors for excessive caloric intake.

KEY POINT

- Bulimia nervosa is characterized by frequent episodes (≥1 per week) of binge eating followed by inappropriate compensatory behaviors (self-induced vomiting or misuse of laxatives, diuretics, and enemas) due to fear of weight gain.

Bibliography

Attia E. In the clinic. Eating disorders. Ann Intern Med. 2012 Apr 3; 156(7):ITC4-1-16. [PMID: 22473445]

Item 11   Answer: D

Educational Objective: Manage otitis media with effusion.

This patient has otitis media with effusion (OME), and clinical observation is the most appropriate next step in management. OME is defined as fluid in the middle ear but without signs of infection. It is associated with eustachian tube dysfunction, which impairs drainage and causes retention of fluid in the middle ear, and frequently occurs following an upper respiratory tract infection or with exacerbation of seasonal allergies, as in this patient. Patients with OME frequently present with symptoms of aural fullness and hearing loss, and examination shows clear or yellowish fluid present behind a retracted tympanic membrane. Most cases of OME will resolve without treatment over the course of 12 weeks. Although many patients with OME are treated with decongestants, antihistamines, or nasal glucocorticoids, evidence of effectiveness is very limited. However, treatments focused on symptoms associated with underlying conditions that may be contributing to eustachian tube dysfunction and OME, such as the nasal congestion with seasonal allergies in this patient, would be reasonable.

Acute otitis media is characterized by fluid and inflammation in the middle ear accompanied by symptoms of infection. Although evidence to guide treatment of acute otitis media in adults is lacking, oral antibiotics such as amoxicillin, along with analgesics and decongestants, are the mainstays of therapy. This patient has no evidence of infection, and antibiotic therapy is therefore not indicated.

Otitis externa is inflammation of the external ear canal and may present either acutely or chronically. Examination shows inflammation of the external ear canal, and treatment may be with a combined antibiotic and glucocorticoid–containing ototopical agent such as combination neomycin, polymyxin B, and hydrocortisone. In this patient with no evidence of external ear canal inflammation on examination, neomycin, polymyxin B, and hydrocortisone ear drops are not indicated.

Although symptoms of OME will resolve in most patients within 12 weeks, those with persistent symptoms beyond that time period who have not responded to other interventions may be considered for myringotomy with tympanostomy tubes. It would be premature to pursue this treatment at this point in this patient's course.

KEY POINT

- Most cases of otitis media with effusion resolve spontaneously; observation and symptomatic treatment of conditions contributing to eustachian tube dysfunction are appropriate.

Bibliography

Harmes KM, Blackwood RA, Burrows HL, et al. Otitis media: diagnosis and treatment. Am Fam Physician. 2013;88:435-40. Erratum in: Am Fam Physician. 2014;89:318. [PMID: 24134083]

Item 12   Answer: D

Educational Objective: Treat a patient with neuropathic pain.

A lidocaine patch is the most appropriate treatment in this patient with neuropathic pain. Topical lidocaine in the form of either a patch or the less expensive cream has been shown in randomized controlled trials to be very effective in treating postherpetic neuralgia and diabetic peripheral neuropathy. It has also been shown to be better tolerated and to have fewer side effects than systemic therapies. Similarly, topical capsaicin is an effective topical therapy for neuropathic pain. In patients with pain amenable to localized therapy, and particularly in those in whom systemic treatment may be problematic, such as this patient with cognitive impairment and an increased risk for falls, a topical agent that avoids central nervous system toxicity is preferable as first-line therapy.

Fentanyl is a potent opioid that is indicated only in patients who are opioid tolerant due to chronic treatment, and this patient has not been taking opioids regularly. Furthermore, fentanyl carries the same risk of delirium as other opioids and would therefore not be an appropriate choice based on her previous episodes of opioid-associated delirium.

Gabapentin is first-line therapy for systemic neuropathic pain conditions that affect large portions of the body that are difficult to treat topically. However, dizziness and drowsiness are major adverse effects of gabapentin and might increase this patient's risk of falls and worsen her cognitive function. This patient has localized pain, which is better suited to topical therapy; therefore, gabapentin would be considered second-line therapy.

Tramadol binds to opioid receptors in the central nervous system and can cause adverse reactions similar to those of other opioid medications, which this patient does not tolerate. Tramadol also has a wide range of potential drug–drug interactions and a significant side effect profile, making it a poor choice for older patients. It would therefore not be an appropriate choice for treating this patient's pain, which is amenable to topical treatments.

KEY POINT

- Topical lidocaine is effective in the treatment of postherpetic neuralgia.

Bibliography

Dubinsky RM, Kabbani H, El-Chami Z, Boutwell C, Ali H; Quality Standards Subcommittee of the American Academy of Neurology. Practice parameter: treatment of postherpetic neuralgia: an evidence-based report of the Quality Standards Subcommittee of the American Academy of Neurology. Neurology. 2004 Sep 28;63(6):959-65. [PMID: 15452284]

Item 13   Answer: D

Educational Objective: Diagnose uveitis.

This patient has uveitis, which is inflammation involving the middle structures of the eye (iris, ciliary body, and choroid).

It usually presents with unilateral eye pain, redness, and photophobia. The characteristic finding on physical examination is circumferential redness around the border of the sclera and cornea (corneal limbus), termed ciliary flush, which represents dilated conjunctival vessels. Pupillary miosis is also often seen. Slit lamp examination commonly reveals inflammatory ("flare") cells in the anterior chamber. Uveitis can either be idiopathic or occur as part of an underlying systemic condition, such as autoimmune disorders, arthritides associated with HLA-B27 antigen, infection (syphilis, tuberculosis, herpes simplex virus), malignancy, and sarcoidosis. This patient has symptoms suggestive of ankylosing spondylitis, including fatigue and low back pain that awakens her from sleep and improves with activity and NSAID therapy. Ankylosing spondylitis is a systemic condition that may be associated with uveitis.

Corneal ulcers are caused by trauma, contact lens wear, herpes simplex virus infection, bacterial infection, and connective tissue disorders (ankylosing spondylitis). Although corneal ulcers can occur in the setting of ankylosing spondylitis, this patient's ciliary flush is more characteristic of uveitis.

Patients with episcleritis typically present with redness, irritation, and tearing but not significant ocular pain. Additionally, the redness seen in episcleritis is usually more widespread rather than limited to the perilimbic region of the involved eye, making this an unlikely diagnosis in this patient.

Scleritis can be associated with autoimmune disorders; however, it typically presents bilaterally, involves redness across the entire sclera, and does not present with ciliary flush.

KEY POINT

- Uveitis is characterized by unilateral eye pain, photophobia, and ciliary flush; it is commonly associated with autoimmune disorders, arthritides associated with HLA-B27 antigen, infection, malignancy, and sarcoidosis.

Bibliography

Bal SK, Hollingworth GR. Red eye. BMJ. 2005 Aug 20;331(7514):438. [PMID: 16110072]

Item 14   Answer: B

Educational Objective: Treat an overweight patient with pharmacologic therapy.

The most appropriate management is to treat this overweight patient with orlistat. Pharmacologic therapy may be used as an adjunct to diet, physical activity, and behavioral treatments in patients with a BMI of 30 or higher or in patients with a BMI of 27 or higher with overweight- or obesity-associated comorbidities. In light of this patient's dieting attempts (including with dietician-monitored diets), physical activity, and behavioral therapy without sustained

weight loss, she should be considered for pharmacologic treatment, and the most appropriate pharmacologic agent for this patient is orlistat. Orlistat is an inhibitor of gastric and pancreatic lipases. Taken three times per day (during or up to 1 hour after meals), orlistat results in malabsorption of approximately 30% of ingested fat. Twelve months of orlistat treatment at doses of 120 mg three times per day or 60 mg (available over the counter) three times per day results in a mean weight loss of 3.4 kg or 2.5 kg (7.5 lb or 5.5 lb), respectively, compared with placebo. Orlistat also reduces BMI, waist circumference, blood pressure, blood cholesterol level, and risk for type 2 diabetes mellitus. Loose stool is a common side effect of orlistat; however, this may not be a major concern for this patient given her chronic constipation.

Lorcaserin, a brain serotonin 2C receptor agonist, acts as an appetite suppressant. It should be used with caution in patients taking medications that increase serotonin levels, such as sertraline. Therefore, this patient should not be prescribed lorcaserin.

Combination low-dose phentermine (a sympathomimetic drug) and low-dose topiramate (an antiepileptic drug) has demonstrated efficacy in reducing weight, possibly by suppressing appetite, altering taste, and increasing metabolism. However, phentermine-topiramate is contraindicated in patients with glaucoma; thus, it should not be prescribed in this patient.

Referral for bariatric surgery is indicated in all patients with a BMI of 40 or higher and in patients with a BMI of 35 or higher with obesity-related comorbid conditions. This patient does not meet the criteria for bariatric surgery.

KEY POINT

- Pharmacologic therapy may be used as an adjunct to diet, physical activity, and behavioral treatments in patients with a BMI of 30 or higher or in patients with a BMI of 27 or higher with overweight- or obesity-associated comorbidities.

Bibliography

Yanovski SZ, Yanovski JA. Long-term drug treatment for obesity: A systematic and clinical review. JAMA 2014 Jan 1;311(1):74-86. [PMID: 24231879]

Item 15   Answer: B

Educational Objective: Counsel a high-risk older driver.

The patient should be advised to retire from driving. The American Medical Association recommends that physicians assess older patients for physical or mental impairments that might adversely affect driving abilities. Assessing the older driver is complex and relies heavily on physician clinical judgment in addition to evaluation of underlying conditions that pose a risk to safe driving. Risk factors that increase the likelihood of an adverse driving event include cognitive dysfunction, caregiver report of unsafe skills, history of citations or accidents, driving fewer than 60 miles per week, alcohol or medications that affect the central nervous system, emotional aggression or impulsivity, impaired mobility (including neck range of motion, range of motion of the extremities, and coordination), visual impairment, and medical disorders that predispose to loss of consciousness. The more risk factors the patient has, the higher the risk of an adverse driving event. This patient has four of these risk factors (cognitive dysfunction, driving fewer than 60 miles per week, caregiver concern, and impaired vision), none of which may be easily reversed. Therefore, given her level of risk, she should be advised to discontinue driving.

Patient self-rating of driving skill has been shown to be unhelpful in assessing driving risk. Caregiver report of driving ability is more reliable. Although this patient is confident in her driving abilities, her daughters' report of "near misses" should be taken into account along with the patient's risk factors for an adverse driving event.

This patient is being seen by an ophthalmologist for her vision loss, which has been stable and meets the minimum limits for the ability to drive. Although her ophthalmologist is able to render an opinion on the status and prognosis of her vision loss, the assessment of the ability to drive safely is complex and multifactorial, of which visual function is only one element. Therefore, the ability of a patient to drive safely should be made by the clinician who has knowledge of these different factors and is able to evaluate them in the overall context of the patient.

Although neuropsychiatric testing may provide greater detail regarding this patient's mild cognitive dysfunction, it is unlikely to change the recommendation to retire from driving considering the multitude of risk factors in addition to her cognitive dysfunction.

KEY POINT

- Older adult patients who have multiple risk factors for an adverse driving event, such as cognitive dysfunction, caregiver report of unsafe skills, history of citations or accidents, impaired mobility, and visual impairment, should be advised to retire from driving.

Bibliography

Iverson DJ, Gronseth GS, Reger MA, Classen S, Dubinsky RM, Rizzo M; Quality Standards Subcommittee of the American Academy of Neurology. Practice parameter update: evaluation and management of driving risk in dementia: report of the Quality Standards Subcommittee of the American Academy of Neurology. Neurology. 2010 Apr 20;74(16):1316-24. [PMID: 20385882]

Item 16   Answer: C

Educational Objective: Manage medically unexplained symptoms with cognitive-behavioral therapy.

This patient with medically unexplained symptoms (MUS) would benefit most from cognitive-behavioral therapy (CBT). She presents with many of the common symptoms seen in patients with MUS, and her symptoms are significantly affecting her quality of life. She has undergone extensive and

costly medical evaluation with normal results, and several medications have been tried without benefit. Although it is tempting for the patient and the physician to think that additional testing or medications will elucidate a previously undiscovered diagnosis, this is rarely the case. This pattern of care often leads to iatrogenic injury, excess health care costs, and patient dissatisfaction. Goals of care should be shifted away from medical diagnosis toward addressing the impact of the patient's symptoms on her life. CBT involves educating the patient so that she understands the plan of care and its purpose, obtaining and reinforcing a commitment from the patient for the chosen plan of care, setting and reviewing mutually chosen patient goals, and negotiating new plans and therapy as needed. CBT has been shown to be effective in patients with MUS. Although CBT is generally performed by trained therapists, the internist can reinforce the basic principles of CBT at each follow-up visit.

Ordering further diagnostic testing, such as a brain MRI, when there is no strong clinical suspicion of disease is inappropriate. Despite this patient's various neurologic symptoms, she has no focal neurologic findings and no indication for brain imaging.

Patients with MUS may have underlying depression; however, this patient reports no depressed mood or affect, anhedonia, or problems with concentration. Additionally, a previous trial of a selective serotonin reuptake inhibitor was unsuccessful. Therefore, treatment with another antidepressant medication is not indicated.

Frequently, the patient with MUS will request referral to a specialist, or the internist will contemplate referral due to frustration or uncertainty. In this patient, referral to another physician risks further fragmentation of care and duplicate or more invasive testing, neither of which is indicated.

Regularly scheduled visits with an internist, accompanied by targeted physical examinations, are essential in the patient with MUS. Randomized trials suggest that this care plan may improve patients' physical functioning. Additionally, recent evidence suggests that telephone contact may be an effective substitute for face-to-face visits. An interval of 6 months between follow-up visits is too long to effectively manage this patient with MUS.

KEY POINT

- Cognitive-behavioral therapy may be beneficial in managing medically unexplained symptoms and should be considered in place of additional testing.

Bibliography

Kent C, McMillan G. A CBT-based approach to medically unexplained symptoms. Adv Psychiatr Treat. 2009 Feb 27;15(2):146-151.

Item 17   Answer: C

Educational Objective: Evaluate a palpable breast mass in a postmenopausal woman.

This woman should undergo a diagnostic core needle biopsy of the palpable breast mass to obtain a tissue diagnosis.

Although mammography is indicated with a newly detected breast lump to assist in evaluation, it has false-negative rates of between 10% and 20% even if a standardized reporting system, such as the Breast Imaging Reporting and Data System (BI-RADS), suggests a negative finding as in this patient with a BI-RADS category of 1, indicating that no radiographic masses, architectural disturbances, or suspicious calcifications are present. Therefore, biopsy is required for a palpable breast mass even if a mammogram is negative or nondiagnostic, as in this patient. Fine needle aspiration cytology is also an option, but evidence indicates slightly better sensitivity and specificity with larger bore core biopsy needles.

Breast MRI may further define the characteristics of the mass but would not provide adequate information to obviate the need for a definitive tissue diagnosis.

Conservative management, with re-evaluation at a follow-up visit in 4 weeks or resuming regular mammographic screening, is not appropriate in a postmenopausal woman with a palpable breast mass, which requires further, immediate evaluation.

KEY POINT

- Biopsy is required for a palpable breast mass even if a mammogram is negative or nondiagnostic.

Bibliography

Harvey JA, Mahoney MC, Newell MS, et al. ACR appropriateness criteria: palpable breast masses. J Am Coll Radiol. 2013 Oct;10(10):742-9.e1-3. [PMID: 24091044]

Item 18   Answer: C

Educational Objective: Evaluate a patient with disequilibrium.

This older patient is experiencing disequilibrium, or unsteadiness with walking or standing, and is likely to benefit from physical therapy. She is lightheaded and dizzy without presyncope, syncope, orthostasis, or vertigo. Disequilibrium frequently presents in frail elderly patients who have multiple sensory deficits (such as impaired visual or auditory acuity and impaired proprioception), motor weakness, joint pain, psychiatric disease, orthostasis, medication side effects, or neuropathic and cerebellar diseases affecting balance and gait. Frequently more than one cause can be identified in a specific patient. Multidisciplinary efforts (physical therapy, visual and auditory screening followed by correction of impairment, and mobility aids that stabilize ambulation) can produce improvement in functional status.

A CT scan of the head is unlikely to be helpful in delineating a cause of dizziness as this patient's neurologic examination is normal and she has no history of falls or head trauma that would put her at risk for a subdural hematoma. CT scans of the head have limited ability to image the posterior fossa and cerebellum, so if a central cause of this patient's symptoms were suspected, MRI of the brain would be the preferred test.

The diagnostic yield of 24- to 48-hour ambulatory electrocardiographic monitoring in uncovering significant cardiac arrhythmias responsible for generalized weakness and dizziness would be low in this patient without a history or symptoms of cardiac disease.

This patient should be evaluated by a physical therapist for the most appropriate gait aid. She currently is unable to use a cane effectively, and she likely will need further evaluation and training in using the best assistive device. A walker should not be provided without additional evaluation.

KEY POINT

- Management of disequilibrium involves physical therapy, visual and auditory screening followed by correction of impairment, and mobility aids that stabilize ambulation; extensive imaging and testing is unnecessary.

Bibliography

Barin K, Dodson EE. Dizziness in the elderly. Otolaryngol Clin North Am. 2011 Apr;44(2):437-54, x. [PMID: 21474016]

Item 19   Answer: D

Educational Objective: Manage postoperative anemia in a patient with cardiovascular disease.

No transfusion or further diagnostic testing is necessary for this patient with postoperative anemia and cardiovascular disease. He had a considerable decline in hemoglobin level, but this is consistent with the amount of blood loss noted in surgery (1200 mL). Moreover, this degree of blood loss after multilevel spine fusion is not atypical. Multiple studies have demonstrated that a conservative approach to perioperative blood management is as good as or superior to a liberal approach (such as maintaining a hemoglobin level of >10 g/dL [100 g/L]). This approach has been demonstrated even in patients with known cardiac disease or risk factors for cardiac disease. Current guidelines recommend transfusing red blood cells if a patient has symptoms attributable to anemia or a hemoglobin level less than 7 to 8 g/dL (70-80 g/L).

Intravenous iron is typically indicated in patients who are unable to take oral iron or unable to take in adequate amounts of oral iron in the presence of ongoing chronic blood loss, and in patients with kidney failure and anemia. However, this patient with mild anemia and likely normal iron stores may not require iron therapy for postoperative anemia and does not have a clear indication for parenteral iron if therapy were needed.

Transfusion of one unit of packed red blood cells (pRBCs) is not indicated because the patient does not have a clear indication for transfusion. If transfusion were indicated, the number of units administered should be based upon the target hemoglobin level and if active blood loss is present. One unit of pRBCs usually raises the hemoglobin level by 1 g/dL (10 g/L).

A frequent practice of clinicians is to order no less than two units of pRBCs at a time. This is based on the erroneous assumption that "more is better," and that the transfusion

CONT.

risks of giving two units is no greater than for one unit. Such practices result in unnecessary depletion of the blood supply and double the risk of transfusion adverse effects because each unit carries its own potential for complications.

KEY POINT

- For patients with cardiovascular disease and postoperative anemia, transfusion of red blood cells is recommended if the patient has symptoms attributable to anemia or a hemoglobin level less than 7 to 8 g/dL (70-80 g/L).

Bibliography

Hogshire LC, Patel MS, Rivera E, Carson JL. Evidence review: periprocedural use of blood products. J Hosp Med. 2013 Nov;8(11):647-52. [PMID: 24124069]

Item 20   Answer: A

Educational Objective: Diagnose acromioclavicular joint degeneration.

This patient's presentation is most consistent with acromioclavicular joint degeneration. Acromioclavicular joint degeneration typically presents with pain located on the superior aspect of the shoulder, although pain may be poorly localized in some patients. On examination, there may be tenderness to palpation of the acromioclavicular joint as well as pain with arm adduction across the body (cross-arm test) and with shoulder abduction beyond 120 degrees. Plain radiographs can reveal degenerative changes of the acromioclavicular joint, although radiography is usually unnecessary. First-line therapy consists of NSAIDs and activity modification.

Patients with adhesive capsulitis typically report decreased range of motion and pain with movement in all directions. On examination, there is loss of both active and passive range of motion with all cardinal shoulder movements and tenderness at the insertion of the deltoid tendon. Plain radiographs are typically normal.

Patients with rotator cuff tears typically have pain with shoulder abduction, internal rotation, or external rotation, depending on the tendon(s) involved. However, a key distinguishing feature of a full-thickness rotator cuff tear is loss of strength. A positive drop-arm test is suggestive of a supraspinatus tear. The absence of weakness and the patient's negative drop-arm test argue against the presence of a rotator cuff tear.

Supraspinatus tendinitis is characterized by pain with active shoulder abduction and a positive painful arc. Internal and external rotation may also elicit pain with involvement of other rotator cuff tendons. Pain is typically elicited with active but not passive range of motion.

KEY POINT

- Acromioclavicular joint degeneration typically presents with pain located on the superior aspect of the shoulder, tenderness to palpation of the acromioclavicular joint, and pain with shoulder adduction and abduction beyond 120 degrees.

Bibliography

Armstrong A. Evaluation and management of adult shoulder pain: a focus on rotator cuff disorders, acromioclavicular joint arthritis, and glenohumeral arthritis. Med Clin North Am. 2014 Jul;98(4):755-75, xii. [PMID: 24994050]

Item 21   Answer: D

Educational Objective: Manage breaking bad news to a patient.

The physician should state that the cancer has returned. Physicians often have difficulty imparting bad news to patients and worry that they will diminish patient hope or leave patients emotionally inconsolable. The SPIKES (Setting, Perception, Invitation, Knowledge, Empathy, Strategize) framework provides a schema for disclosing critical information in a way that allows patients to hear information while supporting their emotional reactions, thereby maintaining hope. In this case, the provider has already addressed the S, P, and I steps of the SPIKES protocol and is at the point of imparting knowledge (K). When delivering the news, it is important for the physician to use short, declarative sentences without jargon or euphemisms. This approach may seem blunt; however, it provides an unambiguous message, thereby improving patient comprehension. After the physician delivers the bad news, the physician will empathically address emotion during step E of SPIKES, preventing the delivery from seeming detached or cold. In the last step of SPIKES, the physician and patient strategize new goals as a method of maintaining hope.

Recounting previous events during bad news delivery, such as explaining the planned surveillance strategy, creates a long-winded response with extraneous information that masks the actual news. There is a high risk that the patient will not hear or understand what is being conveyed. Furthermore, this response attempts to "sugarcoat" the bad news (the patient's cancer has recurred) by implying that it is actually good news (the recurrence was identified). Bad news cannot be turned into good news; the physician can only mitigate the consequences of the bad news. Tempering the delivery of bad news in this way further increases the risk that patients will not understand the news they have been given.

Couching a response in euphemisms (in this case, the word "lesion") is not appropriate. Euphemisms add a layer of uncertainty in communication, increasing the risk of misunderstanding and delaying truth-telling. There is no doubt that this patient has recurrent prostate cancer, and the physician should communicate this in clear terms.

Telling the patient that the cancer has returned but that there are therapeutic options is also not appropriate. In this response, the term "cancer" is used, but it is immediately followed by an attempt to "fix" the situation. This type of "fixing" response is particularly attractive to many providers, who view it as a means of preventing the patient from losing hope. This response bypasses addressing the emotion that bad news generates (step E in SPIKES), which may make the conversation less messy for the physician; however, processing an emotional response to bad news is a necessary stage for patients before they can strategize next steps. Furthermore, providing a solution before the patient has had a chance to strategize based on personal hopes and goals does not allow the patient to fully participate in the decision-making process.

KEY POINT

- The SPIKES (Setting, Perception, Invitation, Knowledge, Empathy, Strategize) protocol can be used to break bad news to patients while maintaining patient hope.

Bibliography

Evans WG, Tulsky JA, Back AL, Arnold RM. Communication at times of transitions: how to help patients cope with loss and re-define hope. Cancer J. 2006 Sep-Oct;12(5):417-24. [PMID: 17034677]

Item 22   Answer: C

Educational Objective: Screen for lung cancer in a former smoker.

In patients who are at high risk for lung cancer, annual low-dose CT is recommended to screen for lung cancer. High-risk patients are adults aged 55 to 80 years with a 30-pack-year or more smoking history, including former smokers who have quit in the last 15 years. Candidates for screening should have a reasonable life expectancy and be willing to undergo curative lung surgery. The U.S. Preventive Services Task Force (USPSTF) recommends that screening be discontinued once a person has not smoked for 15 years or develops a health problem that substantially limits life expectancy or the willingness to have curative lung surgery. A large randomized controlled trial, the National Lung Screening Trial (NLST), found a 20% reduction in lung cancer mortality in patients who were screened with low-dose CT compared with those screened with chest radiography. The number of high-risk patients needed to screen with low-dose CT to prevent one lung cancer death was 320. Potential harms related to screening include a high false-positive rate, radiation exposure, potential for discovering incidental findings, risks associated with follow-up, and overdiagnosis. Twenty-four percent of those screened with low-dose CT had a positive screening, and 96% of those cases were false-positive results.

The greatest risk factors for the development of abdominal aortic aneurysm (AAA) are age, male sex (men outnumber women by up to 6:1), and a history of smoking. The USPSTF recommends one-time screening for AAA with abdominal ultrasonography in all men aged 65 to 75 years who have smoked at least 100 cigarettes in their lifetime and selective screening in men in this age group who have never smoked. Men in this category might include those with a first-degree relative who required repair of an AAA or died of a ruptured AAA. This patient should be screened for AAA when he is 65 years of age.

Plain chest radiography is not recommended to screen for lung cancer in any population.

Routine spirometry is not recommended in asymptomatic individuals, including asymptomatic smokers, to screen for chronic obstructive lung disease.

KEY POINT

- Screening for lung cancer with annual low-dose chest CT is recommended for high-risk patients, defined as adults aged 55 to 80 years with a smoking history of 30-pack-years or more, including former smokers who have quit in the last 15 years.

Bibliography

National Lung Screening Trial Research Team, Aberle DR, Adams AM, et al. Reduced lung-cancer mortality with low-dose computed tomographic screening. N Engl J Med. 2011 Aug 4;365(5):395-409. [PMID: 21714641]

Item 23   Answer: D

Educational Objective: Treat cauda equina syndrome.

The patient has signs and symptoms consistent with cauda equina syndrome, and an emergent surgical evaluation should be obtained. Cauda equina syndrome is an uncommon but potentially catastrophic condition that is caused by compression and ischemia of some or all of the 18 descending nerve roots that make up the cauda equina, with resulting neurologic impairment. Causes may be benign (such as degenerative changes, disk herniation, spondylosis, and other structural abnormalities of the spine; infection; or bleeding) or malignant (with multiple myeloma, lymphoma, and prostate cancers being the most commonly associated cancers). Classic clinical findings include acute low back pain, radicular pain, paresthesias or anesthesia in the perineal and upper thigh regions (termed "saddle anesthesia" due to its distribution in an area where a saddle would contact the body when riding a horse), urinary retention, fecal incontinence, lower extremity weakness, and decreased or absent distal reflexes. However, all of these features are uncommonly present early in the syndrome. For example, pain is the most common early symptom and may precede other neurologic findings; bowel and bladder dysfunction are usually late manifestations and do not occur in all patients. Early detection and surgical treatment offer the best chance of avoiding permanent neurologic damage, requiring careful evaluation of patients who might have this condition. Although this patient has incomplete clinical findings, rapid imaging and surgical evaluation are indicated.

Treatment with either epidural or high-dose glucocorticoids would be of unclear benefit in this patient because there is no definite evidence of an inflammatory disorder, and there is also no evidence suggesting that an acute compressive lesion would respond to glucocorticoids.

Examination of the cerebrospinal fluid would not be expected to be helpful in most patients with cauda equina syndrome and is not necessary to establish the diagnosis.

KEY POINT

- Urgent evaluation for surgical decompression is required in all patients with findings of cauda equina syndrome, characterized by acute low back pain, radicular features, saddle anesthesia, urinary retention, absence of reflexes, and decreased anal tone.

Bibliography

Gitelman A, Hishmeh S, Morelli BN, et al. Cauda equina syndrome: a comprehensive review. Am J Orthop (Belle Mead NJ). 2008 Nov;37(11): 556-62. [PMID: 19104682]

Item 24   Answer: D

Educational Objective: Treat erectile dysfunction in an obese patient.

Lifestyle modification, including weight loss, is the most appropriate next step in the management of this patient who has erectile dysfunction (ED) and is obese. First-line treatments for ED include lifestyle modification (weight loss, exercise, smoking cessation), psychotherapy as needed, and phosphodiesterase type 5 (PDE-5) inhibitors. Randomized controlled trials have shown that obese men who lose weight through dietary changes and exercise experience significant improvement in erectile function compared with obese men who do not lose weight. This patient's sedentary lifestyle has likely contributed to his obesity. He would likely experience improved erectile function as a result of substantial weight loss through healthy diet and exercise. After discussion with the patient, a decision can be made about whether to institute lifestyle changes alone or to combine lifestyle changes with a PDE-5 inhibitor.

Intraurethral alprostadil is more effective than PDE-5 inhibitors at treating ED. However, compliance with intraurethral alprostadil is low, and it is not considered a first-line treatment for ED.

Although it is important to inquire about that status of romantic relationships in patients with sexual dysfunction, this patient reports that his marriage is satisfying; therefore, marriage counseling would not be indicated.

It would be inappropriate to prescribe venlafaxine for depression in this patient who reports that his mood is excellent. Furthermore, venlafaxine is associated with sexual dysfunction.

KEY POINT

- First-line therapy for erectile dysfunction includes lifestyle modification (weight loss, exercise, smoking cessation), psychotherapy as needed, and phosphodiesterase type 5 inhibitors.

Bibliography

Esposito K, Giugliano F, Di Palo C, et al. Effect of lifestyle changes on erectile dysfunction in obese men: a randomized controlled trial. JAMA. 2004 Jun 23;291(24):2978-84. [PMID: 15213209]

Item 25   Answer: B

Educational Objective: Treat hyperlipidemia in a patient with atherosclerotic cardiovascular disease and risk factors for statin-associated adverse effects.

The most appropriate treatment for this patient is moderate-intensity statin therapy, such as with rosuvastatin. This patient has peripheral arterial disease, a form of clinical atherosclerotic cardiovascular disease (ASCVD), and therefore meets the criteria for one of four patient groups that have been shown to benefit from the treatment of hyperlipidemia with statin therapy. Patients with clinical ASCVD benefit most from high-intensity statin therapy; however, for those with risk factors for statin-associated adverse effects, moderate-intensity therapy is recommended. This patient is best treated with a moderate-intensity statin because he has three such risk factors: age older than 75 years, chronic kidney disease, and use of a medication known to interact with statins (diltiazem).

The use of high-intensity rosuvastatin in this patient has significant potential to cause adverse effects, including myopathy and liver dysfunction. In this patient, the risks associated with high-dose statin therapy outweigh the potential benefits, especially since moderate-intensity statin therapy can reduce the LDL cholesterol level 30% to 49% and provide secondary prevention of cardiovascular events.

Niacin monotherapy has not been shown to reduce the incidence of cardiovascular events and is not considered first-line therapy for the prevention of ASCVD. Niacin and other nonstatin drugs are only recommended for patients who have severe hypertriglyceridemia, do not respond to statin therapy, or have a history of statin intolerance.

Providing no additional treatment in this patient with ASCVD would be inappropriate. Current American College of Cardiology/American Heart Association guidelines recommend statin therapy for all patients with clinical ASCVD, regardless of LDL cholesterol levels, to reduce the risk of cardiovascular events.

KEY POINT

- In patients with clinical atherosclerotic cardiovascular disease and risk factors for statin-associated adverse effects, moderate-intensity statin therapy is recommended.

Bibliography

Stone NJ, Robinson JG, Lichtenstein AH, et al; American College of Cardiology/ American Heart Association Task Force on Practice Guidelines. 2013 ACC/ AHA guideline on the treatment of blood cholesterol to reduce atherosclerotic cardiovascular risk in adults: a report of the American College of Cardiology/American Heart Association Task Force on Practice Guidelines. Circulation. 2014 Jun 24;129(25 Suppl 2):S1-45. Erratum in: Circulation. 2014 Jun 24;129(25 Suppl 2):S46-8. [PMID: 24222016]

Item 26   Answer: D

Educational Objective: Recognize relative risk as the standard outcome measure for a cohort study.

In this cohort study, the standard outcome measure is relative risk. Cohort studies are a type of observational study that examines the outcomes of patients with different exposures or risks. This study investigated the outcomes (erectile function scores) of two groups of men who had received radiation therapy for prostate cancer, one of which was exposed to tadalafil and one of which was not.

Relative risk is the ratio of the probability of developing a specific outcome (in this case, erectile function score) in a group with an exposure or risk factor present (treatment with tadalafil) to the probability of developing the specific outcome in a group without the exposure or risk factor present (no treatment with tadalafil). A relative risk that is greater than or less than 1 indicates a more likely or less likely outcome, respectively, of the measured variable in the exposure or risk factor group compared with the group without the exposure or risk factor present.

Confidence intervals are a method for indicating the range in which a value derived from a study is likely to lie, with 95% being the usual calculated range. Whereas a P value is calculated to assess whether a trial result is likely to have occurred simply by chance, confidence intervals provide a range of possible effect size compatible with the data. Confidence intervals may be calculated for most statistical reporting measures but are not themselves used as an outcome measure for evaluating study results.

The number needed to treat (NNT) is an estimate of the number of patients who must receive an intervention to cause one patient to experience the beneficial outcome of interest. The NNT has become a standard reporting measure for randomized controlled trials. It is calculated by taking the inverse of the absolute risk change between study groups. The concept of NNT has been applied to cohort studies to suggest the magnitude of effect of an exposure (sometimes referred to as number needed to be exposed); however, because cohort studies are observational and not experimental trials, the calculation of similar measures for cohort studies is statistically more difficult than in experimental studies. Additionally, the accuracy of these measures for cohort studies is less clear. Therefore, relative risk remains the main outcome measure used for cohort studies.

The odds ratio is conceptually similar to relative risk, but rather than comparing the ratio of rates of occurrence of an event between study groups, the odds ratio compares the odds (the ratio of the probability that the event will happen to the probability that the event will not happen) between study groups. The odds ratio is required for studies using retrospective data, such as case-control studies in which the groups being compared may not have a similar risk for the condition. Case-control studies compare the outcomes of patients with a disease (cases) to those without a disease (controls). Because all of the patients in this study had prostate cancer treated with radiation therapy (a cohort) and a specific subsequent exposure or risk was evaluated, it is not a case-control study and an odds ratio would not be the standard outcome measure.

KEY POINT

- Cohort studies investigate the outcomes of similar patients with different exposures; the standard outcome measure for a cohort study is relative risk.

Bibliography
Guyatt GH, Haynes RB, Jaeschke RZ, et al. Users' Guides to the Medical Literature: XXV. Evidence-based medicine: principles for applying the Users' Guides to patient care. Evidence-Based Medicine Working Group. JAMA. 2000 Sep 13;284(10):1290-6. [PMID: 10979117]

Item 27   Answer: C

Educational Objective: Diagnose hearing loss in an older patient.

This older patient should be evaluated for hearing loss with the whispered voice test. Hearing loss is common in older adults, and it results in significant impairment in quality of life and potentially leads to depression and social isolation. Because patients may experience difficulties in understanding and communication, hearing loss is frequently misdiagnosed as cognitive dysfunction. There is some evidence that hearing aids in older patients improve not only hearing but also quality of life; therefore, patients who have cognitive or affective concerns that may be related to hearing should be screened for hearing loss. No one screening test has been shown to be superior to another. Whispered voice test, finger rub test, hearing loss questionnaire, and hand-held audiometry are all reasonable screening tests. Many patients with significant hearing loss deny any hearing deficits and can compensate for their hearing loss in a quiet office environment; therefore, a patient's perception of his or her own hearing or the patient's ability to carry on a normal conversation in the office setting should not be considered as evidence of adequate hearing. Patients who test positive or who report hearing loss should be referred for formal audiologic testing and consideration of amplification with hearing aids.

This patient has stable mild cognitive dysfunction that is not interfering with his executive functioning. His social functioning is impaired, but hearing loss has not been ruled out as the cause of his social impairment. As such, medication for dementia, such as donepezil, is not currently indicated.

Social isolation is a symptom of depression; however, this patient was appropriately screened with the two-question method ("During the past month, have you been bothered by feeling down, depressed, or hopeless?" and "During the past month, have you been bothered by little interest or pleasure in doing things?"), which has a 97% sensitivity for identifying depression in older adults. A more extensive screen for depression, such as the PHQ-9, is not likely to add helpful information in this patient.

A diagnosis of hearing loss and its correction would be missed with clinical observation alone.

KEY POINT

- Older patients who present with symptoms of a mood disorder or cognitive dysfunction should be screened for hearing loss.

Bibliography
Moyer VA; U.S. Preventive Services Task Force. Screening for hearing loss in older adults: U.S. Preventive Services Task Force recommendation statement. Ann Intern Med. 2012 Nov 6;157(9):655-61. [PMID: 22893115]

Item 28   Answer: C

Educational Objective: Diagnose sacroiliitis.

This patient most likely has sacroiliitis, or inflammation of the sacroiliac (SI) joints. SI joints are true synovial joints between the sacrum and ilium of the pelvis. The SI joint may be involved as part of a systemic inflammatory syndrome such as spondyloarthritis, particularly ankylosing spondylitis, but may also be involved as an isolated musculoskeletal condition. Biomechanical factors that predispose to SI joint injury include repetitive torsional forces or unidirectional pelvic shear forces, as might occur with stepping off of a curb. Patients with leg length discrepancies or those with other conditions that may alter pelvic mechanics, such as pregnancy, scoliosis, or lumbar fixation, may also be at increased risk. The diagnosis of sacroiliitis is supported by the posterior location of this patient's hip pain and a positive FABER test, in which the hip is Flexed, ABducted, and Externally Rotated and gentle downward pressure is applied to the knee. This test has a high specificity for sacroiliitis and a somewhat lower sensitivity. Therapy for sacroiliitis is similar to that for other joint pain, including rest, anti-inflammatory medications, and possibly physical therapy. A number of additional treatments, including glucocorticoid injections, are used in patients who do not respond to conservative therapy.

Hip joint osteoarthritis causes pain directly in the hip joint that frequently radiates to the groin. Range of motion of the hip is usually limited and reproduces the pain. This patient's pain does not radiate, and his range of motion is normal, making this a less likely diagnosis.

Piriformis syndrome results from compression or limitation of the sciatic nerve by the piriformis muscle. It typically causes symptoms similar to sciatic nerve compression in the lumbosacral spine, with pain, tingling, and numbness that radiate into the leg, findings that are not present in this patient.

Trochanteric bursitis classically causes lateral hip pain over the greater trochanteric bursa, which is located over the greater trochanter lateral to the hip joint. Pain associated with trochanteric bursitis may radiate to the buttock or knee and is often worse when lying on the affected side. It does not affect range of motion. Trochanteric bursitis can be differentiated from hip joint pain based on its characteristic location relative to the pain associated with sacroiliitis.

KEY POINT

- Sacroiliitis is characterized by tenderness to palpation of the sacroiliac joint, pain that is reproduced with the FABER (Flexion, ABduction, External Rotation) test, and no pain with passive range of motion of the hips.

Bibliography

Byrd JW. Evaluation of the hip: history and physical examination. N Am J Sports Phys Ther. 2007 Nov;2(4):231-40. [PMID: 21509142]

Item 29   Answer: D

Educational Objective: Manage a patient who has undergone direct-to-consumer genetic testing.

In this patient who has no family history of breast or ovarian cancer, no further testing is necessary, despite the results of the direct-to-consumer genetic test. Direct-to-consumer genetic testing, though attractive to patients, is fraught with many potential drawbacks, including the uncertain validity of the tests themselves. This form of testing relies on a case-control–based approach. Single-nucleotide polymorphisms (SNPs) that are disproportionately found in affected individuals with a specific disease are identified, and odds ratios indicating the influence of particular SNPs on the pretest likelihood for the disease are calculated. Unfortunately, most SNPs have very low odds ratios and contribute only a small proportion to total disease burden. This approach also does not capture the complex interaction between genetic influences on development of disease or the effect of other factors, such as environmental exposures, among other potentially confounding issues. Therefore, a positive result with this type of testing frequently does not indicate an increased probability of having the disease but may cause unnecessary patient concern and anxiety.

Additionally, given the lack of pretest counseling, an essential component of proper genetic testing in which the basic concepts of genetic testing and interpretation can be explained, patient misinterpretation of test results is especially likely. It is essential that this patient be educated about the implications of her test results, including the limitations. This patient should be informed that her risk of developing breast cancer is not 52.5% and is instead much lower. Even if the results of this test were found to be valid, her lifetime risk of developing breast cancer would increase from 12.4% (the lifetime risk for women born in the United States who are considered to be at average risk) to approximately 19%.

According to the U.S. Preventive Services Task Force (USPSTF), *BRCA* genetic testing should be limited to patients whose family history indicates a possible familial inheritance as seen by the presence of *BRCA*-related malignancies. There is no such indication of a familial pattern of disease in this patient; therefore, *BRCA* genetic testing would not be indicated.

Breast MRI is a highly sensitive study for detection of breast cancers and other breast pathology. However, its appropriate use as a screening tool is evolving, with variable recommendations existing for use in patients considered at high risk for breast cancer. This patient does not have a clear increased risk based on her history or the results of her direct-to-consumer genetic testing. Therefore, initiating screening MRI in this patient would not be appropriate.

Breast self-examination has not been shown to be a reliable method for detection of breast cancer in average-risk women or in those at increased risk, and the USPSTF advises against its use for screening. It would therefore not be an appropriate management recommendation for this patient.

- Direct-to-consumer genetic tests have questionable clinical validity and may lead to patient misinterpretation of test results and unnecessary anxiety.

Bibliography

Bellcross CA, Page PZ, Meaney-Delman D. Direct-to-consumer personal genome testing and cancer risk prediction. Cancer J. 2012 Jul-Aug;18(4): 293-302. [PMID: 22846729]

Item 30   Answer: D

Educational Objective: Treat dyspnea at the end of life.

The most appropriate treatment of this patient's dyspnea is oral morphine. Dyspnea is common in many chronic progressive diseases near the end of life, and systemic opioids are the standard of care for refractory dyspnea in advanced disease. Although opioids have been shown to be very effective in treating dyspnea, the exact mechanisms underlying this benefit have not been well defined. Potential mechanisms of action that reduce dyspnea include altering central perception of dyspnea or modulating the activity of peripheral receptors in the lung that contribute to the sensation of dyspnea.

Many physicians worry about depressing respiratory drive with opioids in patients with end-stage disease and dyspnea. In fact, numerous studies have shown that opioids, when dosed and titrated appropriately, do not hasten death, do not raise P_{CO_2}, and do not lead to respiratory failure, but do effectively manage the sensation of dyspnea. Accordingly, a consensus statement issued by the American College of Chest Physicians states that systemic opioids, dosed and titrated appropriately, are effective and safe for dyspnea in the setting of advanced disease. The dose is generally titrated to achieve the lowest effective dose needed to adequately treat a patient's dyspnea. This patient's emphysema is already being maximally medically managed without improvement of symptoms; therefore, she should receive oral morphine.

Nebulized lidocaine is sometimes used in suppressing intractable cough, but it has no role in treating dyspnea.

Nebulized morphine is often prescribed for relief of dyspnea. However, a meta-analysis showed that nebulized morphine had no benefit compared with nebulized saline in the treatment of dyspnea, and it should not supplant the use of systemic opioids to treat dyspnea.

Dyspnea often produces anxiety in patients, and benzodiazepines may have a role in the treatment of patients with both dyspnea and anxiety. Additionally, studies show that benzodiazepines can be helpful when added to opioids, but opioids remains first-line treatment for dyspnea. This patient does not have anxiety; therefore, lorazepam is not indicated.

- Systemic opioids are the standard of care for refractory dyspnea in advanced disease.

Bibliography

Mahler DA, Selecky PA, Harrod CG, et al. American College of Chest Physicians consensus statement on the management of dyspnea in patients with advanced lung or heart disease. Chest. 2010 Mar;137(3): 674-91. [PMID: 20202949]

Item 31   Answer: A

Educational Objective: Manage diabetes mellitus medications in the preoperative setting.

The most appropriate management of this patient's insulin prior to surgery is to administer insulin glargine as usual and withhold the scheduled insulin lispro. Preoperative management of diabetes mellitus requires determination of the patient's medical regimen, recent glycemic control, stress/duration of surgery, and anticipated duration of periprocedural fasting. In most cases, long-acting insulins (glargine and detemir) should be continued uninterrupted at the same dose unless a patient has risk factors for hypoglycemia or is undergoing a procedure requiring a prolonged period without enteral nutrition. Conversely, scheduled short-acting insulins such as lispro should be withheld during the fasting state because their purpose is to suppress postprandial hyperglycemia. In this case, the patient does not require a prolonged procedure or extended period of fasting. He also has no risk factors for hypoglycemia, and his average glucose level is higher than goal. Therefore, continuation of long-acting insulin while withholding scheduled short-acting insulin affords the best approach to glycemic control in the immediate perioperative period.

Continuing insulin lispro along with insulin glargine increases the risk for hypoglycemia during the fasting state. Short-acting insulins should be withheld when a patient is not taking anything by mouth unless the patient requires correction doses for significant hyperglycemia (plasma glucose level >200 mg/dL [11.1 mmol/L]).

Continuous insulin infusion is usually reserved for patients with uncontrolled hyperglycemia, with metabolic acidosis, or who are undergoing high-risk procedures (such as cardiac surgery). This patient has an acceptable plasma glucose level and is undergoing intermediate-risk surgery.

No insulin therapy increases the risk of significant hyperglycemia in this patient under physiologic stress. Therefore, treatment is indicated to prevent significant increases in the plasma glucose level.

- Continuation of long-acting insulin while withholding scheduled short-acting insulin during fasting affords the best approach to glycemic control in the immediate perioperative period.

Bibliography

Inzucchi SE. Management of hyperglycemia in the hospital setting. N Engl J Med. 2006 Nov 2;355(18):1903-11. [PMID: 17079764]

Item 32   Answer: C

Educational Objective: Treat bipolar I disorder.

Treatment with the atypical antipsychotic drug quetiapine is appropriate for this patient with bipolar I disorder, which is defined as one or more manic episodes. A manic episode is characterized by at least 7 days of severe, abnormally expansive, euphoric, or irritable mood associated with at least three of the following symptoms (four if irritable mood only): grandiosity or inflated self-esteem, pressured speech, flight of ideas, distractibility, increased goal-directed activity or psychomotor agitation, excessive involvement in pleasurable activities with high potential for adverse consequences (for example, spending sprees or sexual encounters), and lessened need for sleep. Dysfunction is substantial. The episode is not attributable to the physiologic effects of a substance or to another medical condition. Most patients with bipolar I disorder experience depressive episodes and are at an increased risk for suicide. Periods of depression are more frequent than periods of mania or hypomania in patients with bipolar disorder.

In selecting therapy for patients with bipolar disorder, it is paramount to identify the patient's current phase of illness. For the manic or hypomanic phase of illness, there are 10 different treatments, including one typical antipsychotic agent, lithium, two antiepileptic agents, and six atypical antipsychotic agents. Patients presenting in the depressive phase of illness have two treatment options (quetiapine monotherapy or combination olanzapine-fluoxetine). Different treatment options are available for patients in the maintenance phase of illness. Because identifying the patient's phase of illness and determining complex treatment choices are required, it is paramount that psychiatrists are involved in the care of patients with bipolar disorder.

This patient has acute depression. FDA-approved pharmacologic treatments for bipolar depression are quetiapine alone and combination olanzapine-fluoxetine. Patients with bipolar depression treated with quetiapine should be monitored for hypersomnolence, weight gain, tardive dyskinesia, and hyperglycemia. Lamotrigine is FDA approved for maintenance treatment of bipolar I disorder. Lamotrigine can be prescribed for patients taking quetiapine who experience unacceptable side effects or no improvement of depression.

Antidepressant monotherapy is not recommended (nor FDA approved) for depressed patients with bipolar disorder given lack of efficacy and risk for switching affected patients to hypomania or mania. Therefore, this patient should not receive desipramine, paroxetine, or venlafaxine.

KEY POINT

- FDA-approved pharmacologic treatments for bipolar depression are quetiapine monotherapy and combination olanzapine-fluoxetine.

Bibliography

Frye MA. Clinical practice. Bipolar disorder—a focus on depression. N Engl J Med. 2011 Jan 6;364(1):51-9. [PMID: 21208108]

Item 33   Answer: B

Educational Objective: Manage suspected severe obstructive sleep apnea in the postoperative setting.

This patient should keep the head of his bed elevated at 30 degrees. He is at high risk for obstructive sleep apnea (OSA) as evidenced by his STOP-BANG score of 6 (snoring, observed apneic episodes, hypertension, BMI >35, age >50 years, and male gender). Patients with a STOP-BANG score greater than or equal to 5 have an increased risk for severe OSA and postoperative morbidity. Conservative postoperative measures that may reduce the risk of pulmonary complications from suspected OSA include nonsupine positioning (keeping the head of the bed at 30 degrees), careful use of sedatives and opioids, and continuous pulse oximetry.

Nasogastric intubation is not appropriate in this patient because it is not known to alter risk of complications from possible OSA postoperatively. Nasogastric tubes are associated with an increased risk of aspiration and pneumonia. Good evidence supports the selective use of nasogastric intubation for the same indications as in the nonoperative setting (for example, severe gastric distention and intractable large-volume emesis).

The patient has no wheezing, dyspnea, or other evidence of small airway obstruction. Therefore, he has no indication for the use of albuterol.

Continuous positive airway pressure (CPAP) ventilation is not indicated at this time. The patient is alert, breathing comfortably, and oxygenating well. Furthermore, his pain is well controlled, so he will not require high doses of systemic opioids. The American Society of Anesthesiology recommends only initiating CPAP for patients at risk for OSA who develop hypoxia or apneic episodes. At least one study has suggested that empiric use of CPAP for all patients at risk for OSA did not improve outcomes and increased length of hospital stay.

KEY POINT

- Conservative postoperative measures that may reduce the risk of pulmonary complications from suspected obstructive sleep apnea include nonsupine positioning, careful use of sedatives and opioids, and continuous pulse oximetry.

Bibliography

American Society of Anesthesiologists Task Force on Perioperative Management of Patients with Obstructive Sleep Apnea. Practice guidelines for the perioperative management of patients with obstructive sleep apnea: an updated report by the American Society of Anesthesiologists Task Force on Perioperative Management of Patients with Obstructive Sleep Apnea. Anesthesiology. 2014 Feb;120(2):268-86. [PMID: 24346178]

Item 34   Answer: E

Educational Objective: Manage preoperative evaluation in a patient undergoing low-risk surgery.

This patient is scheduled for cataract extraction, which is a low-risk surgical procedure and requires no specific diagnostic studies for preoperative evaluation. For these and other low-risk invasive procedures, including hernia repairs and superficial surgeries, routine preoperative diagnostic testing is very low yield and unlikely to affect perioperative management. In such situations, diagnostic testing should only be ordered if it is otherwise indicated outside of the preoperative context (such as ordering a urinalysis in a patient with dysuria).

Preoperative chest radiography rarely adds useful information in the evaluation of patients at risk for perioperative pulmonary complications. At least four systematic reviews and guidelines recommend against routine preoperative chest radiography in patients without suspicion of intrathoracic disease.

Routine assessment of blood counts or coagulation parameters is not indicated for most surgical procedures, including low-risk eye surgery. Evaluation for adequate hemostasis requires only a thorough history and physical examination except for procedures in which even a small amount of bleeding could be catastrophic (for example, intracranial surgery). A leukocyte count is indicated only if there is a concern for bone marrow abnormalities or infection. Hemoglobin and hematocrit are reasonable to obtain in patients with findings suggestive of anemia or undergoing large blood loss surgery (such as total hip arthroplasty).

Electrocardiography is not routinely indicated for any surgery and should only be obtained prior to low-risk surgery if there is concern for new or evolving cardiac disease. According to the American College of Cardiology/American Heart Association guidelines, patients with coronary artery disease, arrhythmias, or coronary artery disease equivalents should have electrocardiography performed within 30 days of non–low-risk surgery.

Serum electrolytes and creatinine measurements are not necessary before low-risk surgery unless the patient has signs or symptoms suggestive of active disease that would affect these values (such as vomiting or diarrhea). Even for patients with chronic diseases or medications that may affect kidney function or electrolytes, assessment before low-risk procedures is necessary only if there has been a significant change in the patient's status (such as a recent increase in diuretic dose).

KEY POINT

- Routine preoperative diagnostic testing is generally not recommended for healthy patients undergoing low-risk surgery.

Bibliography

Keay L, Lindsley K, Tielsch J, Katz J, Schein O. Routine preoperative medical testing for cataract surgery. Cochrane Database Syst Rev. 2012 Mar 14;3:CD007293. [PMID: 22419323]

Item 35   Answer: A

Educational Objective: Evaluate a breast mass in a young woman.

The most appropriate management of this woman's breast mass is diagnostic ultrasound. Although up to 90% of breast masses are benign cysts or fibroadenomas, neither the history nor the physical examination can definitively rule in or rule out underlying malignancy with accuracy. Therefore, a palpable mass requires further evaluation with either mammography or ultrasonography; in this 29-year-old woman, a diagnostic ultrasound is the most appropriate next step as it is more sensitive than mammography in younger women. Ultrasonography can effectively determine whether the lesion is solid or cystic, delineate its contours, and can help determine whether additional evaluation with biopsy is indicated.

Mammography, whether digital or film, is less sensitive in women younger than 35 years because of increased breast density. Therefore, ultrasonography is the most appropriate initial imaging choice for this patient.

Aspiration biopsy should not be the next step in this young woman at low risk for breast cancer. She has no family or personal history of breast cancer, has no history of thoracic irradiation, and is not obese. Ultrasonography is the most sensitive and noninvasive way to determine whether or not a biopsy is necessary.

There is no need to stop hormonal contraception in a young woman at risk for pregnancy in the absence of neoplasia or a high risk for neoplasia. One of the therapeutic benefits of combined hormonal contraception is a reduction in prevalence of breast cysts. Given the individualized risk stratification for this young woman, with low risk for breast malignancy, it is reasonable to continue her method of contraception until there is definition of the breast mass.

A palpable breast mass requires further evaluation at any age. The history and physical examination are unlikely to rule out malignancy, and a malignant lesion must be ruled out.

KEY POINT

- A palpable breast mass always requires further evaluation with either mammography or ultrasonography; ultrasonography is a more sensitive test in women younger than 35 years.

Bibliography

Onstad M, Stuckey A. Benign breast disorders. Obstet Gynecol Clin North Am. 2013 Sep;40(3):459-73. [PMID: 24021252]

Item 36   Answer: B

Educational Objective: Treat systemic exertion intolerance disease (formerly known as chronic fatigue syndrome) with cognitive-behavioral therapy.

The most appropriate next step in the management of this patient who meets the clinical criteria for systemic exertion intolerance disease (SEID), formerly known as chronic fatigue syndrome, is cognitive-behavioral therapy (CBT). She has severe fatigue that has persisted for more than 6 months, is not due to ongoing exertion, is not relieved by rest, and is interfering with pre-illness daily activities. Additionally, the fatigue is accompanied by unrefreshing sleep, difficulty concentrating, myalgia, and arthralgia. The physical examination is normal, and an extensive evaluation for a secondary underlying medical condition, including sleep disorders, was normal. Further diagnostic testing is not indicated, and efforts should now be concentrated on evidence-based management. The two treatment strategies that have been shown to be of greatest benefit in the management of these patients are CBT and graded exercise programs. Improvements in fatigue and physical function have been demonstrated in several randomized controlled trials. CBT, usually performed by trained clinicians, is designed to assist patients in modifying their illness beliefs and supporting behaviors and to incorporate effective coping strategies into daily life.

Approximately 70% of patients with SEID meet criteria for depression, anxiety, or dysthymia. However, this patient does not meet the current DSM-5 criteria for either depression or anxiety. Citalopram, or any other antidepressant, is unlikely to be of major benefit in this patient.

In short-term (4-week) studies, methylphenidate did improve fatigue in 30% of patients with SEID, although long-term effectiveness and potential adverse effects associated with long-term use are unknown. Additionally, in this patient of childbearing age with hypertension, the short- and long-term risks of this medication would be increased. Therefore, methylphenidate would not be the next best step in management.

Although several viruses have been implicated in the development of SEID, no precise cause has been established, and antiviral medications, such as valacyclovir, have not demonstrated any clear benefit.

KEY POINT

- Cognitive-behavioral therapy and graded exercise programs have been shown to improve fatigue and physical functioning in patients with systemic exertion intolerance disease.

Bibliography

White PD, Goldsmith KA, Johnson AL, et al; PACE trial management group. Comparison of adaptive pacing therapy, cognitive behaviour therapy, graded exercise therapy, and specialist medical care for chronic fatigue syndrome (PACE): a randomized trial. Lancet. 2011 Mar 5;377(9768):823-36. [PMID: 21334061]

Item 37   Answer: C

Educational Objective: Manage contraception in a young woman with complex migraine.

The most appropriate contraceptive method to recommend to this woman is an intrauterine device (IUD), along with condom use to reduce risk from sexually transmitted infections. Evidence shows that IUDs can be offered to nulliparous or multiparous women across the entire reproductive span, with high rates of continuation and efficacy. There is no evidence of increased risk of pelvic inflammatory disease, infection, or infertility with IUDs. There are two types of IUDs available, one that is hormone free, and one that

contains levonorgestrel. The levonorgestrel IUD generally causes significant diminution of menstrual bleeding, although endometrial response is variable. Given that this patient did not tolerate progestin well, the hormone-free IUD is a reasonable choice also.

In choosing contraception, patient preference, acceptability, concurrent medical conditions, and prior response to other methods should be considered. Because of her migraine with visual aura, this patient should not be treated with an estrogen-containing contraceptive. Although the absolute risk of venous thromboembolism or stroke in young women is low, this risk is increased by a history of migraine with visual aura when estrogen-containing preparations are used. Therefore, either an estrogen-progestin oral contraceptive or a vaginal ring is contraindicated.

This patient also indicated that she experienced unpredictable breakthrough bleeding with depot medroxyprogesterone acetate injections, which is a common side effect. Other progestin-only methods, including implantable inserts and pills, although frequently inducing periods of amenorrhea, may all be associated with breakthrough or irregular bleeding and may be less desirable for this patient.

KEY POINT

- Due to increased stroke risk, combined hormonal contraception containing estrogen is contraindicated in women with a history of migraines preceded by visual aura.

Bibliography

Curtis KM, Tepper NK, Jamieson DJ, Marchbanks PA. Adaptation of the World Health Organization's Selected Practice Recommendations for Contraceptive Use for the United States. Contraception. 2013 May;87(5):513-6. [PMID: 23040134]

Item 38   Answer: B

Educational Objective: Recognize types of bias that affect screening tests.

Length-time bias is the most likely explanation for the positive outcome of the study. The apparent benefits of early diagnosis and intervention on screen-detected cases compared with cases detected by disease symptoms and signs are almost always more favorable than the true effects seen when the outcomes of an overall screened population are compared with an overall population that is not screened for the disease. This difference is caused by several types of bias that tend to occur when examining the effectiveness of screening studies, one of which is length-time bias. Because indolent disease has a longer latent period than more aggressive forms of disease (which are more likely to be detected with onset of symptoms), indolent disease is more likely to be detected by screening. Length-time bias occurs when there is overrepresentation of indolent (low-grade) disease in the screen-detected cohort and overrepresentation of aggressive disease in the symptom-detected (non-screened) cohort, as was the case in this hypothetical study. This makes the screen-detected cohort, with more indolent disease, falsely appear to have a better prognosis than the patients who present with symptoms and signs in the non-screened cohort. A drastic type of length-time bias is termed over-diagnosis and occurs when a disease that is so indolent that it would not otherwise have been clinically significant during a patient's lifespan is detected through screening.

Contamination bias occurs when the control group is unintentionally exposed to the intervention, which biases the estimate toward the null hypothesis. Contamination bias was unlikely in this case as there was little crossover between groups.

Observer bias occurs when knowledge of the hypothesis or intervention received influences data recording, which would not be expected to be an influence in this study in which the researchers were blinded.

Selection bias refers to systematic error in a study resulting from the manner in which the subjects are selected for the study. It can influence the results when the characteristics of the subjects selected for a study differ systematically from those in the target population or when the study and comparison groups are selected from different populations. An example is volunteer bias, in which patients who seek participation in a screening study are often healthier than those who do not undergo screening. Because the patients in this study were randomly selected from the general population, this would not be a likely cause of significant bias.

KEY POINT

- Randomized controlled trials of screening tests may be affected by length-time bias, which occurs when there is overrepresentation of indolent disease in the screen-detected cohort and overrepresentation of aggressive disease in the symptom-detected (non-screened) cohort.

Bibliography
Berry DA. Failure of researchers, reviewers, editors, and the media to understand flaws in cancer screening studies: application to an article in Cancer. Cancer. 2014 Sep 15;120(18):2784-91. [PMID: 24925345]

Item 39   Answer: A
Educational Objective: Manage prepatellar bursitis.

The most appropriate next step in management of this patient is to aspirate the bursal fluid collection for diagnostic and therapeutic purposes. Bursal fluid aspiration and analysis should be performed in all patients who present with prepatellar bursitis. Aspiration is necessary to definitively distinguish the cause of prepatellar bursitis (namely, trauma, gout, and infection). Gram stain and culture of the bursal fluid should be obtained and analyzed for leukocyte count and for the presence of crystals. An extremely elevated leukocyte count (>50,000/μL [50 × 10^9/L]) should raise suspicion for septic bursitis, although a lower count does not entirely eliminate this possibility.

Compression is indicated only after bursal fluid aspiration has been performed. Dressings should be worn for 24 to 48 hours, and patients should be advised to avoid applying direct pressure to the bursa. Once the compression dressing is removed, patients should be advised to wear a neoprene sleeve.

Glucocorticoid injection into the fluid collection is not indicated for patients presenting with acute prepatellar bursitis. Instead, glucocorticoid injection should be reserved for chronic prepatellar bursitis that has a noninfectious cause or that is postinfectious (negative cultures have been obtained after antibiotic administration).

Imaging, either with plain radiography or ultrasonography, is not usually required for the diagnosis of prepatellar bursitis. Plain radiography may show soft-tissue swelling on lateral views but rarely aids in establishing the correct diagnosis. Ultrasonography will show a fluid collection but will not help identify the cause. Therefore, plain radiography or ultrasonography is not indicated in this patient.

KEY POINT

- Bursal fluid aspiration should be performed for both therapeutic and diagnostic purposes in all patients who present with prepatellar bursitis.

Bibliography
Baumbach SF, Lobo CM, Badyine I, Mutschler W, Kanz KG. Prepatellar and olecranon bursitis: literature review and development of a treatment algorithm. Arch Orthop Trauma Surg. 2014 Mar;134(3):359-70. [PMID: 24305696]

Item 40   Answer: A
Educational Objective: Manage the risk of perioperative adrenal insufficiency in a patient on chronic glucocorticoid therapy.

The most appropriate management on the morning of surgery is for the patient to take her current morning prednisone dose of 5 mg. For patients on chronic glucocorticoids, appropriate medical management is crucial to prevent complications such as organ transplant rejection and adrenal insufficiency. Evidence to guide decision making is sparse; a recent Cochrane review found the available data insufficient to provide recommendations. Despite this, expert advice provides a fair consensus to inform clinical decision making. For patients taking low doses of prednisone (<10 mg/d), stress dosing of glucocorticoids typically is not required, even before high-risk surgical procedures (such as intrathoracic surgery). Instead, patients should take their usual glucocorticoid dose on the morning of surgery. This patient is scheduled for a low-risk procedure (carpal tunnel release) and is on a low dose of prednisone; therefore, taking the usual dose of prednisone on the morning of surgery is the most appropriate management.

Doubling the patient's usual prednisone dose is not the most appropriate choice because she is undergoing a low-risk procedure with minimal risk of perioperative adrenal insufficiency. Increasing her prednisone would only increase her risk of other complications, such as hyperglycemia.

Intravenous hydrocortisone is not necessary for this patient due to her low daily dose of prednisone and the low-risk nature of the procedure. Empiric intravenous hydrocortisone is reasonable for patients with primary adrenal insufficiency or for those on high doses of glucocorticoids (equivalent of prednisone ≥10 mg/d) who are undergoing higher risk surgeries. In those circumstances, intravenous hydrocortisone, 50 to 100 mg, is administered shortly before anesthesia induction and then continued every 8 hours for up to 48 hours after surgery.

Although the patient is on a low dose, withholding prednisone for the procedure is not recommended because interrupting therapy might cause unnecessary fluctuations in her immunosuppression or glucocorticoid levels without a clear benefit to her surgical outcome.

KEY POINT

- For patients taking low doses of glucocorticoids, stress dosing typically is not required; patients should take their usual glucocorticoid dose on the morning of surgery.

Bibliography

Njoke MJ. Patients with chronic endocrine disease. Med Clin N Am. 2013 Nov;97(6):1123-37. [PMID: 24182723]

Item 41   Answer: C

Educational Objective: Evaluate decision-making capacity in a patient with mild dementia.

This patient has the capacity to make a decision about the proposed procedure; therefore, the physician should proceed with coronary angiography. Informed consent includes a discussion of the information that a reasonable patient would want to know about his or her illness (proposed diagnostic and treatment plans, the risks and benefits of the proposed plans, and any alternatives), an assessment of patient understanding, and the acceptance or refusal of the treatment. The patient must have decision-making capacity and make each decision of his or her own free will for consent to be considered valid. A patient (for example, one with mild dementia) may have the capacity to make some decisions but not other more complex ones. The graver the consequences of the decision, the greater the capacity required. Decision-making capacity exists when a patient demonstrates an ability to understand relevant information, appreciate the situation and its possible consequences, manipulate information rationally, and make a reasoned choice. Despite this patient's mild dementia, he fulfills these standards and therefore has the capacity to make a decision regarding the procedure.

There is no need to wait for the patient's wife to consent to the procedure. Indeed, waiting for his wife to arrive and delaying treatment increases the patient's risk for harm.

A Mini-Mental State Examination is unnecessary. It will likely confirm the diagnosis of mild dementia but will not help in assessing the patient's decision-making capacity. A diagnosis of dementia or a mental illness does not necessarily mean that a patient is incapable of making health care decisions. The clinician must assess whether or not the patient's decision appears consistent with his or her values and goals of care. If it does, it can probably be accepted as valid.

It is unnecessary to obtain a second opinion to assess this patient's decision-making capacity. The core components of decision-making capacity are understanding the situation at hand, understanding the risks and benefits of the decision being made, and the ability to communicate a decision. The patient has demonstrated these core elements.

KEY POINT

- Decision-making capacity exists when a patient demonstrates an ability to understand relevant information, appreciate the situation and its possible consequences, manipulate information rationally, and make a reasoned choice.

Bibliography

Leo RJ. Competency and the capacity to make treatment decisions: a primer for primary care physicians. Prim Care Companion J Clin Psychiatry. 1999 Oct;1(5):131-141. [PMID: 15014674]

Item 42   Answer: A

Educational Objective: Diagnose epididymitis.

The most likely diagnosis in this patient is epididymitis, which causes pain superolateral to the testicle and results from inflammation of the epididymis. Symptom onset in epididymitis is usually subacute, although in some patients the pain may develop relatively acutely or may be more chronic in nature. Examination is remarkable for pain that is relieved by testicular elevation. Epididymitis most commonly has an infectious cause and has a bimodal age distribution of men younger than 35 years and older than 55 years of age. Patients younger than 35 years are more likely to have sexually transmitted etiologies such as chlamydia or gonorrhea, whereas the causes in older patients are usually *Escherichia coli*, Enterobacteriaceae, or *Pseudomonas* species. This patient's presentation includes young age, history of unprotected sexual activity, subacute onset of symptoms, lower urinary tract symptoms, bogginess and pain to palpation over the superior pole of the testis, and pain relief with elevation of the testis, all clinical findings consistent with epididymitis.

Testicular torsion presents acutely along with nausea and vomiting. Unlike in this patient, the testicle would be high riding and transversely oriented, with pain that worsens with manual elevation. Doppler ultrasonography to assess blood flow is sensitive (82%) and specific (100%) in making the diagnosis of testicular torsion.

Dysuria, frequency, and urgency may accompany epididymitis and suggest the possible presence of a urinary tract infection. However, the presence of testicular bogginess and pain on examination with a lack of significant pyuria on urinalysis does not support the diagnosis of urinary tract infection.

Varicocele does not present with subacute onset, lower urinary tract symptoms, and epididymal swelling and pain. Furthermore, physical examination would reveal a characteristic "bag of worms" consistency with palpation of the scrotal contents that increases with standing and decreases when supine.

KEY POINT

- Epididymitis causes subacute pain in the superolateral testis, is often associated with lower urinary tract symptoms, and is relieved by testicular elevation.

Bibliography

Tracy CR, Steers WD, Costabile R. Diagnosis and management of epididymitis. Urol Clin North Am. 2008 Feb;35(1):101-8. [PMID: 18061028]

Item 43   Answer: B

Educational Objective: Treat stress urinary incontinence in a woman.

Pelvic floor muscle training (PFMT) is most appropriate for this patient. The involuntary loss of urine with sneezing, coughing, laughing, or physical exertion is consistent with stress incontinence. Stress incontinence is thought to be related to anatomic changes in which the support structures of the urethra are weakened (through age, pregnancy and childbirth, or repetitive pelvic floor stress), decreasing the ability of the urethra to maintain adequate pressure to prevent incontinence. Treatment for stress incontinence begins with conservative measures. In this patient, the first-line therapeutic option is bladder training using PFMT in conjunction with weight loss counseling. These measures decrease bladder pressure and increase the pressure generated by the urethra and surrounding tissues.

Weight loss in overweight and obese women generally improves urinary control. An 8% decrease in BMI has been shown to reduce incontinence by 50%. PFMT in women involves learning repetitive exercises (Kegel exercises) to strengthen the voluntary urethral sphincter and levator ani muscles. Outcomes are improved when PFMT is combined with biofeedback and when skilled physical therapists direct the training. Adherence remains an issue, as PFMT must be done repetitively and consistently for best results.

Oxybutynin is one of several available anticholinergic agents approved for treating overactive bladder. It is not indicated for treatment of uncomplicated stress incontinence, nor is pharmacotherapy a first-line therapy for this disorder.

Measurement of postvoid residual urine volume is not necessary in this patient whose presentation is consistent with stress incontinence. Clinical evaluation and history, including the patient's report of frequency, severity, pre-cipitants, and impact on quality of life, are adequate for discriminating among types of incontinence and for making nonsurgical treatment decisions. Voiding diaries are useful in defining symptoms.

Prompted voiding and scheduled toileting may help older patients with functional urinary incontinence. Providing assistance and scheduled toileting are effective for patients who have impaired mobility or cognition, neither of which is present in this patient.

Urodynamic studies are not indicated in women with uncomplicated stress urinary incontinence. Compared with diagnosing the patient based on symptom report, evidence-based reviews indicate that urodynamic studies do not better predict response to treatment.

KEY POINT

- Pelvic floor muscle training, along with other conservative measures such as weight loss, is first-line therapy for women with stress urinary incontinence.

Bibliography

Qaseem A, Dallas P, Forciea MA, et al; Clinical Guidelines Committee of the American College of Physicians. Nonsurgical management of urinary incontinence in women: a clinical practice guideline from the American College of Physicians. Ann Intern Med. 2014 Sep;161(6):429-40. [PMID: 25222388]

Item 44   Answer: B

Educational Objective: Screen for cervical cancer in a young woman.

This patient should receive a Pap smear in 2 years. According to the U.S. Preventive Services Task Force and the American Congress of Obstetricians and Gynecologists, women aged 21 to 65 years should be screened for cervical cancer every 3 years with cytology (Pap smear). Performing screening more frequently adds little benefit while significantly increasing harms. Harms can include evaluation and treatment of transient lesions as well as false-positive screening results, which may lead to unnecessary colposcopies and emotional distress. Screening for cervical cancer is not recommended in women younger than 21 years, women age 65 years and older who are not at high risk and have had adequate prior Pap smears, and women who have had a hysterectomy with removal of the cervix with no previous history of a precancerous lesion. This patient had a normal Pap smear 1 year ago; therefore, she will be due for her next Pap smear in 2 years.

Owing to poor specificity, screening with human papillomavirus (HPV) DNA testing alone is not recommended. HPV testing is not recommended in women younger than 30 years, as HPV is not only highly prevalent but is also more likely to resolve without treatment in this age group. In women aged 30 to 65 years who want to lengthen the screening interval, a combination of cytology and HPV testing can be performed every 5 years. Women should be informed that there is an increased likelihood of receiving a positive screening result with HPV testing and cytology than with cytology alone. A positive HPV test result likely requires additional immediate testing and also involves more frequent surveillance.

All females aged 11 to 26 years should be vaccinated against HPV. HPV vaccination status does not alter recommendations for cervical cancer screening.

KEY POINT

- Women aged 21 to 65 years should be screened for cervical cancer every 3 years with cytology (Pap smear); in women aged 30 to 65 years who want to lengthen the screening interval, a combination of cytology and human papillomavirus testing can be performed every 5 years.

Bibliography

Moyer VA; U.S. Preventive Services Task Force. Screening for cervical cancer: U.S. Preventive Services Task Force recommendation statement. Ann Intern Med. 2012 Jun 19;156(12):880-91, W312. Erratum in: Ann Intern Med. 2013 Jun 4;158(11):852. [PMID: 22711081]

Item 45   Answer: B

Educational Objective: Treat hyperlipidemia in a patient with diabetes mellitus and elevated cardiovascular risk.

The most appropriate treatment for this patient is high-intensity statin therapy, such as with atorvastatin. Strong evidence indicates that statins are effective in both primary and secondary prevention of atherosclerotic cardiovascular disease (ASCVD). According to the American College of Cardiology/American Heart Association guidelines, this patient with diabetes and no clinical ASCVD meets the criteria for one of four patient groups that have been shown to benefit from the treatment of hyperlipidemia with statin therapy. For patients 40 to 75 years of age with diabetes mellitus and an LDL cholesterol level of 70 to 189 mg/dL (1.8-4.90 mmol/L), intensity of statin therapy is dictated by the estimated 10-year risk for ASCVD as determined by the Pooled Cohort Equations. High-intensity statin therapy (for example, atorvastatin, 40-80 mg/d, or rosuvastatin, 20-40 mg/d) is recommended for all patients with a 10-year ASCVD risk of 7.5% or higher, and moderate-intensity therapy is indicated for patients with a risk of less than 7.5%. This patient's 10-year ASCVD risk exceeds 7.5%; therefore, high-intensity therapy is recommended.

Significant reductions in cardiovascular events have not been clearly demonstrated with fibrate monotherapy, rendering gemfibrozil an inferior choice for this patient with elevated risk for clinical ASCVD. Fibrates are indicated for patients with triglyceride levels greater than 500 mg/dL (5.65 mmol/L), patients with hypertriglyceridemia-induced pancreatitis, and patients who have an inadequate response to statin therapy.

Moderate-intensity statin therapy (for example, simvastatin, 20-40 mg/d; atorvastatin, 10-20 mg/d; or rosuvastatin, 5-10 mg/d) is not appropriate for this patient with

diabetes, elevated 10-year risk for ASCVD, other cardiovascular risk factors (family history of premature cardiovascular disease), and no contraindications to high-intensity therapy. Moderate-intensity statin therapy is an acceptable alternative to high-intensity therapy in patients who tolerate statins poorly or have risk factors for statin-associated adverse effects (impaired kidney or liver function, history of muscle disorders, use of drugs affecting statin metabolism [calcium channel blockers, fibrates, protease inhibitors, amiodarone, macrolide antibiotics], and age greater than 75 years). Because none of these factors are present in this patient, high-intensity statin therapy would be the optimal therapeutic approach given his risk profile.

Therapeutic lifestyle changes are a cornerstone of treatment for hyperlipidemia and should be encouraged in all patients; however, additional treatment with statins is indicated in this patient with an elevated 10-year risk of ASCVD and diabetes.

KEY POINT

- In adults 40 to 75 years of age with diabetes mellitus, an LDL cholesterol level of 70 to 189 mg/dL (1.8-4.90 mmol/L), and an estimated 10-year atherosclerotic cardiovascular disease risk of 7.5% or higher, high-intensity statin therapy is recommended.

Bibliography

Stone NJ, Robinson JG, Lichtenstein AH, et al; American College of Cardiology/American Heart Association Task Force on Practice Guidelines. 2013 ACC/AHA guideline on the treatment of blood cholesterol to reduce atherosclerotic cardiovascular risk in adults: a report of the American College of Cardiology/American Heart Association Task Force on Practice Guidelines. Circulation. 2014 Jun 24;129(25 Suppl 2): S1-45. Erratum in: Circulation. 2014 Jun 24;129(25 Suppl 2):S46-8. [PMID: 24222016]

Item 46   Answer: D

Educational Objective: Manage cardiac testing in an asymptomatic patient with low cardiovascular risk.

This patient needs no further testing. Although he is obese and has a history of hypertension, he is at low risk for cardiovascular disease. Risk assessment for atherosclerotic cardiovascular disease (ASCVD) has traditionally been with the Framingham risk score, although the American College of Cardiology/American Heart Association Pooled Cohort Equations, a new method for assessment that includes additional variables for risk stratification, is increasingly being used. With this method, a 10-year risk of ASCVD of less than 5% is considered low risk, 5% to below 7.5% is considered intermediate risk, and 7.5% and above is designated as high risk. This patient has a calculated 10-year risk of 3.2%, making him at low risk for ASCVD. Therefore, no additional testing is indicated at present.

Patients at low risk for cardiovascular disease, such as this one, do not benefit from aggressive risk factor modification and therefore would not benefit from screening using nontraditional risk factors, such as coronary artery calcium scoring. The U.S. Preventive Services Task Force (USPSTF) concludes that there is insufficient evidence to assess the balance of benefits and harms for using nontraditional risk factors to screen asymptomatic, intermediate-risk patients without a history of coronary heart disease. Nontraditional risk factors include ankle-brachial index, CT to assess coronary artery calcification, high-sensitivity C-reactive protein, carotid intima-media thickness, homocysteine, and lipoprotein(a) level. Furthermore, the Society of Cardiovascular Computed Tomography, through the Choosing Wisely campaign, advises against ordering coronary artery calcium scoring for screening purposes in asymptomatic individuals who are at low risk for cardiovascular disease except for those with a family history of premature coronary artery disease.

The USPSTF and the American College of Physicians recommend against resting or exercise electrocardiography (ECG) for cardiovascular disease screening in asymptomatic adults who are at low risk for cardiovascular events. This patient is asymptomatic and is at low risk for cardiovascular disease; therefore, resting and exercise ECG are not indicated. For individuals at intermediate risk for cardiovascular disease, the USPSTF concludes that there is insufficient evidence to assess the balance of benefits and harms for screening with resting or exercise ECG.

KEY POINT

- In asymptomatic patients at low risk for cardiovascular disease, cardiac testing is unnecessary.

Bibliography

Chou R, Arora B, Dana T, Fu R, Walker M, Humphrey L. Screening Asymptomatic Adults for Coronary Heart Disease With Resting or Exercise Electrocardiography: Systematic Review to Update the 2004 U.S. Preventive Services Task Force Recommendation. Rockville (MD): Agency for Healthcare Research and Quality (US); 2011 Sep. Available at www.ncbi.nlm.nih.gov/books/NBK63671/. [PMID: 21977523]

Item 47 Answer: D

Educational Objective: Reduce fall risk in an older patient with vitamin D supplementation.

Vitamin D should be prescribed for this older patient with a high risk for falls. Vitamin D has neuromuscular benefits beyond its role in bone health. Several randomized controlled trials and meta-analyses have shown vitamin D supplementation to significantly decrease the risk for falls in older community-dwelling adults, even in those with normal vitamin D levels. The mechanism of vitamin D supplementation in preventing falls is unclear, although changes in bone mineral density and muscle function have been proposed as contributing factors. With an excellent safety profile, low cost, and a number needed to treat of 15, vitamin D supplementation is an underutilized therapy for fall prevention. The American Geriatrics Society recommends 800 units daily for this purpose.

Compression stockings are used in some patients with orthostatic hypotension to prevent pooling of blood in dependent areas. However, compression stockings are difficult to use, making adherence challenging, and other potential adverse effects such as skin breakdown may occur. Therefore, compression stockings would not be indicated to decrease falls in this patient without evidence of orthostatic hypotension.

Hip protectors are mechanical devices intended to decrease the risk of fractures if falls occur; they do not prevent the falls themselves. Multiple studies have shown that adherence with this intervention is low and there is no compelling evidence that they are effective in preventing hip fractures. Hip protectors would therefore not be indicated in this patient.

Mineralocorticoid supplementation can be helpful in ameliorating orthostasis; however, there is no evidence that this patient's falls are due to orthostatic symptoms. Consequently, there is no indication that mineralocorticoid supplementation would be helpful.

KEY POINT

- Vitamin D supplementation decreases fall risk in older adults, irrespective of vitamin deficiency.

Bibliography

Panel on Prevention of Falls in Older Persons, American Geriatrics Society and British Geriatrics Society. Summary of the updated American Geriatrics Society/British Geriatrics Society clinical practice guideline for prevention of falls in older persons. J Am Geriatr Soc. 2011 Jan;59(1):148-57. [PMID: 21226685]

Item 48 Answer: C

Educational Objective: Diagnose depression in the setting of terminal illness.

This patient's sense of guilt is indicative of pathologic depression. Although anticipatory grief may be common at the end of life, depression is never normal in dying patients. However, it can be very challenging to differentiate normal grief from depression in terminally ill patients. Validated depression screening tools, such as the PHQ-9, rely heavily on the presence of symptoms associated with functions necessary to maintain life (historically termed vegetative symptoms) such as changes in appetite, sleep, and energy level, which are common and expected in patients with advanced illness. This makes these instruments more difficult to interpret when assessing for depression. Many patients with terminal illness, such as this one, verbalize thoughts of death or express a desire for hastened death. Persistent, pervasive thoughts of suicide, which are not seen in this patient, are not normal and should be addressed promptly and aggressively when present. Guilt or self-blame is unique to depression and not seen in normal grief. Other symptoms unique to depression include hopelessness, helplessness, and worthlessness. When differentiating depression from grief, it is important to assess for these symptoms, as depression is highly treatable even in terminally ill patients.

Adjustment disorder with depressed mood occurs in patients who do not meet the criteria for major depression but have a depressed mood. Symptoms begin within

3 months of a stressful event and do not last longer than 6 months. This patient's guilt is indicative of depression, not an adjustment disorder.

Anticipatory grief occurs in patients and loved ones as they mourn the many losses leading up to an expected death. Such grief is waxing and waning in nature, with periods of sadness interspersed with periods of joy.

Grieving that lasts for more than 12 months (6 months in children); is associated with persistent yearning, sorrow, or preoccupation with the deceased; disrupts normal function or social relationships; and is out of proportion to cultural norms is considered pathologic and is termed persistent complex bereavement disorder, formerly complicated grief disorder. Persistent complex bereavement disorder occurs in loved ones after a death, not in the patient who is dying.

KEY POINT

- In a terminally ill patient, feelings of guilt, hopelessness, helplessness, and worthlessness may distinguish depression from anticipatory grief.

Bibliography
Swetz KM, Kamal AH. In the clinic. Palliative care. Ann Intern Med. 2012 Feb 7;156(3):ITC2-1-TC2-16. [PMID: 22312158]

Item 49   Answer: E

Educational Objective: Evaluate a patient for hypogonadism.

A repeat testosterone level is appropriate for this older patient with fatigue, weakness, and erectile dysfunction (ED). Men with specific signs and symptoms of androgen deficiency should be evaluated by measuring morning total testosterone level as the initial diagnostic test. Men with low or low-normal testosterone levels should have confirmatory testing before initiating testosterone therapy, and further evaluation of the cause of hypogonadism should be pursued before treatment is started, if indicated. If the repeat serum total testosterone level is more equivocal (200-350 ng/dL [6.9-12.1 nmol/L]) or if a sex hormone–binding globulin abnormality is likely in the patient being evaluated, a serum free testosterone level by equilibrium dialysis or a calculated serum free testosterone level can determine whether hypogonadism is truly present.

When hypogonadism is confirmed, the next step is to determine whether the patient has primary or secondary hypogonadism by measuring the luteinizing hormone (LH) and follicle-stimulating hormone (FSH) levels. Primary hypogonadism is indicated by supranormal LH and FSH levels. If secondary hypogonadism is confirmed by inappropriately normal or low LH and FSH levels, measurement of the serum prolactin level to evaluate for hyperprolactinemia and iron saturation level (transferrin saturation and ferritin levels) to exclude hemochromatosis should be performed to assess for the possible cause. In addition, the presence of any additional pituitary hormone deficiencies should be assessed.

An MRI of the pituitary gland should be ordered to exclude hypothalamic or pituitary masses as the cause of decreased gonadotropin production and secretion if any symptoms consistent with mass effect are present, including headaches, visual field changes, a serum total testosterone level less than 150 ng/dL (5.2 nmol/L), an increased prolactin level, or any additional pituitary hormonal deficiencies.

Testosterone replacement in older men should be given only in the setting of hypogonadism that is based on symptoms (such as decreased libido and generalized muscle weakness) and morning serum total testosterone levels lower than 200 ng/dL (6.9 nmol/L) on at least two separate occasions. Therefore, this patient needs confirmation on repeat testing before considering testosterone replacement therapy.

KEY POINT

- Men with low or low-normal testosterone levels should have confirmatory morning serum total testosterone testing before initiating testosterone therapy, and further evaluation of the cause of hypogonadism should be pursued before treatment is started.

Bibliography
Heidelbaugh JJ. Management of erectile dysfunction. Am Fam Physician. 2010 Feb 1;81(3):305-12. [PMID: 20112889]

Item 50   Answer: C

Educational Objective: Diagnose plantar fasciitis.

The most likely diagnosis is plantar fasciitis. The pain associated with plantar fasciitis is typically sharp in character and present with the first few steps taken after prolonged inactivity, such as upon awakening in the morning or after sitting for an extended period of time. Plantar fasciitis has a peak incidence between the ages of 40 and 60 years. Risk factors include obesity, pes planus, and a sedentary lifestyle. On examination, there is pain with palpation of the medial calcaneal tubercle where the plantar fascia inserts. Pain is also typically elicited with passive dorsiflexion of the toes (Windlass test).

Achilles tendinopathy is typically associated with posterior heel pain, stiffness, and tenderness approximately 2 to 6 cm proximal to the Achilles tendon insertion. Pain usually develops after there is a rapid increase in exercise level. Pain is generally burning, worsens with activity, and improves with rest.

Heel pad syndrome involves localized inflammation of the soft tissues overlying the heel and is often caused by walking barefoot on hard surfaces. It presents with pain in the middle of the heel that is reproducible on examination, and atrophy of the heel fat pad may occur. Neither of these findings is present in this patient.

Stress fractures typically produce pain in individuals who dramatically increase their physical activity or who exercise repetitively with insufficient rest. The pain associated with a stress fracture of the tarsal navicular bone is usually located on the dorsal midfoot with occasional radiation into the medial arch, which is not present in this patient.

- Plantar fasciitis is characterized by pain and tenderness near the medial plantar heel surface that usually occurs with the first few steps taken after prolonged inactivity.

Bibliography

Young C. In the clinic. Plantar fasciitis. Ann Intern Med. 2012 Jan 3;156(1 Pt 1): ITC1-1-ITC1-15. [PMID: 22213510]

Item 51   Answer: D

Educational Objective: Treat subacute, nonspecific low back pain.

This patient with subacute low back pain would most likely benefit from a trial of massage therapy. Back pain is classified as acute (lasting <4 weeks), subacute (lasting 4-12 weeks), or chronic (lasting >12 weeks); therefore, this patient's clinical findings are consistent with a subacute process. The overall prognosis for most forms of musculoskeletal back pain without neurologic or systemic findings is excellent, and 90% of patients recover within 6 weeks with self-care (remaining active and application of superficial heat) and pharmacologic therapies (acetaminophen or NSAIDs). Patients who do not improve in that time frame may benefit from additional therapeutic interventions, such as spinal manipulation or massage therapy. Massage therapy has been shown to be an effective intervention in patients with subacute or chronic back pain symptoms and would therefore be an appropriate treatment to recommend to this patient. Patients should also be informed that most low back pain resolves spontaneously without intervention.

Bed rest had been historically recommended as a treatment for back pain but has been shown to decrease functional recovery and increase pain levels in many patients. Based on these data, patients with low back pain, such as this one, should be encouraged to maintain their daily activities, if possible.

Despite their anti-inflammatory effect, systemic glucocorticoids (such as prednisone) have not proved effective in treating low back pain when used either for brief treatment periods or longer courses.

Lumbar support has not been demonstrated to be effective in treating low back pain, even in physically active patients. It would therefore not be an appropriate treatment for this patient.

- Massage therapy for low back pain is likely to be helpful in patients with subacute or chronic symptoms and no abnormal neurologic findings.

Bibliography

Furlan AD, Imamura M, Dryden T, Irvin E. Massage for low-back pain. Cochrane Database Syst Rev. 2008 Oct 8;(4):CD001929. [PMID: 18843627]

Item 52   Answer: B

Educational Objective: Continue β-blockers in the perioperative period.

This patient should take his β-blocker, metoprolol, the morning of surgery. He takes three chronic medications, of which two are normally taken in the morning. All medications should be continued uninterrupted throughout surgery unless potential adverse effects from continuation outweigh benefits. Not only is metoprolol important for treatment of his hypertension, but withdrawal of β-blockade in the perioperative setting may cause tachycardia and increased myocardial oxygen demand. The American College of Cardiology (ACC) and the American Heart Association (AHA) provide a level 1 recommendation for the continuation of β-blockers throughout the perioperative period. Thus, metoprolol should be taken the morning of surgery.

Metformin has the potential for causing lactic acidosis and inducing hypoglycemia if taken during fasting. Therefore, it should not be taken on the morning of surgery. Some experts advise withholding this medication for 24 to 48 hours before surgery, although data for the specific withholding timeframe are limited.

The ACC and AHA recommend that for patients currently taking a statin and scheduled for noncardiac surgery, the statin should be continued. This recommendation is based on several systematic reviews that found an association between perioperative statin use and a reduction in postoperative acute coronary syndrome and mortality. This patient should resume his statin therapy in the evening following his operation, maintaining his usual schedule.

- Perioperative β-blockade should be continued uninterrupted in patients who are already taking a β-blocker.

Bibliography

Wijeysundera DN, Duncan D, Nkonde-Price C, et al; ACC/AHA Task Force Members. Perioperative beta blockade in noncardiac surgery: a systematic review for the 2014 ACC/AHA guideline on perioperative cardiovascular evaluation and management of patients undergoing noncardiac surgery: a report of the American College of Cardiology/American Heart Association Task Force on Practice Guidelines. Circulation. 2014 Dec 9;130(24):2246-64. [PMID: 25085964]

Item 53   Answer: A

Educational Objective: Diagnose an anterior cruciate ligament tear.

The most likely diagnosis is an anterior cruciate ligament tear. Anterior cruciate ligament injury usually occurs when a person rapidly decelerates and pivots but may also develop following direct trauma that results in knee hyperextension. A complete tear should be suspected when a popping sound is reported and the patient reports pain and knee instability. The characteristic examination finding is a large effusion with increased laxity seen with both the anterior drawer and Lachman tests. In this patient, the sudden onset of knee pain, swelling, and instability; the mechanism of injury (a noncontact injury that occurred with deceleration and pivoting); and the increased laxity observed on examination with both the anterior drawer and Lachman tests all suggest a complete anterior cruciate ligament tear.

Lateral collateral ligament tears result from laterally directed (varus) forces on the knee and are associated with lateral knee pain, swelling, and instability. On examination, there is lateral joint line tenderness and increased laxity with varus-directed forces. Knee effusions are commonly seen. Although this patient has swelling and instability, which could be consistent with a lateral collateral ligament tear, he does not have lateral joint line tenderness and increased laxity with varus-directed forces, which argue against a lateral collateral ligament tear.

Medial collateral ligament tears occur as a result of a contact injury from a medially directed (valgus) force. Patients with medial collateral ligament tears typically present with medial knee pain and joint instability. On examination, there is medial joint line tenderness and increased laxity with valgus stress testing, which are not seen in this patient. A palpable knee effusion is also commonly present.

Patients with meniscal tears are typically able to bear weight immediately after the injury and are often able to continue participating in the activity they were doing before the injury, unlike this patient. Additionally, patients with meniscal tears will frequently report a locking or catching sensation. On examination, abnormal responses may be seen with both the Thessaly and medial-lateral grind tests. Knee effusions may or may not be present.

KEY POINT

- An anterior cruciate ligament tear is characterized by pain and knee instability that occur after a person rapidly decelerates and pivots; examination findings include a large effusion with increased laxity seen with both the anterior drawer and Lachman tests.

Bibliography
Solomon DH, Simel DL, Bates DW, Katz JN, Schaffer JL. The rational clinical examination. Does this patient have a torn meniscus or ligament of the knee? Value of the physical examination. JAMA. 2001 Oct 3;286(13): 1610-20. [PMID: 11585485]

Item 54　　Answer:　A
Educational Objective: Recognize anchoring as a source of cognitive error.

The care team demonstrated anchoring, a diagnostic cognitive error that results from "locking" onto features of a patient's initial presentation and providing treatment for that diagnosis despite the appearance of new clinical information. In this patient, the care team anchored on the initial history and radiographic findings of constipation and failed to recognize or act upon additional clinical clues, including fever, leukocytosis, and worsening abdominal

pain despite treatment, related to the correct diagnosis of cholecystitis.

Confirmation bias involves using or interpreting information (for example, diagnostic studies) in a way that confirms a current hypothesis. This cognitive error results from the tendency to look for evidence that confirms a suspected diagnosis rather than considering evidence that refutes that diagnosis and may lead to another diagnostic option. Because of anchoring to the initial diagnosis, the care team did not seek additional clinical evidence that could be interpreted to support that diagnosis.

Framing bias is a form of cognitive error that occurs when the way clinical information is presented, or "framed," affects decisions based on that information. An example is the perception of increased effectiveness of a specific therapy when the benefit of treatment is reported in relative instead of absolute terms, since relative benefits frequently appear larger than absolute benefits. Similarly, clinical decisions based on cardiovascular risk may differ if the assessed risk is based on an annual event rate compared with a cumulative 10-year risk. Framing bias does not appear to be a significant factor in the outcome of this case.

Triage cueing occurs when the manner in which triage decisions are made influences the evaluation and diagnosis (for example, when a patient with chest pain is admitted to a cardiology service and receives an extensive evaluation for myocardial infarction rather than an evaluation for gastroesophageal reflux). This patient appears to have been appropriately triaged for initial management, but the subsequent changes in his clinical course were not addressed due to anchoring to the initial diagnosis.

KEY POINT

- Anchoring is a diagnostic cognitive error that results from locking onto features of a patient's initial presentation despite the appearance of new clinical information.

Bibliography
Croskerry P. The importance of cognitive errors in diagnosis and strategies to minimize them. Acad Med. 2003 Aug;78(8):775-80. [PMID: 12915363]

Item 55　　Answer:　D
Educational Objective: Treat acute sinusitis.

This patient, who has acute sinusitis, should be managed with supportive care. Acute sinusitis is most commonly caused by viral infections associated with the common cold, and it has a bacterial etiology in only a small percentage of cases. Acute sinusitis is characterized by symptoms of nasal congestion and obstruction; facial pain, pressure, and fullness that generally worsen when bending forward; headache; purulent nasal discharge; and maxillary tooth pain. When caused by viral infection, fever may be present within the first 24 to 48 hours of symptom onset, often associated with other symptoms such as myalgia and fatigue, but temperature normalizes after this time period. Bacterial sinusitis is more likely if there are severe symptoms associated with a high fever for at least 3 or 4 consecutive days following the onset of illness or if symptoms are persistent (lasting more than 10 days). Initial treatment of acute sinusitis is focused on symptom relief with analgesics, decongestants (systemic or topical), antihistamines, intranasal glucocorticoids, and nasal saline irrigation, and these treatment options would be the most appropriate therapy in this patient who does not have findings concerning for a possible bacterial etiology.

Antibiotics are not indicated in this patient at this time. Although more than 90% of cases of acute sinusitis are viral in origin, antibiotics are regularly prescribed for patients presenting with acute sinusitis symptoms. Antibiotics should be reserved for patients with persistent and severe symptoms (such as high fever and marked facial pain), progressively worsening symptoms, or failure to improve after 10 days of supportive care. If antibiotics are indicated, both amoxicillin-clavulanate and doxycycline would be appropriate first-line agents. Although this patient has purulent nasal discharge, the acute nature of the symptoms makes antibiotics inappropriate at this time.

Imaging with plain radiographs or CT is rarely needed in acute sinusitis and does not help in distinguishing a bacterial from viral cause.

KEY POINT

- Intranasal glucocorticoids, antihistamines, and topical decongestants are all appropriate for initial treatment of acute sinusitis; antibiotics should not be used initially.

Bibliography

Chow AW, Benninger MS, Brook I, et al. IDSA clinical practice guideline for acute bacterial rhinosinusitis in children and adults. Clin Infect Dis. 2012 Apr 54(8):e72-e112. [PMID: 22438350]

Item 56   Answer: C

Educational Objective: Treat vasomotor symptoms in a low-risk menopausal woman.

The most appropriate management of this patient is a combination of oral estradiol and progestin. Severe vasomotor symptoms are best treated with systemic hormone therapy. An individualized approach based on personal risk factors (including age, time since menopause, and absence of increased risk for cardiovascular disease, thromboembolism, or breast cancer) suggests that this patient is an appropriate candidate. The absolute risks associated with hormone therapy use in healthy women younger than 60 years are low, as are the risks of adverse cardiovascular events if time since menopause is less than 10 years. Estradiol can be administered orally or transdermally in gel, patch, or spray; progestin is needed to prevent endometrial proliferation in this patient with an intact uterus.

Treatment should begin with the lowest effective dose needed to achieve symptom relief. Systemic hormone therapy treats the symptoms present in this patient, including

severe hot flushes, vaginal atrophy, and mood swings. Dose, duration, and route of systemic hormone therapy should be based on symptom response, individualized risk stratification, and patient preference. Because treatment duration greater than 5 years is associated with increased breast cancer risk, the need for treatment should be reassessed annually.

A patient who is amenorrheic for more than 12 months is, by definition, menopausal. Therefore, measuring a serum follicle-stimulating hormone level will not alter management and represents unneeded and low value care.

Measurement of serum estrogen levels in this patient would not be helpful in guiding therapy. The treatment of vasomotor symptoms in a menopausal patient is based on clinical presentation and response to treatment, and laboratory studies are not routinely indicated before starting therapy.

Low-dose selective serotonin reuptake inhibitors (SSRIs) such as paroxetine have been shown to alleviate vasomotor symptoms. However, nonhormonal agents such as SSRIs or gabapentin will not alleviate this patient's symptoms of vaginal atrophy and dyspareunia.

Vaginal estradiol will alleviate symptoms of vaginal atrophy; however, local therapy will not relieve her severe hot flushes and mood changes. Therefore, systemic hormone therapy is a better choice for this patient.

KEY POINT

- The absolute risks for use of hormone therapy in healthy women younger than 60 years are low, as are the risks of adverse cardiovascular events if time since menopause is less than 10 years.

Bibliography

Manson JE. Current recommendations: what is the clinician to do? Fertil Steril. 2014 Apr;101(4):916-21. [PMID: 24680650]

Item 57   Answer: A

Educational Objective: Use a cause-and-effect (fishbone) diagram to organize results of a root cause analysis.

A cause-and-effect diagram, also known as a fishbone or Ishikawa diagram, should be completed. Root cause analysis is used to discover the factors contributing to an identified problem and involves capturing information from all stakeholders involved, such as by asking each involved individual why he or she believes the problem may be occurring. However, this potentially large amount of information needs to be organized in a logical manner to enable meaningful conclusions to be drawn in order to address the problem. A cause-and-effect diagram is used to organize the root causes of a problem; the problem, or system process, forms the backbone of the diagram, and root causes are branched off (like ribs of a fish). For example, the quality team in this case may complete a root cause analysis to determine why the rate of urinary catheter–associated infections is high

H CONT.

(the backbone). After interviewing the physicians, nurses, desk staff, and patients, potential root causes are identified and recorded (the ribs). Examining these potential causes, such as the absence of a protocol for discontinuing urinary catheters, relative to the problem helps identify the nature of the contributing factors and their location within the care process. Organizing root cause information in this way may provide a clearer assessment of specific system issues and interventions that may help address the problem and effect system change.

A control chart is used in quality improvement to graphically display variation in a process over time and can help determine if variation is from a predictable or an unpredictable cause. Additionally, control charts can be used to determine if an intervention has resulted in a positive change. For example, the rate of medication errors could be tracked before and after the initiation of a computer physician order system to determine if the system has had an impact on reducing errors.

A Pareto chart is another method for organizing root causes by displaying them on a graph in descending order of frequency. Unlike a fishbone diagram that is used to identify potential causative factors of a problem and the potential relationship between different variables, Pareto charts are more helpful in focusing improvement initiatives on the most common root causes of a problem.

Spaghetti diagrams are used to visually display flow through a system. The flows are drawn as lines on a map and look similar to spaghetti noodles. For example, a spaghetti diagram may be used to follow a medication order through a hospital unit from order generation to administration of the medication. The diagram can help highlight inefficiencies or redundancies in a system.

KEY POINT

- A cause-and-effect diagram, also known as a fishbone or Ishikawa diagram, is a quality improvement tool that is used to organize root causes of a problem.

Bibliography

Varkey P, Reller MK, Resar RK. Basics of quality improvement in health care. Mayo Clin Proc. 2007 Jun;82(6):735-9. [PMID: 17550754]

Item 58   Answer: D

Educational Objective: Evaluate perioperative cardiac risk in a patient with no significant risk factors for major adverse cardiac events.

No further diagnostic testing is needed for this patient's preoperative cardiovascular risk assessment. This patient is scheduled to undergo surgery (total knee arthroplasty) and has an indeterminate functional capacity, but he does not have coronary artery disease or its equivalents (chronic kidney disease, cerebrovascular disease, heart failure, or diabetes mellitus). Whether a risk calculator (for example, the American College of Surgeons National Surgical Quality Improvement Program Surgical Risk Calculator) or a

simplified approach to perioperative cardiac risk assessment (such as the Revised Cardiac Risk Index) is used, this patient's risk for major adverse cardiac events would be low. No further diagnostic testing is therefore indicated.

As outlined by the American College of Cardiology/American Heart Association (ACC/AHA) guidelines, non-invasive pharmacologic cardiac stress testing is not appropriate for an asymptomatic patient with low risk of cardiac complications. Such testing is both low yield and prone to false-positive results. Instead, cardiac stress testing may be considered in patients with elevated cardiac risk and poor or indeterminate functional capacity if the results will alter perioperative management.

Resting echocardiography is useful for evaluating structural heart disease (such as valvular disease or cardiomyopathy). It is not an appropriate modality for coronary artery disease assessment. Because this patient has no signs or symptoms of structural heart disease, resting echocardiography is not indicated.

The utility of cardiac biomarkers such as serum troponin in preoperative cardiac risk assessment is still under debate, and ACC/AHA guidelines do not recommend their use in perioperative risk stratification. Even if their use was considered for risk stratification, it would not be appropriate in patients without other cardiac risk factors due to the potential for false-positive results in this population.

KEY POINT

- If a patient has no history, symptoms, or risk factors for coronary artery disease, no preoperative coronary evaluation is necessary.

Bibliography

Fleisher LA, Fleischmann KE, Auerbach AD, et al; American College of Cardiology; American Heart Association. 2014 ACC/AHA Guideline on perioperative cardiovascular evaluation and management of patients undergoing noncardiac surgery: a report of the American College of Cardiology/American Heart Association Task Force on practice guidelines. J Am Coll Cardiol. 2014 Dec 9;64(22):e77-137. [PMID: 25091544]

Item 59   Answer: B

Educational Objective: Evaluate a patient with syncope.

This patient likely experienced an episode of neurally mediated syncope (reflex syncope) and should undergo electrocardiography. Neurally mediated syncope is the most common cause of syncope and is associated with the vagal prodrome of nausea, warmth, and lightheadedness. In addition to a careful history and physical examination (including orthostatic blood pressure and pulse measurement), the European Society of Cardiology and the National Institute for Health and Care Excellence advocate obtaining a 12-lead electrocardiogram (ECG) in patients with syncope. A normal ECG has a high negative predictive value for serious adverse outcomes. If the ECG is normal in this patient with classic symptoms of vasovagal syncope, no cardiac history, and a normal physical examination, including orthostatic vital

H

CONT.

signs, she can be safely discharged home with outpatient follow-up.

Echocardiography is not recommended as part of the initial evaluation of syncope unless there are historical or clinical findings suggestive of structural heart disease, which are not present in this patient.

Cerebrovascular disease is a rare cause of syncope, and the American College of Physicians does not recommend brain imaging with CT or MRI in any patient with simple syncope and a normal neurologic examination, as is the case in this patient.

Although this patient's clinical history is compatible with neurocardiogenic syncope, a resting electrocardiogram is recommended as part of the evaluation of syncope. Therefore, no additional testing would be inappropriate.

KEY POINT

- In addition to a careful history and physical examination including measurement of orthostatic vital signs, electrocardiography should be performed in all patients with syncope.

Bibliography

Task Force for the Diagnosis and Management of Syncope; European Society of Cardiology (ESC); European Heart Rhythm Association (EHRA); Heart Failure Association (HFA); Heart Rhythm Society (HRS), Moya A, Sutton R, Ammirati F, et al. Guidelines for the diagnosis and management of syncope (version 2009). Eur Heart J. 2009 Nov;30(21):2631-71. [PMID: 19713422]

Item 60   Answer: B

Educational Objective: Manage a patient with recent percutaneous coronary intervention who is scheduled for elective noncardiac surgery.

For this patient who underwent percutaneous coronary intervention and stenting with an everolimus-eluting coronary stent 4 months ago, the optimal preoperative management is to delay surgery for at least 8 months. The American College of Cardiology and American Heart Association (ACC/AHA) guideline recommends an optimal delay of elective noncardiac surgery for a minimum of 12 months after placement of a drug-eluting stent (DES) due to the increased risk of cardiovascular complications, regardless of the type of antiplatelet therapy. Although some data suggest 6 months may be sufficient for normalization of risk, the ACC/AHA still advises delaying elective surgery for 12 months after DES placement. The ACC/AHA guideline states that between 6 and 12 months after DES placement, noncardiac surgery can be considered if the benefits outweigh the risks. This requires collaborative decision making with the patient's cardiologist. Patients with percutaneous coronary intervention alone should avoid surgery for 14 days after their intervention, whereas coronary artery bypass grafting and bare metal coronary stenting require a minimum noncardiac surgical delay of 30 days.

Patients with a DES should remain on uninterrupted dual antiplatelet therapy (DAPT) for at least 12 months after

their intervention. The only perioperative exception is for urgently required surgery in which the bleeding risks are deemed too high to justify continuation of DAPT (for example, intracranial surgery). For patients who must undergo noncardiac surgery before the minimum duration DAPT, either continuation of both antiplatelet agents or aspirin alone may be considered based on discussions between all members of the perioperative care team. However, in this patient's case, surgery is elective and optimally should be delayed for a minimum of 12 months total after DES placement.

Antiplatelet management in elective surgical patients with a previous history of coronary intervention who have surpassed the minimum duration of DAPT is also controversial. The ACC/AHA recommends consensus decision making between a patient's clinicians to provide an individualized antiplatelet management plan, whereas the American College of Chest Physicians advises that patients on aspirin who are at moderate to high risk for cardiovascular events should remain on aspirin throughout surgery. Those at moderate to high cardiovascular risk include patients with ischemic heart disease, heart failure, diabetes mellitus, prior stroke, kidney disease, or undergoing vascular procedures.

KEY POINT

- Elective noncardiac surgery should optimally be delayed for 1 year after placement of a drug-eluting stent due to the increased risk of cardiovascular complications, regardless of the type of antiplatelet therapy.

Bibliography

Fleisher LA, Fleischmann KE, Auerbach AD, et al; American College of Cardiology; American Heart Association. 2014 ACC/AHA Guideline on perioperative cardiovascular evaluation and management of patients undergoing noncardiac surgery: a report of the American College of Cardiology/American Heart Association Task Force on practice guidelines. J Am Coll Cardiol. 2014 Dec 9;64(22):e77-137. [PMID: 25091544]

Item 61   Answer: D

Educational Objective: Treat panic disorder.

Treatment with a selective serotonin reuptake inhibitor (SSRI) such as sertraline is appropriate for this patient who meets the diagnostic criteria for panic disorder. Panic disorder is characterized by recurrent, unexpected, and abrupt surges of extreme anxiety that peaks within minutes and is accompanied by four or more of the following symptoms: palpitations, sweating, trembling, dyspnea, choking sensation, chest pain, nausea or abdominal pain, lightheadedness, chills or heat sensations, numbness or tingling, feeling detached from oneself, and fear of losing control or dying. Diagnosis requires that an attack be followed by at least 1 month of worry by the patient that he or she will experience a recurrent attack. Recommended treatment of panic disorder is a combination of cognitive-behavioral therapy and medication because this has been shown to be more effective than either treatment alone. Various forms of pharmacologic treatment for panic disorder are available: SSRIs, serotonin-norepinephrine reuptake inhibitors (SNRIs), benzodiazepines, tricyclic antidepressants, and monoamine oxidase inhibitors. SSRIs, SNRIs, benzodiazepines, and tricyclic antidepressants are equally effective in treating anxiety and reducing frequency of panic attacks. However, SSRIs are the mainstay of pharmacologic treatment for panic disorder because of side effects associated with the other drug classes. The initial SSRI dose should be low and gradually titrated upward, with the goal of elimination of panic attacks. If response is inadequate, then switching to another SSRI or another class of drug is recommended.

Benzodiazepines, such as alprazolam, are not recommended as the first treatment choice for panic disorder because of their side effects, including potential for dependency and withdrawal syndrome. However, benzodiazepines (such as clonazepam) may have a short-term role in combination with an SSRI for initial treatment of panic disorder. Such short-term (but not long-term) combinations result in more rapid resolution of symptoms and elimination of attacks than SSRI treatment alone.

Buspirone is effective in treating generalized anxiety disorder, but not panic disorder.

β-Blockers such as propranolol can reduce situation-specific anxiety symptoms (for example, public speaking) but are not effective as monotherapy for panic disorder.

KEY POINT

- Selective serotonin reuptake inhibitors are the mainstay of pharmacologic treatment for panic disorder.

Bibliography

Katon WJ. Clinical practice. Panic disorder. N Engl J Med. 2006 Jun 1;354(22): 2360-7. [PMID: 16738272]

Item 62   Answer: D

Educational Objective: Evaluate a patient prior to prescribing hormonal contraception.

This woman may be prescribed a combined hormonal oral contraceptive after a negative screening pregnancy test is obtained. A pregnancy test should be obtained prior to initiating contraception if more than 1 week has passed since the last menstrual period, as in this patient.

In healthy women without chronic conditions, few tests are needed before initiation of combined hormonal contraceptives, and this patient has no history of smoking, thromboembolism, or migraine that could influence the choice of contraceptive method. Blood pressure should be measured before initiation of combined hormonal contraceptives. Baseline weight and BMI are useful for monitoring contraceptive users over time. In this patient, no other screening tests are indicated.

Newer-generation oral contraceptives that contain lower dosages and less androgenic hormones have minimized their effect on different lipid parameters. Because lipid changes seen with hormonal contraception are mild,

usually transient, and not clearly associated with increased cardiovascular risk, testing lipid parameters prior to starting treatment is not indicated.

Breast cancer screening with mammography is also not recommended prior to initiation of hormonal contraception. Breast cancer screening should be performed according to recommended guidelines.

In healthy women of reproductive age, a screening pelvic examination or cervical cancer screening is not required prior to initiation of combined hormonal contraceptives in the absence of symptoms or other clinical findings. Cervical cancer screening should follow recommended guidelines, and this patient is up to date with her age-appropriate screening.

Combined hormonal contraceptives, which include pills, transdermal patches, and vaginal rings, can be initiated at any time in the menstrual cycle. Because these are contraceptive methods that depend on consistent and correct use, patient education and engagement are essential. The provision of information about common side effects such as unscheduled bleeding, especially during the first 3 to 6 months of use, has been shown to increase continuation rates. Bleeding irregularities are generally not harmful and usually improve with continued use. The patient should also be counseled regarding the continued need for condom use to reduce risk of sexually transmitted infections and HIV infection.

KEY POINT

- A pregnancy test should be obtained in all women prior to prescribing hormonal contraception if more than 1 week has passed since the last menstrual period.

Bibliography

Division of Reproductive Health, National Center for Chronic Disease Prevention and Health Promotion, Centers for Disease Control and Prevention (CDC). U.S. Selected Practice Recommendations for Contraceptive Use, 2013: adapted from the World Health Organization selected practice recommendations for contraceptive use, 2nd edition. MMWR Recomm Rep. 2013 Jun 21;62(RR-05):1-60. [PMID: 23784109]

Item 63   Answer: B

Educational Objective: Treat upper respiratory tract infection.

This patient should be treated with a combination antihistamine and decongestant, such as chlorpheniramine-pseudoephedrine. This otherwise healthy nonsmoker has acute cough most likely caused by viral upper respiratory tract infection. His examination findings do not implicate lower respiratory tract infection, and there is no evidence of reactive airways disease. The treatment of acute viral upper respiratory tract infections is based on symptoms. First-generation antihistamine and decongestant preparations (such as chlorpheniramine-pseudoephedrine), inhaled ipratropium, and cromolyn sodium may be used to decrease sneezing and rhinorrhea.

Routine antibiotic treatment of uncomplicated viral upper respiratory tract infections in immunocompetent patients is ineffective, associated with many adverse effects, contributes to antibiotic resistance, and represents low value care; it is therefore not recommended. The purulent nature of this patient's sputum does not reliably differentiate between bacterial and viral causes of infection, and he should not be prescribed an antibiotic.

Codeine is less useful as a cough suppressant in acute cough, as in this patient. Studies suggest, however, that opioids may decrease cough frequency and severity in patients with chronic cough.

This patient has no wheezing or history of reactive airways disease; therefore, inhaled β_2-agonists, such as albuterol, are not indicated.

KEY POINT

- The treatment of acute cough associated with upper respiratory tract infection is symptomatic; routine antibiotic treatment is not recommended.

Bibliography

Kenealy T, Arroll B. Antibiotics for the common cold and acute purulent rhinitis. Cochrane Database Syst Rev. 2013 Jun 4;6:CD000247. [PMID: 23733381]

Item 64   Answer: B

Educational Objective: Diagnose a suspected full-thickness rotator cuff tear.

The most appropriate next step in management of this patient is to obtain an MRI of the right shoulder. This patient likely has an acute full-thickness tear of the right supraspinatus tendon, as suggested by her inability to abduct her right shoulder beyond 90 degrees, to lower her arm from 90 degrees of abduction (drop-arm test), and to maintain full external rotation when the arm is passively externally rotated at 20 degrees of abduction (external rotation lag test). To confirm the diagnosis in this patient, the most appropriate management would be to obtain a shoulder MRI, as it is a highly accurate and widely available modality for diagnosing full-thickness tears. Musculoskeletal ultrasonography is also highly · sensitive for rotator cuff tears and may be used as a diagnostic study for suspected rotator cuff injuries. In the case of an acute full-thickness tear, immediate surgery is indicated.

Although glucocorticoid injection can lead to short-term pain improvement, the evidence for its use in rotator cuff tears is limited. Such injections may have a negative impact on healthy shoulder tendons, leading to worse surgical outcomes, and should therefore be avoided in patients who are potential surgical candidates.

Physical therapy alone would not be appropriate in this patient with a suspected complete rotator cuff tear who is a surgical candidate, as delayed orthopedic referral (>6 weeks) can lead to suboptimal surgical outcomes.

Although this patient has weakness on examination, she lacks other findings, such as paresthesias or pain in a dermatomal distribution, that suggest a nerve injury and might make a nerve conduction study helpful in diagnosis.

KEY POINT

- MRI is the preferred imaging modality for diagnosing full-thickness rotator cuff tears.

Bibliography

Nam D, Maak TG, Raphael BS, Kepler CK, Cross MB, Warren RF. Rotator cuff tear arthropathy: evaluation, diagnosis, and treatment: AAOS exhibit selection. J Bone Joint Surg Am. 2012 Mar 21;94(6):e34. [PMID: 22438007]

Item 65   Answer: B

Educational Objective: Manage depression that does not respond to full-dose antidepressant monotherapy.

Discontinuation of citalopram and initiation of a different antidepressant such as bupropion is the most appropriate next step in the management of this patient. About 40% of patients with depression do not respond to antidepressant monotherapy. However, patients who do not respond to full-dose antidepressant monotherapy for 6 weeks may respond to switching to a different antidepressant drug, either from the same or a different class, or the addition of a second antidepressant drug.

Available evidence is not convincing regarding the efficacy of liothyronine in combination with, or augmenting, selective serotonin reuptake inhibitor treatment of depression.

Patients who do not respond to full-dose antidepressant monotherapy for 6 weeks may respond to the addition of an antipsychotic drug. The FDA has approved the following combinations of antidepressant and antipsychotic drugs for the treatment of depression: aripiprazole or quetiapine extended-release added to any antidepressant, and olanzapine added to fluoxetine. However, olanzapine monotherapy is not an appropriate treatment for this patient.

Electroconvulsive therapy may be appropriate for patients with depression refractory to multiple antidepressant drugs (or intolerance of such drugs), with or without psychotherapy, and patients with severe life-threatening depression (for example, suicidal ideation and catatonia).

Most patients with depression are treated with either antidepressant drugs or psychotherapy; a minority receive combined therapy. However, in a recent meta-analysis, pharmacotherapy combined with psychotherapy was more effective than pharmacotherapy alone in the treatment of depression. In addition to switching to a different antidepressant or adding a second antidepressant or an antipsychotic agent, clinicians should consider psychotherapy for depressed patients who do not respond to antidepressant drug monotherapy.

- Patients refractory to full-dose antidepressant mono-therapy within 6 weeks may respond to a change in therapy, which may include replacement with another antidepressant, either from the same or a different class, or the addition of a second antidepressant.

Bibliography

Gaynes BN, Dusetzina SB, Ellis AR, et al. Treating depression after initial treatment failure: directly comparing switch and augmenting strategies in STAR*D. J Clin Psychopharmacol. 2012 Feb;32(1):114-9. [PMID: 22198447]

Item 66   Answer: A

Educational Objective: Recognize unprofessional physician conduct on social media.

The physician should meet with the colleague to advise that she remove the inappropriate content. The use of social media has grown dramatically in recent years and has changed how people communicate and interact with each other. Although social media can be useful for improving patient care and advocacy, its use creates challenges for professionalism. Physicians should manifest online activity that reflects standards of professional behavior, and they should strive to keep their social and professional online presences separate and conduct themselves professionally in both spheres. Furthermore, physicians should be aware that all posted content is generally public and permanent, and they must assume that patients will be able to view social media postings. In this case, the physician should meet with the colleague to express concerns about the social media postings and why the postings do not reflect standards of professionalism; may diminish patients' trust in the doctor, her group, and the profession; and should be removed if possible.

At this stage, it is unnecessary to report the concern to the head physician of the practice; the colleague will likely respond favorably to discreet feedback. If she does not, escalation to involve the practice leadership would be indicated.

Commenting on the colleague's social media page about the unprofessional content is an inappropriate means of providing feedback.

The physician should not disregard the inappropriate social media posts, even if none of the content can be linked to individual patients.

- Physicians should keep their social and professional online presences separate and conduct themselves professionally in both spheres.

Bibliography

Mostaghimi A, Crotty BH. Professionalism in the digital age. Ann Intern Med. 2011 Apr 19;154(8):560-2. [PMID: 21502653]

Item 67   Answer: D

Educational Objective: Manage chronic cough due to gastroesophageal reflux disease.

The most appropriate management of this patient with chronic cough is an empiric trial of a proton pump inhibitor. In general, an algorithmic approach to chronic cough (cough of greater than 8 weeks' duration) leads to successful outcomes in more than 90% of patients. Patients with chronic cough, especially smokers, should undergo chest radiography. If the chest radiograph does not reveal a potential cause of cough, the physician should consider upper airway cough syndrome, asthma, nonasthmatic eosinophilic bronchitis, and gastroesophageal reflux disease (GERD) and begin a stepwise approach for evaluation and treatment. The definitive diagnosis may be suggested by history and physical examination findings and confirmed by successful empiric treatment. This obese patient with a 15-pack-year history has chronic cough and symptoms typical of GERD (heartburn, cough that is worsened after a large meal). Additionally, his tobacco use, alcohol use, and caffeine intake are risk factors for GERD. Initiating a proton pump inhibitor such as omeprazole is the next most appropriate step and can be started without 24-hour esophageal pH monitoring. All patients with chronic cough who smoke should also receive tobacco cessation counseling.

A combination antihistamine and decongestant is helpful in patients with cough due to upper airway cough syndrome; however, this patient does not present with symptoms or signs of upper airway cough syndrome (allergic symptoms or postnasal drip).

In the presence of a normal chest radiograph, bronchoscopy is unlikely to be of benefit and should be reserved for second-line testing if the patient's symptoms fail to improve after several months of optimized therapy with a proton pump inhibitor.

Echocardiography is helpful in evaluating left ventricular function or valvular heart disease as a cause of cough; however, in the absence of symptoms (shortness of breath, paroxysmal nocturnal dyspnea) or physical examination findings (crackles, S_3, edema, murmur), an echocardiogram is unnecessary and represents low value care.

- Proton pump inhibitor therapy can be initiated without 24-hour esophageal pH monitoring in patients with chronic cough who have a normal chest radiograph and symptoms suggestive of gastroesophageal reflux disease.

Bibliography

Chang AB, Lasserson TJ, Gaffney J, Connor FL, Garske LA. Gastro-oesophageal reflux treatment for prolonged non-specific cough in children and adults. Cochrane Database Syst Rev. 2011 Jan 19;(1):CD004823. [PMID: 21249664]

Item 68   Answer: C

Educational Objective: Screen for atrial fibrillation during the physical examination.

Palpating the pulse to screen for atrial fibrillation should be included in this patient's physical examination. Palpating the pulse has been shown to increase atrial fibrillation case finding among adults age 65 years and older. A cluster-randomized trial of more than 14,000 patients found that detection of new cases of atrial fibrillation was 1.64% per year in patients randomized to receive opportunistic screening (pulse taking and invitation for electrocardiography if the pulse was irregular) compared with 1.04% in patients randomized to receive no active screening.

Abdominal palpation for the detection of abdominal aortic aneurysm (AAA) has been shown to have poor reliability. Ultrasonography is the preferred screening test for detection of AAA because it is noninvasive, easy to implement, and has excellent sensitivity and specificity. The U.S. Preventive Services Task Force (USPSTF) recommends one-time screening for AAA with abdominal ultrasonography in all men aged 65 to 75 years who have smoked at least 100 cigarettes in their lifetime and selective screening in men in this age group who have never smoked.

Carotid artery auscultation of bruits for detection of carotid stenosis has also been shown to have poor accuracy. Although ultrasonography has higher sensitivity and specificity than auscultation, the USPSTF recommends against screening for carotid stenosis in adults, as the harms of screening outweigh the benefits.

The USPSTF recommends against routine testicular examination for the purposes of cancer screening, primarily due to the low incidence and high survival rate of patients with testicular cancer, even when it is clinically detected. Harms associated with testicular cancer screening include false-positive results and unnecessary anxiety.

KEY POINT

- Palpating the pulse has been shown to increase the detection rate of atrial fibrillation among adults age 65 years and older.

Bibliography
Fitzmaurice DA, Hobbs FD, Jowett S, et al. Screening versus routine practice in detection of atrial fibrillation in patients aged 65 or over: cluster randomized controlled trial. BMJ. 2007 Aug 25;335(7616):383. [PMID: 17673732]

Item 69   Answer: D

Educational Objective: Treat trichomoniasis.

The most appropriate additional intervention in this patient is to treat her partner. This patient has the characteristic features of frothy yellow discharge, burning, and dyspareunia associated with infection by *Trichomonas vaginalis* organisms, which are seen on microscopy. Trichomoniasis is the most common curable sexually transmitted infection (STI) worldwide and is evenly distributed among women of all age groups, unlike other STIs that predominate in younger people. It is caused by motile flagellated protozoa that infect the urogenital tract, causing inflammatory vaginitis and urethritis. Treatment with a single 2-g dose of metronidazole is associated with a high rate of cure and should be offered to all symptomatic women. It is important that sexual partners also be treated, even if asymptomatic, because of a high rate of reinfection; documentation of infection is not required before treatment in any partners. Once trichomoniasis is identified, testing for other STIs should be considered in both individuals.

Trichomoniasis has been traditionally associated with a vaginal pH of greater than 4.5 and diagnosed by direct visualization of trichomonads on saline microscopy. However, the specificity of a high vaginal pH and the sensitivity of saline microscopy findings are low. Therefore, point-of-care vaginal swab rapid immunoassays and nucleic acid amplification tests (NAATs) for detection of *T. vaginalis* are increasingly considered to be the gold standard for diagnosis, and particularly when microscopy is not available. NAATs can be performed on a vaginal (or endocervical) swab, urine sample, or liquid-based Pap test specimens. In this patient in whom trichomonads are seen on microscopy, confirmatory testing with another assay is not necessary.

Trichomoniasis causes an inflammatory vaginitis, and cervical contact bleeding may occur due to inflammation from the infection. This inflammation resolves with treatment of the infection, and a follow-up Pap smear to detect cervical pathology would not be required in the absence of additional symptoms or findings.

Treatment of trichomoniasis with single-dose metronidazole is highly effective; therefore, testing for cure is not required in patients whose symptoms have resolved with therapy.

KEY POINT

- Trichomoniasis is characterized by copious, malodorous, pale yellow or gray frothy discharge with vulvar itching, burning, and postcoital bleeding; it is effectively treated with a single dose of metronidazole.

Bibliography
Workowski KA, Bolan GA. Sexually transmitted diseases treatment guidelines, 2015. MMWR Recomm Rep. 2015 Jun 5;64(RR-03):1-137. [PMID: 26042815]

Item 70   Answer: A

Educational Objective: Reduce cardiovascular risk in a patient with metabolic syndrome.

Aspirin is the most appropriate treatment to reduce cardiovascular risk in this patient with metabolic syndrome. According to the International Diabetes Federation and the American Heart Association (AHA), diagnosis of metabolic syndrome is made by the presence of three or more of the following five criteria: (1) increased waist circumference; (2) serum triglyceride level of 150 mg/dL (1.70 mmol/L) or higher (or taking medications for hypertriglyceridemia); (3) HDL cholesterol level lower than 40 mg/dL (1.04 mmol/L) in men and lower than 50 mg/dL (1.30 mmol/L) in women (or taking medication specifically for low HDL cholesterol); (4) blood pressure of 130/85 mm Hg or higher (or taking antihypertensive medications); and (5) fasting plasma glucose level of 100 mg/dL (5.6 mmol/L) or higher (or taking medications for hyperglycemia). The patient meets at least three criteria (elevated triglyceride level, decreased HDL cholesterol level, antihypertensive treatment). Management of patients with metabolic syndrome should focus on optimizing general health and targeting the individual components of the metabolic syndrome. Lifestyle changes include education on the importance of following a heart-healthy diet, implementing a weight loss plan, and exercising for 30 minutes daily at least 5 days per week. Patients with hypertension should be treated aggressively to achieve the blood pressure goals outlined by the Eighth Joint National Committee. Similarly, dyslipidemia should be treated according to American College of Cardiology (ACC) and AHA cholesterol treatment guideline, and hyperglycemia should be managed per guidelines from the American Diabetes Association. Additionally, the AHA recommends low-dose aspirin for patients with metabolic syndrome with a 10-year cardiovascular risk of 10% or higher. This patient's hypertension and hyperlipidemia are being managed; however, he should also be prescribed aspirin based on his increased risk, provided that his risk for bleeding is not increased.

Diltiazem will not provide additional cardiovascular risk reduction in this patient. Moreover, intensification of his hypertension therapy is not indicated, since the blood pressure goal for patients younger than 60 years is a systolic pressure of less than 140 mm Hg and a diastolic pressure of less than 90 mm Hg. The patient's pressures are within this range.

Fenofibrate increases the potential for drug-induced side effects and has uncertain additive cardiovascular risk reduction when used with statins, which are clearly indicated in this patient based on ACC/AHA guidelines. Fibrate therapy is reserved for patients with hyperlipidemia who do not tolerate or do not respond to statin monotherapy, patients who have triglyceride levels higher than 500 mg/dL (5.65 mmol/L), or patients with hypertriglyceridemia-induced pancreatitis.

The role of metformin in the metabolic syndrome has not been clearly defined. It may reduce the incidence of metabolic syndrome in at-risk patients, but healthy lifestyle modifications are equally effective or superior to metformin in reducing cardiovascular risk. Metformin has also not been shown to reduce cardiovascular events in patients without diabetes. Metformin would be a reasonable choice for both treatment of hyperglycemia and improvement of metabolic parameters if this patient did have impaired fasting glucose or impaired glucose tolerance, and it would be the initial drug of choice if the patient develops diabetes.

KEY POINT

- Patients with metabolic syndrome who have a 10-year cardiovascular risk of 10% or higher should be treated with low-dose aspirin for primary prevention of cardiovascular disease.

Bibliography
Blaha MJ, Bansal S, Rouf R, Golden SH, Blumenthal RS, Defilippis AP. A practical "ABCDE" approach to the metabolic syndrome. Mayo Clin Proc. 2008 Aug;83(8):932-41. [PMID: 18674478]

Item 71   Answer: C

Educational Objective: Treat severe menopausal vasomotor symptoms in a woman whose uterus has been removed.

Transdermal estradiol without a progestin is the most appropriate choice for this patient with severe vasomotor symptoms of menopause that are refractory to conservative treatment and are affecting her quality of life. Systemic estrogen improves both hot flushes and genitourinary symptoms. She has had a hysterectomy and therefore does not require the use of a progestin to oppose the proliferative effects of estrogen on the endometrium, making therapy with estrogen alone an appropriate treatment option.

The use of hormones to treat menopausal symptoms requires balancing potential benefits and risks, and an individualized risk profile must be considered. This patient is recently menopausal, younger than 60 years, and does not have a history of thromboembolism or cardiac disease or have an increased risk for breast cancer. Treatment with systemic estrogen would be a reasonable choice and can be administered orally or transdermally by patch, gel, or spray. There is some evidence that transdermal estrogen may be associated with less thromboembolic risk than oral estrogen by avoiding the hepatic first-pass effect. All formulations are equally effective for treating vasomotor symptoms.

Current evidence does not support the use of progestin alone to treat vasomotor symptoms. Although progestins may improve vasomotor symptoms, safety data for progestin alone are lacking. Also, in the Women's Health Initiative, the risk of breast cancer was increased in the estrogen and medroxprogesterone acetate arm, but not in the estrogen-alone arm, raising concern that the risk of breast cancer may be related to progestin use. Therefore, a progestin alone is not the most appropriate choice for the management of vasomotor symptoms.

Vaginal estradiol therapy is useful in treating menopausal genitourinary symptoms, including dryness, itching, dysuria, and dyspareunia. However, local topical treatment does not alleviate vasomotor or other systemic menopausal symptoms. In this patient who has both vaginal symptoms and severe vasomotor symptoms, vaginal treatment alone would not be adequate.

KEY POINT

- In women without a uterus taking systemic estrogen therapy for management of menopausal symptoms, concurrent progestin is not indicated.

Bibliography

ACOG Practice Bulletin No. 141: management of menopausal symptoms. Obstet Gynecol. 2014 Jan;123(1):202-16. [PMID: 24463691]

Item 72   Answer: A

Educational Objective: Adjust medications in a woman who may become pregnant.

Discontinuation of atorvastatin is indicated in this patient who is planning pregnancy. Statin medications should be avoided in pregnancy due to the potential risk for congenital abnormalities. In patients actively planning pregnancy, dyslipidemia is best managed with diet and lifestyle modification for the duration of the pregnancy. Because the effects of statin use during breastfeeding are not known, their use during nursing should be discouraged.

ACE inhibitors and angiotensin receptor blockers are also contraindicated due to potential risk of teratogenicity and should be discontinued in women who are planning pregnancy, as was done in this patient. Her hypertension should be followed and treated, if needed, with another agent known to be safe in pregnancy, such as β-blockers, calcium channel blockers, or methyldopa.

Oral antidiabetic agents should be continued in women contemplating pregnancy to maintain control of diabetes mellitus. Metformin is an FDA pregnancy category B medication (no definitive studies in pregnant women but no animal studies showing risk to the fetus) and is a reasonable option for controlling this patient's hyperglycemia before pregnancy. Evidence suggests that metformin and sulfonylureas are acceptable during pregnancy; however, further management decisions are best made through co-management of medical and obstetric issues with a high-risk obstetrician.

In the treatment of depression, medication discontinuation may not be appropriate in women with a history of major or recurrent depression. Some selective serotonin reuptake inhibitors (SSRIs), including sertraline and fluoxetine, are FDA pregnancy category C (no definitive studies in pregnant women but evidence of potential harm in animal reproduction studies, although potential benefits may warrant use despite potential risks), and their use must be determined on an individual basis. Such agents may be continued if needed, but the risks and benefits of treatment, taking into account severity of depressive symptoms, stage of gestation, and associated circumstances, should be evaluated by a psychiatrist or high-risk obstetrician. SSRIs should not be stopped precipitously.

Because this patient is on a known medication classified as FDA pregnancy category X (atorvastatin), continued treatment with this agent would be inappropriate.

KEY POINT

- Statins, ACE inhibitors, and angiotensin receptor blockers are teratogenic and should be discontinued in women planning pregnancy.

Bibliography

Callegari LS, Ma EW, Schwarz EB. Preconception care and reproductive planning in primary care. Med Clin North Am. 2015 May;99(3):663-82. [PMID: 25841606]

Item 73   Answer: A

Educational Objective: Treat an overweight patient with behavioral therapy.

The most appropriate additional treatment for this patient is behavioral therapy. With a BMI of 29, this patient is overweight, and her waist circumference of 92 cm (36 in) is independently associated with increased cardiovascular risk. According to the American College of Cardiology, American Heart Association, and The Obesity Society, all overweight and obese patients should be offered a comprehensive lifestyle intervention (comprised of diet, physical activity, and behavioral treatments) for weight loss. Behavioral therapy includes providing patients with strategies to facilitate a shift from personal maladaptive eating patterns toward healthful eating and exercise, particularly in this patient who acknowledges eating to reduce stress and suboptimal dietary choices. Such strategies are associated with weight loss and reduced risk for developing diabetes mellitus and hypertension. Although best conducted by a trained therapist, behavioral therapy can be initiated by internists. Specifically, internists can emphasize the behavioral therapy components of self-monitoring, stimulus control, goal setting, and social support. Given this patient's eating patterns and previous dieting attempts, she should be offered behavioral therapy.

Bariatric surgery, such as laparoscopic adjustable gastric banding, should be considered in all patients with a BMI of 40 or higher and in patients with a BMI of 35 or higher with obesity-related comorbid conditions; it is therefore not indicated in this patient.

Pharmacologic agents, such as orlistat or phentermine, are used along with diet, physical activity, and behavioral treatments in patients with a BMI of 30 or higher or in patients with a BMI of 27 or higher with overweight- or obesity-associated comorbidities. This patient does not currently meet the criteria for pharmacologic therapy.

KEY POINT

- All overweight and obese patients should be offered a comprehensive lifestyle intervention for weight loss including diet, physical activity, and behavioral therapy.

Bibliography

Jensen MD, Ryan DH, Apovian CM, et al; American College of Cardiology/American Heart Association Task Force on Practice Guidelines; Obesity Society. 2013 AHA/ACC/TOS guideline for the management of overweight and obesity in adults: a report of the American College of Cardiology/American Heart Association Task Force on Practice Guidelines and The Obesity Society. J Am Coll Cardiol. 2014 Jul 1;63(25 Pt B):2985-3023. Erratum in: J Am Coll Cardiol. 2014 Jul 1;63(25 Pt B): 3029-3030. [PMID: 24239920]

Item 74   Answer: D

Educational Objective: Diagnose somatic symptom disorder.

The patient meets the diagnostic criteria for somatic symptom disorder. These criteria include having at least one somatic symptom causing distress or interference with daily life; excessive thoughts, feelings, and behaviors related to the somatic symptoms; and persistence of somatic symptoms for at least 6 months. Furthermore, potential medical causes must be excluded. She has two somatic symptoms (chest and abdominal pain), which have been present for well over 6 months and have no identifiable organic source despite thorough diagnostic testing. Her missed time from work demonstrates interference with daily functioning, and her frequent utilization of health care resources and daily research of Internet resources are indicative of excessive concern over her symptoms.

Conversion disorder involves one or more symptoms of abnormal sensation or motor function that are not explained by a medical condition and are inconsistent with physical examination findings. This patient's symptoms are somatic rather than neurologic, thus eliminating the possibility of conversion disorder.

Patients with factitious disorder deliberately falsify symptoms or inflict injury upon themselves or another. Although patients with factitious disorder may have no apparent external benefit for their fabricated illness, this patient has no evidence (such as tenderness on abdominal examination) that she is falsifying her symptoms.

Illness anxiety disorder (formerly known as hypochondriasis) is characterized by excessive concern over general health and is associated with undue focus on health-related activities. However, unlike this patient with debilitating somatic symptoms, patients with illness anxiety disorder have minimal or no somatic symptoms.

KEY POINT

- Diagnostic criteria for somatic symptom disorder include having at least one somatic symptom causing distress or interference with daily life; excessive thoughts, feelings, and behaviors related to the somatic symptoms; and persistence of somatic symptoms for at least 6 months.

Bibliography

Dimsdale JE, Creed F, Escobar J, et al. Somatic symptom disorder: an important change in DSM. J Psychosom Res. 2013 Sep;75(3):223-8. [PMID: 23972410]

Item 75   Answer: A

Educational Objective: Treat chronic pain with cognitive-behavioral therapy.

Cognitive-behavioral interventions are some of the most useful tools in helping to manage chronic pain and are consistently recommended in pain management guidelines. There are many different types of cognitive-behavioral interventions, such as cognitive restructuring, relaxation techniques, and mindfulness-based stress reduction, all of which replace maladaptive coping patterns (such as catastrophizing, fear avoidance, and overgeneralizing) with more constructive coping skills. How cognitive-behavioral techniques are incorporated into an individual patient's multimodal management strategy depends on local resources and patient preference; however, numerous studies show that primary care physicians can implement some cognitive-behavioral techniques effectively in the office setting.

The lidocaine patch is an effective topical agent for localized neuropathic pain; however, it would not be an effective option to treat widespread central pain, such as that in this patient with fibromyalgia.

NSAID therapy can be considered for intermittent flares of pain, but it is generally ineffective when used on a scheduled basis for central pain.

There is little evidence supporting the use of opioids in patients with chronic noncancer pain and ample evidence of potential harms of chronic opioid therapy in such patients. Furthermore, there is some weak evidence that opioids may in fact worsen central pain. Therefore, opioids should only be considered as a last resort in certain low-risk patients after all other modalities have failed.

KEY POINT

- Cognitive-behavioral therapy, in which maladaptive coping patterns are replaced with more constructive coping skills, is recommended in the management of chronic pain.

Bibliography

Hooten WM, Timming R, Belgrade M, et al. Institute for Clinical Systems Improvement. Assessment and management of chronic pain. Available at https://www.icsi.org/_asset/bw798b/ChronicPain.pdf. Updated November 2013. Accessed April 24, 2015.

Item 76   Answer: A

Educational Objective: Manage a patient's request for genetic testing.

The most appropriate management of this patient is to obtain a comprehensive three-generation family history that specifically assesses for the presence of breast, ovarian, and other cancers. According to the U.S. Preventive Services Task Force (USPSTF), the decision of whether or not to perform *BRCA* genetic testing should be based on a woman's family history of breast cancer. Family history attributes that suggest an increased likelihood of the presence of a *BRCA* gene mutation include multiple family members with breast cancer, the presence of both breast and ovarian cancer, breast cancer diagnosis before the age of 50 years, breast cancer in one or more male family members, bilateral breast cancer, and Ashkenazi Jewish heritage. Women who are found to be at increased risk for carrying the BRCA1 and BRCA2 gene mutations should be offered genetic counseling and, if appropriate after counseling, BRCA genetic testing. The USPSTF recommends against routine testing for BRCA1 and BRCA2 gene mutations in women who lack a family history suggestive of such mutations.

Ordering screening mammography for this 32-year-old woman is also not appropriate because of her young age. The USPSTF currently recommends biennial screening mammography for women aged 50 to 74 years. Additionally, the USPSTF recommends individualized screening decisions for women younger than 50 years based on patient context and values regarding specific benefits and harms.

According to the USPSTF, performing genetic testing for BRCA1 and BRCA2 gene mutations would not be appropriate before obtaining a comprehensive family history.

Referral for genetic counseling would also be inappropriate at this stage. Referral for genetic counseling should occur if, after obtaining a three-generation family history, BRCA genetic testing is indicated. Genetic counseling should always occur before any genetic test is performed.

KEY POINT

- Genetic testing for BRCA gene mutations should only be performed in patients with a family history that is suggestive of an increased genetic risk.

Bibliography
Moyer VA; U.S. Preventive Services Task Force. Risk assessment, genetic counseling, and genetic testing for BRCA-related cancer in women: U.S. Preventive Services Task Force recommendation statement. Ann Intern Med. 2014 Feb 18;160(4):271-81. [PMID: 24366376]

Item 77   Answer: D
Educational Objective: Prevent falls in a cognitively impaired patient.

There is no specific intervention that would be beneficial in this older patient with cognitive impairment; therefore, continuing this patient's current care is appropriate. In older adults, falls are a source of morbidity, mortality, decreased functionality, and premature institutionalization. Risk factors for falling are myriad and include lower extremity weakness, history of falls, gait or balance deficits, polypharmacy, low vitamin D level, visual impairments, and cognitive impairment. Many risk factors are amenable to remediation; however, there is insufficient evidence to support any specific interventions to reduce fall risk in the cognitively impaired beyond those risk factors that can be treated. This patient is under close supervision and well cared for by her family, and she has no clearly reversible risk factors. Therefore, it is reasonable to continue her current care provided by her family.

Although individualized exercise programs to decrease falls have been shown to be effective in cognitively intact, community-dwelling adults, such exercise programs have not been shown to benefit cognitively impaired individuals. The lack of benefit is speculated to be caused by the cognitively impaired patient's inability to retain and incorporate instructions over time.

Antipsychotic medications, such as risperidone, have not been shown to reduce falls in patients with cognitive deficits. Furthermore, risperidone may induce orthostatic hypotension, which may actually increase this patient's risk of falling.

Although many patients are placed in skilled nursing facilities due to falls, there is no evidence that care in a skilled nursing facility is more likely to reduce falls than conscientious care in the home. This is particularly true in this case in which the patient's daughter is clearly meticulous in the care she provides.

KEY POINT

- No specific interventions have been shown to be beneficial in reducing fall risk in the cognitively impaired patient beyond treating reversible risk factors.

Bibliography
Panel on Prevention of Falls in Older Persons, American Geriatrics Society and British Geriatrics Society. Summary of the updated American Geriatrics Society/British Geriatrics Society clinical practice guideline for prevention of falls in older persons. J Am Geriatr Soc. 2011 Jan;59(1):148-57. [PMID: 21226685]

Item 78   Answer: A
Educational Objective: Administer the seasonal influenza vaccine to a patient with a history of egg allergy.

This patient with a history of egg allergy should receive inactivated influenza vaccine (IIV). Although IIV is prepared using chicken eggs and contains a very small amount of egg protein, it has been shown to be safe in patients who have only experienced hives upon exposure to eggs, according to recommendations released by the Advisory Committee on Immunization Practices (ACIP). As a precaution, however, IIV should be administered in these patients by a health care professional who is trained to recognize the manifestations of egg allergy, and the patient should be observed for 30 minutes or longer for any signs of an adverse reaction. Since this patient has only experienced hives, not anaphylaxis, upon egg exposure, he may receive IIV.

Live attenuated influenza vaccine (LAIV) also contains only a small amount of egg protein; however, it is only approved to be administered to immunocompetent adults aged 49 years and younger without a history of any egg allergies, as it has not been extensively studied in patients with this allergy. Therefore, use of LAIV in this patient would not be appropriate.

Skin testing (either prick or intradermal) with influenza vaccine before vaccine administration is not recommended for patients with egg allergy because the presence of a positive skin test is not predictive of a subsequent systemic reaction. Skin testing with the vaccine may be appropriate for evaluation of patients with possible allergy to the vaccine itself, but not specifically egg allergy.

Influenza vaccination is recommended for all persons aged 6 months and older unless specifically contraindicated. As inactivated influenza vaccine can be safely administered to patients with a history of hives after exposure to egg, it is inappropriate to avoid vaccinating this patient against influenza.

Recombinant influenza vaccine (RIV) is produced using recombinant DNA technology, does not contain egg proteins, and can be used in patients with severe egg allergy (such as those who experience anaphylaxis). However, it would not be necessary in this patient who is a candidate for routine IIV administration.

KEY POINT

- Inactivated influenza vaccine can be safely administered to patients with an egg allergy who have only experienced hives upon exposure to eggs.

Bibliography

Grohskopf LA, Olsen SJ, Sokolow LZ, et al; Centers for Disease Control and Prevention. Prevention and control of seasonal influenza with vaccines: recommendations of the Advisory Committee on Immunization Practices (ACIP)–United States, 2014-15 influenza season. MMWR Morb Mortal Wkly Rep. 2014 Aug 15;63(32):691-7. [PMID: 25121712]

Item 79   Answer: D

Educational Objective: Recommend appropriate pharmacologic treatment for smoking cessation.

Varenicline will most likely give this patient the greatest chance of success in quitting smoking. A recent Cochrane meta-analysis showed that varenicline increased the odds of quitting smoking compared with placebo (OR, 2.88; 95% CI, 2.40-3.47). Although concerns have been raised regarding varenicline use and an increase in cardiovascular events, the FDA noted that the benefits outweigh potential risks in terms of cardiovascular risk.

Varenicline is more effective than bupropion (OR, 1.59; 95% CI, 1.29-1.96). Additionally, there is also concern that bupropion can lower seizure threshold and thus would not be the best option for this patient who has a history of seizures. Both varenicline and bupropion also have FDA warnings highlighting the risk of serious neuropsychiatric symptoms in patients using these medications.

Electronic cigarettes (E-cigarettes) may not be effective in reducing smoking cessation rates. In a recent randomized controlled superiority trial, adult smokers were randomly assigned to nicotine E-cigarettes, nicotine patches, or placebo E-cigarettes (no nicotine), with low intensity behavioral support. At 6 months, the risk difference for nicotine E-cigarettes versus nicotine patches was 1.51 (95% CI, 2.49-5.51); for nicotine E-cigarettes versus placebo E-cigarettes, 3.16 (95% CI, -2.29-8.61). There was insufficient statistical power to conclude superiority of nicotine E-cigarettes to

patches or to placebo E-cigarettes. Currently, the role of E-cigarettes in smoking cessation is uncertain.

Varenicline was also found to be more effective than the nicotine patch (OR, 1.51; 95% CI, 1.22-1.87) and nicotine gum (OR, 1.72; 95% CI, 1.38-2.13), and the nicotine inhaler, spray, tablets, or lozenges (OR, 1.42; 95% CI, 1.12-1.79) all used as single agents. Varenicline was not more effective than combination nicotine replacement therapy (OR, 1.06; 95% CI, 0.75-1.48) such as the combination of a rapid-onset nicotine replacement product (for example, nicotine spray or inhaler) with a long-duration nicotine replacement product (for example, a nicotine patch).

KEY POINT

- Varenicline is more effective in achieving smoking cessation than bupropion or single-agent nicotine replacement therapy but not more effective than combination nicotine replacement therapy.

Bibliography

Cahill K, Stevens S, Perera R, Lancaster T. Pharmacological interventions for smoking cessation: an overview and network meta-analysis. Cochrane Database Syst Rev. 2013 May 31;5:CD009329. [PMID: 23728690]

Item 80   Answer: D   H

Educational Objective: Diagnose brainstem stroke in a patient with vertigo.

This patient has acute vestibular syndrome (AVS), which may be caused by brainstem infarction or hemorrhage, and he should undergo MRI of the brain. AVS is characterized by prolonged vertigo of acute onset, spontaneous nystagmus, postural instability, and autonomic symptoms. The symptoms of AVS may mimic vestibular neuronitis; however, in this older patient with vascular disease, diplopia, gait instability, and immediate nystagmus with the Dix-Hallpike maneuver, a central cause of vertigo must first be ruled out. MRI is the initial test of choice in the patient presenting with a suspected central cause of vertigo. Diffusion-weighted MRI of the brain is recommended over CT scanning in evaluation of the posterior fossa as bone-related artifacts lead to inadequate imaging by CT.

This patient does not demonstrate neurologic signs or symptoms in the carotid artery distribution (monocular visual loss, hemisensory or hemimotor findings, apraxia, or problems with speech); therefore, carotid Doppler ultrasonography is not indicated.

A CT scan of the head and lumbar puncture are the tests of choice for the evaluation of subarachnoid hemorrhage, which is usually accompanied by severe headache and does not present with vertigo. In this patient, CT scan would not effectively image the posterior fossa.

KEY POINT

- Central vertigo is suggested by accompanying symptoms of dysarthria, dysphagia, diplopia, weakness, numbness, or ataxia.

Bibliography

Labuguen RH. Initial evaluation of vertigo. Am Fam Physician. 2006 Jan 15;73(2):244-51. Erratum in: Am Fam Physician. 2006 May 15;73(10):1704. [PMID: 16445269]

Item 81   Answer: C

Educational Objective: Manage a patient with a family history suggestive of an inherited disorder.

This patient should be referred for genetic counseling. Huntington disease, a neurodegenerative disorder, is transmitted as an autosomal dominant condition and is caused by cytosine-adenine-guanine trinucleotide repeat expansion in the *HD* gene (also known as the huntingtin or *HTT* gene). This patient has family members in multiple generations who have been diagnosed with Huntington disease, and he has a 50% chance of inheriting the gene from his father. Obtaining presymptomatic genetic testing in this patient would be appropriate; however, testing should only be performed after the patient undergoes genetic counseling. Key components of genetic counseling include informing the patient of the purpose of the test, implications of the test results, alternative testing options (including the option of foregoing testing), and possible risks and benefits of testing.

Although the choreiform movements that are seen in patients with symptomatic Huntington disease can be captured on electromyography, electromyography is not typically used in diagnosing Huntington disease and has no role in presymptomatic testing. Therefore, obtaining an electromyogram in this patient would not be appropriate.

Performing genetic testing without first providing adequate genetic counseling is not an appropriate intervention. It is essential that patients understand all of the ramifications of testing before testing is performed in order to make an educated decision.

It is inappropriate to tell this patient that genetic testing is unnecessary. Genetic testing is clearly warranted if the patient desires it.

KEY POINT

- Patients with a family history suggestive of an inherited disorder should receive genetic counseling before undergoing genetic testing.

Bibliography

Bordelon YM. Clinical neurogenetics: Huntington disease. Neurol Clin. 2013 Nov;31(4):1085-94. [PMID: 24176425]

Item 82   Answer: C

Educational Objective: Facilitate decision-making for a patient who lacks decision-making capacity.

The most appropriate course of action is to ask this patient's surrogates, his children, to relate what decisions the patient would make if he were capable. In the case of a patient who lacks decision-making capacity, a surrogate must guide decision making. If such a patient has an advance directive, the person named in that advance directive is the most appropriate (and legal) surrogate. If the patient's advance directive does not name a surrogate, or if the patient does not have an advance directive, the best surrogate is the person who best knows the patient's health care values, goals, and preferences; however, many U.S. states stipulate a hierarchy of surrogate decision makers in the absence of an advance directive (for example, the patient's spouse, followed by an adult child, and so forth). Surrogate decision making in the absence of an advance directive is common, as only about 20% of U.S. adults have advance directives in place. In the case of this patient, the two surviving adult children are the most appropriate surrogates. They have ethical and legal obligations to make decisions based on their father's health care–related values, goals, and preferences (that is, substituted judgment). The physician should ask what decision their father would make about his care if he were able.

Many surrogates are often aware of patients' values, goals, and preferences; however, if these values, goals, and preferences are unknown, a surrogate should make decisions in the patient's best interests.

A surrogate should not make decisions based on his or her own values, preferences, or what he or she feels is the correct course of action, as these views may differ from those of the patient.

Because nonmedical personnel may not be able to accurately convey specific medical details that might influence decision making, physicians should not defer these discussions to others (for example, social workers). Additionally, engaging in therapeutic decision making is an inherent professional responsibility of the attending physician.

Court-appointed guardians are selected for patients who lack decision-making capacity; whose health care–related values, goals, and preferences are unknown; and for whom no obvious surrogate decision maker exists. In the case of this patient, surrogates are available.

KEY POINT

- When a patient lacks decision-making capacity and does not have an advance directive, a surrogate who best knows the patient's health care values, goals, and preferences must make decisions.

Bibliography

Snyder L; American College of Physicians Ethics, Professionalism, and Human Rights Committee. American College of Physicians Ethics Manual: sixth edition. Ann Intern Med. 2012 Jan 3;156(1 Pt 2):73-104. [PMID: 22213573]

Item 83   Answer: B

Educational Objective: Screen for breast cancer in a patient with high breast density.

This patient with high breast density should receive routine digital screening mammography. High breast density, categorized as either heterogeneously dense breast tissue or extremely dense breast tissue (using the Breast Imaging

Reporting and Data System [BI-RADS] breast density categories) on mammography, imparts an increased risk of breast cancer (relative risk [RR] of 1.2 for heterogeneously dense breast tissue, RR of 2.1 for extremely dense breast tissue). Approximately 50% of women have high breast density, and some states mandate that increased breast density on mammography is directly reported to patients to inform them of this increased risk. High breast density also decreases the sensitivity of mammography to detect small lesions. Although high breast density alone does not necessitate additional or more frequent breast imaging other than routine screening mammography, there is evidence that digital mammography has an increased sensitivity for detecting small lesions in dense breasts compared with film mammography; it is therefore the preferred modality for routine screening, if available.

MRI is not recommended for either primary screening or as a supplemental test for women with increased breast density due to a lack of documented effectiveness and a high false-positive rate leading to unnecessary biopsies.

Breast ultrasonography is recommended by some organizations as supplemental testing in addition to mammography in women with dense breasts. However, no prospective trials of breast ultrasonography as a primary screening modality currently exist, and its role as a supplemental test to mammography has not been clearly defined. It is therefore not recommended as a replacement to digital mammography.

KEY POINT

- Women with high breast density, categorized as either heterogeneously dense breast tissue or extremely dense breast tissue with the Breast Imaging Reporting and Data System (BI-RADS) breast density categories, should undergo routine digital screening mammography.

Bibliography

Wang AT, Vachon CM, Brandt KR, Ghosh K. Breast density and breast cancer risk: a practical review. Mayo Clin Proc. 2014 Apr;89(4):548-57. [PMID: 24684876]

Item 84   Answer: D

Educational Objective: Evaluate lower extremity edema due to chronic venous insufficiency.

No additional testing is indicated in this patient. The patient's isolated bilateral lower extremity edema is most likely due to chronic venous insufficiency, as supported by the otherwise normal examination findings and lack of abnormal laboratory test results, and no further diagnostic studies are indicated. The edema associated with chronic venous insufficiency typically is insidious in onset. It worsens with prolonged standing and is improved with elevating the legs and with walking. Leg discomfort is also often gradual in onset and is described as a tired or heavy sensation in the legs. Other symptoms can include pruritus, skin discoloration, and ulceration. Compression stockings are considered first-line therapy for patients with lower extremity edema due to chronic venous disease. The patient should be instructed to put on these stockings in the morning before edema is present and to wear the stockings as much as possible when he is in a standing position. The stockings can be removed at night.

Obtaining an abdominal/pelvic CT scan in this patient would not be appropriate, as he lacks signs and symptoms that would suggest abdominal or pelvic pathology.

Lower extremity venous duplex ultrasonography is not necessary in this patient who lacks risk factors for deep venous thrombosis (prolonged immobility, known cancer history, or use of predisposing medications) and does not have a clinical picture consistent with bilateral deep venous thrombosis.

In the absence of symptoms and examination findings that suggest heart failure (such as orthopnea, dyspnea, paroxysmal nocturnal dyspnea, elevated central venous pressure, crackles in the lower lung fields, and S_3 and/or S_4 heart sounds), the diagnostic utility of a transthoracic echocardiogram is likely low and therefore not appropriate in this patient.

KEY POINT

- The diagnosis of lower extremity edema due to chronic venous insufficiency usually may be made based on a consistent clinical presentation and minimal laboratory testing.

Bibliography

Trayes KP, Studdiford JS, Pickle S, Tully AS. Edema: diagnosis and management. Am Fam Physician. 2013 Jul 15;88(2):102-10. [PMID: 23939641]

Item 85   Answer: C

Educational Objective: Manage functional incontinence in a frail older woman.

Behavioral therapy utilizing prompted voiding is the most appropriate management of this patient. This patient's incontinence may be due to multiple factors, including structural and functional causes complicated by her cognitive impairment and decreased mobility. Prompted voiding involves regularly asking the patient to report on incontinence, asking the patient if he or she needs to void, providing assistance with access to the bathroom, and praising the patient for continence. This technique has been shown to reduce urinary incontinence in older patients who have caregivers capable of working with them, such as this one, as well as those residing in assisted-care facilities. This intervention is also usually timed so that prompted voiding occurs before accumulation of a large volume of urine in the bladder, reducing the likelihood that incontinence will occur. With active and consistent caregiver involvement, timed and prompted voiding can help achieve improved bladder control.

Antimuscarinic agents are used to decrease urgency, frequency, or incontinence in overactive bladder with urge incontinence. Adverse effects are common, however, including constipation, dry mouth, dizziness, and confusion, and older patients are at greatest risk for adverse consequences. Therefore, an antimuscarinic agent would not be an appropriate therapeutic choice in this older patient with cognitive impairment.

Pelvic floor muscle training is effective in reducing incontinence but requires active participation by the patient. Although training is implemented by physical therapists or advanced practice nurses, both pelvic floor muscle and bladder training require intact cognition and the ability to self-manage and self-sustain a training regimen and are therefore unlikely to be effective in this patient with dementia.

Systemic estrogen therapy has not been shown to alleviate urinary incontinence and may worsen symptoms. It is also associated with increased cardiovascular risks when initiated in women more than 10 years post-menopause.

Attention to skin care and use of absorptive products with frequent changes are extremely important in preventing skin breakdown in older patients with incontinence. A review of modifiable factors is also helpful, including medication use, mobility issues, weight reduction, and caffeine reduction.

KEY POINT

- Behavioral therapy utilizing prompted voiding has been shown to reduce urinary incontinence in older patients with dementia.

Bibliography

Markland AD, Vaughan CP, Johnson TM 2nd, Burgio KL, Goode PS. Incontinence. Med Clin North Am. 2011 May;95(3):539-54. [PMID: 21549877]

Item 86   Answer: D

Educational Objective: Treat an unstageable pressure ulcer in an older patient.

This patient has a sacral decubitus pressure ulcer that is unstageable, and the most appropriate treatment is surgical debridement. Unstageable pressure ulcers are characterized by full-thickness tissue loss in which the base of the ulcer is covered by slough or eschar. The black eschar at the base of the wound prevents adequate evaluation of wound depth and further impairs wound healing. Therefore, this patient should undergo debridement of the eschar to expose healthy, viable tissue in order to assess the depth of the wound, allow for wound staging, and promote healing. Debridement can be accomplished either surgically or with specialized dressings, such as saline wet-to-dry dressings or autolytic dressings.

Lymphomatous invasion of the skin is highly unlikely in this patient without other evidence of active disease following recent treatment; therefore, biopsy is not indicated.

Antibiotics would be indicated in the case of an infected pressure ulcer; however, there is no evidence that this patient's wound is infected at this time. There is no visible drainage or pus, and there is no surrounding erythema to suggest cellulitis. Additionally, he has no systemic signs or symptoms of infection.

The goal environment for ideal wound healing is a moist wound bed that controls excess exudate. The wound bed should be neither too moist (macerated) nor too dry. Leaving a wound open to air to dry is rarely, if ever, appropriate management.

KEY POINT

- Debridement of eschar is necessary in patients with unstageable pressure ulcers to assess the depth of the wound and promote wound healing.

Bibliography

Schiffman J, Golinko MS, Yan A, Flattau A, Tomic-Canic M, Brem H. Operative debridement of pressure ulcers. World J Surg. 2009 Jul;33(7): 1396-402. [PMID: 19424752]

Item 87   Answer: B

Educational Objective: Treat extrapyramidal symptoms in a patient who has schizophrenia.

The most appropriate treatment for this patient with schizophrenia is to switch his chlorpromazine to clozapine. His history and physical examination findings are suggestive of extrapyramidal symptoms, and tardive dyskinesia in particular. Extrapyramidal symptoms are drug-induced disorders of movement that usually occur with agents that block dopamine receptors. Although a number of different drugs may be associated with extrapyramidal symptoms, they are most frequently caused by first-generation antipsychotic medications (such as chlorpromazine) that antagonize D_2 dopamine receptors. Extrapyramidal symptoms typically include akathisia (a sense of motor restlessness with a compelling urge to move that makes it difficult to sit still), dystonia (continuous, involuntary spasms and contractions of major muscle groups), and parkinsonism (tremor, rigidity, and bradykinesia). Tardive dyskinesia is a specific form of extrapyramidal movement disorder that occurs with longer-term use (typically >1 month) of dopamine-blocking agents with variable findings of orofacial dyskinesia, facial grimacing, athetotic (slow, writhing) movements, and tics. Extrapyramidal symptoms are more common with first-generation antipsychotic agents compared with second-generation antipsychotic medications. Thus, switching to the second-generation antipsychotic clozapine would be the best option in this patient. A recent meta-analysis showed that clozapine was not only the least likely to cause extrapyramidal symptoms among antipsychotic agents, but was also the most effective drug. This patient also exhibits a significant amount of negative symptoms (flat affect, monotone speech, social withdrawal), which may respond better to a second-generation antipsychotic medication.

Continuing chlorpromazine would be inappropriate in this patient because tardive dyskinesia is a serious manifestation of extrapyramidal symptoms and may become untreatable if prolonged. Thus, the offending agent should be stopped as soon as possible.

Haloperidol has been shown to be significantly more likely to cause extrapyramidal symptoms than any other first-generation or second-generation antipsychotic medication; therefore, switching to haloperidol in this patient would not be appropriate.

Similarly, switching to another first-generation antipsychotic agent, thioridazine, would also likely not address his extrapyramidal side effects associated with therapy.

KEY POINT

- The second-generation antipsychotic agent clozapine is the most appropriate treatment option for patients with schizophrenia who exhibit extrapyramidal symptoms.

Bibliography
Leucht S, Cipriani A, Spineli L, et al. Comparative efficacy and tolerability of 15 antipsychotic drugs in schizophrenia: a multiple-treatments meta-analysis. Lancet. 2013 Sep 14;382(9896):951-62. Erratum in: Lancet. 2013 Sep 14;382(9896):940. [PMID: 23810019]

Item 88   Answer: A

Educational Objective: Treat menopausal genitourinary symptoms.

Estradiol vaginal tablets are the most appropriate treatment for this patient with genitourinary syndrome of menopause, indicated by her history of vaginal dryness, dyspareunia, and by pale mucosa with decreased rugae on physical examination, as well as the vaginal pH greater than 4.5. In menopausal women, low estrogen levels result in physiologic changes in the urogenital tissues that may result in genitourinary symptoms. The abnormal vaginal discharge is consistent with atrophic tissue friability.

Menopausal genitourinary symptoms that do not respond to vaginal lubricants are best treated with topical low-dose vaginal estradiol, which is available as vaginal tablets or a cream. Low-dose vaginal formulations are not absorbed systemically to a significant degree, and therefore, oral progestin is not needed when administering these topical agents. Estrogen-containing pliable polymer vaginal rings are also available, but only the low-dose ring is appropriate for treatment of menopausal genitourinary symptoms.

Bacterial vaginosis is commonly characterized by a malodorous thin gray discharge, with a positive whiff test and clue cells on saline microscopy. The absence of these findings argues against this diagnosis, and treatment for bacterial vaginosis with metronidazole vaginal gel would not be appropriate.

Miconazole vaginal cream is the treatment for vulvovaginal candidiasis. This patient did not have the white discharge and pruritus that are associated with a yeast infection, and the wet mount was negative for hyphae. Therefore, this would not be an appropriate treatment for this patient.

When genitourinary symptoms are the primary concern in a menopausal woman, low-dose vaginal estradiol is the therapeutic standard. Systemic hormone therapy can be used selectively to treat moderate to severe systemic vasomotor symptoms, but for this patient, systemic hormone therapy is not indicated.

KEY POINT

- Menopausal genitourinary symptoms that do not respond to vaginal lubricants are best treated with topical low-dose vaginal estradiol.

Bibliography
Management of symptomatic vulvovaginal atrophy: 2013 position statement of The North American Menopause Society. Menopause. 2013 Sep;20(9):888-902. [PMID: 23985562]

Item 89   Answer: B

Educational Objective: Treat acute pain in a patient at the end of life.

This patient with acute severe pain should be treated with hydromorphone. The opioid analgesic hydromorphone is a very effective pain medication. It is preferred over morphine in the setting of kidney failure because it is metabolized primarily by the liver and is less likely to lead to the accumulation of potentially toxic metabolites. When a parenteral route of medication administration is indicated, such as when titrating medication for acute pain, either intravenous or subcutaneous routes are acceptable. The intravenous route results in a faster onset of action, although the medication wears off faster; the subcutaneous route has only a slightly slower onset of action, but the effect may last longer. Absorption and effect are very reliable with both routes of administration. Although the intravenous route tends to be more commonly used, subcutaneous administration is a reasonable alternative in hospitalized patients who may not be good candidates for intravenous medications or may not wish intravenous access, as may occur in patients receiving comfort care measures.

Fentanyl transdermal patches should only be used in patients who already have some degree of opioid tolerance, and this patient is opioid naïve. Additionally, the onset of action for a fentanyl patch is 12 to 18 hours, far too long for a patient with acute severe pain.

Morphine is contraindicated in the setting of significant kidney failure (estimated glomerular filtration rate <30 mL/min/1.73 m²), even at the end of life, due to the accumulation of toxic metabolites that may cause neurotoxicity with symptoms of delirium, myoclonus, and seizure.

This patient has no bowel sounds on examination, and it is unclear whether she would absorb oral medication, such as tramadol. Additionally, oral medications have a longer onset of action than either intravenous or subcutaneous routes. In the setting of acute severe pain, a parenteral route with more reliable absorption and shorter onset of action is more appropriate.

KEY POINT

- Morphine should be avoided in the setting of kidney failure.

Bibliography
Swetz KM, Kamal AH. In the clinic. Palliative care. Ann Intern Med. 2012 Feb 7;156(3):ITC2-1-TC2-16. [PMID: 22312158]

Item 90   Answer: B

Educational Objective: Report an impaired colleague to the appropriate authorities.

The physician should report his colleague's behavior to the colleague's supervisor. Physicians may be reluctant to report colleagues suspected of impairment because of discomfort associated with "speaking up," fears of retaliation, and desire to protect colleagues. However, physicians have a duty to speak up, as an impaired and disruptive colleague's behaviors may harm patients, negatively affect team morale, and impede learning. This physician's colleague manifests multiple behaviors suggestive of impairment, including frequent absences, altered mood, lapses in judgment, and changes in clinical performance. Since the physician has already directly confronted his colleague and his concerns were dismissed, he should report the impaired colleague to the appropriate supervisor.

Asking other physicians if they have made similar observations delays the reporting process and does not relieve the observing physician of his responsibility of reporting the suspected impaired colleague.

Physicians should not review the medical records of patients who are not under their care; therefore, the observing physician should not review the colleague's patient care notes for evidence of negligent care. Conducting such record reviews delays and does not relieve the observing physician of his responsibility of reporting the suspected impaired colleague. Additionally, assuming the observing physician is not the colleague's personal physician, it would be unethical and illegal (breach of confidentiality) for the observing physician to review the colleague's medical record to determine if there might be a medical or psychiatric reason for his behavior, even under circumstances of possible impairment.

The observing physician has a professional and ethical responsibility to report the impaired colleague. Taking no further action may result in patient harm.

KEY POINT

- Physicians have a duty to "speak up" about impaired and disruptive colleagues in order to protect patient welfare.

Bibliography

Topazian RJ, Hook CC, Mueller PS. Duty to speak up in the health care setting: a professionalism and ethics analysis. Minn Med. 2013 Nov;96(11):40-3. [PMID: 24428018]

Item 91   Answer: D

Educational Objective: Evaluate syncope with appropriate use of tilt-table testing.

The most appropriate diagnostic study is tilt-table testing. Tilt-table testing may be helpful in patients with reflex syncope triggered by standing, patients in high-risk settings (for example, construction workers, surgeons) with unexplained episodes of syncope, patients with recurrent syncopal episodes in the absence of organic heart disease, or patients with recurrent episodes in the presence of heart disease

when cardiac causes of syncope are excluded. Given that this patient's syncope is triggered by prolonged standing in the operating room, occurs in a high-risk setting (posing a significant occupational hazard), and occurs in the absence of organic heart disease, she should undergo tilt-table testing. Although the sensitivity, specificity, and reproducibility of the tilt-table test are low, in this setting it may be helpful in elucidating the diagnosis and in differentiating orthostatic hypotension from neurocardiogenic syncope.

The American College of Physicians and other groups do not recommend brain imaging, either with CT or MRI, in the setting of witnessed syncope without seizure activity or other neurologic symptoms because the likelihood of a central nervous system cause of the syncope is extremely low and patient outcomes are not improved with further neurologic testing. This patient did not exhibit seizure activity, and her neurologic examination is normal; therefore, brain MRI is not indicated.

Echocardiography is recommended in the evaluation of syncope if structural heart disease is suspected. However, a cardiac cause of syncope is extremely low in this patient who has no history of structural or ischemic heart disease, no symptoms suggesting heart disease, no murmur on examination, and a normal 12-lead electrocardiogram.

The diagnostic yield of 24- to 48-hour electrocardiographic monitoring is very low (1%-2%) unless there are frequent syncopal episodes over a short period of time. Because this patient has already undergone 24-hour ambulatory electrocardiographic monitoring with normal results and her episodes occur every few months, it is unlikely that 48-hour ambulatory electrocardiographic monitoring will be diagnostically helpful. If arrhythmias were strongly suspected, an implantable loop recorder would be a more appropriate diagnostic option for this patient.

Since this patient has had three separate episodes of syncope that occur in high-risk situations, further diagnostic evaluation to determine the cause of the syncope and guide therapy should be pursued.

KEY POINT

- Tilt-table testing is helpful in evaluating reflex syncope triggered by standing, unexplained episodes of syncope in a high-risk setting, recurrent episodes of syncope in the absence of organic heart disease, or recurrent episodes of syncope in the presence of heart disease when cardiac causes are excluded.

Bibliography

Forleo C, Guida P, Iacoviello M, et al. Head-up tilt testing for diagnosing vasovagal syncope: a meta-analysis. Int J Cardiol. 2013 Sep 20;168(1): 27-35. [PMID: 23041006]

Item 92   Answer: B

Educational Objective: Diagnose generalized anxiety disorder.

The most likely diagnosis is generalized anxiety disorder (GAD). The DSM-5 diagnostic criteria for GAD are as follows: 1) excessive anxiety or worry about a number of events or activities (for example, school or work) occurring more days than not for at least 6 months; 2) the patient recognizes it is difficult to control the worry; 3) the anxiety or worry is associated with at least three of the following symptoms: restlessness, easy fatigability, difficulty concentrating, irritability, muscle tension, and sleep disturbance; 4) the anxiety, worry, or symptoms cause impairment at school, work, or other settings and cannot be attributable to medical or other psychiatric conditions, medications, or substance use. A useful tool for identifying and assessing the severity of GAD is the Generalized Anxiety Disorder 7 (GAD-7) assessment tool that rates seven items on a scale of 0 to 3 based on increasing severity. A score of 5 to 9 indicates mild anxiety, 10 to 14 moderate anxiety, and 15 to 21 severe anxiety. This patient meets the DSM-5 criteria, and his GAD-7 score of 13 is consistent with this diagnosis. Treatment options include psychotherapy and medications. Cognitive-behavioral therapy is the most effective psychotherapy for GAD and in trials has been shown to be as effective as medications.

Symptoms of GAD overlap with those of attention-deficit/hyperactivity disorder. However, the main symptoms that this patient is experiencing are worry and anxiety with associated physical symptoms.

Patients with GAD may manifest symptoms of depression; indeed, patients with anxiety disorders may also experience depression. However, the main symptoms that this patient is experiencing are not related to mood, but rather to worry and anxiety.

This patient is not manifesting symptoms of obsessive-compulsive disorder (such as recurrent and persistent thoughts or impulses), making this diagnosis unlikely.

KEY POINT

- Generalized anxiety disorder is characterized by excessive anxiety and worry about various events or activities occurring most days for at least 6 months, with difficulty controlling worrying.

Bibliography
Patel G, Fancher TL. In the clinic. Generalized anxiety disorder. Ann Intern Med. 2013 Dec 3;159(11):ITC6-1-ITC6-12. [PMID: 24297210]

Item 93   Answer: A

Educational Objective: Manage hepatitis B virus vaccination in a patient with an interrupted vaccine series.

This patient should receive a third dose of the hepatitis B virus (HBV) vaccine to complete the vaccine series. HBV vaccination is indicated in this patient who is traveling to China, an area with a hepatitis B surface antigen (HBsAg) prevalence of 5% to 7%. Typically, the vaccine series is administered as a three-dose regimen over a 6-month time period, with doses administered at 0, 1, and 6 months. Administration of the entire series in accordance with the recommended

schedule leads to seroconversion and adequate immunity in more than 95% of persons. This patient has only received two doses over a period of 9 months; consequently, the series is considered to be interrupted. When a vaccine series is interrupted, the most appropriate approach is to resume rather than restart the series, as development of immunity is progressive and giving doses at longer-than-recommended intervals does not usually decrease the final immunologic response. Therefore, the third dose of the HBV vaccine should be administered to this patient now.

Serologic testing to determine this patient's immunity against hepatitis B is unnecessary, because this patient has yet to complete the primary HBV vaccine series, and routine postvaccination testing is not recommended by the Centers for Disease Control and Prevention. Postvaccination serologic testing is indicated only in patients whose subsequent management depends on their immunity status. These individuals may include health care and public safety workers, HIV-positive individuals, persons who are receiving chronic hemodialysis, sexual partners of HBsAg-positive individuals, and injection drug users.

Administering only two of the three recommended doses of HBV vaccine decreases the likelihood of seroconversion. Therefore, discontinuing the vaccine series following only two doses would not be appropriate.

KEY POINT

- When a vaccine series is interrupted, the most appropriate approach is to resume rather than restart the series.

Bibliography
Kim DK, Bridges CB, Harriman KH; Centers for Disease Control and Prevention; Advisory Committee on Immunization Practices (ACIP); ACIP Adult Immunization Work Group. Advisory committee on immunization practices recommended immunization schedule for adults aged 19 years or older–United States, 2015. MMWR Morb Mortal Wkly Rep. 2015 Feb 6;64(4):91-2. [PMID: 25654609]

Item 94   Answer: B

Educational Objective: Treat a patient with olecranon bursitis.

The most appropriate treatment for this patient is NSAID therapy. The patient is experiencing olecranon bursitis, most likely from the low-level repetitive trauma of rubbing his elbow against the car armrest. The olecranon bursa is a subcutaneous synovial-lined sac overlying the olecranon process at the proximal aspect of the ulna. It cushions the olecranon and reduces friction between the olecranon and the skin during movement. Because of its superficial location, it is particularly susceptible to inflammation with acute or chronic trauma. Although most cases of olecranon bursitis are noninfectious, they may be caused by bacterial infection, particularly if there is an overlying abrasion or cellulitis. Less commonly, olecranon bursitis may be due to a crystalline process, such as gout. Aspiration is indicated in patients with suspected infectious or crystalline bursitis, or if the swelling is extensive and impairs activity, even if likely benign. Protection of the bursa from further trauma or irritation is the cornerstone of therapy, and treatment with an agent that inhibits inflammation and provides pain relief is usually helpful in decreasing fluid accumulation and providing symptom relief. NSAIDs have both analgesic and anti-inflammatory effects, which is ideal for this purpose. Given the patient's otherwise good health, a short course of NSAID therapy at an anti-inflammatory dose will provide maximal benefit with relatively little risk.

Intrabursal glucocorticoid injections may reduce swelling in bursitis. However, there is not strong evidence of effectiveness when used in superficial areas such as the olecranon bursa, and there is significant risk of side effects, including skin atrophy, development of a draining sinus tract, and infection. Additionally, glucocorticoids provide no analgesia. They are therefore used only in severe or refractory cases of olecranon bursitis.

Topical lidocaine and tramadol are analgesic agents and do not have anti-inflammatory effects. They will provide some pain relief but will not reduce the swelling of the bursitis. Topical analgesics may have value in minimizing systemic drug exposure; however, this would not be a major issue for this patient.

KEY POINT

- Physical protection of the bursa and NSAID therapy are effective treatments for noninfectious olecranon bursitis.

Bibliography

Baumbach SF, Lobo CM, Badyine I, Mutschler W, Kanz KG. Prepatellar and olecranon bursitis: literature review and development of a treatment algorithm. Arch Orthop Trauma Surg. 2014 Mar;134(3):359-70. [PMID: 24305696]

Item 95   Answer: D

Educational Objective: Evaluate a patient with medically unexplained symptoms.

This patient with medically unexplained symptoms (MUS) should not undergo repeated or additional testing. Repeated physical examinations and appropriate laboratory and ancillary testing by internists and specialists over an extended period of time have been unrevealing of significant disease. Without significant change in the clinical picture, no further testing is indicated. The physician should instead focus on establishing and strengthening a therapeutic alliance with the patient using patient-centered methods. Cognitive-behavioral therapy that consists of 1) educating the patient so he or she understands the symptoms, 2) obtaining a commitment from the patient to assume responsibility for his or her improvement, 3) facilitating realistic goals, and 4) negotiating a treatment plan can be helpful in the office setting. A systematic review of 34 randomized controlled trials demonstrated that, in most studies, cognitive-behavioral therapy was effective in treating patients with MUS.

Although this patient may have intolerance to certain foods and believes that dietary manipulation improves her symptoms, she does not have evidence of significant food allergy, which may be manifested as an IgE-mediated allergic reaction or more chronic symptoms isolated to the gastrointestinal tract. She has also been evaluated by an allergist who did not pursue food allergy testing. Therefore, food allergy testing would likely be of low yield in this patient.

Although this patient has chronic low back pain, she is without concerning symptoms or physical examination findings that would warrant further imaging of her lumbosacral spine, and MRI would not be beneficial.

Repeat Lyme disease serologic testing is unwarranted in this patient. Although systemic symptoms and chronic fatigue are often attributed to Lyme infection, this is a very uncommon occurrence and would be extremely unlikely in this patient with no clinical findings and negative serology.

KEY POINT

- Patients with medically unexplained symptoms should not undergo repeated or additional testing if there is no change in the clinical presentation.

Bibliography

Isaac ML, Paauw DS. Medically unexplained symptoms. Med Clin North Am. 2014 May;98:663-72. [PMID: 24758967]

Item 96   Answer: A

Educational Objective: Diagnose syncope due to orthostatic hypotension.

The most likely cause of syncope in this patient is orthostatic hypotension. Syncope is nontraumatic, complete transient loss of consciousness and loss of postural tone. Onset is abrupt and recovery is spontaneous, rapid, and complete. Orthostatic syncope is associated with a decline of 20 mm Hg or more in systolic blood pressure (or ≥10 mm Hg drop in diastolic blood pressure) within 3 minutes of standing. Orthostatic syncope may occur as a result of primary autonomic failure, secondary autonomic failure (due to diabetes mellitus, amyloidosis, spinal cord injuries, or Parkinson disease), hypovolemia, medications (vasodilators, diuretics), or age-associated changes in blood pressure regulation. On examination, this patient has significant orthostasis by blood pressure and pulse measurements. These orthostatic changes may be due to volume contraction secondary to chronically elevated blood glucose levels resulting in an osmotic diuresis, autonomic insufficiency as a consequence of long-standing diabetes, and treatment with a vasodilating blood pressure medication. The initial treatment is hydration with isotonic saline, and further evaluation of his diabetic control and medication regimen is indicated.

The absence of aura, rhythmic involuntary movement, postictal confusion, and tongue biting make seizure an unlikely cause of this patient's syncope.

Although patients with diabetes are at risk for cardiac ischemia, this patient has no cardiac symptoms and has an electrocardiogram without acute changes or evidence of prior myocardial infarction, suggesting against a subclinical ischemic cardiac cause.

Cardiac syncope due to arrhythmia is abrupt in onset and may be accompanied by palpitations, which this patient did not have. Additionally, orthostatic changes or other evidence of volume depletion, as is present in this patient, would not be expected with arrhythmia, ischemia, or seizure.

KEY POINT

- Orthostatic syncope is characterized by a decline of 20 mm Hg or more in systolic blood pressure (or ≥10 mm Hg drop in diastolic blood pressure) within 3 minutes of standing and occurs as a result of autonomic failure, hypovolemia, medication use, or age-associated changes in blood pressure regulation.

Bibliography

Puppala VK, Dickinson O, Benditt DG. Syncope: classification and risk stratification. J Cardiol. 2014 Mar;63(3):171-7. [PMID: 24405895]

Item 97   Answer: C

Educational Objective: Screen for HIV infection.

This patient should be screened for HIV infection. The U.S. Preventive Services Task Force (USPSTF) recommends one-time HIV screening for all adults aged 15 to 65 years. Screening in adolescents younger than 15 years and adults older than 65 years may be indicated depending on individual risk factors. The currently recommended method for initial testing is a combination immunoassay that detects both HIV antibody and p24 antigen, a viral capsid protein that is elevated early in infection. This test replaces the previously used highly sensitive enzyme-linked immunosorbent assay (ELISA) for antibodies directed toward HIV. It is estimated that approximately 25% of persons with HIV infection are unaware of their diagnosis. Initiating antiretroviral therapy in asymptomatic patients compared with those who present clinically is associated with reduced risk for AIDS-related death.

The USPSTF strongly recommends lipid screening in women aged 45 years and older who have risk factors for coronary heart disease (diabetes mellitus, personal history of coronary heart disease or noncoronary atherosclerosis, family history of cardiovascular disease before age 50 years in male relatives or age 60 years in female relatives, tobacco use, hypertension, obesity [BMI ≥30]). Although the optimal screening interval is undetermined, it is reasonable to rescreen every 5 years, or at a shorter interval if the patient's lipid levels are approaching those that would indicate therapy. The 2013 American College of Cardiology/American Heart Association cardiovascular risk guideline indicates that it is reasonable to assess traditional risk factors (including total and HDL cholesterol levels) every 4 to 6 years in adults between the ages of 20 and 79 years who are free from atherosclerotic cardiovascular disease. This patient's lipid levels were normal last year and she is otherwise at low risk

for cardiovascular disease; therefore, she would not benefit from repeat lipid screening.

The USPSTF currently recommends screening for type 2 diabetes mellitus only in asymptomatic adults with sustained blood pressure higher than 135/80 mm Hg; however, a USPSTF draft guideline from 2014 recommends screening for abnormal blood glucose level and type 2 diabetes in adults with risk factors, including age 45 years or older, obesity or overweight, first-degree relative with diabetes, history of gestational diabetes or polycystic ovary syndrome, and certain high-risk ethnic backgrounds (African Americans, American Indians/Alaska Natives, Asian Americans, Hispanics/Latinos, and Native Hawaiians/Pacific Islanders). The American Diabetes Association recommends screening for diabetes in all adults aged 45 years and older and adults younger than 45 years with a BMI of 25 or higher and one risk factor for diabetes. The optimal screening interval is unknown, although the American Diabetes Association recommends screening every 3 years. Because a fasting plasma glucose level was obtained in this patient last year, repeat testing is not necessary at this time.

In women aged 30 to 65 years in whom cytology (Pap smear) and human papillomavirus (HPV) testing are negative, repeat testing is recommended in 5 years. Because a Pap smear and HPV testing were performed in this patient 3 years ago, she should be screened again for cervical cancer in 2 years.

KEY POINT

- HIV screening is recommended for all adults aged 15 to 65 years.

Bibliography

Marrazzo JM, del Rio C, Holtgrave DR, et al; International Antiviral Society-USA Panel. HIV prevention in clinical care settings: 2014 recommendations of the International Antiviral Society-USA Panel. JAMA. 2014 Jul 23-30;312(4):390-409. Erratum in: JAMA. 2014 Jul 23-30;312(4):403. JAMA. 2014 Aug 13;312(6):652. [PMID: 25038358]

Item 98   Answer: C

Educational Objective: Manage an older patient with visual impairment.

This older adult patient with vision difficulties should be referred to an eye professional. Vision impairment is common in older adults, and unlike in younger patients, older patients are more likely to have conditions such as glaucoma, macular degeneration, or diseases of the vitreous body or retina. An undilated ophthalmoscopic examination in the primary care setting is insufficient to diagnose these eye disorders. Evaluation for glaucoma involves measurement of intraocular pressure (tonometry), which is not available in most clinicians' offices, and other conditions involving the vitreous body or retina require eye dilation and examination with a slit lamp to allow for full evaluation. Additionally, the relatively rapid change in this patient's otherwise stable vision is suggestive of an acute or rapidly progressive process. Therefore, timely referral to an eye professional is the most appropriate next step in managing this patient's vision symptoms.

Obtaining an erythrocyte sedimentation rate is necessary in patients with suspected giant cell arteritis; however, this patient does not present with symptoms of headache, muscle aches, or jaw claudication, making the pretest probability of giant cell arteritis very low. Therefore, obtaining an erythrocyte sedimentation rate is not indicated at this time.

Visual screening tests, such as the Snellen eye chart or the pinhole test, are used primarily to assess for presbyopia. Although these tests may be abnormal in this patient, they would not sufficiently evaluate other potentially serious visual conditions that may be present.

KEY POINT

- Visual acuity screening alone is insufficient to adequately assess for eye disorders in older patients.

Bibliography
U.S. Preventive Services Task Force. Screening for impaired visual acuity in older adults: U.S. Preventive Services Task Force recommendation statement. Ann Intern Med. 2009 Jul 7;151(1):37-43, W10. [PMID: 19581645]

Item 99   Answer: B

Educational Objective: Diagnose patellofemoral pain syndrome.

This patient has patellofemoral pain syndrome. Patellofemoral pain syndrome is of unclear etiology but is likely due to several different factors that affect the load distribution underneath the patella, such as deconditioning and patellofemoral malalignment. It is characterized by anterior knee pain that is slow in onset and typically made worse with running, climbing stairs, and prolonged sitting. On examination, there is frequently increased patellar laxity with medial and lateral displacement. Additionally, pain may be reproduced when posteriorly directed pressure is applied to the patella. Treatment is often challenging but generally consists of addressing any identified underlying causes (such as deconditioning), activity modification, and physical therapy.

Iliotibial band syndrome can occur from overuse or from alterations in anatomic alignment or biomechanical function. It typically causes lateral knee pain that is worsened by walking down an incline. On examination, there is frequently tenderness to palpation of the lateral femoral epicondyle, which is approximately 2 to 3 cm proximal to the lateral joint line, accompanied by weakness of the hip abductor muscles and the knee extender and flexor muscles. Pain is reproduced when the examiner repeatedly flexes and extends the supine patient's knee while the examiner's thumb is on the lateral femoral epicondyle (positive Noble test).

Pes anserine bursitis is caused by inflammation of the pes anserine bursa, located at the proximal anteromedial tibia. Bursitis usually develops as the result of overuse or constant friction and stress on the bursa. Pes anserine

bursitis is common in athletes, particularly runners. Tenderness on the anteromedial aspect of the knee about 4 to 5 cm below the joint line is reproduced by palpation.

Prepatellar bursitis is caused by inflammation of the prepatellar bursa, which overlies the anterior surface of the patella. Patients with prepatellar bursitis present with anterior knee pain and swelling. Possible causes include direct trauma, gout, and infection. On examination, a palpable fluid collection is often present.

KEY POINT

- Patellofemoral pain syndrome is characterized by anterior knee pain that is slow in onset and typically made worse with running, climbing stairs, and prolonged sitting.

Bibliography
Collado H, Fredericson M. Patellofemoral pain syndrome. Clin Sports Med. 2010 Jul;29(3):379-98. [PMID: 20610028]

Item 100   Answer: D

Educational Objective: Manage cachexia in a patient with cancer.

The patient's current care should be continued. Anorexia, weight loss, and cachexia reflect a final common pathway during the terminal phase of most disease processes. Assuming potentially reversible conditions (nausea, altered taste, medication side effects, bowel obstruction, dysphagia, psychological comorbidities) have been ruled out, disease-related cachexia is caused by an altered neurohormonal, inflammatory milieu that results in profound alterations in metabolism. These changes lead to a decreased appetite and increased catabolism, leading to progressive weight loss. Educating this patient and her family on the etiology and pathophysiology of cachexia is the primary intervention and may help them to better understand and accept the expected course of the disease.

Only 20% to 30% of patients who take pharmacologic agents, such as dronabinol and megestrol, for cachexia of advanced disease gain any weight at all. For those who do gain weight, there is no improvement in mortality, and the majority of studies of their use in cachexia associated with cancer show no improvement in the quality of life. The role of other agents for treatment of cachexia in advanced disease, including anabolic steroids, medical marijuana and its derivatives, melatonin, and NSAIDs, remains to be defined.

Cachexia cannot be significantly reversed by more aggressive or invasive methods of nutritional support, including enteral (or parenteral) nutrition, and these interventions in the context of cachexia of advanced disease do not improve morbidity or mortality. Additionally, interventions to provide artificial nutrition, such as use of a nasogastric or nasojejunal tube or placement of a percutaneous endoscopic gastrostomy tube, have some associated risk and a potential negative effect on the patient's quality of life.

KEY POINT

- Artificial nutrition and pharmacologic agents do not improve morbidity and mortality or quality of life in cancer patients with cachexia.

Bibliography

Swetz KM, Kamal AH. In the clinic. Palliative care. Ann Intern Med. 2012 Feb 7;156(3):ITC2-1-TC2-16. [PMID: 22312158]

Item 101   Answer: A

Educational Objective: Diagnose a central pain syndrome.

This patient has fibromyalgia, one type of central pain syndrome. Central pain results from dysregulation of sensory processing pathways within the nervous system. This dysregulation amplifies sensory input, resulting in the increased perception of pain. Central pain can be classically neuropathic, such as poststroke pain or post–spinal cord injury pain, or it can be more indistinct, such as in fibromyalgia. The pain is usually constant, with bursts of more severe pain, often exacerbated by cough, temperature changes, movement, or emotions. Central pain syndromes can also evolve out of unrelenting chronic pain when persistent stimulation of peripheral pain receptors results in the upregulation of central pain modulators. It is important to recognize patients who have pain as a result of central mechanisms, as these conditions respond particularly well to multimodal pain management, and neuromodulating medications are more effective for this type of pain than opioids.

The hallmarks of neuropathic pain are stinging, burning, or tingling sensations, none of which are present in this patient. Furthermore, neuropathic pain follows the distribution of the nerves affected. This patient describes widespread pain all over her body that is not compatible with an anatomic nerve distribution.

Nociceptive pain is dull, aching, or throbbing pain caused by tissue injury. It is localized to the site of the injury. This patient has no evidence of tissue injury, and her pain is not localized.

Although psychological conditions can impact how patients experience their pain or can perpetuate pain, they are not thought to be a mechanism of pain generation in and of themselves. Additionally, this patient has no evidence of psychological comorbidity.

KEY POINT

- Central pain varies widely in character and may affect a specific area of the body or occur more diffusely; pain is usually constant, with bursts of more severe pain, often exacerbated by cough, temperature changes, movement, or emotions.

Bibliography

Hooten WM, Timming R, Belgrade M, et al. Institute for Clinical Systems Improvement. Assessment and management of chronic pain. Available at https://www.icsi.org/_asset/bw798b/ChronicPain.pdf. Updated November 2013. Accessed April 24, 2015.

Item 102   Answer: B

Educational Objective: Vaccinate a patient with anatomic asplenia against pneumococcal disease.

This patient who will be undergoing splenectomy should receive the pneumococcal conjugate vaccine (PCV13) now, followed by the pneumococcal polysaccharide vaccine (PPSV23) in 8 weeks. Persons with functional or anatomic asplenia are at risk for infection with encapsulated organisms and therefore should be vaccinated against pneumococcus. There are two pneumococcal vaccines: a polysaccharide vaccine composed of capsular material from 23 pneumococcal subtypes (PPSV23) and a conjugate vaccine containing capsular material from 13 pneumococcal subtypes conjugated to a nontoxic protein (PCV13), which increases its immunogenicity. Both pneumococcal vaccines are recommended in these patients; however, when PCV13 is indicated, it should be given before PPSV23. Therefore, administration of PCV13 would be appropriate now, followed by a single dose of PPSV23 8 weeks later. Administration of a second dose of PPSV23 is recommended 5 years after administration of the first PPSV23 dose for patients aged 19 to 64 years who have functional or anatomic asplenia. Furthermore, individuals who receive PPSV23 before age 65 years should receive an additional dose of PPSV23 at age 65 years provided that at least 5 years have passed since the most recent PPSV23 administration. Therefore, this patient should receive a second dose of PPSV23 at age 40 years and a third dose of PPSV23 once he is 65 years of age, provided that he remains on schedule. No additional doses of PCV13 are required.

According to the Advisory Committee on Immunization Practices, PCV13 and PPSV23 should not be administered together. The minimum acceptable interval between administration of PCV13 and PPSV23 is 8 weeks.

PPSV23 should not be the only pneumococcal vaccine administered in patients with asplenia, as it is significantly less immunogenic than PCV13. PPSV23 is only 60% to 70% effective in preventing invasive pneumococcal disease; however, PCV13 is more than 90% effective.

Several large randomized, multicenter trials have shown a decreased serologic response in patients who received PCV13 after PPSV23 compared with those who received PCV13 first; therefore, administration of PPSV23 now and PCV13 in 8 weeks is not recommended.

KEY POINT

- Patients with functional or anatomic asplenia should receive a dose of pneumococcal conjugate vaccine (PCV13), followed by a dose of pneumococcal polysaccharide vaccine (PPSV23) 8 weeks later.

Bibliography

Centers for Disease Control and Prevention. Use of 13-valent pneumococcal conjugate vaccine and 23-valent pneumococcal polysaccharide vaccine for adults with immunocompromising conditions: recommendations of the Advisory Committee on Immunization Practices. MMWR Morb Mortal Wkly Rep. 2012 Oct 12;61(40):816-9. [PMID: 23051612]

Item 103   Answer: D

Educational Objective: Treat social anxiety disorder.

The most appropriate pharmacologic treatment for this patient with social anxiety disorder is a selective serotonin reuptake inhibitor (SSRI), such as sertraline. Social anxiety disorder is characterized by severe, persistent anxiety or fear of social or performance situations (public speaking, meeting unfamiliar people) lasting at least 6 months. In these situations, affected patients experience anxiety and physical symptoms such as palpitations, dyspnea, and flushing. Patients recognize their anxiety is excessive but nonetheless avoid trigger situations (or endure them with extreme anxiety), resulting in impairments at home, work, and other settings. SSRIs and the serotonin-norepinephrine reuptake inhibitor (SNRI) venlafaxine are first-line therapy for social anxiety disorder. In addition, cognitive-behavioral therapy (CBT) is very effective for social anxiety disorder.

Limited evidence suggests that benzodiazepines, such as clonazepam and diazepam, may be useful in patients with social anxiety disorder and are commonly used in patients with social anxiety disorder who cannot tolerate or do not adequately respond to SSRIs or SNRIs. However, benzodiazepines are not first-line drugs for social anxiety disorder because of their side effects, including potential for dependency and withdrawal syndrome and potential for impairment when mental clarity is important (for example, during a speech).

β-Blockers are useful on an as-needed basis for performance anxiety (for example, propranolol, 10-20 mg, taken orally 60 minutes before a performance or speech). However, this patient's anxiety surrounding social interaction impairs her ability to function effectively in her workplace. Therefore, episodic therapy for performance anxiety would not be appropriate for this patient with an indication for treatment of a more extensive anxiety disorder.

CBT, which seeks to address maladaptive beliefs, anxious feelings, and avoidance behaviors, has been shown to be of benefit and is an alternative approach to pharmacologic therapy. There is limited evidence that combining pharmacologic therapy and CBT is superior to either treatment alone.

KEY POINT

- Selective serotonin reuptake inhibitors and the serotonin-norepinephrine reuptake inhibitor venlafaxine are first-line therapy for patients with social anxiety disorder.

Bibliography

Schneier FR. Clinical practice. Social anxiety disorder. N Engl J Med. 2006 Sep 7;355(10):1029-36. [PMID: 16957148]

Item 104   Answer: C

Educational Objective: Evaluate a patient with asymptomatic severe aortic stenosis undergoing elective noncardiac surgery.

The most appropriate management is to proceed to surgery with anesthesiology consultation. This patient has asymptomatic severe aortic stenosis, a condition that previously had been associated with a high risk of adverse cardiac events. However, advances in anesthetic and surgical techniques have led to a significant decrease in perioperative complications, and newer data indicate only a twofold increase in risk of postoperative myocardial infarction and 30-day mortality. The American College of Cardiology/American Heart Association (ACC/AHA) and American College of Chest Physicians (ACCP) guidelines recommend that elective noncardiac surgery is reasonable to perform in patients with asymptomatic severe aortic stenosis with appropriate intraoperative and postoperative hemodynamic monitoring (as can be determined by anesthesiology consultation). The risks of surgical delay must be weighed against the risks of the procedure. In this patient who meets no criteria for aortic valve replacement and is losing the ability to perform activities of daily living, performance of elective shoulder arthroscopy offers the best balance of risks.

Delaying or foregoing surgery would avoid potential perioperative risks but would also leave the patient with significant disability that could endanger her ability to remain independent in the community.

Dobutamine stress echocardiography is not indicated because the patient underwent an appropriate stress test less than 1 year ago and had no evidence of ischemia or symptoms after achievement of target heart rate and 4 metabolic equivalents (METs).

Repeat echocardiography would provide little additional value because this patient's cardiac structure and function are highly unlikely to have changed in less than 1 year. The ACC/AHA guideline recommends preoperative echocardiography for patients with moderate or worse valvular disease if it has been more than 1 year since the last study or the patient has had a change in clinical status.

KEY POINT

- Elective noncardiac surgery is reasonable to perform in patients with asymptomatic severe aortic stenosis with appropriate intraoperative and postoperative hemodynamic monitoring.

Bibliography

Fleisher LA, Fleischmann KE, Auerbach AD, et al; American College of Cardiology; American Heart Association. 2014 ACC/AHA guideline on perioperative cardiovascular evaluation and management of patients undergoing noncardiac surgery: a report of the American College of Cardiology/American Heart Association Task Force on practice guidelines. J Am Coll Cardiol. 2014 Dec 9;64(22):e77-137. [PMID: 25091544]

Item 105   Answer: C

Educational Objective: Treat drug-induced lower extremity edema.

The most appropriate next step in management is to switch amlodipine to lisinopril. Based on the normal physical examination findings and laboratory test results, this patient most likely has drug-induced edema caused by the calcium channel blocker amlodipine. Peripheral edema is a common side effect of calcium channel blockers, occurring in up to 25% of patients who take these medications. The risk of developing edema appears to be both dose and treatment duration dependent, with high doses and long treatment times associated with an increased incidence. Drug-induced edema typically resolves after withdrawal of the offending drug. Therefore, the first step in the management of this patient is to discontinue amlodipine and switch to an alternative antihypertensive agent, such as lisinopril.

Compression stockings may help to reduce this patient's edema; however, compression stockings may not be needed if his edema is due to his medication and an acceptable agent could be substituted for amlodipine in his antihypertensive therapy. Additionally, compliance with wearing compression stockings is often low due to the difficulty that patients experience in donning and removing the stockings.

Lower extremity venous duplex ultrasonography may be used in evaluating for the presence of venous thrombosis; however, this patient's clinical presentation and lack of calf tenderness are not consistent with a deep venous thrombosis. Therefore, venous duplex ultrasonography is not necessary or cost effective in this patient.

Diuretics are often used to treat generalized edema caused by cirrhosis or heart failure, as these conditions are associated with total body volume overload. However, the mechanism of lower extremity edema in this patient is associated with the vasodilatory properties of the medication and not volume overload. Therefore, diuretics are only minimally helpful in treating edema caused by calcium channel blockers. Additionally, diuretics may lead to electrolyte abnormalities and kidney dysfunction.

KEY POINT

- Treatment of drug-induced lower extremity edema is discontinuation of the offending agent.

Bibliography
Makani H, Bangalore S, Romero J, et al. Peripheral edema associated with calcium channel blockers: incidence and withdrawal rate–a meta-analysis of randomized trials. J Hypertens. 2011 Jul;29(7):1270-80. [PMID: 21558959]

Item 106　　　Answer:　　E
Educational Objective: Manage cyclic mastalgia.

The most appropriate management for this patient's breast pain is use of a support bra. Breast pain is common among women and is categorized primarily as cyclic and noncyclic. This patient has cyclic mastalgia, which is bilateral and worsens in the days before menses and then abates. A well-fitting support bra has been shown to alleviate discomfort for many women. Reassurance and education are important, and women are often greatly relieved to hear that breast pain is rarely a symptom of malignancy.

In the absence of palpable abnormalities, skin changes, or other pathologic findings, diagnostic imaging is not indicated. There is no role for ultrasound in the management of cyclic mastalgia.

There is no clear evidence that the exclusion of methylxanthines present in tea, coffee, cola and chocolate improves symptoms. Similarly, placebo-controlled trials have failed to support the efficacy of vitamins A, B, and E for treating breast pain.

Combined hormonal contraception is not effective in treating cyclic mastalgia and may even be associated with increased breast tenderness.

Medical treatment for cyclic mastalgia is generally reserved for women with severe and persistent pain that has not responded to conservative measures and interferes with quality of life. Danazol is FDA approved for the treatment of cyclic mastalgia, but side effects are frequent and limit its use. Danazol would not be appropriate for this patient before conservative measures are tried.

KEY POINT

- Cyclic mastalgia is initially treated conservatively; measures include education, reassurance, and use of a well-fitting support bra.

Bibliography
Onstad M, Stuckey A. Benign breast disorders. Obstet Gynecol Clin North Am. 2013 Sep;40(3):459-73. [PMID: 24021252]

Item 107　　　Answer:　　C
Educational Objective: Manage cardiac syncope with appropriate inpatient cardiac monitoring in a high-risk patient.

This patient should undergo inpatient cardiac monitoring because of his clinical history and presentation consistent with cardiogenic syncope. His loss of consciousness was abrupt, without prodrome except for palpitations, and occurred while seated, all of which are characteristics consistent with the presentation of cardiogenic syncope. Additionally, he is at high risk for ischemic cardiac disease based on his risk factors, including hypertension, hyperlipidemia, diabetes mellitus, tobacco use, and left bundle branch block noted on electrocardiogram. Cardiac syncope is associated with a high mortality rate (1-year mortality rate of 18%-33%), whereas the risk for negative outcomes with most other causes of syncope is markedly lower. Therefore, patients with syncope of possible cardiac etiology, such as this one, should be admitted to the hospital for further monitoring and evaluation.

Several risk stratification tools are available to assist in making admission decisions in patients with syncope. The Risk Stratification of Syncope in the Emergency Department (ROSE) index is a validated tool that identifies specific independent predictors for severe outcomes at 1 month (myocardial infarction, life-threatening arrhythmia, pulmonary embolism, stroke, intracranial or subarachnoid hemorrhage, or pacemaker insertion). These predictors are elevated B-type natriuretic peptide concentration ($\geq$300 pg/mL), bradycardia (≤50 beats/minute), fecal occult blood in patients with suspected gastrointestinal bleeding, anemia (hemoglobin level ≤9 g/dL [90 g/L]), chest pain, electrocardiogram with Q waves (not in lead III), and oxygen saturation less than 94% on ambient air. Other high risk factors include age greater than 65 years; abnormal ECG; history of heart failure, ischemic heart disease, or ventricular arrhythmias; or lack of warning signs or symptoms. In patients with these clinical findings, many of which are present in this patient, inpatient monitoring and evaluation are recommended.

As this patient with a history suggestive of cardiac syncope is at high risk for adverse events, outpatient evaluation with event monitoring would not be appropriate.

Implantable loop recorders are best reserved for patients with unexplained recurrent syncope, which is not present in this patient. Inpatient monitoring and further cardiac evaluation for ischemia are the most appropriate next steps in management.

Criteria for pacemaker insertion in a patient with syncope include symptomatic bradycardia or asystolic pauses. This patient currently only has mild bradycardia, which would not be the cause of his syncope, and a pacemaker is not indicated at this time. He should be monitored for further decline in heart rate and symptoms or for the development of advanced-degree block and other symptomatic arrhythmias. This should initially take place in the inpatient setting.

KEY POINT

- Patients with syncope who have identified clinical risk factors for adverse outcomes should undergo inpatient monitoring and evaluation.

Bibliography
Ebell MH. Risk stratification of patients presenting with syncope. Am Fam Physician. 2012 Jun 1;85(11):1047-52. [PMID: 22962874]

Item 108   Answer: A

Educational Objective: Manage a patient with rotator cuff tendinitis.

This patient most likely has rotator cuff tendinitis (specifically, supraspinatus tendinitis). He has pain with overhead activities, a painful arc, and pain with active abduction on examination, all of which are consistent with this diagnosis. Additionally, he works as a painter, a profession that frequently involves overhead activities that predispose patients to developing rotator cuff tendinitis. Given the patient's presentation and examination findings, it is appropriate to diagnose the patient without further testing. Initial therapy typically includes rest, avoidance of aggravating activities, NSAIDs, and physical therapy that strengthens the rotator cuff muscles and improves flexibility.

When the diagnosis is unclear or if concern exists for a rotator cuff tear, imaging of the shoulder should be obtained. MRI is the preferred imaging modality (>90% sensitivity), although ultrasonography, in experienced hands, is also an option. This patient has no evidence of a rotator cuff tear, as his strength is preserved and he has negative drop-arm, external rotation lag, external rotation resistance, and internal rotation lag tests, all of which argue against a full-thickness tear. Therefore, MRI of the left shoulder is unnecessary in this patient.

Referral for orthopedic surgery would be premature prior to a trial of conservative measures for 6 to 9 months.

In the absence of trauma and tenderness to palpation of bony structures, obtaining shoulder radiographs is likely to be of limited value and is unnecessary in this patient.

KEY POINT

- Imaging of the shoulder is typically not needed to diagnose rotator cuff tendinitis but should be considered if a full-thickness rotator cuff tear is suspected or if there is diagnostic uncertainty.

Bibliography
Hermans J, Luime JJ, Meuffels DE, Reijman M, Simel DL, Bierma-Zeinstra SM. Does this patient with shoulder pain have rotator cuff disease?: The Rational Clinical Examination systematic review. JAMA. 2013 Aug 28;310(8):837-47. [PMID: 23982370]

Item 109   Answer: D

Educational Objective: Evaluate acute, nonspecific low back pain.

This patient with nonspecific low back pain does not require additional testing. In patients presenting with low back pain, the history and physical examination should focus on determining the likelihood of a specific underlying condition causing the back pain and identifying any neurologic involvement that may be present. In patients in whom low back pain cannot be attributed to a specific disease or spinal abnormality (defined as nonspecific low back pain), the American College of Physicians and other organizations recommend against imaging or obtaining other diagnostic studies routinely. Such testing should be reserved for patients in whom a serious underlying condition is suspected, those with severe or progressive neurologic deficits, or patients who do not have symptom improvement after 4 to 6 weeks of conservative management. As this patient's pain meets the definition of nonspecific low back pain, no additional imaging or testing is indicated before initiating therapy.

An erythrocyte sedimentation rate is a marker of inflammation and is indicated only if a systemic inflammatory process or infectious cause of low back pain is suspected, neither of which is suggested in this patient.

Ankylosing spondylitis is a spondyloarthritis with systemic features that typically presents with low back pain, morning stiffness, and sacroiliitis; extra-articular manifestations may include uveitis. HLA-B27 testing can be useful in the appropriate clinical scenario to support the diagnosis of ankylosing spondylitis; however, HLA-B27 can be positive in other disease processes as well. This patient has no additional symptoms associated with his back pain and no suggestive findings on examination, making the diagnosis of ankylosing spondylitis unlikely.

Radiography of the lumbar spine is indicated only if fracture, degenerative arthritis, or an inflammatory process such as ankylosing spondylitis is suspected, none of which are likely diagnostic considerations in this patient.

KEY POINT

- Imaging or other diagnostic tests should not be routinely obtained in patients with nonspecific low back pain.

Bibliography

Chou R, Qaseem A, Snow A, et al. Diagnosis and treatment of low back pain: a joint clinical practice guideline from the American College of Physicians and the American Pain Society. Ann Intern Med. 2007 Oct 2;147(7): 478-91. [PMID: 17909209]

Item 110   Answer: D

Educational Objective: Treat mild lower urinary tract symptoms caused by benign prostatic hyperplasia.

This patient with mild lower urinary tract symptoms (LUTS) caused by benign prostatic hyperplasia (BPH) should be conservatively managed with observation. The main purpose of treating LUTS from presumed BPH is to reduce bothersome symptoms. The American Urological Association Symptom Index (AUA-SI) score is a validated questionnaire used to determine the severity of and to monitor LUTS. The questionnaire assesses frequency, nocturia, weak stream, hesitancy, intermittency, incomplete emptying, and urgency, with each question graded on a 5-point scale from 0 (not present) to 5 (almost always present). The total score is interpreted as follows: 1-7 (mild), 8-19 (moderate), and 20-35 (severe). This patient's AUA-SI score of 4 indicates mild symptoms. The AUA currently suggests a treatment approach that is based on AUA-SI score severity. Mild LUTS from BPH can be addressed by observation. Conservative measures that may help patients with mild symptoms include reducing fluid intake, timed voiding (every 3 hours while awake), limiting caffeine and alcohol, modifying medications, improving mobility, and avoiding bladder irritants.

Urinalysis is the only test indicated for all patients with LUTS that is believed to be secondary to BPH. However, this patient's urinalysis, which shows only 2 leukocytes/ hpf, does not clearly indicate the presence of a urinary tract infection, and his clinical presentation is not suggestive of chronic prostatitis. Therefore, antibiotic therapy with ciprofloxacin is not indicated.

5-α Reductase inhibitors, such as finasteride, are indicated in patients with large prostates (40 mL), elevated prostate-specific antigen levels, and/or severe symptoms of BPH. Finasteride is not indicated in this patient with mild symptoms.

α-Blockers, such as tamsulosin, are first-line therapy for treating BPH. However, observation without medical therapy would be the most appropriate first-line approach in this patient with mild BPH.

KEY POINT

- In patients with mild lower urinary tract symptoms caused by benign prostatic hyperplasia, observation with conservative therapy measures is appropriate.

Bibliography

Beckman TJ, Mynderse LA. Evaluation and medical management of benign prostatic hyperplasia. Mayo Clin Proc. 2005 Oct;80(10):1356-62. [PMID: 16212149]

Item 111   Answer: B

Educational Objective: Identify mood disorder as a cause of erectile dysfunction.

This patient has erectile dysfunction (ED) secondary to a mood disorder, most likely major depressive disorder. Characteristic features of inorganic (psychological) ED are sudden onset of symptoms and persistence of nocturnal or morning erections, which indicates that the anatomic and physiologic mechanisms for erection are intact. This patient has guilt, low energy, and decreased interest, all of which are symptoms of depression. Patients with inorganic ED can be reassured that their condition is likely to resolve with time and effective treatment of their mood disorder.

This middle-aged man is not likely to have hypogonadism. His testicles are of normal volume, and he reports continued sexual desires. One of the earliest symptoms of hypogonadism is substantial reduction or absence of sexual thoughts.

This patient has poor sleep; however, he is not overweight and reports no snoring, gasping, apnea, or daytime somnolence. Depression is the most likely cause for this patient's fatigue, given his guilt, anhedonia, and inorganic ED.

Although an early sign of prolactinoma is ED, the persistence of nocturnal and morning erections in this patient makes an organic cause unlikely. Additionally, he lacks other symptoms of prolactinoma, such as headache, visual changes, or decreased body and facial hair.

KEY POINT

- Characteristic features of inorganic erectile dysfunction are sudden onset of symptoms and persistence of nocturnal or morning erections.

Bibliography

Beckman TJ, Abu-Lebdeh HS, Mynderse LA. Evaluation and medical management of erectile dysfunction. Mayo Clin Proc. 2006 Mar;81(3): 385-90. [PMID: 16529142]

Item 112   Answer: C

Educational Objective: Recognize threats to the validity of a study.

The validity of this study could be improved by measuring the outcomes of both study groups concurrently.

Validity, or the trustworthiness of a study's results, can be threatened by many factors, including errors in sampling, measurement, and data analysis. Systematic error results from bias that influences the study findings in a certain direction. Systematic error must be addressed by eliminating sources of bias, and doing so is a primary goal of study design. Seasonal variation in asthma symptoms is widely recognized, and in this study, the separation of study groups into summer and winter months is a systematic error that could account for the different peak-flow rates and quality-of-life scores between groups. This represents a potentially significant bias that could threaten the validity of the study outcomes. Therefore, this study could be improved by measuring outcomes for both study groups at the same time of year in order to eliminate this potential source of bias.

Including patients with COPD in the study would not improve the study's validity regarding the impact of meditation on the outcomes of patients with asthma.

Increasing the sample size and precision of measures would be effective in reducing the impact of random errors, but not systematic errors.

KEY POINT

- Systematic error threatens the validity of a study and must be addressed by eliminating bias.

Bibliography
Guyatt GH, Haynes RB, Jaeschke RZ, et al. Users' Guides to the Medical Literature: XXV. Evidence-based medicine: principles for applying the Users' Guides to patient care. Evidence-Based Medicine Working Group. JAMA. 2000 Sep 13;284(10):1290-6. [PMID: 10979117]

Item 113   Answer: D

Educational Objective: Diagnose vestibular neuronitis.

This patient has vestibular neuronitis, which is manifested by acute, severe, and persistent nonpositional peripheral vertigo. Vestibular neuronitis may follow a viral upper respiratory tract infection and is thought to be caused by postviral inflammation of the vestibular portion of cranial nerve VIII. Symptoms may be severe and prolonged. Nausea and vomiting are common. When the Dix-Hallpike maneuver is performed on this patient, the results are consistent with peripheral vertigo, with nystagmus that is provoked after a brief latency period and is relatively severe and short in duration (<1 minute).

Benign paroxysmal positional vertigo (BPPV), the most common cause of vertigo, is classically precipitated by head movement and is caused by otoliths that perturb the labyrinthian sensory receptors. In a patient with BPPV, episodes of vertigo generally last less than 1 minute.

Brainstem infarction or hemorrhage as well as cerebellar infarction or hemorrhage cause vertigo of central origin. In central vertigo, there is no latency in the occurrence of nystagmus with the Dix-Hallpike maneuver. Compared with the findings in a patient with peripheral vertigo, the nystagmus generally lasts longer than 1 minute and symptoms are less severe. Based on the history and physical examination, this patient's presentation is inconsistent with brainstem infarction.

Labyrinthitis is similar to vestibular neuronitis in etiology and presentation except that in labyrinthitis patients exhibit hearing loss. Hearing is preserved in this patient, making labyrinthitis an unlikely diagnosis.

KEY POINT

- Vestibular neuronitis is characterized by acute, severe, and persistent nonpositional peripheral vertigo.

Bibliography
Huh YE, Kim JS. Bedside evaluation of dizzy patients. J Clin Neurol. 2013 Oct;9(4):203-13. [PMID: 24285961]

Item 114   Answer: D

Educational Objective: Manage risk for cardiovascular disease and cancer in a healthy patient.

No vitamin supplementation is indicated to reduce the risk for cardiovascular disease and cancer in this patient. Although one third of U.S. adults use supplemental vitamins, the U.S. Preventive Services Task Force (USPSTF) has concluded that there is insufficient evidence to assess the balance of benefits and harms of vitamin use, including use of vitamin A, vitamin C, and antioxidant combinations, in the prevention of cardiovascular disease and cancer. This recommendation applies to multivitamin preparations and to single- or paired-vitamin preparations, with the exception of vitamin E and β-carotene. Because of potential adverse effects associated with their use, the USPSTF specifically recommends against the use of vitamin E and β-carotene for these purposes. This patient should be advised that taking supplemental vitamins or minerals will not lower his risk for cardiovascular disease and cancer. Instead, he should continue to consume a balanced diet that includes fruits and vegetables and to exercise regularly.

Vitamin supplementation should be used in treating known deficiencies or in clinical situations in which it has been shown to be effective, such as vitamin D supplementation in patients with osteoporosis.

KEY POINT

- Vitamin supplementation, either with a multivitamin or with a single- or paired-vitamin preparation, has not been shown to reduce the risk for cardiovascular disease or cancer.

Bibliography
Moyer VA; U.S. Preventive Services Task Force. Vitamin, mineral, and multivitamin supplements for the primary prevention of cardiovascular disease and cancer: U.S. Preventive services Task Force recommendation statement. Ann Intern Med. 2014 Apr 15;160(8):558-64. [PMID: 24566474]

Item 115   Answer: C
Educational Objective: Diagnose scleritis.

This patient most likely has scleritis. Scleritis is inflammation of the fibrous layers of the eye underlying the episclera and conjunctiva and overlying the choroid. Patients may present with severe, continuous, boring ocular pain that radiates to the surrounding facial areas, redness, photophobia, and tearing. It most commonly affects both eyes and is frequently worse at night, and because of traction of the extraocular muscles on the sclera, pain is often worse with eye movement. Vision may be normal, but impairment may result from inflammatory involvement of adjacent ocular structures or loss of globe integrity. Roughly 50% of patients with scleritis have an underlying systemic disease, such as an inflammatory connective tissue disorder (rheumatoid arthritis) or infection (tuberculosis). Because scleritis can be a sight-threatening condition, it requires urgent referral to an ophthalmologist for further evaluation and treatment.

The episclera is a vascular fibroelastic structure superior to the sclera. Inflammation of the episclera, or episcleritis, is less commonly associated with pain or photophobia, as seen in this patient, but more commonly with redness, irritation, and tearing. This history is usually most helpful in differentiating scleritis from episcleritis, as they may be difficult to distinguish by physical examination alone. Episcleritis is also uncommonly associated with risk for visual impairment.

Keratoconjunctivitis sicca (dry eye) includes symptoms of dryness, irritation, and burning. This patient does not have a presentation consistent with dry eye.

Patients with subconjunctival hemorrhage present with blotchy redness (from extravascular blood) that is typically confined to one area of the conjunctiva. Subconjunctival hemorrhage is painless, occurs spontaneously, and resolves within several weeks. This patient's severe eye pain, diffuse redness, and persistence of symptoms argue against the diagnosis of subconjunctival hemorrhage.

KEY POINT
- Scleritis, painful inflammation of the fibrous layers of the eye underlying the episclera and conjunctiva, is often associated with systemic diseases including inflammatory connective tissue disorders and infections.

Bibliography
Bal SK, Hollingworth GR. Red eye. BMJ. 2005 Aug 20;331(7514):438. [PMID: 16110072]

Item 116   Answer: B
Educational Objective: Diagnose borderline personality disorder.

This patient has borderline personality disorder (BPD). Features of BPD include interpersonal hypersensitivity (for example, intense and unstable relationships and intense efforts to avoid abandonment), difficulty controlling emotions such as anger, impulsive or destructive behavior (for example, spending money or promiscuous sex), recurrent suicidal gestures, and unstable self-image. BPD can be misdiagnosed as depression or bipolar disorder. About 6% of primary care patients have BPD. The mainstay of treatment for BPD is psychotherapy. Pharmacologic treatment of BPD is adjunctive to psychotherapy. There are no FDA-approved medications for personality disorders; medications are used to relieve symptoms (for example, mood stabilizers for mood swings and impulsivity).

Patients with bipolar disorder report different neurovegetative symptoms than patients with BPD, such as a decreased need for sleep and waking with increased energy; they report an increase in activities but may move from one thing to another without completing tasks and may become more social or hypersexual but without indication of interpersonal loss. The patient's speech is often loud and full of jokes and puns, and he or she may be distractible, responding to irrelevant stimuli. Patients with BPD tend to behave angrily, impulsively, or self-destructively in the context of real or perceived interpersonal loss, whereas no such pattern is apparent in those with bipolar disorder.

Depressed mood, anhedonia, lack of motivation, lack of energy or mood reactivity, overeating, and oversleeping are typical characteristics of a depressive disorder. BPD depressions are often characterized by feelings of emptiness; patients' mood often improves after being reunited with a "lost" partner or finding a new loved one.

Generalized anxiety disorder (GAD) is characterized by excessive anxiety and worry about various events or activities on most days for at least 6 months, with difficulty controlling worrying. Associated symptoms include fatigue, irritability, restlessness, insomnia, and difficulty concentrating. Such patients often have comorbid anxiety disorders, depression, or substance abuse. Patients with GAD often have somatoform symptoms, which can make them high utilizers of health care resources. This patient does not exhibit any of these symptoms, making this diagnosis unlikely.

KEY POINT
- Features of borderline personality disorder include interpersonal hypersensitivity, difficulty controlling emotions such as anger, impulsive and destructive behavior, recurrent suicidal gestures, and unstable self-image.

Bibliography
Gunderson JG. Clinical practice. Borderline personality disorder. N Engl J Med. 2011 May 26;364(21):2037-42. [PMID: 21612472]

Item 117   Answer: B
Educational Objective: Evaluate cardiovascular risk in a patient with erectile dysfunction before initiating therapy.

The most appropriate next step in management is a cardiac stress test for this patient with erectile dysfunction (ED) and symptoms indicative of cardiovascular disease.

First-line therapy for ED includes lifestyle modification (smoking cessation, exercise, and weight loss) and phosphodiesterase type 5 (PDE-5) inhibitor therapy. ED and cardiovascular disease share many risk factors (diabetes mellitus, hyperlipidemia, and hypertension), and ED is itself a cardiac risk factor that independently predicts mortality and confers a risk similar to that of moderate smoking. Therefore, it is important to assess cardiovascular risk and safety for sexual activity before initiating a PDE-5 inhibitor. This can generally be accomplished using guidelines established by the Third Princeton Consensus Conference. This patient has new-onset exertional dyspnea and fatigue that resolve with rest, raising the possibility of ischemic heart disease. Consequently, this patient should undergo cardiac stress testing, especially before considering medical therapy for ED.

Patients with symptoms of ischemic heart disease should undergo exercise stress testing before initiating a PDE-5 inhibitor such as tadalafil. If stress testing demonstrates that the patient can achieve 5 to 6 metabolic equivalents without ischemia, the patient is at low risk for cardiovascular events with PDE-5 inhibitor therapy and sexual activity. Also, this patient is already taking the α-blocker tamsulosin and has a low-normal blood pressure. PDE-5 medications and α-blockers should be combined with caution due to the risk of profound hypotension.

This patient does not require a psychiatric evaluation because he has no obvious symptoms of mood disorder. Features of his sexual history that point against mood disorder are intact interpersonal relationships, strong libido, gradual onset of erectile dysfunction, and loss of nocturnal erections.

Nearly one third of obese men will have improvement in ED symptoms simply by exercising regularly and losing weight. Attempts should therefore be made to lower the BMI below 30. However, weight loss is not the most appropriate next step in management in this mildly overweight patient who may have untreated coronary artery disease.

KEY POINT

- Because erectile dysfunction shares many risk factors with atherosclerotic cardiovascular disease and itself is an independent risk factor, an assessment of the patient's cardiovascular risk should be made before prescribing a phosphodiesterase type 5 inhibitor for treatment of erectile dysfunction.

Bibliography

Nehra A, Jackson G, Miner M, et al. The Princeton III Consensus recommendations for the management of erectile dysfunction and cardiovascular disease. Mayo Clin Proc. 2012 Aug;87(8):766-78. [PMID: 22862865]

Item 118   Answer: B
Educational Objective: Recognize autism spectrum disorder.

This patient meets criteria for autism spectrum disorder (ASD). ASD encompasses a group of heterogeneous conditions characterized by (1) persistent deficits in communication and social interaction associated with impairment in function and (2) repetitive behaviors that are inflexible and nonfunctional and interests that are often restricted. This patient's persistent problems with social communication and interaction, including difficulty with relationships and reading body language, adherence to routines, and repetitive behaviors, are consistent with this diagnosis. The DSM-5 has eliminated the subclassifications of autism (including Asperger syndrome) and merged all related entities into ASD.

Antisocial personality disorder is characterized by lack of remorse and disregard for others. Patients with this disorder usually have no regard for right and wrong. Although this patient has difficulty with social relationships, his symptoms are not consistent with antisocial personality disorder.

Although this patient's insistence on turning the light off and on three times and lining up his shoelaces nightly may be classified as obsessions, his difficulty with social relationships and communication make his clinical findings more consistent with autism than obsessive-compulsive disorder.

Social anxiety disorder is characterized by severe and persistent anxiety regarding social situations, including public speaking and meeting new people. Patients with this disorder may also have difficulty with social relationships accompanied by significant, often debilitating, anxiety. However, patients with social anxiety disorder do not have the restricted or repetitive behaviors that are associated with autism, as seen in this patient.

KEY POINT

- Autism spectrum disorder encompasses a group of heterogeneous conditions characterized by restrictive, repetitive behaviors and interests and persistent deficits in communication and social interaction associated with impairment in function.

Bibliography

Lai MC, Lombardo MV, Baron-Cohen S. Autism. Lancet. 2014 Mar 8;383(9920):896-910. [PMID: 24074734]

Item 119   Answer: B
Educational Objective: Prevent recurrent vulvovaginal candidiasis.

The most appropriate recommendation for this patient is extended-course antifungal treatment to decrease the risk of recurrent vulvovaginal candidiasis (VVC). Although VVC is common, complicated VVC is recurrent (defined as four or more episodes in 1 year), characterized by more severe symptoms, or may be due to non-albicans candida such as *Candida glabrata*. Complicated infection may develop in women who are pregnant, have uncontrolled diabetes mellitus, or are immunosuppressed but may also occur in patients without associated medical issues, such as this one. In women with complicated VVC, more sustained treatment of a recurrent infection may be needed to achieve symptom relief and cure. Extended-course antifungal therapy appears to decrease the risk of recurrence, and there is minimal evidence suggesting that more prolonged treatment increases the level of fungal resistance to antimicrobial agents. However, the optimal antifungal regimen and time frame have not been defined.

The role of sexual activity in recurrent VVC is unclear, and there is equivocal evidence that treatment of a sexual partner for *Candida* is of benefit in decreasing the risk of recurrent infection. Therefore, treating this patient's partner in the absence of symptoms is not recommended.

The probiotic *Lactobacillus* is sometimes taken by patients, either orally or intravaginally, in an attempt to decrease the colonization of the vagina with *Candida*, thereby reducing the risk of recurrent VVC. However, there are few data suggesting that women with VVC are deficient in lactobacilli or that attempting to reduce vaginal *Candida* colonization by this method is effective in decreasing recurrent VVC. It is therefore not recommended as a method of preventing recurrent infection.

Although indwelling contraceptive methods (such as vaginal sponges, diaphragms, and intrauterine devices) have been inconsistently associated with *Candida* colonization, switching to an alternative contraceptive method would not be expected to be of benefit in reducing infections in this patient.

KEY POINT

- Extended-course antifungal agents may be helpful for decreasing the risk of recurrent vulvovaginal candidiasis.

Bibliography
Achkar JM, Fries BC. Candida infections of the genitourinary tract. Clin Microbiol Rev. 2010 Apr;23(2):253-73. [PMID: 20375352]

Item 120   Answer: D
Educational Objective: Diagnose retinal detachment.

This patient most likely has retinal detachment. Retinal detachment, which occurs mainly in patients with myopia, results when the neurosensory layer of the retina separates from the retinal pigment epithelial layer and choroid. The characteristic features of retinal detachment are floaters, flashes of light (photopsias), and squiggly lines, followed by a sudden, peripheral visual field defect that resembles a black curtain and progresses across the entire visual field. The most common type of retinal detachment is posterior vitreous detachment (PVD), which typically occurs in persons aged 50 to 75 years. Symptoms usually progress over a period of 1 week to 3 months and can lead to blindness. Patients with retinal detachment should be urgently evaluated by an ophthalmologist.

Age-related macular degeneration (AMD) is a leading cause of blindness in older patients. In dry AMD, extracellular material (drusen) is deposited in the macular region of one or both eyes. Patients often report a gradual loss of vision. In wet AMD, patients with pre-existing dry AMD will progress to develop new vessel growth under the retina. Bleeding and exudation from these vessels result in sudden (or rapid onset over weeks), painless blurring or warping of central vision. Wet AMD results in severe vision loss. This patient's peripheral vision loss and the presence of floaters and photopsias are not consistent with AMD.

Patients with branch retinal vein occlusion, which is caused by arterial compression of the retinal vein, are typically asymptomatic. Funduscopic examination may reveal an afferent pupillary defect, congested retinal veins, scattered retinal hemorrhages, and cotton wool spots in the region of occlusion, which are not present in this patient.

Central retinal artery occlusion (CRAO) is caused by vasospasm or emboli. Patients with CRAO are usually elderly and present with profound and sudden vision loss. Findings on funduscopic examination include afferent pupillary defect and cherry red fovea that is accentuated by a pale retinal background, both of which are absent in this patient.

KEY POINT

- Retinal detachment, which occurs mainly in patients with myopia, is characterized by floaters, photopsias, and squiggly lines, followed by a sudden, peripheral visual field defect that resembles a black curtain and progresses across the peripheral field of vision.

Bibliography
Lee E, Dogramaci M, Williamson T. Displacement of the retina. Ophthalmology. 2012 Jan;119(1):206.e1; author reply 206-7. [PMID: 22214956]

Item 121   Answer: D
Educational Objective: Diagnose spinal stenosis.

Spinal stenosis is the most likely cause of this patient's symptoms. Spinal stenosis results from narrowing of the spinal canal, usually due to degenerative arthritis of the spine that causes mechanical compression and ischemia of the lumbosacral spine nerve roots. Clinical manifestations of spinal stenosis are progressively worsening low back discomfort and severe leg pain that tends to be minimized when the low back is flexed (leading patients to lean forward) and worsened with spinal extension (such as when standing and walking up steps). Plain radiographs may reveal degenerative changes or alterations in the mechanical structure of the lumbosacral spine; however, CT may be more helpful in defining bony changes, and MRI is the study of choice for evaluating the neural structures in the low back. It is important to note that spinal stenosis may be incidentally detected in a substantial number of asymptomatic patients who have imaging for other reasons, and the degree of stenosis does not predict development of symptoms. Therefore, this finding alone does not require further evaluation in the absence of symptoms or possibly associated clinical findings.

Compression fractures may cause low back pain and, if severe, may cause nerve compression and radiculopathy.

However, this patient does not have clear risk factors for compression fracture (such as trauma, glucocorticoid use, or osteoporosis), and the symptoms associated with compression fracture tend to be of acute onset (and not progressive, as in this patient) with significant point tenderness over the spine at the level of the fracture. Additionally, the symptoms associated with compression fracture tend to be less positional than those seen in spinal stenosis.

Hip osteoarthritis may be worsened with walking, and pain may radiate posteriorly toward the low back and groin region. However, it would not explain this patient's lower extremity symptoms and other positional findings.

Symptoms associated with spinal stenosis are sometimes termed pseudoclaudication because they worsen with ambulation and improve with rest, similar to claudication due to peripheral arterial disease. However, these conditions are usually distinguished by the fact that vascular claudication symptoms do not tend to worsen with standing or spinal extension. Additionally, this patient has no clear risk factors for peripheral arterial disease.

KEY POINT

- Spinal stenosis is characterized by pseudoclaudication and severe leg pain that is absent when seated and may be relieved when leaning forward.

Bibliography
Berger D. Leg discomfort: beyond the joints. Med Clin North Am. 2014 May;98(3):429-44. [PMID: 24758955]

Item 122   Answer: D
Educational Objective: Manage a patient with medically unexplained symptoms.

The most appropriate management of this patient who has had extensive evaluation of multiple nonspecific symptoms and has been appropriately diagnosed with medically unexplained symptoms (MUS) is regular visits with her internist. Consistent, regularly scheduled follow-up visits with brief focused history and physical examination, rather than ad hoc, unscheduled visits for crisis management, are the cornerstone of management. Regular visits allow for growth of the physician-patient relationship and the ability to discuss the diagnosis and specific symptoms with the patient and anticipate potential problems and issues. This patient's symptoms are persistent but not progressive, and there are no accompanying pathologic findings on examination or with previous diagnostic testing. Additionally, her symptoms have adversely affected her quality of life, and previous trials of antidepressant medication have been unsuccessful. Although co-management with a psychiatrist can be beneficial in the care plan of some patients with MUS, the internist assumes the central role, and this would be the most appropriate approach to managing this patient.

Long-acting benzodiazepines are not recommended in patients with MUS because they have not been proved beneficial in treating symptoms, and the sedative effects and risk for dependence outweigh any potential benefits.

Neuropsychological testing is generally performed to further evaluate cognitive dysfunction and is unnecessary in this patient who has clinically normal cognitive function.

Physical therapy may be beneficial in the patient with prominent musculoskeletal symptoms. However, these symptoms are absent in this patient, and physical therapy should not supplant the central role of regularly scheduled visits with the internist.

KEY POINT

- Consistent, regularly scheduled follow-up visits with brief focused history and physical examination are the cornerstone of management of patients with medically unexplained symptoms.

Bibliography
Isaac ML, Paauw DS. Medically unexplained symptoms. Med Clin North Am. 2014 May;98:663-72. [PMID: 24758967]

Item 123   Answer: C
Educational Objective: Treat a patient with alcohol withdrawal.

Lorazepam is the most appropriate treatment for this patient with alcohol withdrawal and chronic liver disease. Alcohol withdrawal symptoms can start within 4 hours to several days after the last drink. Alcohol activates the same receptor as γ-aminobutyric acid, which is the major inhibitory neurotransmitter in the brain, causing central nervous system depression. If ethanol has been present frequently enough in a heavy drinker to develop tolerance and dependence, sudden withdrawal creates a state of central nervous system hyperactivity, which can be life threatening. Early symptoms include agitation, tremulousness, headache, and symptoms of autonomic hyperactivity (fever, diaphoresis, tachycardia, and hypertension). As withdrawal becomes more severe, patients may experience seizures and/or hallucinations, usually within 12 to 24 hours of abstinence. Delirium tremens is a systemic syndrome characterized by hypertension, tachycardia, diaphoresis, fever, disorientation, and hallucinations. Onset is usually 48 to 96 hours after the last drink and sometimes persists for many days. Benzodiazepines are the treatment of choice for alcohol withdrawal. Thiamine, glucose, and folate are supplemented routinely, and nutrition should be instituted early.

All benzodiazepines appear similarly efficacious in reducing signs and symptoms of alcohol withdrawal. Longer-acting agents, such as chlordiazepoxide, may be more effective in preventing seizures but can pose a risk for excess sedation in older adults and patients with marked liver disease, such as this patient. Short-acting benzodiazepines, such as lorazepam, are preferred to long-acting benzodiazepines in patients with liver disease because short-acting benzodiazepines cause less metabolite buildup in the liver. In this patient, benzodiazepines will not only help to control

CONT.

his current symptoms but will also help to prevent him from progressing to severe alcohol withdrawal.

Clonidine and β-blockers such as propranolol have been used as an adjunctive therapy in alcohol withdrawal because they reduce withdrawal symptoms related to autonomic hyperactivity. However, there is little evidence that either of these medications reduce or prevent seizures and delirium.

KEY POINT

- Benzodiazepines are the treatment of choice for alcohol withdrawal.

Bibliography

Kosten TR, O'Connor PG. Management of drug and alcohol withdrawal. N Engl J Med. 2003 May 1;348(18):1786-95. [PMID: 12724485]

Item 124   Answer: D

Educational Objective: Evaluate an obese patient.

The most appropriate cardiovascular risk stratification strategy for this obese patient is to measure waist circumference. The American Heart Association, American College of Cardiology, and The Obesity Society (AHA/ACC/TOS) guideline for the management of overweight and obesity recommends screening for overweight and obesity by calculating BMI at annual visits or more frequently. Additionally, the guideline recommends measuring waist circumference at the level of the iliac crest in overweight and obese patients. (Measuring waist circumference in patients with a BMI >35 is unnecessary, as the waist circumference will likely be elevated.) Central adiposity (waist circumference >102 cm [40 in] in men and >88 cm [35 in] in women) is associated with an increased risk for hypertension, type 2 diabetes mellitus, and coronary heart disease, independent of BMI. Together, BMI and waist circumference can be used to risk stratify patients.

Exercise stress testing is typically indicated for evaluation of chest pain in symptomatic individuals. This patient is asymptomatic and likely at low risk for coronary heart disease. Therefore, there are no indications for stress testing.

Although the patient reports occasional snoring, he does not report nonrestorative sleep or daytime hypersomnolence, which would be suggestive of obstructive sleep apnea. Therefore, overnight oximetry or polysomnography is not indicated.

Screening resting electrocardiography should not be performed in this patient. The American College of Physicians specifically recommends against screening asymptomatic low-risk adults for ischemic heart disease with resting or stress electrocardiography, stress echocardiography, or stress myocardial perfusion imaging. Instead, clinicians should address modifiable cardiovascular risk factors, such as obesity, smoking, hypertension, hyperlipidemia, and diabetes, and encourage healthy diet and levels of exercise.

Along with a history and physical examination, the AHA/ACC/TOS obesity guideline recommends performing clinical and laboratory assessments, including measuring blood pressure, fasting plasma glucose level, and fasting lipid

levels, in overweight and obese patients to assess for cardiovascular risk factors and obesity-associated comorbidities.

KEY POINT

- Central adiposity increases risk for hypertension, type 2 diabetes mellitus, and coronary heart disease; in obese and overweight patients, measuring waist circumference is a cost-effective way to risk stratify patients.

Bibliography

Jensen MD, Ryan DH, Apovian CM, et al; American College of Cardiology/American Heart Association Task Force on Practice Guidelines; Obesity Society. 2013 AHA/ACC/TOS guideline for the management of overweight and obesity in adults: a report of the American College of Cardiology/American Heart Association Task Force on Practice Guidelines and The Obesity Society. J Am Coll Cardiol. 2014 Jul 1;63(25 Pt B):2985-3023. Erratum in: J Am Coll Cardiol. 2014 Jul 1;63(25 Pt B):3029-3030. [PMID: 24239920]

Item 125   Answer: C

Educational Objective: Monitor statin therapy in an asymptomatic patient with hyperlipidemia.

A fasting lipid panel is the most appropriate laboratory test for this patient. He has a history of atherosclerotic cardiovascular disease and is being treated with high-intensity statin therapy in accordance with the American College of Cardiology/American Heart Association cholesterol treatment guideline. Before initiating statin therapy, a fasting lipid panel, including total cholesterol, triglyceride, HDL cholesterol, and LDL cholesterol levels, should be obtained. Although therapy is not adjusted to achieve specific LDL cholesterol targets, a repeat fasting lipid panel is appropriate 1 to 3 months after initiation of statin therapy to determine medication adherence and effectiveness of treatment, which is defined as a reduction in the LDL cholesterol level of 50% or more from the pretreatment baseline. Further monitoring of statin therapy should be individualized, but in patients on a stable dose, the guidelines recommend retesting at 3- to 12-month intervals.

Alanine aminotransferase level should be measured before initiating therapy to rule out undiagnosed liver disease; however, based on the low risk of hepatotoxicity, the FDA no longer suggests measurement of hepatic enzymes during statin therapy. If the patient experiences symptoms suggestive of liver dysfunction, including fatigue, anorexia, jaundice, nausea, or abdominal pain, assessment of hepatic aminotransferases would be appropriate.

Baseline assessment of creatine kinase level is useful in patients with a family history of myopathy or risk factors for statin-induced myopathy (for example, concomitant therapy with medications that alter statin metabolism). Routine creatine kinase assessment is low yield and cost ineffective, as the incidence of myopathy is relatively rare. For this patient without symptoms or risk factors for myopathy, neither initial creatine kinase measurement nor testing during statin therapy is indicated.

Elevated high-sensitivity C-reactive protein level is a risk factor for cardiovascular disease and may be useful in patients for whom the best therapeutic approach for hyperlipidemia is uncertain. However, this patient has a clear indication for high-intensity statin therapy based on his clinical atherosclerotic cardiovascular disease. Therefore, high-sensitivity C-reactive protein testing is not indicated.

KEY POINT

- A repeat fasting lipid panel should be obtained 1 to 3 months after initiation of statin therapy to determine medication adherence and effectiveness of treatment.

Bibliography

Stone NJ, Robinson JG, Lichtenstein AH, et al; American College of Cardiology/American Heart Association Task Force on Practice Guidelines. 2013 ACC/AHA guideline on the treatment of blood cholesterol to reduce atherosclerotic cardiovascular risk in adults: a report of the American College of Cardiology/American Heart Association Task Force on Practice Guidelines. Circulation. 2014 Jun 24;129(25 Suppl 2):S1-45. Erratum in: Circulation. 2014 Jun 24;129(25 Suppl 2):S46-8. [PMID: 24222016]

Item 126   Answer: D

Educational Objective: Manage cervical cancer screening in an older woman.

Cervical cancer screening, including Pap smears and human papillomavirus (HPV) testing, should be discontinued in this patient. Screening for cervical cancer can be stopped in women age 65 years and older who have had adequate prior screening, which consists of three consecutive negative Pap smears or two consecutive negative Pap smears plus HPV tests within the last 10 years. The most recent testing should be within the last 5 years. This patient meets these criteria with consistently negative Pap smear screenings, with the latest being 2 years ago. The American Cancer Society recommends that screening not continue in women over age 65 years, even in those who have a new sexual partner. Women who have had a hysterectomy with removal of the cervix for benign reasons (no history of high-grade precancerous lesions or cervical cancer) should not be screened regardless of age. This includes women who have had a hysterectomy with removal of the cervix during surgery for ovarian or endometrial cancer, as they are not considered to be at high risk for cervical cancer.

In women age 65 years and older who are at high risk for cervical cancer, including immunocompromised women (such as those with HIV infection), women with in utero exposure to diethylstilbestrol (DES), and women who have had previous treatment of a high-grade precancerous lesion, screening should continue.

KEY POINT

- Screening for cervical cancer can be stopped in women age 65 years and older who have had three consecutive negative Pap smears or two consecutive negative Pap smears plus human papillomavirus test results within the last 10 years, with the most recent test performed within 5 years.

Bibliography

Moyer VA; U.S. Preventive Services Task Force. Screening for cervical cancer: U.S. Preventive Services Task Force recommendation statement. Ann Intern Med. 2012 Jun 19;156(12):880-91, W312. Erratum in: Ann Intern Med. 2013 Jun 4;158(11):852. [PMID: 22711081]

Item 127   Answer: D

Educational Objective: Treat chronic neurogenic neck pain.

This patient should be treated with gabapentin. Her history and physical examination findings are consistent with chronic neurogenic neck pain. Features that support this diagnosis are the quality of the pain (burning and tingling), radiation to the arms, limited range of motion of the neck, and reproduction of pain with compression of the spinal nerves via the Spurling test. The findings of normal upper extremity muscle strength, the absence of upper extremity hyperreflexia and spasticity, and her imaging results make spinal cord involvement unlikely, as does the lack of evidence of a systemic process such as malignancy. Patients with chronic neurogenic neck pain frequently do not respond to analgesics, such as acetaminophen, or anti-inflammatory medications, such as NSAIDs. However, they may respond to agents such as gabapentin and tricyclic antidepressants.

Muscle relaxants such as cyclobenzaprine are sometimes used in patients with neck and back pain, particularly if muscle spasm is present. However, muscle relaxants tend to be more effective for acute than chronic pain and have considerable side effects, such as sedation. Additionally, although benzodiazepines such as diazepam have muscle relaxant properties, they have not been shown to be superior to nonbenzodiazepine muscle relaxants and also have greater potential for abuse. Therefore, they are often reserved for use in patients with muscle spasm in whom other muscle relaxants have failed. Muscle relaxant therapy, particularly with a benzodiazepine, would not be indicated in this patient without evidence of significant muscle spasm associated with her neck pain.

Data supporting the effectiveness of epidural glucocorticoid injections for chronic neurogenic neck pain are limited and inconsistent. Although they are occasionally used in patients with chronic pain refractory to other therapies, the FDA has issued a drug safety communication about epidural injection of glucocorticoids due to the potential for rare but serious adverse effects. Therefore, this would not be an appropriate intervention in this patient who has not been treated with other interventions for her pain.

Laboratory tests, such as erythrocyte sedimentation rate, are also not indicated in the absence of clinical evidence of a systemic disorder that might be the cause of neck pain. This patient is otherwise healthy, and there is no clear need for laboratory testing as part of the evaluation of her neck pain.

KEY POINT

- Patients with chronic neurogenic neck pain may respond to agents such as gabapentin and tricyclic antidepressants.

Bibliography

Newman JS, Weissman BN, Angevine PD, et al; Expert Panel on Musculoskeletal Imaging. ACR Appropriateness Criteria®: chronic neck pain. American College of Radiology Web site. Available at https://acsearch.acr.org/docs/69426/Narrative/. Accessed June 5, 2015.

Item 128   Answer: A

Educational Objective: Manage surrogate decision making in a patient without decision-making capacity.

The surrogate decision maker's understanding of this patient's medical condition and previously expressed health care wishes and values should be evaluated. For the patient who lacks decision-making capacity, the surrogate decision maker should not make decisions based on his or her own values and preferences. Rather, the surrogate has ethical and legal obligations to make decisions that are based on the patient's health care values, goals, and preferences (the concept of substituted judgment). If these values, goals, and preferences are unknown, the surrogate should make decisions based on what he or she considers to be the best interests of the patient. In this case, the patient's daughter may think that the patient's prognosis is poor and may be acting based on that misconception. The patient's daughter should be engaged in a discussion to evaluate her understanding of the patient's condition and to clarify the patient's health care preferences in order to ensure that the decision is consistent with the patient's previously expressed wishes.

Obtaining a court-appointed guardian is not indicated in this case in which the patient clearly stated her views in her advance directive and subsequent care decisions will be made by a duly appointed surrogate based on the patient's wishes. The most appropriate approach is to explore the daughter's understanding of her mother's medical condition as well as her understanding of her mother's previously expressed health care wishes and values.

The patient's daughter's refusal of further treatment should not be summarily accepted. Rather, the physician should determine the daughter's understanding of the proposed treatment plan and suggest a treatment recommendation that does not conflict with the patient's previously expressed wishes. If the surrogate's decisions seem inconsistent with the patient's values or previous directives, the clinician should proceed with extreme caution. Ethics consultations are helpful in reconciling these conflicts.

KEY POINT

- A surrogate decision maker has ethical and legal obligations to make decisions that are based on the patient's health care values, goals, and preferences.

Bibliography

Snyder L; American College of Physicians Ethics, Professionalism, and Human Rights Committee. American College of Physicians Ethics Manual: sixth edition. Ann Intern Med. 2012 Jan 3;156(1 Pt 2):73-104. [PMID: 22213573]

Item 129   Answer: A

Educational Objective: Evaluate a study using absolute risk reduction.

According to this study, the absolute risk reduction (ARR) in mortality from a myocardial infarction (MI) after taking a statin medication for 5 years is 4%.

The effectiveness of different therapeutic interventions is frequently reported as relative or absolute risk differences between study groups. Relative comparisons compare the rates of events, such as death or complications, in two study groups, and the differences between groups is usually reported as relative risk (RR), odds ratio, or hazard ratio. Absolute comparisons, however, represent the absolute (that is, total) difference in outcomes between the experimental and control groups. Absolute measures may also be used to calculate the number needed to treat (NNT), an estimate of the number of patients needing to be exposed to an intervention to expect the studied outcome to occur. To perform calculations for diagnostic tests and medical therapeutics, it is useful to create a table (shown):

	Disease	
	Yes	No
Exposed	a	b
Not exposed	c	d

The data extracted from this study are shown:

	Death from Myocardial Infarction	
	Yes	No
Statin	53	1000
Placebo	93	1000

ARR can then be calculated as follows:

Control event rate (CER) $= c/(c+d) = 93/(93+1000) = 0.085$

Experimental event rate (EER)

$= a/(a+b) = 53/(53+1000) = 0.050$

$ARR = CER - EER = 0.085 - 0.050 = 0.035$

$NNT = 1/0.035 = 29$

Relative risk reduction (RRR) can be calculated as follows:

$RR = EER/CER = 0.050/0.085 = 0.59$

$RRR = 1 - RR = 1 - 0.59 = 0.41$

A disadvantage of relative comparisons is the potential for exaggerated outcomes, especially if the outcomes are uncommon. For example, although statin medications were associated with a 41% RRR in mortality from MI, the ARR was only 4%.

KEY POINT

- A disadvantage of relative comparisons is the potential for exaggerated outcomes, especially if the outcomes are uncommon; absolute risk reduction can provide a more realistic estimate of risk than relative risk reduction.

Bibliography

Barratt A, Wyer PC, Hatala R, et al; Evidence-Based Medicine Teaching Tips Working Group. Tips for learners of evidence-based medicine: 1. Relative risk reduction, absolute risk reduction and number needed to treat. CMAJ. 2004 Aug 17;171(4):353-8. [PMID: 15313996]

Item 130   Answer: C
Educational Objective: Diagnose sexual interest/arousal disorder.

This woman most likely has sexual interest/arousal disorder. She reports persistent lack of interest and decreased receptiveness to sexual activity over the past 2 years, and these issues have caused her personal distress. Sexual dysfunction comprises various sexual problems with overlapping biologic, psychological, and interpersonal components. Rather than discrete diagnostic categories, the DSM-5 categorizes female sexual dysfunction into broad domains that allow for increased complexity within a diagnosis. Sexual interest/arousal disorder is characterized by the presence of at least three of the following symptoms: lack of sexual interest, lack of sexual thoughts or fantasies, decreased initiation of sexual activity or decreased responsiveness to partner's initiation attempts, reduced excitement or pleasure during sexual activity, decreased response to sexual cues, or decreased sensations during sexual activity; the presence of associated personal distress is required for diagnosis. Furthermore, a diagnosis of sexual dysfunction requires a duration of at least 6 months to distinguish transient sexual difficulties from more persistent dysfunction.

Genitopelvic pain/penetration disorder is characterized by persistent urogenital pain associated with intercourse that is not related exclusively to inadequate lubrication or vaginismus. Physiologic conditions that may cause dyspareunia and pelvic pain include interstitial cystitis, pelvic adhesions, infection, and endometriosis. This patient's absence of sexual pain and lack of other associated symptoms and signs make this disorder unlikely.

Orgasmic disorder is the persistent or recurrent delay or absence of orgasm following a normal excitement phase. In this patient, the distress is associated with a lack of interest and decreased libido, rather than lack of orgasm, so this is a less likely diagnosis.

Vulvodynia is a syndrome of persistent vulvar or vestibular discomfort or burning pain, generally occurring in the absence of clinically identifiable findings. The pain is marked and chronic, but variable in terms of severity, constancy, and provocative features. Its etiology is unknown. In this patient, pain is not a symptom, so this is not a correct diagnosis.

KEY POINT

- Sexual interest/arousal disorder is characterized by a lack of sexual interest or arousal; symptoms must be present for at least 6 months and must cause the patient personal distress.

Bibliography

Latif EZ, Diamond MP. Arriving at the diagnosis of female sexual dysfunction. Fertil Steril. 2013 Oct;100(4):898-904. [PMID: 24012196]

Item 131   Answer: D
Educational Objective: Exclude hypertrophic cardiomyopathy in a high school athlete.

No further testing is required in this patient. For persons undergoing a preparticipation sports evaluation, current American Heart Association guidelines consist of a 12-step clinical history and physical examination focused on cardiovascular screening. The elements of this examination include obtaining a family history for evidence of heart disease or premature death, evaluating the patient for cardiac-related symptoms (such as unexplained near-syncope/syncope or exertional dyspnea or fatigue), and performing a physical examination. Physical examination findings in patients with hypertrophic cardiomyopathy (HCM) usually include a systolic crescendo-decrescendo murmur frequently heard best at the left lower sternal border, which is due to left ventricular outflow tract obstruction. The murmur of HCM is augmented by maneuvers that decrease venous return (Valsalva) and is diminished by those that increase preload (leg elevation, hand-grip). Additional testing, with either cardiovascular imaging or electrocardiography, is not indicated in the absence of suspicious symptoms, physical findings, or family history. Therefore, no further testing is indicated in this patient with normal findings on physical examination and no suspicious symptoms or historical findings.

Because HCM is the most common cause of sudden cardiac death in persons younger than age 35 years, especially during athletic training and competition, evaluating for this diagnosis is often the focus of a preparticipation sports evaluation. However, the routine use of electrocardiography, echocardiography, or electrocardiographic stress testing to exclude HCM in the United States is probably impractical, lacks proven cost-effectiveness, and would require considerable infrastructure that currently does not exist. Additionally, such screening also could potentially cause harm to many young athletes because of false-positive results that would lead to unnecessary further evaluation, anxiety, and possibly unwarranted disqualification from sports. These guidelines differ from recommendations in Europe, where a 12-lead electrocardiogram is often incorporated into preparticipation sports evaluations. Focused screening is indicated only for first-degree relatives of patients with HCM, with the timing of screening intervals based on age, aerobic activity, family history, and clinical suspicion. Screening in these individuals includes electrocardiography and an imaging study in addition to a comprehensive history and physical examination.

KEY POINT

- In the absence of suspicious symptoms, physical examination findings, or family history in a patient undergoing a preparticipation sports evaluation, additional testing with either cardiovascular imaging or electrocardiography to exclude hypertrophic cardiomyopathy is not indicated.

Bibliography

Maron BJ, Thompson PD, Ackerman MJ, et al; American Heart Association Council on Nutrition, Physical Activity, and Metabolism. Recommendations and considerations related to preparticipation screening for cardiovascular abnormalities in competitive athletes: 2007 update: a scientific statement from the American Heart Association Council on Nutrition, Physical Activity, and Metabolism: endorsed by the American College of Cardiology Foundation. Circulation. 2007 Mar 27;115(12):1643-55. [PMID: 17353433]

Item 132   Answer: D

Educational Objective: Monitor a patient with chronic noncancer pain on opioid therapy.

This patient's long-term opioid therapy should be monitored with surveillance of a prescription monitoring program, if available. Prescription monitoring programs are state-run systems that gather information on controlled substance prescriptions from pharmacies and prescribers, allowing prescribers to view a patient's controlled substance history and to monitor controlled substance use. This information is helpful in documenting adherence and for early detection of possible abuse.

Although there is little to no evidence supporting the use of long-term opioid therapy for chronic noncancer pain, there are substantial documented risks, even in patients who are compliant and whose medication is prescribed within recommended guidelines. As such, the decision to treat patients with long-term opioid therapy should be made with great care. Although the evidence that shows improved outcomes with various risk mitigation strategies is weak, most guidelines strongly recommend employing a risk assessment tool (such as the DIRE [Diagnosis, Intractability, Risk, and Efficacy] score), baseline urine drug screening, and written treatment agreements. Guidelines also agree that adherence monitoring in the form of regular surveillance of prescription monitoring programs should be performed to reduce prescription drug abuse. With continuous adherence monitoring, opioid therapy can be maintained in appropriate populations with improvement in physical functional status and minimal adverse effects.

Documentation of opioid side effects (cognitive impairment, sedation, constipation, falls), absence of aberrant opioid behavior (lost prescriptions, early refill requests, multiple concurrent opioid providers or "doctor shopping," consistently missed appointments, or erratic follow-up), and

the patient's enduring functional improvement is recommended at every visit in order to justify the ongoing benefit of continued opioid therapy.

Experts recommend frequent and regularly scheduled office visits indefinitely as long as the patient remains on opioid therapy. Follow-up functional assessment twice yearly in a patient being started on long-term opioid therapy would not be adequate to monitor medication adherence, appropriateness of dosing, or potential side effects. Converting to as-needed follow-up after 3 months also would not be appropriate.

Guidelines recommend baseline and periodic urine drug testing to assess adherence, but there is no recommendation that it be performed at every visit.

KEY POINT

- In patients on long-term opioid therapy for chronic noncancer pain, adherence monitoring in the form of regular surveillance of prescription monitoring programs should be performed to reduce prescription drug abuse.

Bibliography

Manchikanti L, Abdi S, Atluri S, et al; American Society of Interventional Pain Physicians. American Society of Interventional Pain Physicians (ASIPP) guidelines for responsible opioid prescribing in chronic non-cancer pain: Part 2–guidance. Pain Physician. 2012 Jul;15(3 Suppl):S67-116. [PMID: 22786449]

Item 133   Answer: E

Educational Objective: Treat hyperlipidemia in a patient with low risk for atherosclerotic cardiovascular disease.

Therapeutic lifestyle modification is the most appropriate therapy for this patient. Lifestyle modification is an essential element of treatment for all patients with elevated lipid parameters but is the primary therapy in those with hyperlipidemia without clinical atherosclerotic cardiovascular disease (ASCVD), diabetes mellitus, elevation of LDL cholesterol greater than 190 mg/dL (4.92 mmol/L), or elevated 10-year risk for developing ASCVD. The 2013 American Heart Association/American College of Cardiology lifestyle management guideline strongly recommends that adults who would benefit from LDL cholesterol lowering (1) consume a diet that emphasizes vegetables, fruits, and whole grains, and limits intake of sweets and red meats; (2) aim for a dietary intake of 5% to 6% of calories from saturated fat; and (3) reduce the percentage of calories from saturated fat and *trans* fat. Moderate-strength recommendations include performing aerobic physical activity (three to four sessions per week, with an average of 40 minutes per session, and involving moderate- to vigorous-intensity physical activity) to lower LDL cholesterol level, non-HDL cholesterol level, and blood pressure.

Ezetimibe is not recommended as first-line therapy for hyperlipidemia in patients with an indication for treatment, as there are insufficient data on the efficacy of ezetimibe in reducing ASCVD risk. There is also no indication for its use in patients at low risk.

In patients without clinical ASCVD or diabetes, statin therapy is typically reserved for those with an LDL cholesterol level of 190 mg/dL (4.92 mmol/L) or higher or an estimated 10-year risk of ASCVD of 7.5% or higher. The benefits of statin therapy in healthy patients with an LDL cholesterol level lower than 190 mg/dL (4.92 mmol/L) are not established. In this patient, treatment with neither high-intensity statin therapy nor moderate-intensity statin therapy would be appropriate.

Although niacin has several favorable effects on lipids, it is less effective than statin drugs in preventing ASCVD and is also not recommended as first-line therapy for patients with an indication for treatment. It would also not be appropriate treatment for this patient who does not have a clear indication for pharmacologic lipid-lowering therapy.

KEY POINT

- In patients with hyperlipidemia but without clinical atherosclerotic cardiovascular disease (ASCVD), diabetes mellitus, an LDL cholesterol level of 190 mg/dL (4.92 mmol/L) or higher, or elevated 10-year risk for developing ASCVD, therapeutic lifestyle modification is the primary intervention for prevention of ASCVD.

Bibliography

Eckel RH, Jakicic JM, Ard JD, et al; American College of Cardiology/American Heart Association Task Force on Practice Guidelines. 2013 AHA/ACC guideline on lifestyle management to reduce cardiovascular risk: a report of the American College of Cardiology/American Heart Association Task Force on Practice Guidelines. Circulation. 2014 Jun 24;129(25 Suppl 2):S76-99. Erratum in: Circulation. 2014 Jun 24;129(25 Suppl 2):S100-1. [PMID: 24222015]

Item 134   Answer: D

Educational Objective: Manage disclosure of a medical error to an affected patient.

The attending physician's colleague should be informed of the medical error, and steps should be taken to prevent future errors. Physicians are ethically and legally obligated to disclose medical errors to patients. Medical errors do not necessarily represent unethical behavior, negligence, or malpractice; however, failure to disclose errors may. Nondisclosure, if discovered, damages trust, engenders patient and family anger, and increases the likelihood of legal action. In contrast, full disclosure facilitates informed decision making about future care. Patients who are informed of medical errors and receive authentic apologies are more likely to be forgiving and work with involved caregivers. In this case, the colleague who erred in prescribing trimethoprim-sulfamethoxazole should be held accountable for the error. However, informing the colleague of the error is not the patient's responsibility. Instead, the attending physician has this responsibility and should hold the colleague accountable (for example, by taking steps to prevent future errors).

Although the pharmacy shares responsibility for the error, assigning blame at this stage (before an investigation is held) is inappropriate.

The attending physician should not offer to transfer the patient's care to a physician at another hospital unless a trusting and therapeutic relationship with the patient no longer exists or the patient desires the transfer.

KEY POINT

- Physicians are ethically and legally obligated to disclose medical errors to patients.

Bibliography

Snyder L; American College of Physicians Ethics, Professionalism, and Human Rights Committee. American College of Physicians Ethics Manual: sixth edition. Ann Intern Med. 2012 Jan 3;156(1 Pt 2):73-104. [PMID: 22213573]

Item 135   Answer: D

Educational Objective: Manage perioperative anticoagulation in a patient on chronic warfarin therapy who has a low annual risk of thromboembolism.

This patient should stop warfarin 5 days before his umbilical hernia repair surgery but requires no bridging anticoagulation. He is scheduled for an invasive procedure with a moderate or high risk of bleeding and therefore requires discontinuation of warfarin for surgery. Cessation of warfarin 5 days before surgery is typically sufficient to assure a normalized INR for the procedure. For patients requiring stoppage of chronic anticoagulation, the necessity of bridging anticoagulation must then be determined based on the patient's thromboembolic risk. Contemporary mechanical aortic valve prostheses have a low (<5%) annual risk of thromboembolism, and guidelines recommend no anticoagulation bridging for patients with these prostheses if they are in sinus rhythm and have no additional risk factors for arterial thromboembolism. Perioperative aspirin continuation in a patient whose only indication for antiplatelet therapy is a mechanical valve prosthesis is a matter of debate. The American College of Chest Physicians and the American College of Cardiology/American Heart Association both suggest that aspirin be continued throughout surgery in any patient in whom the antithrombotic benefits outweigh the bleeding risks. If aspirin is continued, the additional bleeding risk it confers should be factored into the decision making regarding bridging anticoagulation.

Both intravenous unfractionated heparin and therapeutic-dose subcutaneous enoxaparin are not appropriate in this patient. Either is an acceptable form of bridging anticoagulation for patients at intermediate or high risk of thromboembolism, but for patients with low thromboembolism risk, the potential bleeding complications of bridging outweigh the possible thromboembolism prevention. For bridging-eligible patients, low-molecular-weight heparin (LMWH) is often preferred because it can be administered in the outpatient setting and does not require laboratory monitoring; however, no evidence suggests any difference in outcomes with LMWH or unfractionated heparin.

Prophylactic-dose subcutaneous enoxaparin is only an acceptable choice for perioperative anticoagulation bridging in intermediate-risk (5%-10% annual rate of thromboembolism) patients on warfarin for a history of venous thromboembolism. For other chronic anticoagulation indications (atrial fibrillation and mechanical heart valves), no data are available to suggest a benefit from prophylactic-dose LMWH.

KEY POINT

- Bridging anticoagulation is not indicated for patients who stop chronic warfarin therapy before surgery and have a low annual risk of thromboembolism.

Bibliography

Baron TH, Kamath PS, McBane RD. Management of antithrombotic therapy in patients undergoing invasive procedures. N Engl J Med. 2013 May 30;368(22):2113-24. [PMID: 23718166]

Item 136   Answer: D

Educational Objective: Treat upper airway cough syndrome due to allergic rhinitis.

The most appropriate treatment for this patient is an intranasal glucocorticoid. This patient has chronic cough (cough of more than 8 weeks' duration) due to upper airway cough syndrome (UACS) associated with allergic rhinitis. UACS is associated with conditions that cause excessive mucus production in the upper airways and postnasal drip, triggering cough. Allergic rhinitis is a frequent cause of UACS and is likely in this patient with evidence of seasonal allergies (clear nasal drainage, postnasal drip) and symptoms that are worse in high allergy seasons (fall and spring). Patients with UACS due to allergic rhinitis respond well to intranasal glucocorticoids, and these agents are considered first-line therapy.

Antibiotics are not indicated in this patient who has no clinical evidence of acute or chronic bacterial sinusitis.

First-generation antihistamine and decongestant therapy is recommended for patients with UACS due to nonallergic rhinitis. Since this patient's presentation is typical of seasonal allergies, intranasal glucocorticoids are a better option. Additionally, the systemic side effects associated with oral medications do not occur with intranasal administration.

Although cough can be a manifestation of asthma, this patient had no reports of wheezing, even with exercise, and physical examination did not reveal the presence of wheeze or airflow limitation. Therefore, inhaled bronchodilators are not indicated.

KEY POINT

- Intranasal glucocorticoids are first-line therapy for patients with upper airway cough syndrome due to allergic rhinitis; antibiotics should not be used without clear evidence of bacterial infection.

Bibliography

Wallace DV, Dykewicz MS, Bernstein DI, et al; Joint Task Force on Practice; American Academy of Allergy; Asthma Immunology; American College of Allergy; Asthma and Immunology; Joint Council of Allergy, Asthma and Immunology. The diagnosis and management of rhinitis: a updated practice parameter. J Allergy Clin Immunol. 2008 Aug;122(2 Suppl):S1-84. Erratum in: J Allergy Clin Immunol. 2008 Dec;122(6):1237. [PMID: 18662584]

Item 137   Answer: D

Educational Objective: Treat obesity with lifestyle modification.

This patient should be advised to reduce his caloric intake to maintain a deficit of 500 kcal/d. With a BMI of 36, this patient meets the criterion for obesity (BMI greater than or equal to 30). Furthermore, his waist circumference is higher than 102 cm (40 in), which is independently associated with increased cardiovascular risk. Treatment of overweight and obese patients should begin with establishing a weight loss goal and individualized treatment plan. A reasonable goal is weight loss of 0.5 to 1.0 kg (1.1-2.2 lb) per week to achieve a total weight loss of 10%. The mainstay of obesity treatment is lifestyle modification that includes diet for weight loss, increased physical activity, and behavioral therapy. In addition to increasing physical activity and behavioral therapy (aimed at avoiding fast food and inappropriate snacking), this patient should be prescribed a diet that maintains a 500-kcal/d deficit. Maintaining a continuous negative energy balance of 500 kcal/d results in a weight loss of about 0.5 kg (1.1 lb) per week. Involving dieticians, exercise therapists, and behavioral therapists increases the chances of success.

Bariatric surgery, such as laparoscopic adjustable gastric banding or sleeve gastrectomy, should be considered in all patients with a BMI of 40 or higher and in patients with a BMI of 35 or higher with obesity-related comorbid conditions. This patient does not meet the criteria for bariatric surgery at this time.

Pharmacologic treatment is preferably used as an adjunctive therapy in patients with a BMI of 30 or higher or in patients with a BMI of 27 or higher with overweight- or obesity-associated comorbidities who have not achieved significant weight loss with comprehensive lifestyle interventions. Orlistat is an inhibitor of gastric and pancreatic lipases that leads to malabsorption of approximately 30% of ingested fat. It is available both over the counter and by prescription. If lifestyle interventions are ineffective in obesity treatment, a pharmacologic agent such as orlistat can be added to, not substituted for, those lifestyle interventions.

Lorcaserin is another effective weight loss agent that acts as an appetite suppressant by stimulating serotonin 2C receptors in the brain. However, it would not be a preferable next step in management prior to initiation of comprehensive lifestyle interventions.

KEY POINT

- The mainstay of obesity treatment is lifestyle modification that includes diet for weight loss, increased physical activity, and behavioral therapy.

Bibliography

Jensen MD, Ryan DH, Apovian CM, et al; American College of Cardiology/American Heart Association Task Force on Practice Guidelines; Obesity Society. 2013 AHA/ACC/TOS guideline for the management of overweight and obesity in adults: a report of the American College of Cardiology/American Heart Association Task Force on Practice Guidelines and The Obesity Society. J Am Coll Cardiol. 2014 Jul 1;63(25 Pt B):2985-3023. Erratum in: J Am Coll Cardiol. 2014 Jul 1;63(25 Pt B):3029-3030. [PMID: 24239920]

Item 138   Answer: C

Educational Objective: Evaluate a patient with benign prostatic hyperplasia.

Obtaining a urinalysis is the most appropriate next step in the management of this patient with benign prostatic hyperplasia (BPH), a common cause of lower urinary tract symptoms (LUTS). Most men age 60 years and older have LUTS of varying degree associated with prostate enlargement. Symptoms may be mild and include decreased urinary stream, incomplete bladder emptying, urinary frequency, and nocturia. Severe symptoms may include urinary retention, urgency, and incontinence. Diagnosis of BPH in most cases is by history and physical examination, with exclusion of other potential causes of LUTS, which may include malignancy (prostate, bladder), infection (prostatitis, sexually transmitted infections), neurologic causes (spinal cord injury, stroke, Parkinson disease), medical conditions (poorly controlled diabetes mellitus, hypercalcemia), and behavior (alcohol or caffeine intake, excessive water consumption). When these other causes are not highly suspected, only a urinalysis is recommended to exclude infection (bacteria and pyuria), malignancy (hematuria), or postobstructive nephropathy (active urine sediment). Prostate-specific antigen testing is not routinely indicated for diagnosis or following the course of BPH because it may be inconsistently elevated due to prostate hypertrophy, and increased levels of prostate-specific antigen associated with BPH do not reliably correlate with LUTS.

An increased postvoid residual urine volume, determined by catheterization or ultrasonography, is supportive of the presence of BPH but is not required for diagnosis. It has also been used as an indicator of significant obstruction to inform decisions regarding the need for surgical intervention in BPH, although there is not significant evidence that the postvoid residual volume is a reliable predictor of surgical outcomes. Because this patient has no evidence of significant urinary retention, measurement of postvoid residual volume is not indicated.

Prostate ultrasonography is an effective method for measuring prostate volume or evaluating other prostate abnormalities such as nodules. However, volume measurement by ultrasonography is not required for diagnosis of BPH, and this patient has no other indication for prostate imaging.

Urine flow studies are an accurate means of determining bladder outlet obstruction. However, this study is usually reserved for patients with atypical symptoms in whom the diagnosis of BPH is unclear or if there is concern for other urinary tract flow problems in addition to BPH. Because this patient has mild, typical symptoms consistent with BPH, urine flow studies are not indicated.

KEY POINT

- In patients with usual symptoms of benign prostatic hyperplasia (BPH), a careful history and physical examination can usually render the diagnosis; a urinalysis is also indicated in evaluating BPH to exclude infection, malignancy, or postobstructive nephropathy.

Bibliography

Beckman TJ, Mynderse LA. Evaluation and medical management of benign prostatic hyperplasia. Mayo Clin Proc. 2005 Oct;80(10):1356-62. [PMID: 16212149]

Item 139   Answer: B

Educational Objective: Treat a patient with chronic insomnia.

This patient with chronic insomnia should undergo counseling regarding sleep hygiene. Insomnia is defined as the inability to initiate or maintain adequate sleep and is a common disorder. It can lead to daytime somnolence, work absenteeism, motor vehicle accidents, poor general health, functional impairment, and impaired quality of life. The initial management of insomnia focuses on implementing good sleep hygiene, which refers to the optimization of the environmental and behavioral factors associated with sleep. Patients should be advised to establish a regular relaxing bedtime routine; associate the bed and bedroom with sleep; avoid increasingly common disruptors of sleep such as cell phone, television, or computer use in the bedroom; adhere to a stable bed time and arising time; and keep the room quiet and dark.

Alcohol disrupts continuous sleep; however, this patient's modest alcohol use is unlikely to be contributing to his chronic and progressive insomnia.

Antidepressant therapy may improve sleep difficulties in the depressed patient. In addition, some antidepressants, including trazodone, doxepin, and mirtazapine, have sedative side effects, which can be used to advantage in a depressed patient with significant insomnia. Doxepin, in doses lower than needed for an antidepressant effect, is the only antidepressant agent approved for the treatment of insomnia. This patient does not manifest other symptoms of depression, and treating insomnia in the absence of depression with antidepressant agents other than doxepin is not indicated.

Zolpidem is a short-acting nonbenzodiazapine that is used in the treatment of insomnia. Because of potential adverse effects, the use of pharmacologic agents such as zolpidem should be considered only after attempts at behavioral therapy and other nonpharmacologic interventions have failed.

- The initial treatment of insomnia focuses on implementing good sleep hygiene, which refers to the optimization of the environmental and behavioral factors associated with sleep.

Bibliography

Masters PA. In the clinic. Insomnia. Ann Intern Med. 2014 Oct 7;161:ITC1-15. [PMID: 25285559]

Item 140   Answer: D

Educational Objective: Manage cerumen impaction.

Clinical observation is the most appropriate management of this patient. Cerumen, or ear wax, is secreted in the lateral third aspect of the external auditory canal and serves as a protective lining against water damage and infection. Cerumen is normally progressively removed from the ear by epithelial migration and movement of the soft tissues of the lateral ear canal by normal motions such as chewing. Cerumen may accumulate if there is excessive production or interference with this normal removal process. Cerumen impaction is an accumulation of cerumen that causes symptoms or blocks visualization of the tympanic membrane. Guidelines suggest that treatment of cerumen impaction is indicated only in symptomatic patients or if the tympanic membrane needs to be visualized. Since this patient's impacted cerumen was found incidentally and he has no hearing loss, tinnitus, or ear pain, clinical observation is all that is needed at this time.

Ceruminolytic agents, manual removal, and irrigation are all effective means to remove cerumen in symptomatic patients. No ceruminolytic agent has been shown to be superior to any other. Manual removal does not subject the ear canal to moisture, so it may be associated with lower rates of infection. However, manual removal requires operator skill and a cooperative patient, with the potential for mechanical injury to the ear canal and tympanic membranes. Vacuum devices that extract cerumen with suction are available and avoid many of the complications of irrigation or manual cerumen removal.

KEY POINT

- Treatment of cerumen impaction is indicated only in symptomatic patients or if the tympanic membrane needs to be visualized.

Bibliography

Roland PS, Smith TL, Schwartz SR, et al. Clinical practice guideline: Cerumen impaction. Otolayngol Head Neck Surg. 2008 Sep;139(3 Suppl 2):S1-S21. [PMID: 18707628]

Item 141   Answer: D

Educational Objective: Manage the gastrointestinal side effects of opioid therapy.

The most appropriate management of this patient is to add a scheduled stimulant laxative, such as senna. Opioid-induced constipation is nearly universal in patients on regularly scheduled opioid therapy. Unlike other side effects of opioid medications such as nausea or somnolence, tolerance to constipation does not develop over time. Therefore, all patients on scheduled opioids should be prescribed a scheduled stimulant laxative, such as senna or bisacodyl. If this therapy does not adequately control opioid-associated constipation, osmotic agents (polyethylene glycol powder, sorbitol, lactulose) can be added.

Stool softeners, such as docusate, are inadequate to manage opioid-induced constipation when given alone. However, stool softeners may be given along with a stimulant laxative to further aid in preventing constipation in patients on chronic opioid therapy. Similarly, fiber supplements or other bulking agents are ineffective in managing opioid-induced constipation.

Methylnaltrexone, an injectable peripheral opioid antagonist, is very effective in treating opioid-induced constipation without adversely affecting analgesia. However, it is reserved for opioid-induced constipation that has failed to respond to an aggressive laxative regimen, and as such, it is considered second-line therapy. This patient has not had a trial of aggressive laxative therapy; therefore, methylnaltrexone is not yet indicated.

KEY POINT

- All patients on scheduled opioid therapy should be prescribed a scheduled stimulant laxative.

Bibliography

Swetz KM, Kamal AH. In the clinic. Palliative care. Ann Intern Med. 2012 Feb 7;156(3):ITC2-1-TC2-15. [PMID: 22312158]

Item 142   Answer: C

Educational Objective: Manage postoperative venous thromboembolism prophylaxis in a patient with abdominal cancer.

Prophylactic-dose enoxaparin for up to 28 days after surgery is the most appropriate management for venous thromboembolism (VTE) prophylaxis for this patient. He just underwent major abdominal surgery to resect a malignancy. The VTE risk in patients following abdominal cancer surgery is particularly high due to the prothrombotic state caused by a neoplasm and the immobility caused by major abdominal surgery. Unless bleeding risk is considered prohibitive, these patients should receive pharmacologic VTE prophylaxis. Current American College of Chest Physicians (ACCP) guidelines recommend the use of prophylactic-dose low-molecular-weight heparins for up to 28 days after surgery. This patient had relatively low blood loss with only a small decline in his hemoglobin level and has no other known risk factors for severe bleeding. Therefore, his bleeding risk is not high. Because of this, use of prophylactic-dose enoxaparin for 1 month after surgery is the most appropriate management.

Intermittent pneumatic compression devices do not provide sufficient VTE prophylaxis in patients who have undergone abdominal surgery and have other risk factors such as cancer. They are appropriate to use if a patient has an elevated bleeding risk, but this patient has no evidence of bleeding or risk factors for bleeding (for example, concomitant antiplatelet therapy).

Aspirin is not an acceptable choice for VTE prophylaxis following abdominal surgery. ACCP guidelines only recommend aspirin as an option after hip or knee arthroplasty, and in that situation, it should be continued for 35 days after surgery. Data on the most effective dose of aspirin for major orthopedic surgery VTE prophylaxis are sparse.

Prophylactic-dose enoxaparin limited to the duration of hospitalization is not considered to be a sufficient duration of therapy.

Similar to aspirin, therapeutic warfarin is a VTE prophylaxis option recommended only for major orthopedic surgery (hip or knee replacement or hip fracture repair).

KEY POINT

- The most appropriate venous thromboembolism prophylaxis in patients who have undergone cancer surgery is prophylactic-dose low-molecular-weight heparin for up to 28 days after surgery.

Bibliography
Douketis JD, Spyropoulos AC, Spencer FA, et al; American College of Chest Physicians. Perioperative management of antithrombotic therapy: Antithrombotic Therapy and Prevention of Thrombosis, 9th ed: American College of Chest Physicians Evidence-Based Clinical Practice Guidelines. Chest. 2012 Feb;141(2 Suppl):e326S-50S. Erratum in: Chest. 2012 Apr;141(4):1129. [PMID: 22315266]

Item 143   Answer: D
Educational Objective: Initiate palliative care in an appropriate patient.

Palliative care should be initiated now in this patient with serious, life-limiting illness. Palliative care focuses on achieving individualized goals of therapy and coordinating management of care to achieve those goals. Historically, palliative care was equated only with end-of-life care or considered appropriate only when other, potentially curative therapies had failed. However, contrary to this view, palliative care may be provided concurrently with life-prolonging therapies or with therapies with curative intent. It may be appropriately accessed at any time during a patient's illness, from diagnosis to death. Ideally, palliative care is initiated early and integrated throughout the disease trajectory to help optimize the focus of care on the patient's values and goals of treatment, an important aspect of managing complex and serious disease. Provision of early palliative care has been shown to result in prolonged life of higher quality. For example, patients with metastatic non–small cell lung cancer randomized to early palliative care had improved quality of life, less aggressive care at the end of life, and lived on average 2.7 months longer than those patients randomized to standard care (median survival 11.6 months versus 8.9 months). This is a survival benefit comparable to first-line chemotherapy in patients with non–small cell lung cancer. It

is a common and unfortunate misconception that palliative care decreases life expectancy.

Hospice is a specialized type of palliative care that is reserved for patients in the terminal phase of their disease, arbitrarily defined as the last 6 months of life. Since this patient is interested in pursuing life-prolonging treatment, initiation of hospice care would not be appropriate.

Although one of the main goals of palliative care is aggressive symptom management, uncontrolled symptoms are not a requirement for palliative care involvement. Palliative care has much to offer patients outside of the domain of symptom management, including care coordination, help in establishing goals of care and navigating complex decision making, and assistance with coping. Therefore, there is no need to wait until the patient has pain or completes active treatment before accessing palliative care.

KEY POINT

- Palliative care that is initiated early and integrated throughout the disease trajectory results in prolonged life of higher quality in patients with serious illness when compared with patients who do not receive palliative care.

Bibliography
Temel JS, Greer JA, Muzikansky A, et al. Early palliative care for patients with metastatic non-small-cell lung cancer. N Engl J Med. 2010 Aug 19;363(8):733-42. [PMID: 20818875]

Item 144   Answer: C
Educational Objective: Manage transition of care in an older patient who requires posthospital rehabilitation.

The most appropriate management of this patient is short-term rehabilitation at a skilled nursing facility (SNF). The purpose of rehabilitation is to maximize functional recovery and independence. Older patients such as this one often require posthospital rehabilitation due to deconditioning associated with acute medical or surgical illness. Rehabilitation can be provided in many different settings, and the optimal type and location of rehabilitation depends on the medical needs of the patient and his or her ability to participate in rehabilitation activities. This patient requires the assistance of another person for safety in accomplishing basic activities of daily living, such as transfers and toileting, and although her family is supportive, they would not be able to provide the level of care needed. Additionally, this patient is actively participating in therapy and making progress; however, she is unable to tolerate intensive rehabilitation services (usually defined as 3 hours per day, 5 days per week) at this time. For these reasons, this patient would be better suited to lower-intensity rehabilitation at a SNF, most of which are able to provide these services.

Rehabilitation services can be provided on an outpatient basis, either in the patient's own home if the patient is homebound or at an outpatient rehabilitation clinic in

CONT.

patients who are more functional. However, because this patient's family is not able to provide adequately extensive care in the home, rehabilitation services in this setting are not appropriate.

Long-term acute care hospitals (LTACHs) are designed to accommodate complex, high-intensity care needs for patients who require frequent physician input but no longer require standard hospitalization. Patients who require care at an LTACH include those with ongoing mechanical ventilation weaning, complex wound care needs, or multiple intravenous therapies. Although LTACHs may provide rehabilitation services, this is not their primary function. This patient does not require the level of medical care provided in an LTACH, and the focus of her care should be on rehabilitation.

Free-standing rehabilitation hospitals or units provide specialized, high-intensity rehabilitation under the direction of physiatrists. They have specific admission criteria, one of which is usually the ability to participate in 3 hours of therapy per day during the week, which this patient would not tolerate.

KEY POINT

- In older patients who require posthospital rehabilitation but cannot tolerate active, intensive therapy (3 hours per day, 5 days per week), rehabilitation services may be performed in a skilled nursing facility.

Bibliography

Kane RL. Finding the right level of posthospital care: "We didn't realize there was any other option for him". JAMA. 2011 Jan 19;305(3):284-93. [PMID: 21245184]

Item 145   Answer: A

Educational Objective: Treat moderate dry age-related macular degeneration with high-dose antioxidants to prevent progression to advanced disease.

This patient with moderate dry age-related macular degeneration (AMD) should be treated with antioxidant vitamins and zinc, using the Age-related Eye Disease Study 2 (AREDS2) formulation. AMD is a degenerative disease of the macula that results in loss of central vision. Dry AMD is typically seen as subretinal deposits of yellowish or white extracellular material (drusen) and atrophy of the retinal pigment epithelium. Wet AMD is characterized by growth of abnormal blood vessels (neovascularization) into the subretinal space. Although dry AMD is more common, wet AMD is associated with a greater risk of vision loss. The Age-related Eye Disease Study (AREDS) found that daily high doses of vitamins C and E, β-carotene, and the minerals zinc and copper (the AREDS formulation) slowed the progression of moderate dry AMD (defined as extensive intermediate size drusen or at least one large lesion, or significant retinal pigment epithelium atrophy in one or both eyes) to advanced AMD. A second randomized trial, AREDS2, focused on whether the

AREDS formulation could be improved with the addition of omega-3 fatty acids and/or certain antioxidants (lutein and zeaxanthin) and the subtraction of β-carotene. Although omega-3 fatty acids did not provide any additional benefit, lutein and zeaxanthin were found to be an appropriate substitute for β-carotene. Since β-carotene has been associated with an increased risk of lung cancer, particularly in smokers and former smokers, the AREDS2 formulation is a more appropriate choice for this patient with a significant smoking history; the AREDS formulation would be an appropriate choice for nonsmokers.

Laser therapy has not been shown to be beneficial in patients with dry AMD and may be detrimental by increasing rates of neovascularization. Laser therapy may have a very limited role in treating selected patients with wet AMD, but it would not be an appropriate therapy in this patient.

Vascular endothelial growth factor inhibitors are an established therapy for wet AMD due to their inhibitory effect on neovascularization, but they do not have a role in treating dry AMD.

Clinical observation without treatment with antioxidant vitamins would not be appropriate in this patient with moderate dry AMD given the established benefit of antioxidants in reducing the risk of developing more advanced and potentially sight-threatening disease.

KEY POINT

- High-dose antioxidant vitamins are indicated to prevent the progression of moderate dry age-related macular degeneration (AMD) to advanced AMD.

Bibliography

Aronow ME, Chew EY. Age-related Eye Disease Study 2: perspectives, recommendations, and unanswered questions. Curr Opin Ophthalmol. 2014 May;25(3):186-90. [PMID: 24614146]

Item 146   Answer: D

Educational Objective: Manage a patient's refusal of life-prolonging treatment.

Hemodialysis should be withheld in this patient who has refused treatment. Patients have the right to refuse any treatment, including those that are life prolonging. A patient's decision to refuse life-prolonging treatments is not necessarily irrational; rather, it is often based on the patient's health care values, goals, and preferences in the context of the perceived benefits and burdens of the proposed treatment. In these cases, the physician's duty is to understand the rationale for the decision and ensure that it is informed. This patient has provided informed refusal for hemodialysis, and her decision should be respected.

A psychiatric evaluation is not necessary in this case because the patient has demonstrated all three elements of decision-making capacity: understanding of her current situation, understanding of the risks and benefits of her decision, and the ability to communicate her decision. In addition, her decision appears well aligned with her underlying beliefs. Psychiatrists may be helpful in determining decision-making capacity in situations in which there is a question about the patient's ability to make decisions or apparent misalignment between the decision and underlying beliefs. Additionally, a psychiatrist cannot determine if a patient is competent, as this is a legal decision made by the courts.

If a physician begins or continues a treatment that a patient has refused, the physician, regardless of his or her intent, is committing battery. Overriding this patient's refusal of hemodialysis is unethical and illegal.

There is no evidence that this patient lacks decision-making capacity; therefore, there is no need to refer to the patient's advance directive and ask the son to make a decision regarding his mother's hemodialysis.

KEY POINT

- In the case of a patient who refuses life-prolonging treatment, the physician's duty is to understand the rationale for the decision and ensure that it is informed; provided that the decision meets these criteria, the physician must honor it.

Bibliography

Snyder L; American College of Physicians Ethics, Professionalism, and Human Rights Committee. American College of Physicians Ethics Manual: sixth edition. Ann Intern Med. 2012 Jan 3;156(1 Pt 2):73-104. [PMID: 22213573]

Item 147   Answer: A
Educational Objective: Diagnose Achilles tendinopathy.

This patient most likely has Achilles tendinopathy, which classically presents with burning heel pain and stiffness that worsen with activity and improve with rest. As there is no inflammation seen on histopathologic examination, use of the term tendinopathy is preferred to tendinitis. On examination, there is frequently tenderness to palpation approximately 2 to 6 cm proximal to the Achilles tendon insertion on the calcaneus. Symptoms typically begin after an individual increases his or her level of physical activity, as is the case with this patient.

This patient has no evidence of Achilles tendon rupture, which usually but not always presents with the sudden onset of heel pain while the patient is participating in a strenuous activity. Patients may also report hearing a popping sound. On examination, a palpable Achilles tendon defect may be present, and there is usually a positive Thompson test.

High ankle sprains typically result from excessive dorsiflexion or eversion that causes injury to the tibiofibular syndesmotic ligaments connecting the distal tibia and fibula. Unlike in this patient, pain is typically elicited by medial-lateral compression of the leg at the mid-calf level (squeeze test) or by having the patient cross his legs with the mid-calf of the painful leg resting on the other knee (crossed-leg test).

Tarsal tunnel syndrome is caused by compression of the posterior tibial nerve as it passes within the tarsal tunnel below the medial malleolus. It is characterized by pain and paresthesias in the medial ankle that extend into the midfoot. Symptoms commonly worsen with standing, walking, and running. On examination, pain can be elicited by tapping on the posterior tibial nerve along its course.

KEY POINT

- Achilles tendinopathy classically presents with burning heel pain and stiffness that worsen with activity and improve with rest.

Bibliography

Roche AJ, Calder JD. Achilles tendinopathy: a review of the current concepts of treatment. Bone Joint J. 2013 Oct;95-B(10):1299-307. [PMID: 24078523]

Item 148   Answer: D
Educational Objective: Treat genitourinary syndrome of menopause.

The most appropriate management of this woman with dyspareunia due to genitourinary syndrome of menopause is topical vaginal estradiol. Symptoms of atrophic vaginitis affect 10% to 40% of postmenopausal women and include vaginal dryness, dyspareunia, vulvovaginal irritation, and itch. The associated dyspareunia may lead to avoidance of sexual activity due to discomfort. Treatment for genitourinary syndrome of menopause may include hormone-free vaginal moisturizers, which may control symptoms in some women. If symptoms persist with lubricant use, topical estradiol is useful in alleviating vaginal symptoms. A low-dose tablet containing 25 µg of 17-β estradiol is available; it is generally inserted nightly for 2 weeks and then twice weekly on nonconsecutive nights to restore vaginal epithelium. Concurrent progestin is generally not indicated for women with an intact uterus who use low-dose vaginal estrogen alone, as systemic absorption is minimal.

Several classes of medication may exacerbate vaginal dryness, including antiestrogens (tamoxifen, aromatase inhibitors), progestins, antihistamines, and anticholinergics. However, ACE inhibitors, such as benazepril, are not associated with vaginal dryness.

Systemic estrogen therapy with a patch, gel, or tablet may be used in conjunction with vaginal estrogen to treat vasomotor symptoms or for other indications, along with concurrent progestin treatment in patients with an intact uterus. Moderate to severe vasomotor symptoms can be treated with systemic hormone therapy in the appropriate risk-stratified patient; however, this patient's hot flush symptoms are tolerable and do not warrant systemic hormone therapy.

This patient's decreased interest in sexual intercourse is likely related to her dyspareunia and not decreased libido. Additionally, topical or systemic testosterone is not currently FDA approved for treatment of decreased libido in women, and its use for this purpose is discouraged by the Endocrine Society until long-term safety data can be established.

- Vaginal estrogen therapy is effective in treating women who have moderate to severe symptoms of genitourinary syndrome of menopause that have not responded to lubricants.

Bibliography

Management of symptomatic vulvovaginal atrophy: 2013 position statement of The North American Menopause Society. Menopause. 2013 Sep; 20(9):888-902; quiz 903-4. [PMID: 23985562]

Item 149   Answer: D

Educational Objective: Diagnose the cause of tinnitus.

This patient has sensorineural hearing loss, which is the most common cause of continuous, high-pitched tinnitus. Sensorineural hearing loss results from decreased sound perception due to disorders of the cochlea or acoustic nerve. Risk factors include age (presbycusis), exposure to loud noise, and ototoxic medications. Given this patient's age, chronic and bilateral symptoms, past sound exposure, and difficulty hearing when background noise is present, sensorineural hearing loss is the most likely cause of his tinnitus. Evaluation for hearing loss in the office may be accomplished by the whispered voice test, in which the examiner stands at arm's length behind the patient and the patient occludes the untested ear canal. The examiner then whispers six sets of three letter or number combinations to the patient; failure to repeat at least three of the six sets correctly constitutes a positive result.

Acoustic neuroma (or vestibular schwannoma) is a Schwann cell–derived tumor that arises from the vestibular portion of cranial nerve VIII and may cause sensorineural hearing loss and tinnitus. However, acoustic neuromas are rarely bilateral or cause symmetric hearing loss, such as that seen in this patient, making this an unlikely diagnosis.

Meniere disease is typically characterized by the triad of sensorineural hearing loss, tinnitus, and vertigo. Although this patient has evidence of sensorineural hearing loss and tinnitus, which frequently accompany one another, he does not have vertigo. Therefore, Meniere disease is much less likely.

Otosclerosis is a cause of conductive hearing loss resulting from bony changes in the middle ear. Although usually also of progressive onset, otosclerosis results in loss of ability to hear low-pitched sounds without tinnitus. Conductive hearing loss can be distinguished in the office from sensorineural hearing loss by using the Weber and Rinne tests.

- Sensorineural hearing loss is the most common cause of continuous, high-pitched tinnitus; risk factors include age, exposure to loud noise, and ototoxic medications.

Bibliography

Walling AD, Dickson GM. Hearing loss in older adults. Am Fam Physician. 2012 Jun 15;85(12):1150-6. [PMID: 22962895]

Item 150   Answer: D

Educational Objective: Diagnose primary open angle glaucoma.

This patient has primary open angle glaucoma (POAG). Patients with POAG present with bilateral peripheral visual loss that occurs gradually and painlessly. Findings on examination are increased cup:disc ratio, vertical extension of the central cup, and disc hemorrhages. Testing shows an elevation of intraocular pressure (generally considered >22 mm Hg) and loss of peripheral visual field depth. The primary treatment for POAG is lowering the intraocular pressure with medications. β-Blockers have traditionally been used as first-line therapy, although prostaglandins are increasingly being used for this purpose. Other medication options include α-adrenergic agonists, cholinergic agents, and topical carbonic anhydrase inhibitors, and although effective, they are associated with more ocular side effects than β-blockers or prostaglandins. Other interventions include laser therapy and surgical therapy, such as iridectomy or trabeculectomy.

Ophthalmic or posterior ciliary artery occlusion (sometimes referred to as arteritic anterior ischemic optic neuropathy) is the most common cause of permanent vision loss in patients with giant cell arteritis, as the ophthalmic artery and the posterior ciliary artery (a branch of the ophthalmic artery from the internal carotid artery) serve as the main arterial supply to the optic nerve. Giant cell arteritis is unlikely in this patient due to his younger age, chronic symptoms, bilateral involvement, and the absence of systemic symptoms such as fatigue, fever, or weight loss.

Optic neuritis is an inflammatory, demyelinating condition, most commonly occurring in the setting of multiple sclerosis, which typically presents with rapid onset (hours to days) of eye pain (particularly with movement) and monocular visual loss. This diagnosis is not supported by this patient's clinical setting or presentation.

Papilledema, or swelling of the optic disc, results from increased intracranial pressure. Papilledema may be seen with any entity that causes increased intracranial pressure, including intracranial mass lesions, cerebral edema, and cerebrospinal fluid production or resorption abnormalities. Findings on funduscopic examination include venous engorgement, blurring of the optic margins, and elevation of the optic disc, none of which are seen in this patient.

- Findings of primary open angle glaucoma include increased cup:disc ratio, vertical extension of the central cup, disc hemorrhages, and increased intraocular pressure.

Bibliography

Weinreb RN, Aung T, Medeiros FA. The pathophysiology and treatment of glaucoma: a review. JAMA. 2014 May 14;311(18):1901-11. [PMID: 24825645]

Item 151   Answer: C

Educational Objective: Treat insomnia in a patient in whom sleep hygiene techniques are ineffective.

The most appropriate next step in the management of this patient is to recommend sleep restriction counseling. Insomnia is the inability to initiate or maintain adequate sleep, and it may be acute or chronic. This patient's symptoms have been persistent. The initial step in the evaluation of a patient with insomnia is a thorough history and physical examination. When there is no evidence of stimulant use, sleep-disordered breathing, restless legs syndrome, hypothyroidism, depression, or other chronic medical problems that might impair sleep (COPD, heart failure, osteoarthritis), initial treatment should focus on sleep hygiene and, if unsuccessful, a trial of sleep restriction. Sleep restriction limits and then gradually increases the time in bed for sleep. It utilizes the concept of sleep efficiency (total sleep time divided by total time in bed). The patient calculates the average total sleep time per night, and then he or she spends that amount of time in bed, keeping the arising time constant. For example, if a patient determines that his total time asleep is 6 hours per night and he sets his waking time as 6:00 AM, his bedtime would be 12:00 AM, even if he is feels tired before that time. The time in bed gradually increases by 15 minutes as long as the sleep efficiency is greater than 85%. This patient has implemented good sleep hygiene techniques (avoiding daytime napping, limiting caffeine and alcohol, keeping the bedroom quiet and dark, and avoiding the use of electronic devices in bed) without achieving significant benefit. Sleep restriction should be initiated next in this patient.

Diphenhydramine, an over-the-counter sedating antihistamine, is commonly used to treat insomnia. It induces sedation; however, its resultant anticholinergic side effects, daytime somnolence, and cognitive impairment limit its overall safety and benefit. In most patients, nonpharmacologic interventions are preferred for treatment of insomnia, particularly chronic insomnia. If pharmacologic therapy is needed, diphenhydramine is not generally recommended due to its significant side effect profile.

In general, a regular exercise regimen can help improve sleep. However, vigorous exercise before bedtime should be avoided because it may impair the ability to fall asleep.

Zolpidem, a short-acting nonbenzodiazepine selective γ-aminobutyric acid (GABA) agonist, is prescribed for the treatment of short-term or situational insomnia. It may have fewer side effects than older prescription sleep aids, but cognitive impairment, rebound insomnia, dependency, sedation, and, rarely, sleep driving, eating, and walking have been reported. In this patient, sleep restriction should be tried before pharmacologic therapy.

KEY POINT

- In patients with insomnia in whom sleep hygiene techniques are ineffective, sleep restriction may be beneficial; sleep restriction limits and then gradually increases the time in bed for sleep.

Bibliography
Masters PA. In the clinic. Insomnia. Ann Intern Med. 2014 Oct 7;161:ITC1-15. [PMID: 25285559]

Item 152   Answer: A

Educational Objective: Diagnose allergic conjunctivitis.

This patient most likely has allergic conjunctivitis, which typically presents with eye redness, itching, and tearing, often in conjunction with allergy symptoms following allergen exposure. Eye findings are typically bilateral, and chemosis (conjunctival edema) and a watery, nonpurulent discharge are often seen on examination. Treatment of allergic conjunctivitis includes allergen avoidance and other nonpharmacologic interventions, such as cool topical compresses and artificial tears. Discontinuing contact lens use is also usually recommended for symptomatic patients. Pharmacologic treatment may include over-the-counter antihistamine/vasoconstrictor eye drops, oral antihistamines, or topical antihistamines (olopatadine ophthalmic 0.1%, ketotifen ophthalmic).

Bacterial conjunctivitis tends to be an acute process, commonly occurring in one eye. Patients frequently report redness, itching, and a mucopurulent discharge that causes crusting in the morning but also persists during the day. Bacterial conjunctivitis is commonly caused by infection with *Staphylococcus aureus*, *Streptococcus pneumoniae*, *Haemophilus influenzae*, or *Moraxella catarrhalis*. It tends to be very contagious, and treatment is topical antibiotics. This patient's watery eye discharge is not consistent with bacterial conjunctivitis.

Blepharitis is a diffuse inflammation of the sebaceous glands or lash follicles of the eyelids. Common causes are *S. aureus* infection, rosacea, and seborrheic dermatitis. This patient does not have evidence of seborrheic dermatitis, which, if present, would predispose her to blepharitis.

Viral conjunctivitis is usually an acute process associated with antecedent upper respiratory tract infection. It is commonly caused by one of several types of adenovirus and is often seen following exposure to infected persons. One eye is frequently involved, although the other eye may become involved following the first. Symptoms include itching, foreign body sensation, and a watery or mucoid discharge with crusting of the eyelids following sleep. Treatment is supportive, including cold compresses and artificial tears. This patient's symptoms and clinical course make viral conjunctivitis less likely.

KEY POINT

- Allergic conjunctivitis, which occurs following exposure to an allergen, is characterized by bilateral eye redness, chemosis, itching, and tearing.

Bibliography
Bal SK, Hollingworth GR. Red eye. BMJ. 2005 Aug 20;331(7514):438. [PMID: 16110072]

Item 153   Answer: A

Educational Objective: Prevent stroke with statin therapy following a transient ischemic attack.

High-intensity statin therapy (atorvastatin, 40-80 mg/d; rosuvastatin, 20-40 mg/d) is appropriate in this patient who experienced a transient ischemic attack, a clinical manifestation of atherosclerotic cardiovascular disease (ASCVD). In addition to aspirin and treatment of other cardiovascular risk factors (hypertension, diabetes mellitus, smoking), statin therapy should be initiated for its well-established benefits in treating blood cholesterol levels to reduce future cardiovascular events. Even with concomitant hypertriglyceridemia, high-intensity statin therapy is still the primary treatment for patients with clinical ASCVD, unless patients have risk factors for statin-related adverse effects.

Moderate-intensity statin therapy (atorvastatin, 10-20 mg/d; simvastatin, 20-40 mg/d; fluvastatin, 40 mg twice daily; lovastatin, 40 mg/d; pitavastatin, 2-4 mg/d; pravastatin, 40-80 mg/d; rosuvastatin, 5-10 mg/d) is not the first choice for patients with clinical ASCVD due to the superior benefits of high-intensity statin therapy in this population. If the patient had risk factors for statin-related adverse effects, such as age older than 75 years or kidney or hepatic dysfunction, moderate-intensity statin therapy is an appropriate second-line treatment.

Fibrates are effective in treating hypertriglyceridemia; however, fibrate monotherapy, such as with fenofibrate, is not an acceptable initial choice for secondary prevention in patients with clinical ASCVD. Although treatment of hyperlipidemia no longer focuses on a specific LDL cholesterol target, the primary goal of treatment remains lowering LDL cholesterol, and statins have been shown to be effective at reducing LDL cholesterol levels and recurrent cardiovascular events. Only if triglyceride levels exceed 500 mg/dL (5.65 mmol/L) or the patient has a history of hypertriglyceridemia-induced pancreatitis should fibrate therapy be considered.

Studies have demonstrated that there is no additional ASCVD risk reduction with the use of combination therapy (statin plus nonstatin drugs). Nonstatin medications also have significant potential to cause adverse effects. Therefore, combination therapy is reserved for those with inadequate response or poor tolerance to statin therapy.

KEY POINT

- High-intensity statin therapy is indicated for secondary prevention in patients with clinical atherosclerotic cardiovascular disease.

Bibliography

Stone NJ, Robinson JG, Lichtenstein AH, et al; American College of Cardiology/American Heart Association Task Force on Practice Guidelines. 2013 ACC/AHA guideline on the treatment of blood cholesterol to reduce atherosclerotic cardiovascular risk in adults: a report of the American College of Cardiology/American Heart Association Task Force on Practice Guidelines. Circulation. 2014 Jun 24;129(25 Suppl 2): S1-45. Erratum in: Circulation. 2014 Jun 24;129(25 Suppl 2):S46-8. [PMID: 24222016]

Item 154   Answer: A

Educational Objective: Treat a patient at high risk for group A streptococcal pharyngitis.

This patient is at high risk for group A streptococcal (GAS) pharyngitis and should be treated with penicillin. Pharyngitis most frequently has viral causes (up to 80% of cases). However, GAS pharyngitis, which accounts for approximately 15% of cases, should be detected to prevent potentially serious complications, such as acute rheumatic fever. Diagnosis and treatment of patients with GAS pharyngitis is aided by the four-point Centor criteria: (1) fever, (2) absence of cough, (3) tonsillar exudates, and (4) tender anterior cervical lymphadenopathy. Patients who meet the four criteria, such as this one, are at highest risk and can be treated empirically with antibiotics. Penicillin is the first-line agent; a macrolide antibiotic is indicated for penicillin-allergic patients.

Rapid streptococcal antigen test or GAS throat culture is indicated to confirm the diagnosis in patients who meet two or three Centor criteria. Rapid antigen detection testing for GAS has a specificity of greater than 95% and a sensitivity of 85% to 95%. Antibiotics should be initiated only if either test is positive.

If one Centor criterion is present, reassurance and symptomatic treatment is recommended.

KEY POINT

- A patient at high risk for group A streptococcal pharyngitis based on the Centor criteria should be treated with empiric antibiotics.

Bibliography

Weber R. Pharyngitis. Prim Care. 2014 Mar;41:91-8. [PMID: 24439883]

Item 155   Answer: B

Educational Objective: Manage a patient's request to withdraw life-prolonging treatment.

This patient's request for implantable cardioverter-defibrillator (ICD) deactivation should be carried out. Patients have the right to refuse or request the withdrawal of any treatment, even those that are life prolonging (that is, death inevitably follows withdrawal of the treatment). In these circumstances, the physician's duty is to understand the reasons for the request and to ensure that the request is informed. Patients who have ICDs may experience uncomfortable shocks during the dying process, and in order to avoid shocks, some patients request ICD deactivation. This patient understands the consequences of ICD deactivation, and her request should be fulfilled. In caring for a patient at the end of life, withdrawing a treatment that is perceived by the patient as burdensome or may cause discomfort (in this case, ICD shocks) is consistent with comfort care.

No treatment has unique moral status; that is, there is no treatment that must always be administered or must be continued once started. Because this patient has demonstrated clear and consistent decision-making capacity, it is unethical to refuse to comply with her wishes and continue the ICD.

It is ethically and legally permissible for physicians to withhold or withdraw treatments from patients who no longer want them without need for a psychiatric evaluation, provided the patient demonstrates clear and consistent decision-making capacity. In addition, a psychiatric evaluation cannot determine a patient's competence, as that is a legal determination made in a court of law.

It is illegal to invoke this patient's power of attorney and advance directive, as these only go into effect at a time when the patient herself is unable to make her own decisions. As long as the patient is awake and demonstrates decision-making capacity, her decisions override those of her power of attorney and those outlined in her advanced directive.

KEY POINT

- Patients with intact decision-making capacity have the right to request the withdrawal of any treatment, even those that are life prolonging.

Bibliography

Lampert R, Hayes DL, Annas GJ, et al; American College of Cardiology; American Geriatrics Society; American Academy of Hospice and Palliative Medicine; American Heart Association; European Heart Rhythm Association; Hospice and Palliative Nurses Association. HRS expert consensus statement on the management of cardiovascular implantable electronic devices (CIEDs) in patients nearing end of life or requesting withdrawal of therapy. Heart Rhythm. 2010 Jul;7(7):1008-26. [PMID: 20471915]

Item 156   Answer: B

Educational Objective: Administer the tetanus, diphtheria, and acellular pertussis vaccine during pregnancy.

This pregnant patient should receive the tetanus, diphtheria, and acellular pertussis (Tdap) vaccine now. To decrease the burden of pertussis in infants (who are at the greatest risk for the disease), the Advisory Committee on Immunization Practices (ACIP) recommends that pregnant women receive a single dose of the Tdap vaccine during each pregnancy, regardless of when they last received either the tetanus and diphtheria (Td) or Tdap vaccine. Because maternal immunity wanes over time, administering the Tdap vaccine between 27 and 36 weeks' gestation is thought to provide optimal protection against pertussis for the infant throughout the newborn period, during which time the child is solely dependent upon maternal antibodies for protection, by boosting the mother's antibody levels. The Td and Tdap vaccines do not contain live elements and are considered safe to administer to pregnant women, as there is no evidence to suggest an increased rate of adverse events in this population.

Although the Tdap vaccine can be given at any point during a woman's pregnancy, administering the vaccine between 27 and 36 weeks' gestation is thought to confer maximal antibody protection to newborn infants. It is not advisable to wait until after 36 weeks of pregnancy.

The Td vaccine does not provide protection against pertussis and therefore should not be given either now or after 36 weeks' gestation.

Withholding vaccination against tetanus, diphtheria, and acellular pertussis during pregnancy is inappropriate. Although this patient received the Tdap vaccine during her first pregnancy, that vaccination is unlikely to provide sufficient protection for her second child at the time of delivery, as antibody levels wane significantly during the first year after vaccination.

KEY POINT

- Pregnant women should receive a single dose of the tetanus, diphtheria, and acellular pertussis (Tdap) vaccine between 27 and 36 weeks' gestation during each pregnancy, regardless of when they last received either the tetanus and diphtheria (Td) or Tdap vaccine.

Bibliography

Centers for Disease Control and Prevention (CDC). Updated recommendations for use of tetanus toxoid, reduced diphtheria toxoid, and acellular pertussis vaccine (Tdap) in pregnant women–Advisory Committee on Immunization Practices (ACIP), 2012. MMWR Morb Mortal Wkly Rep. 2013 Feb 22;62(7):131-5. [PMID: 23425962]

Item 157   Answer: D

Educational Objective: Evaluate a patient with systemic exertion intolerance disease (formerly known as chronic fatigue syndrome).

No further testing is indicated in this patient who meets the clinical criteria for systemic exertion intolerance disease (SEID), previously termed chronic fatigue syndrome. He has fatigue that has persisted for more than 6 months that is not due to exertion and is not relieved by adequate sleep. He also experiences unrefreshing sleep, muscle pain, joint pain without synovitis, headaches, and recurring sore throat.

There is no specific objective laboratory test to diagnose SEID, and since the presenting symptoms are nonspecific, it remains a diagnosis of exclusion. Recommended value-based screening tests include complete blood count, glucose levels, and thyroid function tests. If indicated by the history and physical examination, electrolytes, calcium level, serum creatinine level, hepatic enzyme levels, liver chemistry tests, and antinuclear antibody test may be performed. This patient has undergone evaluation for underlying medical conditions in which fatigue is a common symptom, and all test results were normal. At present, no further testing is indicated, and attention should be directed to management with either graded exercise or cognitive-behavioral therapy.

Although Lyme disease and Epstein-Barr virus have been implicated in the development of SEID, no single infectious cause has been definitively linked. An Epstein-Barr virus titer would not be indicated, as this test is nondiagnostic and not value based. Additionally, antiviral treatment has been shown to be ineffective. Lyme disease testing is also unwarranted because this patient's nonspecific symptoms are not consistent with Lyme disease. Additionally, the pretest probability of Lyme disease is low, and testing for Lyme antibodies is not recommended by the American College of Rheumatology.

Repeat HIV testing in this patient would be low value care. He had a recent negative HIV test and has not had high-risk exposure since that time.

KEY POINT

- There is no specific objective laboratory test to diagnose systemic exertion intolerance disease (formerly known as chronic fatigue syndrome); recommended value-based tests to rule out this disease include complete blood count, glucose level, and thyroid function tests.

Bibliography
Yancey JR, Thomas SM. Chronic fatigue syndrome: diagnosis and treatment. Am Fam Physician. 2012 Oct 15;86(8):741-6. [PMID: 23062157]

Item 158 Answer: C
Educational Objective: Diagnose otosclerosis as a cause of conductive hearing loss.

This patient most likely has otosclerosis, a form of conductive hearing loss. Otosclerosis is caused by abnormal bone hardening and growth in the middle ear that disrupts sound transmission from the middle ear to the inner ear. Diagnostic clues in this patient include gradual onset, difficulty hearing low-pitched sounds, and no history of exposure to loud noises. When the Weber test is performed on this patient, the tuning fork is heard more loudly on the left, indicative of conductive hearing loss in the left ear. Treatment of otosclerosis is amplification or surgical stapedectomy, in which a portion of the stapes is removed and replaced with a prosthesis to improve conductive hearing.

Drug-induced hearing loss, a form of sensorineural hearing loss, can be caused by ototoxic medications, including aminoglycosides, chemotherapeutic agents, aspirin, antimalarial agents, and loop diuretics. The dose of aspirin this patient is taking would not be high enough to cause ototoxicity.

Meniere disease is classically a triad of sensorineural hearing loss, tinnitus, and vertigo. This patient does not have either tinnitus or vertigo.

Presbycusis, another form of sensorineural hearing loss, is age-related hearing loss and is typically symmetric and affecting high frequencies. Although this patient is older, his hearing loss is asymmetric and low frequency, which is less consistent with presbycusis.

KEY POINT

- Otosclerosis is a form of conductive hearing loss characterized by gradual onset, difficulty hearing low-pitched sounds, and no history of exposure to loud noises.

Bibliography
Walling AD, Dickson GM. Hearing loss in older adults. Am Fam Physician. 2012 Jun 15;85(12):1150-6. [PMID: 22962895]

Item 159 Answer: A
Educational Objective: Treat a patient with medically complicated obesity.

This patient with medically complicated obesity should be referred for bariatric surgery. He has multiple obesity-associated comorbidities including hypertension, inadequately controlled type 2 diabetes mellitus, obstructive sleep apnea, and bilateral knee osteoarthritis. In light of his previously unsuccessful weight loss attempts with diet and pharmacologic agents, he should be referred for bariatric surgery. Referral for bariatric surgery should be considered in all patients with a BMI of 40 or higher and in patients with a BMI of 35 or higher with obesity-related comorbid conditions, such as this patient. The goal of bariatric surgery is weight loss that prevents and treats obesity-associated complications. Candidates should be evaluated by a multidisciplinary team with medical, surgical, nutritional, and psychiatric expertise.

The evidence for the use of hypnosis for weight loss in obese patients is unclear.

Lorcaserin, a brain serotonin 2C receptor agonist, acts as an appetite suppressant. It should be used with caution in patients taking medications that increase serotonin levels, such as paroxetine. Therefore, lorcaserin should be avoided in this patient. Additionally, he has already tried a different pharmacologic agent (orlistat) without sustained weight loss.

Diet for weight loss is one of the key components of obesity treatment. There are many diets available, from high-protein, high-fat diets to very-low-fat diets. They differ in their palatability and ability to suppress appetite in individual patients; however, when effective, these diets achieve the same outcome: calorie deficits that result in weight loss. However, given this patient's failure to achieve sustained weight loss in the past with multiple dietary interventions, another dieting attempt in this patient will likely be unsuccessful. He should continue dietary, lifestyle (physical activity), and behavioral therapy measures following bariatric surgery.

KEY POINT

- Referral for bariatric surgery should be considered in all patients with a BMI of 40 or higher and in patients with a BMI of 35 or higher with obesity-related comorbid conditions.

Bibliography
Jensen MD, Ryan DH, Apovian CM, et al; American College of Cardiology/ American Heart Association Task Force on Practice Guidelines; Obesity Society. 2013 AHA/ACC/TOS guideline for the management of overweight and obesity in adults: a report of the American College of Cardiology/American Heart Association Task Force on Practice Guidelines and The Obesity Society. J Am Coll Cardiol. 2014 Jul 1;

63(25 Pt B):2985-3023. Erratum in: J Am Coll Cardiol. 2014 Jul 1;63(25 Pt B):3029-3030. [PMID: 24239920]

Item 160   Answer: B

Educational Objective: Manage polypharmacy in an older patient.

This older patient's clinical findings are most likely the result of adverse medication effects related to polypharmacy, and her drug regimen requires adjustment. She has significant medical comorbidities and is taking numerous drugs. Administration of multiple medications increases the risk for inappropriate use, drug-drug interactions, adverse reactions, poor adherence, and medication errors. This patient is taking two anticholinergic agents (oxybutynin for urinary incontinence and the over-the-counter antihistamine loratadine). The American Geriatrics Society Beers Criteria recommend against the use of anticholinergic agents in older patients because they can cause confusion, urinary retention, constipation, and dry mouth. She is also on the proton pump inhibitor omeprazole without an apparent indication for treatment. In addition, the risk-to-benefit ratio of using a lipid-lowering agent to confer long-term benefits must be reassessed in very elderly adults. Prescriptions for statins are frequently carried over from previous years, but statin use results in additional cost, extra pills, and increased risk for drug-drug interactions. Lastly, parameters for blood pressure control are less stringent in older adults, and, in this patient, antihypertensive agents should be reassessed, as her hypertension is overtreated. Ongoing review of the indications, risks, benefits, and dosing of all drugs in older patients is recommended.

This patient has a history of mild chronic kidney disease; however, with normal volume status, normal electrolytes, and a minimal change in her serum creatinine level, she does not have evidence of significant worsening of her kidney function. This would make acute kidney injury an unlikely cause of her current clinical findings.

Infections are a frequent cause of systemic symptoms, including weakness, dizziness, anorexia, and altered mental status in older patients, with pneumonia and urinary tract infection being the most common types. However, this patient has no clinical findings consistent with pneumonia given her normal oxygenation, leukocyte count, and chest radiograph, or suggestion of urinary tract infection with a normal urinalysis. Therefore, the absence of evidence of infection makes this an unlikely cause of her current clinical findings.

KEY POINT

- Administration of multiple medications, especially in older patients, increases the risk for inappropriate use, drug-drug interactions, adverse reactions, and medication errors.

Bibliography

Maher RL, Hanlon J, Hajjar ER. Clinical consequences of polypharmacy in elderly. Expert Opin Drug Saf. 2014;13(1):57-65. [PMID: 24073682]

Item 161   Answer: B

Educational Objective: Manage sexual side effects in a patient taking a selective serotonin reuptake inhibitor.

The norepinephrine and dopamine reuptake inhibitor bupropion is the most appropriate alternative treatment recommendation for this patient with depression. The most widely prescribed antidepressant drugs are selective serotonin reuptake inhibitors (SSRIs), which have excellent safety profiles compared with tricyclic antidepressant drugs. She has responded well to treatment with the SSRI citalopram, with improved clinical symptoms and objective scoring on the PHQ-9. However, sexual side effects are common with SSRIs. Bupropion is an appropriate alternative agent for an overweight patient experiencing sexual side effects with an SSRI because it is an effective antidepressant, has a low rate of sexual side effects, and is not associated with weight gain.

Tricyclic antidepressants are also effective antidepressant agents but are associated with both sexual side effects and weight gain; therefore, amitriptyline would not be a good alternative treatment choice for this patient.

Buspirone is approved for the treatment of anxiety disorders, but not depression. Although there is some evidence suggesting that buspirone, when added to SSRI treatment for depression, may augment the antidepressant effect and counter sexual side effects caused by SSRIs, it would not be an appropriate substitution as a single agent in this patient.

Although mirtazapine is associated with a low rate of sexual side effects, this agent stimulates appetite and is associated with weight gain. Mirtazapine is an appropriate antidepressant for patients with anorexia and weight loss due to depression.

KEY POINT

- The norepinephrine and dopamine reuptake inhibitor bupropion is an appropriate alternative antidepressant for patients who experience sexual side effects from selective serotonin reuptake inhibitor therapy.

Bibliography

Bostwick JM. A generalist's guide to treating patients with depression with an emphasis on using side effects to tailor antidepressant therapy. Mayo Clin Proc. 2010 Jun;85(6):538-50. [PMID: 20431115]

Item 162   Answer: D

Educational Objective: Evaluate a study using number needed to treat.

The number needed to treat (NNT) is 10. Numbers needed are estimates of the number of patients who must receive an intervention to cause one patient to experience the outcome being studied; if beneficial, it is termed the NNT, and if detrimental, the number needed to harm (NNH). Numbers needed are useful indicators of the clinical impact of an intervention because they provide a sense of magnitude expected from the intervention. If available, NNT and NNH for the same intervention provide a convenient method for evaluating the benefits and harms of an intervention, which is immensely valuable for high value care decision making.

The NNT is calculated by taking the reciprocal of the absolute risk reduction (ARR). In this study, the risk of developing prostate cancer in the control (placebo) group can be calculated as:

$$\text{Absolute risk (AR)} = \text{(patients with event in group)} / \text{(total patients in group)}$$
$$AR = 300/(300 + 700) = 300/1000 = 0.30$$

The risk of developing prostate cancer in the group treated with finasteride can be calculated as:

$$AR = 200/(200 + 800) = 200/1000 = 0.20$$

The ARR is the difference in rates of events between the treatment group and control group, which is 0.10 for this study. The NNT is therefore 1/0.10, or 10. This indicates that 10 patients would need to be treated with finasteride for 7 years to prevent one case of prostate cancer.

KEY POINT

- The number needed to treat, which is the number of patients required to receive an intervention in order for one patient to benefit from it, is the reciprocal of the absolute risk reduction.

Bibliography
Cook RJ, Sackett DL. The number needed to treat: a clinically useful measure of treatment effect. BMJ. 1995;310(6977):452-4. Erratum in: BMJ 1995;310(6986):1056. [PMID: 7873954]

Item 163   Answer: A
Educational Objective: Evaluate perioperative cardiovascular risk in a patient with cardiac risk factors but good functional capacity.

For this patient with known coronary artery disease (CAD) but normal cardiac function scheduled for intermediate-risk surgery (defined as a risk of cardiac death or nonfatal myocardial infarction of 1%-5%), electrocardiography is indicated according to the current American College of Cardiology/American Heart Association (ACC/AHA) guideline. Due to the patient's CAD, the baseline electrocardiogram may be abnormal but probably would not alter preoperative management. Instead, the electrocardiogram guides postoperative medication management by identifying conduction disturbances (such as QT-interval prolongation) and is useful as a comparison should the patient develop postoperative cardiac symptoms.

The ACC/AHA guideline does not support noninvasive coronary evaluation (either pharmacologic or exercise stress testing) in this patient. Regardless of cardiac risk factors, no further coronary evaluation is advised for patients with an exercise capacity greater than or equal to 4 metabolic equivalents (METs), and climbing a flight of stairs meets that criterion. In patients with an exercise capacity less than 4 METs, coronary evaluation is indicated if the estimated risk of perioperative major adverse cardiac events is greater than or equal to 1%. Due to its superior prognostic value, exercise testing is preferred to pharmacologic stress testing unless contraindicated by patient factors.

A resting echocardiogram only provides diagnostic information about structural heart disease and is not an appropriate form of noninvasive coronary evaluation. Therefore, preoperative echocardiography is not indicated in this patient without evidence of significant structural heart disease.

KEY POINT

- In patients with cardiac risk factors undergoing elevated-risk procedures, preoperative coronary evaluation is not required if the patient has a good functional capacity ($\geq$4 metabolic equivalents).

Bibliography
Fleisher LA, Fleischmann KE, Auerbach AD, et al; American College of Cardiology; American Heart Association. 2014 ACC/AHA guideline on perioperative cardiovascular evaluation and management of patients undergoing noncardiac surgery: a report of the American College of Cardiology/American Heart Association Task Force on practice guidelines. J Am Coll Cardiol. 2014 Dec 9;64(22):e77-137. [PMID: 25091544]

Item 164   Answer: B
Educational Objective: Treat underlying depression in a patient with medically unexplained symptoms.

The most appropriate treatment for this patient with medically unexplained symptoms (MUS) is citalopram. This patient has a 3-year history of multiple nonspecific symptoms with an extensive negative evaluation, consistent with the presentation of MUS. Patients with MUS frequently have primary or secondary underlying depression, which may be overlooked during the unsuccessful quest for a unifying or previously undiagnosed organic illness. This patient meets the criteria for depression; he has depressed mood and affect for more than 6 months accompanied by hypersomnia and hopelessness. Antidepressant therapy, such as with the selective serotonin reuptake inhibitor (SSRI) citalopram, is the most appropriate treatment at this time. A systematic review of 94 randomized controlled trials found improvement in symptoms in patients with MUS who were treated with antidepressants.

Although the patient experiences anxiety at night and is unable to sleep well, alprazolam, a benzodiazepine, is a poor choice for chronic management of his anxiety. Alprazolam is associated with sedation, impaired cognition, and a high risk of dependence. This patient's primary symptoms of depression and anxiety will most likely respond to an SSRI.

Lithium would be appropriate if the patient had symptoms consistent with bipolar disorder. This patient has no history of bipolar disorder, and he is not manifesting any symptoms of mania.

Methylphenidate is a central nervous system stimulant that is used in the treatment of attention-deficit/hyperactivity disorder and narcolepsy. It may be used off label for the treatment of depression in adults who are terminally ill or receiving palliative care. First-line treatment of this patient with underlying depression is an SSRI.

KEY POINT

- Antidepressant therapy has been found to improve symptoms in patients with medically unexplained symptoms and primary or secondary underlying depression.

Bibliography

Edwards TM, Stern A, Clarke DD, Ivbijaro G, Kasney LM. The treatment of patients with medically unexplained symptoms in primary care: a review of the literature. Ment Health Fam Med. 2010 Dec;7(4):209-21. [PMID: 22477945]

Item 165   Answer: C
Educational Objective: Diagnose orbital cellulitis.

This patient has orbital cellulitis, which is inflammation of the structures of the orbit, including the extraocular muscles and orbital fat. Orbital cellulitis often results from a contiguous dental or sinus infection, as was likely present in this patient. Clinical characteristics of orbital cellulitis include eyelid swelling, ophthalmoplegia, pain with eye movement, and occasionally proptosis. Because it is a deep infection and involves critical structures, rapid diagnosis and treatment are necessary to preserve vision and prevent extension to central nervous system structures. CT is used to evaluate the extent of infection and to exclude abscess, which may need surgical drainage. This patient requires hospitalization and intravenous antibiotics.

Blepharitis is inflammation of the sebaceous glands or lash follicles of the eyelid, which can progress to conjunctivitis or keratitis. It usually presents with findings limited to the eyelid, although patients may complain of a gritty, burning sensation in the eye. Blepharitis is not associated with the key findings of orbital cellulitis.

Endophthalmitis is inflammation of the aqueous and vitreous humors. Symptoms may include visual loss, photophobia, and ocular pain and discharge. It is usually caused by bacterial or fungal infection following surgery, especially for cataracts. Other causes are globe trauma and foreign bodies.

Preseptal cellulitis is inflammation that is limited to the areas of the eyelids and facial tissues that are anterior to the orbital septum. It is more common than orbital cellulitis in adults and can usually be differentiated from orbital cellulitis by pain localized to the anterior tissues without ophthalmoplegia, pain with eye movement, or proptosis, which this patient has. Therefore, it is a less likely diagnosis in this patient.

KEY POINT

- Orbital cellulitis often occurs in the setting of recent dental or sinus infection; characteristic findings include eyelid swelling, ophthalmoplegia, pain with eye movement, and occasionally proptosis.

Bibliography

Gelston CD. Common eye emergencies. Am Fam Physician. 2013 Oct 15;88(8):515-9. [PMID: 24364572]

Item 166   Answer: A
Educational Objective: Evaluate anovulatory bleeding in a premenopausal woman.

The most appropriate next step for this woman with intermittent heavy vaginal bleeding is referral for endometrial biopsy. Her bleeding is characteristic of an anovulatory pattern based on the unpredictable occurrence of bleeding of variable flow and duration. In women with prolonged anovulation, there is loss of normal hormonal flux with exposure to unopposed estrogen without the normal endometrial protective effect of progesterone. This increases the risk for endometrial hyperplasia and endometrial malignancy. Additional risk factors for endometrial cancer in premenopausal women include obesity, nulliparity, age 35 years or older, diabetes mellitus, family history of colon cancer, infertility, and treatment with tamoxifen. In women younger than 35 years of age with anovulatory bleeding and no other risk factors for endometrial cancer, hormonal therapy for anovulation is appropriate. However, in women younger than 35 years of age with risk factors, or any patient with anovulatory bleeding 35 years of age or older, endometrial biopsy should be performed to exclude significant endometrial pathology. Because this patient is 40 years of age and has an additional risk factor for endometrial cancer (nulliparity), endometrial biopsy is the most appropriate next step in management.

A follicle-stimulating hormone (FSH) level can be used to evaluate ovarian dysfunction, but levels vary depending on menstrual phase, age, medications, and hormonal disorders. FSH level can be used to confirm menopausal status if a woman has been amenorrheic for longer than 12 months. However, a single FSH level can be misleading during perimenopause because levels may vary. In this patient, who is premenopausal, measurement of the FSH level is of limited use.

In a woman of reproductive age with abnormal vaginal bleeding, the first test to be performed is always a urine pregnancy test, which is a sensitive qualitative measure of β-human chorionic gonadotropin level and was already obtained in this patient. There is no further gain from obtaining a serum β-human chorionic gonadotropin level, which is a quantitative measure but adds no further value in this diagnostic evaluation.

Transvaginal ultrasonography may have a role in evaluation of postmenopausal bleeding to assess for endometrial thickness, but it is not useful in assessing bleeding in premenopausal women due to significant variations in endometrial thickness caused by hormonal fluctuation. It is therefore not used routinely for evaluation of premenopausal bleeding unless a structural uterine abnormality that may be contributing to bleeding is suspected.

KEY POINT

- In women with anovulatory bleeding with risk factors for endometrial cancer, endometrial biopsy should be performed to exclude significant endometrial pathology.

Bibliography

Sweet MG, Schmidt-Dalton TA, Weiss PM, et al. Evaluation and management of abnormal uterine bleeding in premenopausal women. Am Fam Physician. 2012 Jan 1;85(1):35-43. [PMID: 22230306]

Item 167   Answer: D

Educational Objective: Recognize the indications for imaging studies in the diagnosis of neck pain.

Symptomatic care is indicated in this patient. Most patients with neck pain do not require diagnostic imaging. Imaging is indicated for neck pain following trauma or if a structural abnormality, such as a compression fracture, is suspected. Imaging may also be indicated in patients who have weakness or clinical evidence of spinal cord involvement as a cause of neck pain. Additionally, imaging may be useful in those with a clinical presentation suggestive of malignancy or infection as a cause of neck pain. This patient has no history of trauma, weakness, or findings suggestive of a spinal cause of her pain. Despite her history of breast neoplasm, she has not had evidence of recurrence and has no other symptoms or findings suggestive of metastatic disease (such as point tenderness to palpation over the spine). Her otherwise normal presentation does not support a systemic process such as infection. Therefore, imaging in this patient would not be expected to be of benefit. Instead, the focus should be on symptomatic treatment of her neck pain using usual therapeutic modalities including mobilization, exercise, and analgesic agents.

CT myelography involves injection of nonionic water-soluble contrast agents into the spinal canal followed by a CT scan. Because of the effectiveness of other imaging modalities, myelography is usually limited to specific situations in which it may provide more helpful information than other studies, such as multilevel disk abnormalities or radiculopathies, fragmented disks, and patients who have had spinal surgery. This patient has no clear indication for this form of imaging.

MRI of the cervical spine best delineates the spinal cord and nerve roots, intervertebral disks, surrounding soft tissue, ligamentous structures, and vertebral arteries, but it is not indicated in this patient who has no neurologic signs or findings suggestive of abnormalities of these structures.

Plain radiography of the cervical spine is useful in evaluating the bony structures of the spine and is therefore helpful in excluding fracture in patients with trauma or who are suspected of having other bony abnormalities, such as compression fractures, metastatic disease, or infection affecting

the spine. However, this patient has no history suggestive of an abnormality likely to be detected with plain radiography.

KEY POINT

- Most patients with neck pain do not require diagnostic imaging.

Bibliography

Cohen SP. Epidemiology, diagnosis, and treatment of neck pain. Mayo Clin Proc. 2015 Feb;90(2):284-99. [PMID: 25659245]

Item 168   Answer: B

Educational Objective: Manage colorectal cancer screening in an average-risk patient.

The most appropriate screening strategy for this patient is yearly fecal immunochemical testing (FIT). Annual stool testing for occult blood using either high-sensitivity guaiac fecal occult blood testing (gFOBT) or FIT is an acceptable colon cancer screening strategy in average-risk patients. Randomized controlled trials have shown statistically significant reductions in colorectal cancer incidence (17%-20%) and mortality (15%-33%) with regular gFOBT screening. Limitations of gFOBT screening include low sensitivity for advanced adenomas (11%-41%), diet and medication interactions that may produce false-positive or false-negative results, and the need for appropriate diagnostic follow-up (that is, colonoscopy) if test results are positive to achieve maximum benefit. FIT uses specific antibodies to detect globin in the stool and is generally considered to be a more sensitive study than guaiac-based testing. In cross-sectional studies, FIT sensitivity has ranged from 60% to 85% for colorectal cancer and 25% to 50% for advanced adenomas. Pretest dietary restrictions are not necessary. As with gFOBT, FIT requires appropriate diagnostic follow-up for positive results.

The U.S. Preventive Services Task Force (USPSTF) recommends screening all adults aged 50 to 75 years for colorectal cancer with one of several different methods: high-sensitivity fecal occult blood testing (gFOBT or FIT) every year, flexible sigmoidoscopy every 5 years, combined flexible sigmoidoscopy every 5 years with high-sensitivity fecal occult blood testing every 3 years, or colonoscopy every 10 years. The American Cancer Society (ACS), U.S. Multi-Society Task Force on Colorectal Cancer, and American College of Radiology (ACR) colorectal cancer screening guideline includes additional screening options: CT colonography (every 5 years) and stool DNA testing (interval unknown). Since publication of the guideline, the ACS has recommended that stool DNA testing occur every 3 years. As these are newer tests with many areas of uncertainty, they are not currently recommended by the USPSTF. The ACS/U.S. Multi-Society Task Force/ACR guideline also recommends preference to cancer prevention tests (colonoscopy, flexible sigmoidoscopy, double contrast barium enema, or CT colonography) over cancer detection tests (gFOBT or FIT) when resources are available.

The USPSTF recommends flexible sigmoidoscopy every 5 years with gFOBT or FIT every 3 years, not yearly. Randomized controlled trials have consistently demonstrated a mortality benefit for distal, but not proximal, colorectal cancer of 30% to 50% with flexible sigmoidoscopy.

In patients at average risk, colonoscopy can be performed every 10 years. Observational studies have shown that colonoscopy provides significant mortality benefit for both distal and proximal colorectal cancer. Colonoscopy is the preferred test of the American College of Gastroenterology.

KEY POINT

- All adults aged 50 to 75 years should be screened for colorectal cancer using high-sensitivity fecal occult blood testing every year, flexible sigmoidoscopy every 5 years, combined flexible sigmoidoscopy every 5 years with high-sensitivity fecal occult blood testing every 3 years, or colonoscopy every 10 years.

Bibliography

Lieberman DA. Clinical practice. Screening for colorectal cancer. N Engl J Med. 2009 Sep 17;361(12):1179-87. [PMID: 19759380]

Index

A

NAME AND ADDRESS (Please complete.)

Last Name _____ First Name _____ Middle Initial

Address

Address cont.

City _____ State _____ ZIP Code

Country

Email address

B

Order Number

(Use the Order Number on your MKSAP materials packing slip.)

C

ACP ID Number

(Refer to packing slip in your MKSAP materials
for your ACP ID Number.)

ACP ®
American College of Physicians
Leading Internal Medicine, Improving Lives

**Medical
Knowledge
Self-Assessment
Program** ® **17**

TO EARN *AMA PRA CATEGORY 1 CREDITS* ™ YOU MUST:

1. Answer all questions.
2. Score a minimum of 50% correct.

==

TO EARN *FREE* INSTANTANEOUS *AMA PRA CATEGORY 1 CREDITS* ™ ONLINE:

1. Answer all of your questions.
2. Go to **mksap.acponline.org** and enter your ACP Online username and password to access an online answer sheet.
3. Enter your answers.
4. You can also enter your answers directly at **mksap.acponline.org** without first using this answer sheet.

To Submit Your Answer Sheet by Mail or FAX for a $15 Administrative Fee per Answer Sheet:

1. Answer all of your questions and calculate your score.
2. Complete boxes A–F.
3. Complete payment information.
4. Send the answer sheet and payment information to ACP, using the FAX number/address listed below.

COMPLETE FORM BELOW ONLY IF YOU SUBMIT BY MAIL OR FAX

Last Name _____ First Name _____ MI

Payment Information. Must remit in US funds, drawn on a US bank.

The processing fee for each paper answer sheet is $15.

☐ Check, made payable to ACP, enclosed

Charge to ☐ **VISA** ☐ **MasterCard** ☐ **AMERICAN EXPRESS** ☐ **DISCOVER**

Card Number _____

Expiration Date _____ / _____ Security code (3 or 4 digit #s) _____
　　　　　　　　MM　　　YY

Signature _____

Fax to: 215-351-2799

Mail to:
Member and Customer Service
American College of Physicians
190 N. Independence Mall West
Philadelphia, PA 19106-1572

1 Ⓐ Ⓑ Ⓒ Ⓓ Ⓔ
2 Ⓐ Ⓑ Ⓒ Ⓓ Ⓔ
3 Ⓐ Ⓑ Ⓒ Ⓓ Ⓔ
4 Ⓐ Ⓑ Ⓒ Ⓓ Ⓔ
5 Ⓐ Ⓑ Ⓒ Ⓓ Ⓔ

6 Ⓐ Ⓑ Ⓒ Ⓓ Ⓔ
7 Ⓐ Ⓑ Ⓒ Ⓓ Ⓔ
8 Ⓐ Ⓑ Ⓒ Ⓓ Ⓔ
9 Ⓐ Ⓑ Ⓒ Ⓓ Ⓔ
10 Ⓐ Ⓑ Ⓒ Ⓓ Ⓔ

11 Ⓐ Ⓑ Ⓒ Ⓓ Ⓔ
12 Ⓐ Ⓑ Ⓒ Ⓓ Ⓔ
13 Ⓐ Ⓑ Ⓒ Ⓓ Ⓔ
14 Ⓐ Ⓑ Ⓒ Ⓓ Ⓔ
15 Ⓐ Ⓑ Ⓒ Ⓓ Ⓔ

16 Ⓐ Ⓑ Ⓒ Ⓓ Ⓔ
17 Ⓐ Ⓑ Ⓒ Ⓓ Ⓔ
18 Ⓐ Ⓑ Ⓒ Ⓓ Ⓔ
19 Ⓐ Ⓑ Ⓒ Ⓓ Ⓔ
20 Ⓐ Ⓑ Ⓒ Ⓓ Ⓔ

21 Ⓐ Ⓑ Ⓒ Ⓓ Ⓔ
22 Ⓐ Ⓑ Ⓒ Ⓓ Ⓔ
23 Ⓐ Ⓑ Ⓒ Ⓓ Ⓔ
24 Ⓐ Ⓑ Ⓒ Ⓓ Ⓔ
25 Ⓐ Ⓑ Ⓒ Ⓓ Ⓔ

26 Ⓐ Ⓑ Ⓒ Ⓓ Ⓔ
27 Ⓐ Ⓑ Ⓒ Ⓓ Ⓔ
28 Ⓐ Ⓑ Ⓒ Ⓓ Ⓔ
29 Ⓐ Ⓑ Ⓒ Ⓓ Ⓔ
30 Ⓐ Ⓑ Ⓒ Ⓓ Ⓔ

31 Ⓐ Ⓑ Ⓒ Ⓓ Ⓔ
32 Ⓐ Ⓑ Ⓒ Ⓓ Ⓔ
33 Ⓐ Ⓑ Ⓒ Ⓓ Ⓔ
34 Ⓐ Ⓑ Ⓒ Ⓓ Ⓔ
35 Ⓐ Ⓑ Ⓒ Ⓓ Ⓔ

36 Ⓐ Ⓑ Ⓒ Ⓓ Ⓔ
37 Ⓐ Ⓑ Ⓒ Ⓓ Ⓔ
38 Ⓐ Ⓑ Ⓒ Ⓓ Ⓔ
39 Ⓐ Ⓑ Ⓒ Ⓓ Ⓔ
40 Ⓐ Ⓑ Ⓒ Ⓓ Ⓔ

41 Ⓐ Ⓑ Ⓒ Ⓓ Ⓔ
42 Ⓐ Ⓑ Ⓒ Ⓓ Ⓔ
43 Ⓐ Ⓑ Ⓒ Ⓓ Ⓔ
44 Ⓐ Ⓑ Ⓒ Ⓓ Ⓔ
45 Ⓐ Ⓑ Ⓒ Ⓓ Ⓔ

46 Ⓐ Ⓑ Ⓒ Ⓓ Ⓔ
47 Ⓐ Ⓑ Ⓒ Ⓓ Ⓔ
48 Ⓐ Ⓑ Ⓒ Ⓓ Ⓔ
49 Ⓐ Ⓑ Ⓒ Ⓓ Ⓔ
50 Ⓐ Ⓑ Ⓒ Ⓓ Ⓔ

51 Ⓐ Ⓑ Ⓒ Ⓓ Ⓔ
52 Ⓐ Ⓑ Ⓒ Ⓓ Ⓔ
53 Ⓐ Ⓑ Ⓒ Ⓓ Ⓔ
54 Ⓐ Ⓑ Ⓒ Ⓓ Ⓔ
55 Ⓐ Ⓑ Ⓒ Ⓓ Ⓔ

56 Ⓐ Ⓑ Ⓒ Ⓓ Ⓔ
57 Ⓐ Ⓑ Ⓒ Ⓓ Ⓔ
58 Ⓐ Ⓑ Ⓒ Ⓓ Ⓔ
59 Ⓐ Ⓑ Ⓒ Ⓓ Ⓔ
60 Ⓐ Ⓑ Ⓒ Ⓓ Ⓔ

61 Ⓐ Ⓑ Ⓒ Ⓓ Ⓔ
62 Ⓐ Ⓑ Ⓒ Ⓓ Ⓔ
63 Ⓐ Ⓑ Ⓒ Ⓓ Ⓔ
64 Ⓐ Ⓑ Ⓒ Ⓓ Ⓔ
65 Ⓐ Ⓑ Ⓒ Ⓓ Ⓔ

66 Ⓐ Ⓑ Ⓒ Ⓓ Ⓔ
67 Ⓐ Ⓑ Ⓒ Ⓓ Ⓔ
68 Ⓐ Ⓑ Ⓒ Ⓓ Ⓔ
69 Ⓐ Ⓑ Ⓒ Ⓓ Ⓔ
70 Ⓐ Ⓑ Ⓒ Ⓓ Ⓔ

71 Ⓐ Ⓑ Ⓒ Ⓓ Ⓔ
72 Ⓐ Ⓑ Ⓒ Ⓓ Ⓔ
73 Ⓐ Ⓑ Ⓒ Ⓓ Ⓔ
74 Ⓐ Ⓑ Ⓒ Ⓓ Ⓔ
75 Ⓐ Ⓑ Ⓒ Ⓓ Ⓔ

76 Ⓐ Ⓑ Ⓒ Ⓓ Ⓔ
77 Ⓐ Ⓑ Ⓒ Ⓓ Ⓔ
78 Ⓐ Ⓑ Ⓒ Ⓓ Ⓔ
79 Ⓐ Ⓑ Ⓒ Ⓓ Ⓔ
80 Ⓐ Ⓑ Ⓒ Ⓓ Ⓔ

81 Ⓐ Ⓑ Ⓒ Ⓓ Ⓔ
82 Ⓐ Ⓑ Ⓒ Ⓓ Ⓔ
83 Ⓐ Ⓑ Ⓒ Ⓓ Ⓔ
84 Ⓐ Ⓑ Ⓒ Ⓓ Ⓔ
85 Ⓐ Ⓑ Ⓒ Ⓓ Ⓔ

86 Ⓐ Ⓑ Ⓒ Ⓓ Ⓔ
87 Ⓐ Ⓑ Ⓒ Ⓓ Ⓔ
88 Ⓐ Ⓑ Ⓒ Ⓓ Ⓔ
89 Ⓐ Ⓑ Ⓒ Ⓓ Ⓔ
90 Ⓐ Ⓑ Ⓒ Ⓓ Ⓔ

91 Ⓐ Ⓑ Ⓒ Ⓓ Ⓔ
92 Ⓐ Ⓑ Ⓒ Ⓓ Ⓔ
93 Ⓐ Ⓑ Ⓒ Ⓓ Ⓔ
94 Ⓐ Ⓑ Ⓒ Ⓓ Ⓔ
95 Ⓐ Ⓑ Ⓒ Ⓓ Ⓔ

96 Ⓐ Ⓑ Ⓒ Ⓓ Ⓔ
97 Ⓐ Ⓑ Ⓒ Ⓓ Ⓔ
98 Ⓐ Ⓑ Ⓒ Ⓓ Ⓔ
99 Ⓐ Ⓑ Ⓒ Ⓓ Ⓔ
100 Ⓐ Ⓑ Ⓒ Ⓓ Ⓔ

101 Ⓐ Ⓑ Ⓒ Ⓓ Ⓔ
102 Ⓐ Ⓑ Ⓒ Ⓓ Ⓔ
103 Ⓐ Ⓑ Ⓒ Ⓓ Ⓔ
104 Ⓐ Ⓑ Ⓒ Ⓓ Ⓔ
105 Ⓐ Ⓑ Ⓒ Ⓓ Ⓔ

106 Ⓐ Ⓑ Ⓒ Ⓓ Ⓔ
107 Ⓐ Ⓑ Ⓒ Ⓓ Ⓔ
108 Ⓐ Ⓑ Ⓒ Ⓓ Ⓔ
109 Ⓐ Ⓑ Ⓒ Ⓓ Ⓔ
110 Ⓐ Ⓑ Ⓒ Ⓓ Ⓔ

111 Ⓐ Ⓑ Ⓒ Ⓓ Ⓔ
112 Ⓐ Ⓑ Ⓒ Ⓓ Ⓔ
113 Ⓐ Ⓑ Ⓒ Ⓓ Ⓔ
114 Ⓐ Ⓑ Ⓒ Ⓓ Ⓔ
115 Ⓐ Ⓑ Ⓒ Ⓓ Ⓔ

116 Ⓐ Ⓑ Ⓒ Ⓓ Ⓔ
117 Ⓐ Ⓑ Ⓒ Ⓓ Ⓔ
118 Ⓐ Ⓑ Ⓒ Ⓓ Ⓔ
119 Ⓐ Ⓑ Ⓒ Ⓓ Ⓔ
120 Ⓐ Ⓑ Ⓒ Ⓓ Ⓔ

121 Ⓐ Ⓑ Ⓒ Ⓓ Ⓔ
122 Ⓐ Ⓑ Ⓒ Ⓓ Ⓔ
123 Ⓐ Ⓑ Ⓒ Ⓓ Ⓔ
124 Ⓐ Ⓑ Ⓒ Ⓓ Ⓔ
125 Ⓐ Ⓑ Ⓒ Ⓓ Ⓔ

126 Ⓐ Ⓑ Ⓒ Ⓓ Ⓔ
127 Ⓐ Ⓑ Ⓒ Ⓓ Ⓔ
128 Ⓐ Ⓑ Ⓒ Ⓓ Ⓔ
129 Ⓐ Ⓑ Ⓒ Ⓓ Ⓔ
130 Ⓐ Ⓑ Ⓒ Ⓓ Ⓔ

131 Ⓐ Ⓑ Ⓒ Ⓓ Ⓔ
132 Ⓐ Ⓑ Ⓒ Ⓓ Ⓔ
133 Ⓐ Ⓑ Ⓒ Ⓓ Ⓔ
134 Ⓐ Ⓑ Ⓒ Ⓓ Ⓔ
135 Ⓐ Ⓑ Ⓒ Ⓓ Ⓔ

136 Ⓐ Ⓑ Ⓒ Ⓓ Ⓔ
137 Ⓐ Ⓑ Ⓒ Ⓓ Ⓔ
138 Ⓐ Ⓑ Ⓒ Ⓓ Ⓔ
139 Ⓐ Ⓑ Ⓒ Ⓓ Ⓔ
140 Ⓐ Ⓑ Ⓒ Ⓓ Ⓔ

141 Ⓐ Ⓑ Ⓒ Ⓓ Ⓔ
142 Ⓐ Ⓑ Ⓒ Ⓓ Ⓔ
143 Ⓐ Ⓑ Ⓒ Ⓓ Ⓔ
144 Ⓐ Ⓑ Ⓒ Ⓓ Ⓔ
145 Ⓐ Ⓑ Ⓒ Ⓓ Ⓔ

146 Ⓐ Ⓑ Ⓒ Ⓓ Ⓔ
147 Ⓐ Ⓑ Ⓒ Ⓓ Ⓔ
148 Ⓐ Ⓑ Ⓒ Ⓓ Ⓔ
149 Ⓐ Ⓑ Ⓒ Ⓓ Ⓔ
150 Ⓐ Ⓑ Ⓒ Ⓓ Ⓔ

151 Ⓐ Ⓑ Ⓒ Ⓓ Ⓔ
152 Ⓐ Ⓑ Ⓒ Ⓓ Ⓔ
153 Ⓐ Ⓑ Ⓒ Ⓓ Ⓔ
154 Ⓐ Ⓑ Ⓒ Ⓓ Ⓔ
155 Ⓐ Ⓑ Ⓒ Ⓓ Ⓔ

156 Ⓐ Ⓑ Ⓒ Ⓓ Ⓔ
157 Ⓐ Ⓑ Ⓒ Ⓓ Ⓔ
158 Ⓐ Ⓑ Ⓒ Ⓓ Ⓔ
159 Ⓐ Ⓑ Ⓒ Ⓓ Ⓔ
160 Ⓐ Ⓑ Ⓒ Ⓓ Ⓔ

161 Ⓐ Ⓑ Ⓒ Ⓓ Ⓔ
162 Ⓐ Ⓑ Ⓒ Ⓓ Ⓔ
163 Ⓐ Ⓑ Ⓒ Ⓓ Ⓔ
164 Ⓐ Ⓑ Ⓒ Ⓓ Ⓔ
165 Ⓐ Ⓑ Ⓒ Ⓓ Ⓔ

166 Ⓐ Ⓑ Ⓒ Ⓓ Ⓔ
167 Ⓐ Ⓑ Ⓒ Ⓓ Ⓔ
168 Ⓐ Ⓑ Ⓒ Ⓓ Ⓔ
169 Ⓐ Ⓑ Ⓒ Ⓓ Ⓔ
170 Ⓐ Ⓑ Ⓒ Ⓓ Ⓔ

171 Ⓐ Ⓑ Ⓒ Ⓓ Ⓔ
172 Ⓐ Ⓑ Ⓒ Ⓓ Ⓔ
173 Ⓐ Ⓑ Ⓒ Ⓓ Ⓔ
174 Ⓐ Ⓑ Ⓒ Ⓓ Ⓔ
175 Ⓐ Ⓑ Ⓒ Ⓓ Ⓔ

176 Ⓐ Ⓑ Ⓒ Ⓓ Ⓔ
177 Ⓐ Ⓑ Ⓒ Ⓓ Ⓔ
178 Ⓐ Ⓑ Ⓒ Ⓓ Ⓔ
179 Ⓐ Ⓑ Ⓒ Ⓓ Ⓔ
180 Ⓐ Ⓑ Ⓒ Ⓓ Ⓔ